A PRIMER OF CHEMICAL PATHOLOGY

Evelyn S C Koay

PhD, FAACB, MRCPath
Senior Lecturer (Chemical Pathology)
National University of Singapore
Consultant (Clinical Chemistry)
National University Hospital, Singapore

Noel Walmsley

MBBS, FRCPath, MCB, MAACB, FRCPA
Consultant Chemical Pathologist
ClinPath Laboratories, Adelaide
South Australia
Visiting Specialist in Chemical Pathology
Repatriation General Hospital
Daw Park, South Australia

A PRIMER OF CHEMICAL PATHOLOGY

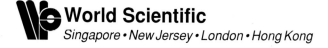

World Scientific
Singapore • New Jersey • London • Hong Kong

Published by

World Scientific Publishing Co. Pte. Ltd.

P O Box 128, Farrer Road, Singapore 912805

USA office: Suite 1B, 1060 Main Street, River Edge, NJ 07661

UK office: 57 Shelton Street, Covent Garden, London WC2H 9HE

First published 1996
First reprint 1997

A PRIMER OF CHEMICAL PATHOLOGY

ISBN 981-02-2449-4
      981-02-2571-7 (pbk)

Printed in Singapore.

Preface

This text is based on the Authors' experience of teaching clinical chemistry to medical students and to postgraduate students taking chemical pathology, clinical chemistry and other medically-related examinations. It covers appropriate basic physiology, pathophysiology, and touches on investigative procedures. The latter is not considered in great detail because this book has been written to complement a text covering this area (*Cases in Chemical Pathology: A Diagnostic Approach, 3rd ed.* Walmsley, Watkinson and Koay, World Scientific Publications, Singapore, 1993).

Readers of *Handbook of Chemical Pathology*, Koay and Walmsley, published in 1989 by PG Publishing, Singapore, will recognise that this text is a revised version of the earlier volume, which we have given a different title in the new edition. In this new edition we have substantially revised and updated each chapter as necessary. The text is now illustrated with many more figures and tables, and is printed in a dual-column format using a smaller font size in the effort to produce a practical study text.

This is indeed a study text and not a reference book. The material is deemed sufficient for undergraduates but should be used as a basic foundation text by postgraduate students.

ESK & RNW
September 1995

Acknowledgements

I thank my coauthor, Noel Walmsley, for his chapters, for creating 89 of the 175 figures in the text, including all but three of the algorithms (flow diagrams) for the evaluation of various conditions, for helping with the computer graphics for another 70 figures, and for the opportunity to collaborate with him on this project.

I gratefully acknowledge Noel's employer, ClinPath Laboratories, Kent Town, South Australia, who own the copyright for the algorithms, for permission to reproduce them, in part or in full. For some other figures, acknowledgement is made in the legends below the corresponding figures, in deference to specific instructions from the respective publishers, and is not repeated here.

I am also deeply indebted to the following colleagues: Associate Professor T.C. Aw for professional support and for liberal use of the department library resources; Misses Loh Sook Keng, Tan Hui Lang and Tok Kwee Lee for their help in producing the gels and slides used in Chapter 12 (Serum and CSF Proteins); Miss Christine Tsiang, Mr Lim Su Thay and Ms Liew Hong Yin for secretarial and administrative assistance. Colleagues at World Scientific Publishing, Singapore, contributed invaluable editorial input and assisted with the cover design; Mr K.P. Yap and Mrs S.C. Lim were particularly helpful.

Last but not least, I thank my family, especially my husband and son, for their selfless forebearance and unstinting support throughout the sixteen months of gestation of the text.

Evelyn Koay

Contents

Chapter 1

Sodium and Water Metabolism

Disorders of salt and water homeostasis result in a variety of clinical syndromes such as dehydration, oedema, hyponatraemia and hypernatraemia. Patients with these disorders require careful clinical evaluation prior to appropriate therapy, and this evaluation will not be satisfactory unless the clinician has an adequate grasp of the physiological principles involved. Furthermore it should be emphasised that in these subjects the most important investigation is the clinical examination, particularly the history and the evaluation of the patient's hydration status. Diagnosis is often made on clinical grounds and laboratory tests should be used to confirm a clinical impression and to uncover specific abnormalities such as hypernatraemia, renal failure and the like.

A number of definitions, which may be new to the reader, are used throughout the chapter and are appropriately dealt with in the body of the text. Two terms which recur are osmolality and tonicity which require some explanation.

Osmolality

The *osmolality* of a fluid is a measure of the total number of particles (ions, molecules) present in solution. It differs from the closely related term, osmolarity, in that it is expressed in millimoles per *kilogram* (concentrations per *mass*) of *solvent* (water in the case of plasma) whilst *osmolarity* is expressed in millimoles per *litre* (concentrations per *volume*) of *solution*. Both osmolality and osmolarity are units of measurement of osmotic effects; however, osmolality is a thermodynamically more precise expression than osmolarity because:

- Solution concentrations expressed on a weight basis are temperature independent, while those based on volume (e.g., osmolarity) will vary with temperature in a manner dependent on the thermal expansion of the solution.

- It is the osmolal, not the osmolar, concentration which exerts an effect across the cell membrane and which is controlled by homeostatic mechanisms. This is because of the volume occupied by the solid phase of plasma (made up mainly of its protein and lipid content) which in normal plasma

is about 7% of the plasma volume. Dissolved particles are confined to the aqueous phase of plasma.

A one osmolal solution is defined to contain 1 osmole/kg water; however, the term milliosmole/kg (mOsm/kg) which should have been used for the relatively low osmolalities of physiological fluids is not an SI unit and mmol/kg is recommended to be used in its stead. The plasma osmolality is normally 295 ± 5 mmol/kg.

As we shall see later, the distribution of water across biological membranes separating different compartments depends on the concentration difference of particles between the two compartments. On a per unit volume basis there will be a larger number of small molecular weight particles which will exert a greater osmotic effect, as compared to bigger particles. Thus the major contributors to plasma osmolality are Na^+, K^+ and their associated anions (mainly Cl^- and HCO_3^-), urea and glucose. Plasma proteins, because of their massive sizes, exert a relatively insignificant osmotic effect, individually or as a group. In practice, plasma osmolality can either be measured or calculated (see below).

Measured plasma osmolality. This is obtained using osmometers which measure colligative properties such as freezing point depression or vapour pressure. It gives a measure of the total osmolality of the solution -- the sum of the osmotic effects exerted by all the ions and molecules present in the solution across a membrane which, unlike biological ones, is permeable to water.

Calculated plasma osmolarity. As sodium is the major cation of the extracellular fluid (interstitial fluid or plasma) its osmolarity can be roughly estimated from the following equation:

$$\text{Calculated ECF osmolarity (mmol/L)} = 2 \times [Na^+]^* + [\text{urea}]^* + [\text{glucose}]^*$$

* (plasma analyte values expressed in mmol/L)

The factor of 2 applied to the $[Na^+]$ allows for its associated anions and assumes complete ionization.

Because of the volume taken up by the solid phase of plasma, the measured plasma osmolality should be higher than its calculated osmolarity value. However, there is usually little difference between the two values due to the incomplete ionization of some of the salts in plasma which reduces the osmotic effect by roughly the same proportion. The calculated parameter is thus a valid approximation of the true plasma osmolality; provided that large quantities of other osmotically active particles are not present in the plasma, the measured and calculated osmolalities should agree within 10 mmol/kg.

If substances other than electrolytes, urea, and glucose (e.g., alcohol, drugs) are present, then the measured osmolality will be much larger than the calculated value, with the difference exceeding 10 mmol/kg. This difference is referred to as an *osmolal gap* (Figure 1.1) -- a high osmolal gap is clinically significant. A high osmolal gap is also found in patients with gross hyperlipidaemia or hyperprotein-aemia, conditions which expand the volume of the solid phase and are associated with pseudohypo-natraemia (page 19).

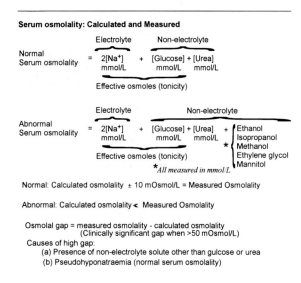

Figure 1.1. Serum osmolality and the osmolal gap.

Tonicity

Urea and a number of other small molecular weight substances (e.g., alcohol, ethylene glycol) are able to diffuse freely across cell membranes -- which are selectively permeable to these compounds in addition

to water -- and do not exert an osmotic gradient across them, and therefore do not induce fluid shifts. Thus the tonicity, often called the *effective osmolality*, of a solution is a measure of only those particles that exert an osmotic effect *in vivo*.

In the case of normal serum the effective osmolality is given by subtracting the urea concentration from the measured osmolality. Values above 300 mmol/kg are abnormal and those above 320 mmol/kg are indicative of clinically significant hyperosmolality.

WATER

In terms of body weight water is the single most abundant body constituent. It is also essential to intermediary metabolism and vital organ functions. Both the total body water balance and the distribution of water among the various body compartments -- intracellular, interstitial, intravascular -- are tightly maintained by homeostatic mechanisms within narrow limits. In particular, it is important to maintain the intravascular (blood) volume because the delivery of substrates to, and the removal of waste products from, the tissues depend on adequate tissue perfusion which, in turn, is governed by cardiac output, vascular resistance, and intravascular volume. Normally cardiac output and vascular resistance remain relatively constant and the major determinant of tissue perfusion is the blood volume.

The blood volume which is a part of, and therefore a function of, the extracellular volume, is primarily determined by the extracellular sodium content (see below). An inbalance between the two may lead to hypernatraemia or hyponatraemia, and changes in plasma osmolality, with consequent movement of water into or out of the vascular compartment. Osmotic and volume disturbances often occur together and hence the importance of always considering both salt and water metabolism when assessing patients with hydration problems.

Homeostasis

In the normal subject the day-to-day fluctuations of the body water content is less than 1%. This is due to a fine balance between intake, controlled by thirst, and output, controlled primarily by the kidney and the hypothalamic hormone, arginine vasopressin (AVP).

Both intake and loss of water are controlled by the osmotic gradient across the cell membranes in the hypothalamic centres that govern the thirst reflex and secretion of AVP. Sodium is the predominant extracellular cation and, with its associated anions, accounts for more than 90% of the osmotic activity of the ECF, which also determines water distribution across cell membranes. Thus the total body water and the distribution of water between the various compartments is determined mainly by the total body sodium content, the bulk of which is extracellular, via its osmotic effect. An important point to note is that the osmotic activity of the ECF is dependent on the *relative* amounts of water and sodium in the ECF, rather than on the absolute quantity of either.

Table 1.1 lists the main factors involved in water homeostasis, several of which (those marked with asterisks) primarily control sodium balance.

Table 1.1. Factors involved in water homeostasis.

Neural factors:	thirst
	*autonomic nervous system
Renal factors:	*glomerular filtration rate
	countercurrent multiplier
	countercurrent exchange
Circulating hormones:	arginine vasopressin
	*atrial natriuretic factor
	*aldosterone
	cortisol
	thyroid hormones

Table 1.2. Total body water content according to sex and age.

	% of body weight
Infants	~70
Young males	~60
Young females	~55
Elderly males	~50
Elderly females	~45

DISTRIBUTION

In the adult male the total body water is about 60% of the body weight (approximately 42 litres in a 70 kg subject). It varies with sex and age, being less in females due to a higher proportion of adipose tissue, and in the elderly (Table 1.2). The distribution in the various body compartments is shown in Table 1.3.

Table 1.3. Water distribution in a healthy young adult male. *(TBw, total body water content)*

	litres	% TBw	% body weight
Total	~42	100	~60
Intracellular	~23	~55	~33
Extracellular	~19	~45	~27
interstitial	~16	~38	~23
plasma	~3	~7	~4

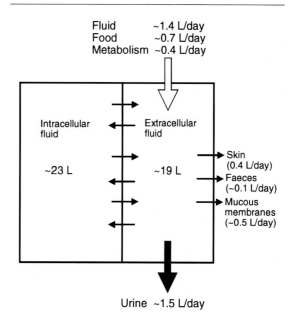

Figure 1.2. Water distribution and balance.

INTAKE

The daily intake of water is variable depending on body losses and psychological factors. An average intake would be around 2.5 litres a day (Figure 1.2). The major factor determining intake is thirst which is under the control of the thirst centre located in the hypothalamus. Normal functioning of this centre is influenced by:

1. ECF tonicity: hypertonicity increases thirst.

2. Blood volume: decreased volume increases thirst.
3. Miscellaneous factors: pain and stress, for example increase thirst.

OUTPUT

A subject is in water balance when total intake and overall loss of body water are approximately equal. Variable amounts of fluid are lost from the skin (sweating) and the mucous membranes (electrolyte-free water in expired air), depending on the environmental temperature and respiratory rate. Neither of these losses can be controlled to meet water requirements. A small amount of water is lost in the faeces (<100 mL/day) but the major loss, and thus control of output, occurs via the kidney.

Renal water excretion (Figure 1.3)

Each day 130-180 litres of water are presented as glomerular filtrate to the proximal renal tubules. Only 1 to 2 litres finally appear as urine. This is due to passive reabsorption of 70-80% in the proximal tubule (obligatory isosmotic water flow, consequent to sodium reabsorption), and further reabsorption in the collecting ducts under the influence of AVP.

The kidney has the ability, on the one hand, to excrete large amounts of dilute urine (up to 20-30 L/day) and, on the other hand, to concentrate the urine to such an extent that the output can fall as low as 0.5 L/day. This ability to dilute and concentrate the urine is due to two mechanisms:

1 The ability to remove electrolytes, particularly NaCl, from the glomerular filtrate to produce a dilute urine.
2 The ability of the collecting ducts to reabsorb water from the luminal fluid.

Dilution of urine. The thick segment of the ascending limb of the loop of Henle (the 'diluting segment') is impermeable to water and, under normal circumstances, actively reabsorbs some 20-30% of the filtered sodium and potassium (and chloride) ions. This results in a dilute urine with an osmolality of 50-100 mmol/kg. The rate of fluid delivery from this segment is about 20 mL/min (~30 L/day) and if this were allowed to pass through the remainder of the nephron unimpeded, homeostasis would be difficult to maintain. Further processing involves further

reabsorption of water in the collecting ducts.

Reabsorption of water from collecting ducts. The collecting ducts are normally impermeable to water but in the presence of AVP the ducts become water permeable and if there is a high interstitial fluid tonicity (osmolality) water can be reabsorbed, resulting in a decreased volume of concentrated urine. The two aspects to this mechanism, AVP and a high interstitial tonicity, require further explanation.

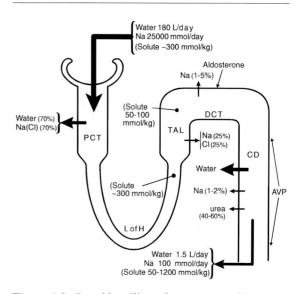

Figure 1.3. Renal handling of water and sodium. *AVP, arginine vasopressin; PCT, proximal convoluted tubule; TAL, thick ascending limb of loop of Henle; DCT, distal convoluted tubule; CD, collecting duct.*

AVP. Arginine vasopressin, commonly known as antidiuretic hormone (ADH), acts on the collecting duct epithelium making it permeable to water, which allows reabsorption of water from the lumen, provided there is an osmotic gradient between the luminal fluid and the renal interstitial tissue.

AVP is a nanopeptide synthesised in the supraoptic and paraventricular nuclei of the hypothalamus and transported along nerve axons to the posterior pituitary where it is stored. It is released into the blood stream in response to a number of stimuli (see below) and acts on the collecting duct epithelium resulting in increased permeability and water reabsorption.

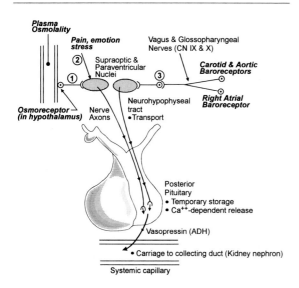

Figure 1.4. Control of ADH secretion and release. Redrawn, with permission of W.B. Saunders, from Andreoti E. The posterior pituitary. In: Wyngaarden JB and Smith LH (eds), *Cecil Textbook of Medicine, 18th edn.* W.B. Saunders, Philadelphia, 1988.

There are two main factors, ECF tonicity and blood volume, as well as a number of miscellaneous stimuli, controlling AVP production and secretion (see also Figure 1.4):

- *Tonicity of ECF:* Osmoreceptors, located in the hypothalamus, respond to an increase in the ECF tonicity by increasing AVP production and secretion. A decrease in tonicity causes the reverse. This is a very sensitive mechanism responding to changes of 1-2% in the plasma tonicity which is equivalent to a change in plasma sodium concentration of only about 3 mmol/L.

- *Blood volume:* Baroreceptors, located in the right atrium and carotid sinus, respond to a decrease in blood volume by stimulating AVP production and release. This mechanism only responds to gross changes, e.g., a 10% change in volume. However, it can override the effect of ECF tonicity on AVP secretion, e.g., in Addison's disease, when the plasma is hypo-osmolal (page 252).

- *Miscellaneous stimulants:* Other factors stimulating AVP release are: (a) stress, e.g., pain and trauma; (b) nausea, e.g., post-surgery, (c) drugs, e.g.,

opiates, barbiturates, chlorpropamide (see page 15). A transient increase in AVP secretion often occurs after surgery due to pain, stress, nausea, and opiate medication. Hypovolaemia due to blood loss could be a further stimulant.

Renal interstitial tonicity. The maintenance of a high interstitial tonicity requires two separate renal mechanisms, the countercurrent multiplier and the countercurrent exchanger.

Countercurrent multiplier: During antidiuresis the renal medulla interstitial fluid can be maintained at a tonicity of ~1200 mmol/kg by a mechanism involving the loop of Henle and the collecting duct which concentrates and traps salt and urea (countercurrent multiplier). The countercurrent exchange system of the vasa recta maintains this tonicity. Four parts of the nephron are involved in the multiplier system (Figure 1.5): descending thin limb, ascending thin limb, thick ascending limb and collecting ducts.

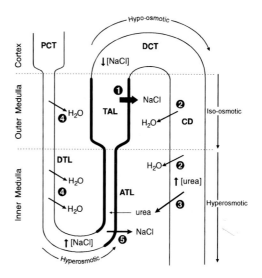

Figure 1.5. The countercurrent multiplier. *See text for details.*

1. The thick ascending limb of the loop of Henle (TAL), which is impermeable to water, actively transports NaCl (as Na^+ and Cl^- ions) out of the lumen into the interstitial tissue which results in:

(a) dilution of urine (osmolality of luminal fluid at the TAL is 50-100 mmol/kg)

(b) increased tonicity of the outer medulla

2 The high medullary tonicity induces water reabsorption from the upper collecting duct (CD) which increases the tubular urea concentration.

3 The inner medullary CD is permeable to urea and it passes along its concentration gradient into the interstitial tissue and increases the tonicity of the inner medulla.

4 The increased medullary interstitial fluid tonicity draws water out of the descending portion of the loop of Henle (DTL) increasing the luminal sodium concentration.

5 The ascending thin limb (ATL) of the loop of Henle is impermeable to water but permeable to NaCl which passes out into the medulla along its concentration gradient.

These five steps result in a high tonicity of the medullary interstitial tissue varying from ~1200 mmol/kg at the renal papillae to just above 300 mmol/kg in the outer medulla. To prevent its dissipation by the medullary blood circulation, a further mechanism to trap the solutes in the medulla is required. This is performed by the countercurrent exchanger.

Countercurrent exchanger. The high solute concentration of the medulla is maintained by the vasa rectae utilising a countercurrent exchanger type of system (Figure 1.6). These blood vessels loop down into the medulla and their descending and ascending limbs are appositioned closely together, enabling exchange of solutes to occur between them as well as with the medullary interstitial tissue.

Isosmotic blood entering the vasa rectae encounters increasingly high interstitial solute concentrations. As the blood flows down the descending limb, NaCl and other solutes enter from the interstitial fluid and water flows out into the interstitial area -- the reverse process of course occurs in the ascending limb; thus the osmolality of blood flowing through these vessels continually equilibrates with that of the outside fluid (Figure 1.6 *Left*).

As hypertonic blood ascends the ascending limb and normal blood enters the descending limb, there is

also an exchange of solute and water between the two limbs -- NaCl and other solutes from the ascending limb enter the blood of the descending limb and water from the descending limb enters the blood of the ascending limb (Figure 1.6 *right*). Thus the solute is trapped in the medullary area and not 'washed out' by the traversing blood vessels, and the medullary solute concentration remains relatively undisturbed.

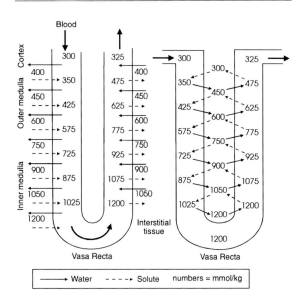

Figure 1.6. The countercurrent exchanger. *See text for details.*

INTRACELLULAR-EXTRACELLULAR DISTRIBUTION

The relative volumes of the intracellular fluid (ICF) and the extracellular fluid (ECF) depend on the tonicity gradient across the cell membranes. If the ICF tonicity is greater than that of the ECF then fluid passes into the cells; in the reverse situation fluid moves out of the cells into the ECF. In the normal subject the intracellular tonicity (due mainly to potassium) and the extracellular tonicity (due mainly to sodium) are similar (around 300 mmol/kg) and large water shifts do not occur.

As the ECF tonicity is due mainly to sodium then the extracellular volume (and intracellular volume) will vary with the total ECF sodium content. Thus, changes in the ECF sodium content will cause changes in water distribution between the two compartments, i.e.,

- An increase in the ECF sodium (increased ECF tonicity) will cause water to come out of cells and cause cellular dehydration.

- A decrease in the ECF sodium (decreased ECF tonicity) will cause water to enter the cells causing overhydration or cellular oedema.

Thus water balance depends on the extracellular sodium content:

1. ↑ ECF sodium → ↑ ECF tonicity →
   (a) ↑ thirst (increased water intake)
   (b) ↑ AVP secretion (increased renal water reabsorption)
   (c) Water shift from ICF to ECF

   a + b + c → ↑ ECF volume and ↓ ICF volume

2. ↓ ECF sodium → ↓ ECF tonicity →
   (a) ↓ thirst (decreased water intake)
   (b) ↓ AVP secretion (increased renal water excretion)
   (c) water shift from ECF to ICF

   a + b + c → ↓ ECF volume and ↑ ICF volume

Thus total body sodium (most of which is in the ECF) can be said to control the extracellular volume (and water balance) and, as will be seen later, the extracellular volume controls the total body sodium (and sodium balance).

SODIUM

From a pathophysiological point of view the function of sodium is to maintain the extracellular and intravascular volumes. A decrease in the total body sodium, which is mainly extracellular, results in a decreased extracellular volume (ECV) and an increased total body sodium is associated with an increased ECV.

Homeostasis

DISTRIBUTION

The total body sodium content is around 3000 to 3500 millimoles with in excess of 90% located in the ECF compartment (Table 1.4) where it determines the volume of this compartment.

Table 1.4. Distribution of sodium.

	Content (mmol)	Concentration (mmol/L)
Total body	~3050	
Intracellular	~250	5-10
Extracellular	~2800	~140
Plasma	~400	~140

INTAKE

On a western diet the daily intake of sodium in food and drink is about 150 to 250 mmol/day, most of which is absorbed. Unlike the thirst mechanism for water there is no well defined 'sodium centre'; however, there appears to be an ill-defined sodium appetite, e.g., subjects with the salt-depleting Addison's disease have a salt-craving. Generally the intake is governed by habit rather than need.

OUTPUT

To maintain sodium balance the intake must equal the output. A small amount of sodium (10-20 mmol/day) is excreted in the sweat and faeces, but almost all of the intake has to be excreted in the urine and the kidney is the main controller of homeostasis.

Renal sodium excretion (Figure 1.3)

Each day some 25000 mmol of sodium ions are filtered by the glomerulus but less than 1% of this (100 to 200 mmol) appears in the urine as a consequence of reabsorption along the nephron. The amount excreted in the urine calculated as a percentage of the amount filtered is termed the *fractional excretion of sodium*

(FE_{Na}). For practical purposes this can be roughly calculated from the sodium and creatinine concentrations of plasma and of a spot (untimed) urine sample collected at the same time as the blood sample.

$$FE_{Na} = \frac{U_{Na}}{P_{Na}} \times \frac{P_{Cr}}{U_{Cr}} \times 100\%$$

where U_{Na} is urinary sodium concentration, P_{Na} plasma sodium concentration, P_{Cr} plasma creatinine concentration, and U_{Cr} urinary creatinine concentration (all in mmol/L).

The normal range of FE_{Na} is less than 1%. Reabsorption of sodium occurs throughout the nephron including the proximal tubule, loop of Henle, distal convoluted tubule and collecting duct areas. The whole of the extracellular sodium content could be lost by passive filtration in little more than an hour, if these absorptive mechanisms fail.

Proximal tubule. About 70 to 75% is actively reabsorbed by an energy dependent process. Water is iso-osmotically absorbed along with sodium and its associated anions so that the fluid entering the loop of Henle has a similar concentration to the original filtrate. A high luminal solute concentration may cause an osmotic diuresis (page 20).

Loop of Henle. In the thick ascending limb 15 to 25% of the filtered sodium ions is reabsorbed. This segment has two unique features:

1. Chloride ions (Cl⁻) are actively reabsorbed with the sodium ions following passively (the reverse of the mechanism in the proximal tubule).

2. This section of the nephron is impermeable to water and the luminal fluid exiting it is diluted to an osmolality of 50 to 100 mmol/kg (hence the term diluting segment).

As mentioned above this part of the nephron is crucial for concentrating and diluting urine (page 5). The reabsorbed sodium and chloride ions not only result in dilution of the filtrate but are also major contributors to the high tonicity of the interstitial medullary tissue, which is necessary for water reabsorption.

Distal convoluted tubule. A variable amount of sodium (1-5%) is reabsorbed in this section under the influence of aldosterone (see below).

Collecting duct. This part of the nephron, also influenced by aldosterone, is responsible for reabsorption of 1-2% of filtered sodium. This section acts as a fine tuner for sodium homeostasis.

CONTROL OF SODIUM EXCRETION

As mentioned above sodium balance is dependent on the rate of renal sodium excretion and this in turn is controlled by the intravascular volume, or more specifically, the effective arterial blood volume (EABV). The EABV describes the 'fullness' of the arterial space and does not necessarily reflect the true blood volume, e.g., an increased blood volume residing in a dilated vascular system can be associated with 'underfilling' of the system.

Specifically, the renal excretion of sodium is controlled by the *glomerular filtration rate (GFR), aldosterone, and atrial natriuretic factor* (Figure 1.7).

GFR. The amount of sodium presented to the tubules depends, in the first instance, on the amount filtered (determined by the renal blood flow and its sodium content) and there is some evidence that the GFR influences the tubular reabsorption rate, e.g., a decreased GFR is associated with sodium retention. Under normal circumstances there is a balance between the amount filtered and the amount reabsorbed (glomerulotubular balance), i.e., increased filtered sodium is balanced by increased tubular reabsorption and *vice versa,* and the FE_{Na} is normally maintained at less than 1%.

Aldosterone. A decrease in the renal blood flow (hypovolaemia, low EABV) causes renin release and subsequently an increased production of angiotensin II which causes vasoconstriction and secretion of aldosterone (page 65). Aldosterone increases the distal renal tubular reabsorption of sodium ions and increases the excretion of potassium and hydrogen ions. The sodium ions enter the tubular cells through specific sodium channels (this mechanism is blocked by amiloride) leaving a negatively charged luminal aspect (due to the retained Cl⁻) which 'encourages' the secretion of the positively charged cellular hydrogen

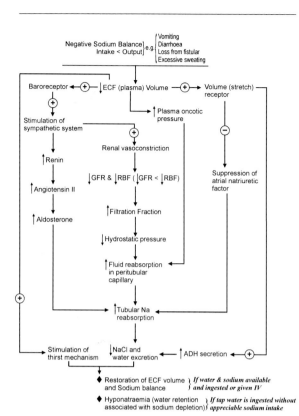

Figure 1.7. Mechanisms responsible for restoring sodium balance and extracellular fluid volume. Redrawn, with permission of W.B. Saunders, from: Klahr S. Structure and function of the Kidneys. In: Wyngaarden JB and Smith LH (eds), *Cecil Textbook of Medicine, 18th edn.* W.B. Saunders, Philadelphia, 1988.

and potassium ions. Sodium ions are then 'pumped' from the cells into the ECF (i.e., back into circulation) in exchange for potassium ions by the mechanisms put in train by aldosterone (page 62).

Atrial natriuretic peptide (ANP). ANP is released from the atrium in response to stretching (e.g., increased blood volume, hypervolaemia); it causes:

- Increased GFR
- Increased glomerular filtration fraction
- Natriuresis

- Kaliuresis
- Diuresis
- Decreased renin and aldosterone secretion

It is unclear how ANP induces natriuresis but the most likely mechanism is variation of the intrarenal blood flow causing increased GFR and increased filtration fraction (constriction of the efferent glomerular arterioles). Its action in inhibiting renin and aldosterone secretion may also be a factor.

From the above it will be appreciated that:

1. *Increased intravascular volume (or effective arterial blood volume) results in* **increased renal sodium excretion** *(decreased aldosterone plus increased ANP).*
2. **Decreased blood volume** *produces* **renal sodium retention** *(increased aldosterone, decreased ANP)*

Abnormalities of Total Body Sodium

Total body sodium content (TB_{Na}), the bulk of which resides in the extracellular compartment, determines the ECF volume and hence directly affects the total body water content. As an increase in sodium generally results in an increase in the ECF (e.g., oedema), and a decrease results in dehydration, the TB_{Na} can be estimated clinically by determining the patient's volume status from the symptoms due to ECV depletion or overloading. Note that if sodium and water are lost or gained in equivalent amounts, the plasma sodium concentration would remain unchanged, despite perturbations of TB_{Na}.

SODIUM DEPLETION

Sodium depletion, which is usually due to excessive loss from the body rather than decreased intake, results in ECF volume depletion and the clinical features reflect this state.

Causes

The basic cause is that sodium intake is inadequate to replace sodium loss, producing a negative sodium balance. The intake can be low, normal, or even

9

increased but if losses exceed the intake, then TB_{Na} depletion will occur.

1. ***Decreased intake in face of normal or increased loss:***
   - dietary deficiency
   - inappropriate iv therapy
2. ***Skin loss:***
   - excessive sweating
   - severe burns
3. ***GIT loss:***
   - vomiting
   - diarrhoea
   - loss from fistulae
4. ***Renal Loss:***
   - Diuretics (including osmotic diuresis)
   - Mineralocorticoid deficiency syndromes:
     Addison's disease, adrenal enzyme defects
   - Tubular disease: salt-losing nephritis

Consequences

The major consequence will be a decreased extracellular volume (ECV) but depending on the cause and severity there may be changes in serum and urinary electrolytes.

Extracellular volume. Sodium depletion is always associated with water depletion and a decreased ECV (dehydration) because:

(a) sodium is lost in the form of body fluids or
(b) if the major cause is inadequate sodium intake the consequent decreased tonicity will result in:
   (i) fluid shift to the intracellular compartment
   (ii) decreased AVP secretion causing increased renal free water excretion.

The clinical manifestations of a decreased ECV depend on the degree of depletion:

- If it is less than 5% body weight there will be minimal signs except perhaps for a modest increase in the pulse rate.

- Losses of 5-10% are associated with an increased pulse rate, orthostatic hypotension and, perhaps, supine hypotension.

- Losses in excess of 10% and approaching 20 to 25% will compromise cardiovascular function,

decrease tissue perfusion and eventually result in shock.

Other variable features are thirst, dry skin and mucous membranes, loss of tissue turgor, and increased plasma urea concentration (prerenal insufficiency, page 78). Haemoconcentration may result in increased plasma protein concentrations and a high packed red cell volume (provided these were not decreased at the beginning of the process).

As dehydration proceeds the urine volume will fall and the patient characteristically passes a small volume of concentrated urine (page 4).

Serum [Na]. The serum sodium concentration is a function of water balance (page 12). In patients with hypovolaemia, depending on the specific circumstance, the level may be increased (hypernatraemia), decreased (hyponatraemia), or normal (eunatraemia). Body fluids generally contain more water relative to sodium (i.e., they are usually hypotonic) and their loss will result, in the first instance, in hypernatraemia (more water is lost than sodium). However, if salt-poor fluids (e.g., tap water) are administered the water lost will be replaced and the serum [Na] returns towards normal. Continued water intake, without sodium intake, can result in hyponatraemia, particularly if there is a defect in renal water excretion (e.g., hypovolaemic stimulation of AVP release, page 5).

Urinary [Na]. If the sodium loss is extrarenal (vomiting, diarrhoea, etc) the kidney will avidly retain sodium (page 17) resulting in a low urinary [Na]. On the other hand, if the kidney is at fault, the urinary [Na] will be high. The urinary handling of sodium is usually evaluated by measuring the sodium concentration on a spot (untimed) urine sample. Levels less than 10 mmol/L indicate the appropriate response of a normal kidney to hypovolaemia; with defective renal function, the urinary [Na] will usually be greater than 20 mmol/L.

Laboratory evaluation

As noted above, sodium depletion may present with hypernatraemia (page 16), or hyponatraemia (page 18) in addition to dehydration which is usually associated with oliguria (page 22) -- see designated pages for evaluation.

SODIUM EXCESS

Excessive total body sodium, which may be due to decreased renal excretion or increased intake or both, results in water retention and an increased extracellular volume. Generally an increased extracellular volume implies renal sodium retention.

Causes

The basic cause is that sodium intake exceeds its excretion, producing a positive sodium balance.

1. *Oral:*
   - excessive dietary sodium
   - ingestion of sea water.
2. *Intravenous :*
   - hypertonic saline/sodium bicarbonate infusions
3. *Renal sodium retention:*
   - renal failure
   - mineralocorticoid excess syndromes**
     Primary: hyperaldosteronism, Cushing's syndrome, steroid therapy
     Secondary: oedematous states (cardiac failure, nephrotic syndrome, cirrhosis)

** The **primary mineralocorticoid excess syndromes** are dealt with in Chapter 4.

Renal failure. In mild renal insufficiency sodium retention usually does not occur unless there is a high salt intake, whilst in chronic renal failure extracellular fluid expansion is common with increases in both intravascular and interstitial compartments, leading to hypertension and oedema, respectively, in most cases.

Congestive cardiac failure. As cardiac output falls there is a fall in blood pressure, tissue perfusion, and the effective arterial blood volume (see page 9). This stimulates renal sodium retention, mainly through the renin-aldosterone system, and water retention follows -- the underperfused kidney cannot excrete the water load -- resulting in an increased intravascular volume which restores cardiac output. As failure declines further there is more salt and water retention which leads to peripheral oedema.

Nephrotic syndrome. The cause of sodium retention is not clear but the suggested sequence of events is:

Renal albumin loss
→ hypoalbuminaemia
→ low plasma colloidal osmotic pressure
→ loss of intravascular fluid to the interstitial fluid compartment
→ decreased intravascular volume
    (decreased effective arterial blood volume)
→ increased renal sodium retention
    (mainly aldosterone-generated)

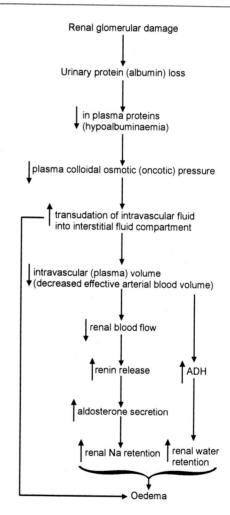

Figure 1.8. Pathogenesis of sodium retention in the nephrotic syndrome. Redrawn from: Schreiner FE. The nephrotic syndrome. In: Strauss MB and Welt LG (eds), *Diseases of the Kidney, 2nd edn.* Little, Brown, Boston, 1971.

11

Hepatic cirrhosis. Cirrhosis is associated with renal sodium retention, ascites, and hypoalbuminaemia. The cause of the sodium retention is unclear but a decreasing intravascular volume secondary to hypo-albuminaemia has been suggested (as for the nephrotic syndrome). However, a low plasma oncotic pressure due to hypoalbuminaemia is unlikely to be the only cause in these subjects because (a) the same degree of hypoalbuminaemia in patients with other conditions (malabsorption, malnutrition) does not always result in sodium retention and oedema, and (b) patients with the rare analbuminaemia condition rarely become oedematous.

Consequences

An increase in the extracellular sodium concentration results in an increase in the extracellular volume. The serum and urinary sodium levels are variable depending on the underlying cause.

Extracellular volume. An increase in the total body sodium will, in the first instance, increase the tonicity of the extracellular fluid which will result in:

(a) Thirst and increased oral water intake
(b) Water egress from the intracellular fluid to the extracellular fluid.
(c) Increased AVP secretion leading to renal water conservation.

(a) + (b) + (c)   →   increased extracellular volume

The retained fluid will be variably distributed between the intravascular space, where it may produce cardiac overload and perhaps hypertension, and the interstitial fluid where it presents as peripheral oedema.

The fluid overload may be 'acute', as in inappropriate intravenous infusions and massive oral salt ingestion, resulting in a rapid increase in the intravascular volume. This may produce cardiac overload and pulmonary oedema. In the 'chronic' situation associated with renal sodium retention peripheral oedema occurs, which in cirrhosis may be associated with ascites. In the primary mineralocorticoid excess syndromes the sodium retention is self-limiting because of the 'escape' phenomenon (page 67) and oedema tends not to occur, although hypertension due to increased intravascular volume may be present.

Serum [Na]. The serum sodium level is generally normal because of the associated water retention. There are two exceptions:

● In the primary mineralocorticoid excess syndromes and renal failure the serum [Na] may be slightly increased or at the upper reference limit.
● The oedematous syndromes may present with hyponatraemia which is due to water retention in excess of sodium retention (cause unclear).

Urinary [Na]. In the oedematous syndromes (renal sodium retention) the urinary sodium output is low and the spot urinary sodium concentration is often less than 10 mmol/L. Acute salt and water retention is associated with high urinary sodium excretion rates and high urinary sodium concentrations. Patients with the mineralocorticoid excess syndromes are generally in sodium balance (escape phenomenon) and the urinary sodium will reflect the intake.

Laboratory evaluation

The evaluation of the oedematous patient is a clinical problem but laboratory tests that may be useful are: liver function tests (cirrhosis), serum and urinary albumin (nephrotic syndrome), blood gases (congestive cardiac failure).

Abnormalities of total body water

Clinically total body water (TB_W) deficiency, or dehydration, presents with the classical picture of thirst, dry skin and mucous membranes, loss of skin turgor, decreased urinary output and circulatory disturbances reflecting a low blood volume (high pulse rate, orthotension, hypotension, shock, etc); the serum [Na] depends on the body sodium content and can be either high, low, or normal. TB_W excess can present as peripheral oedema, pulmonary oedema, ascites, and circulatory overload with cardiac failure.

However, minor degrees of dehydration and water excess can present as euvolaemia, i.e., without clinical evidence of either dehydration or hypervolaemia. In this case the serum [Na] can be useful, e.g., hyponatraemia may indicate overhydration and hypernatraemia, dehydration. Ascribing a definite diagnosis

12

using the serum [Na] criterion, however, can be dangerous because overhydration may be associated with hypernatraemia and dehydration with hyponatraemia. The following sections discuss these issues.

WATER DEFICIENCY

Subjects who present with water deficiency (dehydration) also have varying degrees of sodium depletion because all fluids lost from the body contain sodium.

Causes

The basic cause of water deficiency, which presents as dehydration, is a negative water balance, i.e., input less than output, with the input factor being the major problem as far as water is concerned (losses can be readily replaced if the patient has access to water and the thirst mechanism is intact). On the other hand, sodium is present in significant quantities in all body fluids (including urine) and its deficiency in dehydration states is due mainly to excessive loss from the body rather than inadequate intake. Depending on the amount of concomitant sodium loss, water depletion is usually classified on the basis of the lost fluid into three types: *predominant water depletion, hypotonic fluid loss, and isotonic fluid loss.*

Predominant water depletion. In 'pure' water depletion the problem is inadequate fluid intake (oral or iv) in the face of normal, or increased, renal loss (including diabetes insipidus, osmotic diuresis). It may occur in:

- Subjects too old, too young, or too sick to drink
- Inappropriate iv therapy
- Disturbances of the thirst centre

In these situations the insensitive losses of water in expired air or sweat will contribute considerably to abnormal water balance when homeostatic mechanisms (e.g., the thirst reflex) fail, or in the face of gross depletion, either due to inadequate intake or to excessive loss by other routes.

Hypotonic fluid loss. Dehydration due to loss of fluid containing significant amounts of sodium

(coupled with inadequate fluid intake) may be due to:

- Skin losses: excessive sweating
- Gut losses: vomiting, diarrhoea, drainage into fistulae
- Renal losses: diuretic therapy, Addison's disease, salt-losing nephritis, diabetes insipidus

Isotonic fluid loss. This is unusual but may occur in:

- Loss of blood: haemorrhage, accidents
- Loss of serum: burns
- 'Third space' accumulations: ileus, pancreatitis, peritonitis, crush injury

Consequences

Water depletion is associated with hypovolaemia (dehydration) and various abnormalities of the serum and urinary sodium levels, and the urine osmolality and volume which depend on the route and type of fluid lost.

Pure (predominant) water depletion. In pure water depletion which really means loss of fluid containing very small amounts of sodium (5 to 10 mmol/L), the loss is shared between the intracellular and extracellular compartments and losses have to be substantial before there is any clinical evidence of hypovolaemia (low blood pressure, increased pulse rate). Such patients develop hypernatraemia (due to water loss being greater than sodium loss) which can be quite severe, e.g., 160 to 170 mmol/L, without any evidence of hypovolaemia, i.e., they can appear clinically euvolaemic with normal blood pressure and pulse rate.

If the kidneys are functioning normally (extrarenal causes of water depletion) the urine will be:

- Low in volume
- Highly concentrated (osmolality 600-1000 mmol /kg) due to hypertonicity-induced AVP release**
- Low in sodium (spot [Na] values less than 10 mmol/L) due to renal sodium conservation (mild hypovolaemia)

**In the case of diabetes insipidus the absence of AVP will result in the passage of copious amounts of a very dilute urine (osmolality 50-100 mmol/kg).

13

Isotonic fluid loss infers a loss of fluid with a similar sodium content to that of the ECF ([Na] 140-150 mmol/L, osmolality of ~300 mmol/L). Such fluid losses only involve the extracellular compartment (in the first instance); hence there are no changes in the ECF osmolality (normonatraemia) and no shifts of water from the intracellular compartment. These subjects, depending on the amount lost, will have a decreased ECF volume and a decreased intravascular volume leading to a compromised circulation, and may develop hypotension, an increased pulse rate, etc.

The hypovolaemia stimulates:

(a) renal sodium retention resulting in a low urinary sodium concentration (<10 mmol/L), and

(b) the release of AVP resulting in a high urinary osmolality (higher than the plasma osmolality and usually of the order of 600-1000 mmol/kg).

Hypotonic fluid loss involves fluids of tonicity intermediate between those of isotonic fluids and pure water, e.g., a fluid with a [Na] of ~50 mmol/L. The loss can be considered to consist of two phases, a pure water phase and an isotonic fluid phase. For example, a loss of three litres of fluid with a NaCl content of 50 mmol/L (tonicity of 100 mmol/kg) can be considered to be a loss of two litres of pure water plus one litre of isotonic saline ([Na] 150 mmol/L). Loss of such a fluid would result in:

(a) Loss of one litre from the ECF (isotonic portion), plus,

(b) Loss of two litres shared between the ECF and the ICF (pure water portion).

The difference between hypotonic fluid loss and pure water loss (of the same volume) is the larger decrease in ECF volume, and hence the intravascular volume, in the former resulting in clinical symptoms of hypovolaemia (increased pulse rate, hypotension).

If the loss is extrarenal (vomiting, diarrhoea, etc) the urinary sodium will be low (spot concentration <10 mmol/L) and this will be associated with a low urine volume of fluid which is highly concentrated (urine osmolality 600-1000 mmol/L, urine:serum osmolality ratio of 2-3). On the other hand, if the loss is of renal origin (diuretics, mineralocorticoid deficiency), the urinary sodium may be high (>20 mmol/L).

The patient who has sustained loss of hypotonic fluids can present with *variable serum [Na]* and on the basis of the latter, may be classified as having *hypertonic, isotonic or hypotonic dehydration*. The loss of hypotonic fluid will, in the first instance, result in hypernatraemia because of the relative greater loss of water than of sodium, i.e., the patient will be hypernatraemic (and hypertonic). Hypertonic dehydration stimulates the thirst centre and if the patient has access to water he can replace some of the deficit. If the replacement fluid is tap water (no salt) the additional water will decrease the serum tonicity and the sodium concentration producing normonatraemia (eunatraemia) and often hyponatraemia.

Laboratory evaluation

The water-deficient patient should be evaluated for the presence of oliguria (page 22), hypernatraemia (page 16), and hypovolaemia (page 13), the more common forms of presentation, with the appropriate tests, including serum and urine osmolality, and serum and urine [Na]; the urine volume should be noted as it is an important clue to the diagnosis.

WATER EXCESS

The patient with excessive total body water may present in a variety of ways, but the common ones are peripheral oedema and hyponatraemia. Oedema is always associated with sodium excess. Hyponatraemia, in the context of body water excess, is usually associated with a normal or slightly decreased total body water content (the exception being the occasional finding of hyponatraemia in oedematous conditions, page 18).

Causes

Water excess usually reflects decreased renal water excretion due to increased AVP or AVP-like activity, although theoretically it could be due to increased intake or inadequate excretion or both. A subject with normal renal function can excrete up to 20-30 litres of water daily, e.g., the patient with diabetes insipidus; however, the water excess conditions occur with fluid intakes much less than this (e.g., 2 to 3 litres a day) and thus the primary lesion is an inability of the kidney to excrete a normal water load. Renal water retention can occur as the primary lesion in the absence of salt excess or secondary to the salt excess syndromes.

Sodium retention. See page 10 -- the salt excess syndromes.

Decreased renal water excretion. Antidiuresis is usually due to excessive AVP secretion but it can also be associated with a variety of drugs:

- Syndrome of inappropriate antidiuretic hormone secretion (SIADH)
- Antidiuretic drugs
- Diuretic-related hyponatraemia
- Endocrine disorders

SIADH. This condition, as the name suggests, is due to the continued secretion of AVP (or ADH) in the face of hypotonicity or increased intravascular volume or both, i.e., its secretion is inappropriate in that it occurs under conditions that normally suppress its secretion.

Causes. The commonest cause is the ectopic production of AVP by a malignant tumour, but it can also be produced by a wide variety of conditions:

Tumours
    Carcinoma of bronchus, prostate, pancreas
    Brain tumours: glioma, meningioma
Brain pathology
    Tumours; Trauma/cerebrovascular accidents
    Infections: abscess, meningitis, encephalitis
Pulmonary pathology
    Tumours: bronchial carcinoma
    Infection: tuberculosis, pneumonia
    Pneumothorax
    Hydrothorax
Miscellaneous
    Guillain-Barre syndrome
    Acute alcohol withdrawal

Pathophysiology. The sequence of events is:

$\uparrow$ AVP $\rightarrow$ $\uparrow$ renal water retention $\rightarrow$ $\uparrow$ECV and haemodilution $\rightarrow$ $\downarrow$ serum osmolality and $\downarrow$ serum [Na]; $\downarrow$ urine volume and $\uparrow$ urine osmolality

Hence the characteristic features are a low serum osmolality and a low serum sodium concentration associated with an inappropriately high urine osmolality. The urinary sodium concentration is usually greater than 20 mmol/L which is reflecting a concentrated urine.

From the practical aspect it is important to point out that a number of conditions must be satisfied before making the diagnosis of SIADH. This is to differentiate it from other causes of hyponatraemia which may require different treatment. In addition to low serum sodium and osmolality values, and high urine sodium and osmolality values, the following must be satisfied:

- No evidence of dehydration
- No cardiac, adrenal, pituitary, or thyroid dysfunction
- No drug or diuretic therapy
- Positive response to fluid restriction (<500 mL/day) with normalisation of serum analyte values

A further practical point is that the urine osmolality needs only be inappropriate for a low plasma osmolality, i.e., it does not have to exceed the plasma value (urine values in excess of 200 mmol/kg are deemed inappropriate). As suggested above the usual method of treatment is fluid restriction.

Antidiuretic drugs. There are a wide variety of drugs which can produce a syndrome indistinguishable from SIADH due either to stimulated AVP secretion or potentiation of AVP activity at the renal level.

Drugs that increase AVP secretion
    Hypnotics: barbiturates
    Narcotics: morphine, pethidine
    Hypoglycaemics: chlorpropamide, tolbutamide
    Anticonvulsants: carbamazepine
    Antineoplastics: vincristine, vinblastine, cyclophosphamide
    Miscellaneous: clofibrate, nicotine derivatives

Drugs that potentiate AVP activity
    Hypoglycaemics: chlorpropamide, tolbutamide
    paracetamol
    indomethacin

These drug-related conditions are best referred to as *syndromes of inappropriate antidiuresis* to distinguish them from SIADH. The treatment is to discontinue the drug but if this is not possible fluid restriction may be necessary.

Diuretic-related hyponatraemia. Hyponatraemia is not uncommon in patients on diuretic therapy and it is usually related to hypovolaemia (page 20). However, the occasional patient can present with features similar to SIADH, i.e., instead of being hypovolaemic they are euvolaemic. The characteristic feature is moderate to severe hypokalaemia and potassium depletion (not associated with SIADH), the characteristic patient is over the age of 70 years, and the characteristic diuretic is moduretic although it has also been reported in association with thiazides and frusemide. The exact mechanism is unclear but it has been suggested that potassium depletion sensitises the osmo-receptors causing them to secrete AVP at lower than normal serum osmolality levels.

Endocrine disorders. Hypothyroidism and isolated cortisol deficiency may be associated with a SIADH-like syndrome. Again the cause is unclear but it has been suggested that in hypothyroidism the degradation of circulating AVP is retarded, and that in cortisol deficiency the baroreceptors do not respond appropriately to intravascular pressure changes.

Disturbances of water intake. Compulsive water drinking should not lead to water intoxication if renal function remains intact. Iatrogenic water administration, e.g., excessive fluid infusions following major surgery temporarily suppresses ADH release.

Consequences

Water overload may result in oedema (see above) and hyponatraemia (page 18). The resulting haemodilution will not only result in a decreased serum sodium concentration but also low concentrations of other analytes such as urea, creatinine, proteins, and urate. The low ECF osmolality (tonicity) will be associated with the shift of water into the intracellular compartment producing cellular oedema. In most organs this is inconsequential but it may cause problems in the brain because of the rigid enclosing skull preventing expansion.

Laboratory evaluation

The evaluation of hyponatraemia associated with water overload is discussed on page 19.

Disorders of the serum sodium

At the risk of belabouring the point, we reemphasise that the serum sodium concentration tells the clinician little, or nothing, about the total body sodium; it merely reflects the ratio of sodium to water in the extracellular fluid. Furthermore, if the subject's extracellular sodium content is stable (irrespective of whether it is low, high, or normal) the serum sodium concentration indicates the state of water balance: hypernatraemia suggests a negative balance (input less than output), and hyponatraemia, a positive water balance. To further complicate the picture it is possible, at a given point, to be hypovolaemic and in positive water balance, and *vice versa* (see below).

HYPERNATRAEMIA

Hypernatraemia is generally defined as a serum sodium concentration in excess of 145 mmol/L but for practical and clinical purposes a value in excess of 148 mmol/L is more realistic. As a working proposition it is reasonable to assume that hypernatraemia equals a negative water balance which is due to decreased water intake.

Causes

If at a given point a subject has a stable extracellular sodium content (regardless of the amount) then he will only become hypernatraemic if his extracellular water content falls, changing the ratio between sodium and water. A fall in the body water content will only occur if there is a negative water balance, i.e., if input is less than output.

Given normal circumstances an adult can drink in excess of 20 L of water daily and excrete the same amount to keep in balance (such can occur in diabetes insipidus, page 21). Furthermore, except in severe cholera, there are no common clinical conditions where a patient loses in excess of 20 L a day; hence, provided the patient has access to and can take in water he will not end up in negative water balance because of losses of fluid from the body -- he only acquires a negative water balance (and hypernatraemia) if his water input is not adequate.

For purposes of diagnosis and management, hypernatraemia is usually classified on the basis of the patient's volume status.

Table 1.5. Causes of hypernatraemia.

Pure water depletion (inadequate intake in face of normal losses)
    Subject too old, too young, or too sick to drink
    Access to water denied
    Oesophageal obstructions
    Thirst centre lesions

Sodium and water depletion (hypotonic fluid loss)
    Extrarenal
        GIT: vomiting, diarrhoea
        Skin: excessive sweating
    Renal
        Osmotic diuresis: glucose, mannitol
        Diuretic therapy
        Diabetes insipidus: neurogenic, nephrogenic

Salt gain (without proportional gain in water)
    Iatrogenic: iv hypertonic saline/sodium bicarbonate
    Salt ingestion: intentional, accidental
    Primary mineralocorticoid excess (page 66)

(1) **Euvolaemic hypernatraemia.** These are the patients who are predominantly water depleted because, in the face of *normal fluid losses* from the body, they are unable to take fluid in, i.e., it could be one who is:

    (a) too young, too old, or too sick to drink;
    (b) with no access to water;
    (c) with lesions of the thirst centre;
    (d) with an obstructed oesophagus; or
    (e) receiving inappropriate iv therapy.

As noted above these patients are dehydrated but there is only a mild decrease in the ECV because fluid losses are shared between the intra- and extracellular fluid compartments. If renal function is normal the urine volume will be low and what urine is produced will be very concentrated (of high osmolality). Clinically the subjects do not appear dehydrated or hypervolaemic (oedematous).

(2) **Hypovolaemic hypernatraemia.** This describes patients who, in addition to not taking in adequate fluid, are losing hypotonic fluid from the body, i.e., they are both water and salt depleted but the water depletion is relatively greater than the salt depletion. They are hypovolaemic and present with overt clinical evidence of this condition (high pulse rate, hypotension, etc). If they lose fluid from an extrarenal site they will be passing a small amount of highly concentrated urine with a low sodium content (renal retention of water and sodium stimulated by hypovolaemia). If the origin of the fluid loss is the kidney the urine volume is variable and the urine osmolality is often similar to that of the plasma (urine:plasma osmolality ratio ~1) except in diabetes insipidus in which large volumes of dilute urine are excreted (urine:plasma osmolality <1). Causes of extrarenal and renal losses are given in Table 1.5.

(3) **Hypervolaemic hypernatraemia.** This is the salt-overloaded subject (page 10). Causes include:

    Iatrogenic.   iv hypertonic saline, iv sodium bicarbonate
    Salt ingestion. intentional, accidental, sea water
    Mineralocorticoid excess (primary)

In the first two situations (exogenous salt excess) the negative water balance proposition does not apply; any water ingested or given intravenously will be retained due to renal water retention consequent to hypertonic induction of AVP release. This produces the hypervolaemia which is predominantly intravascular and can result in pulmonary oedema and circulatory overload. Primary mineralocorticoid excess (page 66), although associated with an increased intravascular volume and total body sodium, does not usually present with hypernatraemia because of the proportional retention of water. However, if there is inadequate water intake hypernatraemia will occur.

Consequences

The repercussions of hypernatraemia are those of extracellular hypertonicity, regardless of its cause. The high extracellular tonicity draws fluid out of the intracellular compartment resulting in intracellular dehydration. This is prone to produce intracerebral damage, albeit minor, because as the brain shrinks it pulls away from the rigid skull tearing small blood vessels which pass from the bone to the cerebral tissue.

    If the hypertonicity persists the brain cells compensate by increasing their solute content which draws fluid back into the brain and restores its volume. These additional solutes, called idiogenic molecules, are of uncertain origin but include electrolytes, such as potassium and sodium from the extracellular compartment, and locally produced amino acids, particularly taurine. Although they restore the brain volume, and presumably function, they create another problem which occurs when the tonicity of the extracellular fluid is iatrogenically decreased towards normal by low-solute fluid infusions. Water will now flow into the cell along the concentration gradient producing cerebral oedema. Hence the importance of slowly decreasing a subject's extracellular hypertonicity during treatment so as not to produce rapid fluid shifts. A useful rule-of-thumb is to return the ECF tonicity to normal over the same period of time it took to develop.

Other findings sometimes found and ascribed to hypertonicity are hyperkalaemia (redistribution from cells) and diminished insulin secretion (? cause) resulting in hyperglycaemia.

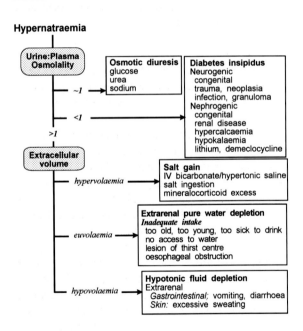

Hypernatraemia

Figure 1.9. Evaluation of hypernatraemia.

Laboratory evaluation

As with hyponatraemia the evaluation of the hypernatraemic patient (Figure 1.9) involves assessment of the hydration status which gives some indication of the type of abnormality -- euvolaemia suggests pure water depletion, hypovolaemia or dehydration indicates hypotonic fluid depletion, and volume overload (hypervolaemia) hints at salt overload. The urine: plasma osmolality ratio is useful to exclude osmotic diuresis (~1.0) and diabetes insipidus (<1.0).

Note: Assessment of the state of hydration of a patient requires some experience -- it depends on observation of the clinical state and on laboratory evidence of haemoconcentration or haemodilution. Both these methods are empirical and crude, and moderate or even quite severe disturbances can occur before they are detected by these clinical or laboratory indices.

HYPONATRAEMIA

Serum sodium concentrations less than 130 mmol/L, except in pseudohyponatraemia (see below), indicate a positive water balance due to decreased renal water excretion. Like hypernatraemia they may be associated with increased, normal, or decreased total body water.

Causes (Table 1.6)

If a subject's extracellular sodium content remains constant, hyponatraemia will only occur if the extracellular water content is increased, i.e., there is a sustained period of positive water balance. This indicates that the subject's water intake is greater than output. As stated earlier a normal adult can drink upwards of 20 L of water daily and stay in water balance, but hyponatraemia occurs in patients on water intakes much less than that (e.g. 2 to 3 litres a day).

Thus it follows that the problem is not excessive intake but decreased water excretion, i.e., excessive AVP or AVP-like activity as described above (page 14). From a diagnostic and laboratory point of view it is useful to classify hyponatraemia on the basis of the patient's serum osmolality, i.e., as eutonic, hypertonic, or hypotonic hyponatraemia.

Eutonic hyponatraemia. Hyponatraemia associated with a normal plasma osmolality is termed *pseudo-hyponatraemia* and usually associated with severe hyperlipidaemia (serum triglycerides >30 mmol/L).

18

Table 1.6 . Causes of hyponatraemia. (TB$_{Na}$, total body sodium content)

Euvolaemic (TB$_{Na}$ normal)
Pseudohyponatraemia (eutonic)
    Hyperlipidaemia
Excess intracellular solute (hypertonic)
    Hyperglycaemia
Acute water overload (hypotonic)
    Rapid water intake PLUS
        Hypovolaemia
        Drugs (page 15)
        Stress: post-surgery, psychogenic
        Endocrine: hypothyroidism, cortisol deficiency
Chronic water overload (hypotonic)
    SIADH (page14)
    Drugs (page 15)
    Renal failure
    Endocrine: hypothyroidism, cortisol deficiency

Hypovolaemic (TB$_{Na}$ decreased)
Extrarenal causes (hypotonic)
    GIT: vomiting, diarrhoea
    Skin: burns
Renal causes (hypotonic)
    Diuretic therapy
    Addison's disease
    Salt-losing nephritis

Hypervolaemic (TB$_{Na}$ increased/Oedematous; hypotonic)
    Cardiac failure
    Nephrotic syndrome
    Liver cirrhosis

This is a laboratory artefact due to the way sodium is measured. Serum contains 94% water and some 6% solids consisting mainly of proteins and lipids; the sodium ions reside only in the water phase. During analysis an aliquot (e.g., 0.1 mL) of serum is taken and its sodium content measured which is then related to the whole serum rather than to the serum water, i.e., it is reported as mmol of sodium per litre of serum. If the solid content of serum is increased, to say 10% by the presence of fat particles, then the aliquot contains less water and proportionately less sodium which upon measurement will be again related to the whole serum. Thus even though the sodium concentration in the serum water phase is normal, the serum sodium concentration will be lower -- hence pseudohyponatraemia.

The osmometer measures the number of particles in the serum water, and because fats and proteins are very large molecules they contribute very little to the overall osmolality, and even concentration changes of several-fold will not significantly affect the osmolality. Thus in pseudohyponatraemia, the serum osmolality remains normal -- eutonic hyponatraemia -- this may be used to exclude or confirm pseudohyponatraemia.

Hypertonic hyponatraemia. A low serum sodium concentration associated with a high serum osmolality usually indicates hyperglycaemia. Severe hyperglycaemia, e.g., >40 mmol/L, can cause hyponatraemia by virtue of its osmotic effect. The high extracellular osmolality (tonicity) draws water out of cells into the extracellular compartment, causing dilutional hypo-natraemia. In such cases, when the glucose is taken up by the cells (e.g., following insulin therapy) the excess extracellular water will pass back to the cells. A useful rule-of-thumb for calculating the *true* serum sodium concentration after the removal of glucose is to divide the serum glucose concentration (in mmol/L) by 4 and add this figure to the measured serum sodium concentration.

Hypotonic hyponatraemia. Patients with hyponatraemia and a low serum osmolality may be *hypervolaemic, euvolaemic, or hypovolaemic.*

Hypervolaemic. This describes the oedematous patients with hyponatraemia (page 20). The commonest cause of hyponatraemia associated with oedema is diuretic therapy. However, a number of untreated oedematous subjects present with hyponatraemia which is presumably due to retention of more water relative to sodium.

Hypovolaemic. They are the subjects who have lost hypotonic fluids by a renal or extrarenal route and thereafter replaced their salt and water loss by drinking pure water, but still remain dehydrated. This is a *depletional hyponatraemia* (not to be confused with dilutional hyponatraemia which is associated with euvolaemia).

Euvolaemic. This describes subjects who are hyponatraemic but who are neither oedematous nor dehydrated. The pathophysiology is water excess due to decreased renal water excretion (*dilutional hypo-natraemia*). This may occur as an acute or chronic process:

Acute water overload: This occurs when there is rapid water intake (oral or more usually iv) in a patient who has a problem excreting water due to:
-   Hypovolaemia (inducing AVP secretion): haemorrhage, burns.
-   Stress: post-surgery, psychogenic (↑ AVP)
-   Drugs (page 15)
-   Endocrinopathies (page 15)

Chronic water overload: SIADH, drug effects, hypothyroidism, cortisol deficiency.

Consequences

Extracellular hyponatraemia (hypotonicity) is associated with water passing into the cells along the concentration gradient producing cellular oedema. This can cause cerebral problems, e.g., confusion, decreased mentation, convulsions, because of the inability of the brain to expand within the bony skull.

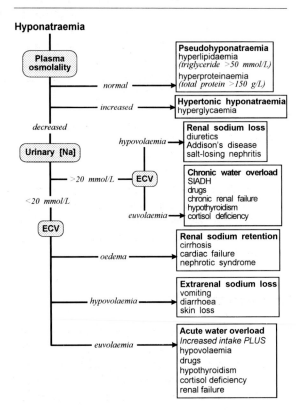

Hyponatraemia

Figure 1.10. Laboratory evaluation of hyponatraemia.

Laboratory evaluation

The most useful and most important procedures in the evaluation of a subject with hyponatraemia is the history (vomiting, diarrhoea, diuretic therapy, etc) and the clinical estimation of the patient's volume status. In the latter the patient will be diagnosed as oedematous (hypervolaemia), dehydrated (hypovolaemia) or neither of these (euvolaemia). Generally this evaluation is straightforward but problems do arise in differentiating between euvolaemia and mild dehydration which can be clinically silent.

From the laboratory point of view the serum osmolality value should be the starting point. From here the evaluation follows logically with the only other test necessary being a sodium concentration on a spot (untimed) sample of urine (Figure 1.10).

Disorders of Renal Water Excretion

An increased urinary output (polyuria) is usually always associated with an increased intake. It may be primarily due to a high fluid intake, or secondary to disorders of AVP production, AVP action at the renal level, or osmotic diuresis. Similarly, a low urine output (oliguria) may reflect a decreased fluid intake or be secondary to renal disease.

POLYURIA

Polyuria is a subjective symptom and difficult to define but a urinary volume in excess of 3 litres a day is a reasonable starting point. It should not be confused with frequency (frequent passage of small amounts of urine but a normal daily output).

Causes

A high urinary volume can be due to increased fluid intake in an otherwise normal subject or to some defect in renal concentrating ability. In order for the kidney to reabsorb water and concentrate the urine the following must be satisfied:

(1) Delivery of a dilute urine to the collecting ducts (i.e., a normal functioning 'diluting' segment)
(2) AVP availability

(3) Normal response of the collecting duct to AVP
(4) High medullary to luminal osmotic gradient in the collecting duct area

Thus polyuria may be the result of:

(1) **Osmotic diuresis:** high luminal concentrations of glucose (diabetes mellitus) and sodium (diuretic therapy) produce a high urine osmolality and inhibit delivery of a dilute urine to the collecting ducts.

(2) **AVP deficiency:**

   (a) neurogenic diabetes insipidus;
   (b) drugs that modify release of ADH (page 15);
   (c) post-surgical stress, hypoxia, hypercapnia (temporary suppression of AVP release).

(3) **Abnormalities of collecting ducts:**

   (a) *Functional:* nephrogenic diabetes insipidus (inborn error of metabolism resulting in ducts being non-responsive to AVP);
   drugs that suppress or inhibit ADH activity at the collecting duct.
   (b) *Structural damage:* pyelonephritis, analgesic nephropathy, hypercalcaemia, hypokalaemia, nephrocalcinosis.

(4) **Loss of medullary tonicity:** Defective reabsorption of sodium and chloride ions by the ascending limb of the loop of Henle due to diuretic therapy will compromise the medullary tonicity (page 5).

From a laboratory diagnosis viewpoint it is convenient to classify the polyurias on the basis of the type of diuresis:

Water diuresis (urine osmolality <200 mmol/kg):

   (1) *High intake* (psychogenic polydipsia)
   (2) *Diabetes insipidus:*
      (i) central or neurogenic
      (ii) nephrogenic.

Solute diuresis (urine osmolality ~300 mmol/kg):

   (1) *Sodium:* high intake, diuretic therapy
   (2) *Glucose:* diabetes mellitus
   (3) *Urea:* hypercatabolic states, renal disease.

Diabetes insipidus (DI). There are two varieties of DI, the *neurogenic and nephrogenic.*

Neurogenic DI: The inability to produce or secrete AVP may be due to hypothalamic or pituitary disease (primary disease, trauma, tumours, infections, etc). The lack of this hormone results in the passage of very large amounts (5 to 20 L/day) of very dilute urine (osmolality 50-100 mmol/kg). It will not result in dehydration or hypernatraemia unless there is an inadequate fluid intake. The disorder responds to exogenous AVP.

Nephrogenic DI: This may be due to an inherited disorder whereby the collecting duct cells will not respond to AVP or it may be due to local mechanisms (structural renal disease, metabolic disorders). It presents with a similar picture to the neurogenic variety but it will not respond to exogenous AVP.

Psychogenic overdrinking. This disorder has similar features to DI -- polydipsia, polyuria with a dilute urine. The difference is the patient's response to dehydration. After overnight fluid restriction a normal subject will concentrate his urine to produce an osmolality greater than 750 mmol/kg; a patient with DI, depending on the degree of defect, will rarely produce a urine osmolality above 400 mmol/kg and often it will be less than 200 mmol/kg. In the case of psychogenic overdrinking there will usually be a normal, or near normal response (urine osmolality >600 mmol/kg) to fluid restriction.

Solute diuresis. In solute diuresis the polyuria is due to osmotic diuresis and hence it can be distinguished from water diuresis by a urine osmolality of around 300 mmol/kg and identification of the offending solute.

Consequences

The clinical consequences, as opposed to the personal and social problems, of polyuria *per se* are minimal. If the oral fluid intake does not keep up with the output, as during illness, then dehydration and hypernatraemia can occur. If the polyuria is longstanding dilation of the ureters may occur.

Laboratory evaluation

Figures 1.11 to 1.13 cover the approach to, and the diagnosis of, the patient with polyuria.

Having determined that polyuria is present the first procedure is to measure the serum and urine osmolalities: if the urine value is similar to the plasma value (± 50 mmol/kg) one should consider solute diuresis; if the urine osmolality is low (e.g., less than 250 mmol/kg) then 'screen' the patient by performing an osmolality on the first urine sample passed on rising in the morning (with no fluids permitted after 9.00 pm). Values in excess of 750 mmol/kg are considered normal. Values less than this may occur if there is pre-existing renal disease or may indicate a renal concentrating defect. In the latter a dehydration-AVP test should be considered.

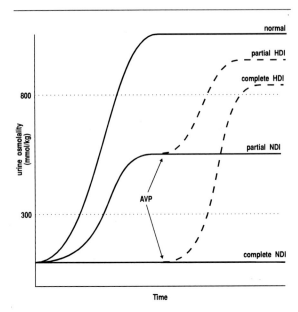

HDI, hypothalamic diabetes insipidus
NDI, nephrogenic diabetes insipidus
AVP, arginine vasopressin

Figure 1.12. Interpretation of dehydration test.

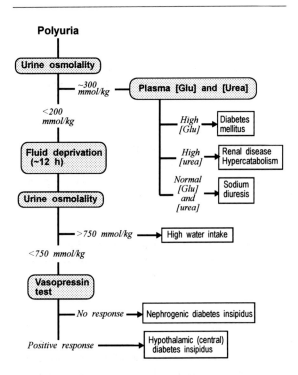

Figure 1.11. Evaluation of polyuria.

There are many ways of performing a dehydration or water deprivation test; the following has been found useful.

1   No water taken from 9.00 pm the night before until conclusion of the test.

2   At 7.00 am the next morning empty bladder and discard urine.

3   Beginning at 8.00 am pass urine hourly (empty bladder completely). Estimate the osmolality and continue in this manner hourly until either the osmolality reaches 750 mmol/L (no abnormality) or until the osmolality reaches a plateau (difference between consecutive estimations of less than 30 mmol/kg).

4   When a plateau is reached take a blood sample for a serum osmolality and administer AVP (5 units of aqueous vasopressin intramuscularly or DDAVP nasally). Exactly one hour later collect urine and estimate the osmolality.

The interpretation of this test is illustrated in Figures 1.11 to 1.13. Some relevant points of note are:

●   Incomplete emptying of the bladder (residual urine interferes with the test) and surreptitious water drinking during the test will invalidate the procedure.

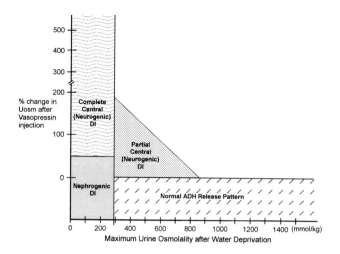

Figure 1.13. The change in urine osmolality following vasopressin administration versus the maximum urine osmolality attained in the water deprivation test. (Adapted from data presented by Miller et al, Ann Internal Med 1970;73:721). DI, diabetes insipidus; ADH, antidiuretic hormone (vasopressin),Uosm,urine osmolality. The triangular area denotes the zone in which most of the results for cases of partial neurogenic diabetes insipidus will fall.

- An otherwise normal subject who has had an excessive fluid intake for a long period may 'wash-out' the renal interstitial osmoles and produce a test result indicating incomplete nephrogenic DI.

- Figures 1.12. and 1.13 are two ways of plotting the results obtained from the water deprivation test. The former plots the representative urine osmolalities attained during the test duration for the various groups, whilst the latter plots the relationship between the percentage changes in urine osmolality after vasopressin administration and the maximal urine osmolality values attained by the different groups of patients following water deprivation.

OLIGURIA

Oliguria, a low urine output, usually indicates renal dysfunction and is usually considered in sections on renal disease. However, it can occur in the absence of renal disease and will be discussed here for the sake of completeness. A definition in terms of urine volume is difficult but an excretion of less than 500-600 mL/day is a useful figure (if the average amount of solute to be cleared by the kidney is 600 mmol and the kidney can concentrate the urine up to a maximum of 1200 mmol/kg, then 500 mL is the minimal amount of urine required).

Causes

A decrease in urine output is usually classified as prerenal, renal, and postrenal depending on the site of the dysfunction.

Prerenal oliguria. In this situation the kidney and urinary apparatus are normal and the decrease is due to a decreased GFR which in turn is due to hypovolaemia, e.g., dehydration, blood loss, serum loss.

Renal oliguria. This indicates that the kidney is at fault (renal disease) but for the sake of completeness, we will add conditions associated with increased AVP activity.

Renal disease: Both acute and chronic renal failure can present with oliguria but they can also be associated with polyuria due to uraemia-induced diuresis (page 21). Acute renal shutdown (acute tubular necrosis) may present with severe oliguria (page 79) and has to be distinguished from prerenal failure.

Increased AVP activity: Increased AVP activity due to SIADH or various drugs (page 5) will decrease urinary output but it may not be sufficient to lower the volume to below 600 mL/day or to be noticed by the patient or clinician as a decreased urinary output.

Postrenal oliguria. This occurs in an otherwise normal patient who has an obstruction to urine outflow. The obstruction can be anywhere from the kidney pelvis to the urethra. The commonest site is the prostatic area (prostatic hyperplasia or malignancy) but stones and strictures may occur at any level. Obstruction at the base of the bladder and all points onwards can produce anuria (no urine) which is uncommon in other conditions associated with a decreased urine output.

Consequences

The clinical repercussions of oliguria depend on the cause. Prolonged obstruction of the ureter will result in dilation of the bladder, the ureters and the kidney pelvis. If it is unrelieved the back pressure on the kidney will destroy the parenchyma and often there is early tubular dysfunction manifested by retention of potassium and hydrogen ions (hyperkalaemic metabolic acidosis, page 51). The consequences of renal disease (page 76), prerenal failure (page 78) and increased AVP activity (page 4) are discussed elsewhere. In all cases, except increased AVP activity, there is an inability of the kidney to clear the blood of urea and, depending on the severity, of creatinine. Hence raised serum urea and creatinine concentrations are common markers of decreased urine output.

Laboratory evaluation

After excluding postrenal obstruction by clinical and radiological means, the problem in oliguria is to distinguish prerenal dysfunction from renal dysfunction (acute tubular necrosis). The most useful procedure is microscopic examination of the urine: acute tubular necrosis (ATN) is associated with haematuria, red blood cells, casts, and cell debris; whereas in prerenal failure the urine is usually 'clean'. Other useful tests are the urinary sodium concentrations (ATN, >20 mmol/L; prerenal, <10 mmol/L) and the fractional excretion of sodium (ATN, >3%; prerenal , <1%). These tests are discussed in more detail on page 79.

REFERENCES/FURTHER READING

Abraham WT, Schrier RW. Edematous disorders: pathophysiology of renal sodium and water retention and treatment with diuretics. Curr Opin Nephrol Hypertension 1993;2:798-805.

Berl T. Treating hyponatremia: damned if we do, damned if we don't. Kidney Internl 1990;37:1006-1018.

Bevilacqua M. Hyponatraemia in AIDS. Baillieres Clinics Endocrinol Metab 1994;8:837-48.

Breyer MD, Ando Y. Hormonal signaling and regulation of salt and water transport in the collecting duct. Annual Rev Physiol 1994;56:711-39.

Gennari FJ. Serum osmolality: uses and limitations. N Engl J Med 1984;310:102-105.

Gunning ME, Brenner BM. Natriuretic peptides and the kidney: current concepts. Kidney Internl (suppl) 1992;38:S127-S133.

Mulloy AL, Caruana RJ. Hyponatremic emergencies. Med Clinics North Am 1995;79:131-53.

Oh MS, Carroll HJ. Disorders of sodium metabolism: hypernatremia and hyponatremia. Critical Care Med 1992;20:94-105.

Schrier RW, Niederberger M. Paradoxes of body fluid volume regulation in health and disease. A unifying hypothesis. West J Med 1994;16:393-408.

Statter MB. Fluids and electrolytes in infants and children. Semin Pediatr Surg 1992;1:208-11.

Turnheim K. Epithelial sodium transport: basic autoregulatory mechanisms. Physiol Res 1994;43:211-218.

Usberti M, Gazzotti RM, Poiesi C, D'Avanzo L, Ghielmi S. Considerations on the sodium retention in nephrotic syndrome.Am J Nephrol 1995;15(1):38-47.

Chapter 2

Potassium

The major portion of the total body potassium (3000-3500 mmol) is intracellular; the potassium concentration ([K]) inside the cells being 120-150 mmol/L. The extracellular fluid (ECF) with a [K] of 3.5-5.0 mmol/L contains only 2-3% of the total content (70-80 mmol), but this potassium is important in the maintenance of cell membrane polarisation. The magnitude of the cell membrane resting potential, 50-90 mV (negative on the inside), is proportional to the concentration of potassium on either side of the membrane; thus changes in the extracellular [K] will affect neuro-muscular activity, e.g., muscle weakness occurs in both hyperkalaemia and hypokalaemia.

In the routine laboratory, potassium status is assessed by estimating the plasma [K]; although this estimation is important from a therapeutic point of view, it does not necessarily give an indication of the total body content. A large potassium deficiency, or excess, may be associated with normal plasma levels and both hyperkalaemia and hypokalaemia can be associated with a normal body potassium content.

Homeostasis

In the normal subject potassium is taken in orally (in the diet) and balance is achieved by excretion in the faeces, the sweat, and the urine. The major excretory path is via the kidney (faecal and sweat losses are relatively insignificant), and it is the proper function of this organ on which potassium homeostasis depends. Of equal importance in homeostasis is the distribution of potassium between the intracellular and extracellular fluid compartments because of the effect on membrane polarisation, and because rapid increases in the ECF potassium content are 'buffered' in the first instance by cellular potassium uptake.

INTAKE

Potassium intake depends on the diet and is of the order of 1-2 mmol/kg/day (50-100 mmol/day). Virtually all is absorbed in the gut with less than 10 mmol/day appearing in the faeces. There is no physiological control over potassium intake.

DISTRIBUTION

The potassium concentration gradient across the cell membrane determines the cell membrane potential and disturbances in the ECF potassium content disturb the ratio more than changes in the intracellular fluid (ICF) potassium content. For example, assuming an ICF potassium of 3400 mmol and an ECF potassium of 70 mmol then the ratio is 48.57:1. If the ICF potassium increases by 7 mmol (10% of ECF potassium) the ratio becomes 48.67:1; when a 7 mmol increase occurs in the ECF the ratio becomes 44.15:1. Hence adjustments in internal balance are critical to defend the subject against hyperkalaemia. This is of particular relevance during eating as a single meal may contain up to 50 mmol of potassium.

Potassium distribution between the ICF and the ECF is maintained by a membrane-associated Na^+-K^+-ATPase pump. Potassium ions and sodium ions diffuse across cell walls and the maintenance of the ionic concentrations on both sides of the cell membrane is controlled by the pumping of K^+ into the cell and Na^+ out of it. The factors which influence potassium transfer across the cell membrane are:

1 **Potassium load.** 50% of any potassium added to the ECF (oral or intravenous) crosses into the cells. The stimulus for this uptake is unclear (? local stimulation of the ATPase mechanism by potassium ions). About 40% of the excess potassium is excreted by the kidneys over 2 to 3 hours.

2 **Insulin.** Insulin directly induces cellular potassium uptake, an action independent of its action on glucose. On the other hand, insulin deficiency results in potassium 'leaking' from cells. The practical application of this mechanism is the use of insulin administration to treat hyperkalaemia.

3 **Catecholamines.** Adrenaline and β-adrenergic

receptor agonists such as salbutamol increase cellular K$^+$ uptake and can result in hypokalaemia. The action is biphasic: administration of adrenalin results in an initial release of K$^+$ from the liver followed by a more sustained uptake.

4 Aldosterone. Although aldosterone increases the uptake of ECF K$^+$ by the distal renal tubular cells, large gut cells, sweat gland cells, and mammary gland cells it probably plays only a minor role in uptake by other cells.

5 ECF hydrogen ion concentration ([H$^+$]). In *alkalaemia* (low ECF [H$^+$]), hydrogen ions tend to diffuse out of cells in exchange for extracellular potassium ions (maintenance of electroneutrality). This can result in hypokalaemia and in addition there is increased renal potassium excretion (see below). Similarly, during *acidaemia* (high ECF [H$^+$]) the cells will 'mop up' extracellular H$^+$, which may be exchanged for intracellular K$^+$. This exchange probably only occurs when the acidosis is of the hyperchloraemic type (e.g., infusion of HCl) because of the difficulty for chloride ions to enter cells. When the acidosis is due to organic acids (lactic acidosis, ketoacidosis), the acid anion, e.g., lactate, is able to cross the cell membrane in tandem with the H$^+$ and thus electroneutrality is maintained without K$^+$ crossing in the opposite direction.

OUTPUT

Under normal circumstances potassium balance is maintained by renal excretion; only a small amount (5-10 mmol/day) is excreted in the sweat and faeces.

Renal potassium excretion

About 700 mmol/day of potassium is filtered by the glomerulus. Most of this (>95%) is reabsorbed in the proximal nephron and the major part of the urinary potassium results from secretion by the distal nephron.

Proximal tubule. About 70% of the filtered potassium is actively reabsorbed by a process that is independent of sodium reabsorption.

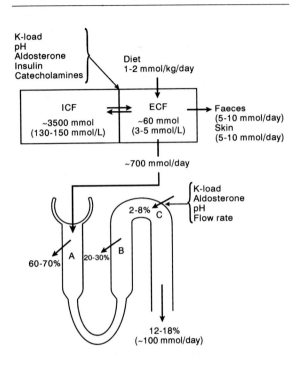

Figure 2.1. Potassium distribution, exchange and homeostasis in an average adult. A, proximal tubule; B, thick ascending limb of Henle; C, collecting duct; ICF, intracellular fluid; ECF, extracellular fluid.

Loop of Henle. In the thick ascending limb (diluting segment) of the loop of Henle 20 to 25% of the filtered potassium is reabsorbed along with sodium consequent to active chloride reabsorption.

Distal tubule and collecting duct. Secretion of K$^+$ occurs in the distal tubule along the electrochemical gradient caused by the active reabsorption of Na$^+$. This is not a 1:1 coupling with sodium ions (Na$^+$ reabsorption can be more than the sum of K$^+$ and H$^+$ secretion and occurs mainly in the distal portion).

Control of potassium excretion

The renal secretion (and excretion) of potassium is governed mainly by two factors: the potassium concentration in the distal renal tubular cells, and the rate of urine flow past these cells.

The intracellular potassium ions rapidly equilibrate with the luminal fluid across the luminal side of the cell membrane. The following relationships apply: an increased cellular [K⁺] associated with a normal flow rate will result in increased secretion (a low [K⁺] with normal flow gives a low excretion); a normal cellular [K⁺] and an increased flow rate produces an increased secretion (a normal [K⁺] and a low flow gives a low excretion).

Cell potassium content. Factors increasing the cellular [K⁺] (and renal excretion) are:

- Increased aldosterone (page 66)
- Alkalaemia (low ECF [H⁺]) due to H⁺-K⁺ exchange across the cell wall. Thus primary metabolic alkalosis is nearly always associated with hypokalaemia due to increased renal potassium excretion.
- Increased potassium load

The reverse situations, hypoaldosteronism, acidaemia, and decreased potassium load result in a low cell [K⁺] and decreased excretion.

Urine flow rate. Factors which increase the urine flow rate and renal potassium excretion are:

- Increased sodium load (sodium diuresis)
- Osmotic diuresis
- Diuretics acting proximal to the distal tubule (sodium diuresis)

A decreased flow rate and potassium retention occur if there is a decreased GFR (dehydration, shock, etc) and in acute renal failure (page 78).

NOTE:

1 The kidney is very good at handling potassium loads, e.g., chronic intakes of 500-1000 mmol/day can be readily excreted (this is not surprising given the high potassium content of most foods). However, the kidney is not so good at conserving potassium and chronic dietary deficiency can result in potassium depletion because of continued excretion.

2 An acute load of potassium is 'buffered' in the first instance by the cells: 50% is taken up by the cells and 40% is excreted by the kidney over the next 2 to 3 hours (hence only 10% is retained in the extracellular fluid). This occurs even in potassium-depleted states, i.e., 50% of replacement potassium is excreted in the urine.

Disordered Potassium Homeostasis

Potassium deficiency is generally due to increased loss in the face of normal or decreased intake (negative potassium balance), and potassium excess usually represents decreased renal potassium excretion in the face of a normal or increased intake (positive potassium balance).

As stated above the plasma [K] does not necessarily reflect the total body potassium content. For example, hypokalaemia can be associated with a normal body potassium content, as in the hypokalaemia associated with salbutamol therapy; and hyperkalaemia, with a low body potassium content, as occurs in diabetic ketoacidosis. The importance of hyper- and hypokalaemia lies in the fact that such conditions represent an abnormal intracellular-extracellular gradient that may require vigorous therapy. From a therapeutic view hypokalaemia is usually associated with potassium deficiency, whilst hyperkalaemia generally implies that potassium has to be removed from the extracellular compartment.

HYPERKALAEMIA

Hyperkalaemia is defined as a plasma potassium value in excess of 5.0 mmol/L (our reference range: 3.5-5.0 mmol/L). It is a common problem presenting in up to 5% of hospital patients although factitious values (haemolysis, etc) are the commonest cause.

Causes/pathophysiology

A useful practical classification is to divide the causes of hyperkalaemia into three groups: pseudohyperkalaemia, increased potassium input into the ECF, and decreased renal excretion (Table 2.1).

Pseudohyperkalaemia. The serum from blood containing large numbers of white cells (leucocytosis)

Table 2.1. Causes of hyperkalaemia.

Pseudohyperkalaemia
    Haemolysis
    Leucocytosis
    Thrombocytosis

Increased intake/load to ECF
Exogenous
    Oral/IV therapy
Endogenous
    Tissue necrosis: crush injury, burns, malignancy

Disturbed intracellular/extracellular distribution
    Acidaemia
    Insulin deficiency: diabetes mellitus
    Drugs: digoxin toxicity, succinylcholine
    Hypertonicity: glucose, sodium
    Hyperkalaemic periodic paralysis

Decreased renal excretion
Renal failure: Acute, Chronic
Drugs
    Potassium-sparing diuretics: amiloride,
        triamterene, spironolactone
    Prostaglandin inhibitors: indomethacin, ibuprofen
    Captopril
    Heparin
Mineralocorticoid deficiency syndromes
    Low cortisol and aldosterone: Addison's disease,
        Adrenal hyperplasia, C21-hydroxylase defect
    Selective aldosterone deficiency:
        Hyporeninaemic hypoaldosteronism
        Prostaglandin inhibition (indomethacin)
Mineralocorticoid resistant syndromes
    Interstitial nephritis
    Sickle cell disease
    Obstructive uropathy
    Systemic lupus erythrematosus
    Amyloidosis
    Pseudohypoaldosteronism

or platelets (thrombocytosis) often has a factitiously high potassium concentration due to release of potassium from these elements during clotting. This can be overcome by taking a fresh sample into heparin and quickly separating the plasma. *In vitro* haemolysis and seepage of potassium from red cells due to delayed separation of the serum (>4 hours) is also a common problem. Pseudohyperkalaemia is the commonest cause of a high serum [K] encountered in the laboratory.

Tissue destruction. Acute tissue necroses (crush injuries, burns, chemotherapy of malignancy) will release large amounts of potassium into the ECF. These patients often have compromised renal function which worsens the hyperkalaemia.

Acidaemia. As stated above acidaemia has the potential to produce hyperkalaemia due to efflux of potassium from cells in exchange for extracellular hydrogen ions. However, this will only occur in 'mineral acidaemia' due to HCl or arginine-HCl infusions. Hyperkalaemia occurring in the organic acidaemias (ketoacidosis, lactic acidosis) is due to other mechanisms, e.g., insulin deficiency in diabetic ketoacidosis (Note: one of the features of lactic acidosis is the usually normal serum potassium level).

Extracellular hypertonicity. Hypertonicity due to high ECF concentrations of sodium or glucose is associated with efflux of potassium from cells which may produce a mild hyperkalaemia.

Hyperkalaemic periodic paralysis. This is a rare inherited condition associated with bouts of muscular paralysis and hyperkalaemia (potassium release from cells). It can be precipitated by exercise, cold exposure, or potassium therapy. The cause is unclear.

Drugs and hyperkalaemia. The drugs that may be associated with hyperkalaemia are the potassium-sparing diuretics, prostaglandin inhibitors, digoxin, succinylcholine, captopril, and heparin.

Potassium-sparing diuretics. Amiloride, spironolactone, and triamterene act on the distal tubule inhibiting sodium reabsorption. This is associated with inhibition of potassium and hydrogen ion excretion and may cause hyperkalaemic hyperchloraemic metabolic acidosis (see Figure 2.3, page 32).

Prostaglandin inhibitors. Normal prostaglandin

metabolism is necessary for the normal secretion of renin and aldosterone and the prostaglandin inhibitor drugs, such as indomethacin and ibuprofen, can produce a syndrome similar to the syndrome of hyporeninaemic hypoaldosteronism (see below).

Digoxin. Hyperkalaemia may be associated with digoxin toxicity (potassium release from cells).

Succinylcholine. This muscle relaxant (used as an anaesthetic) depolarises the muscle cells and allows potassium to escape into the ECF.

Captopril. This agent and other angiotensin-converting enzyme inhibitors have the potential to produce hypoaldosteronism and hence hyperkalaemia. However, hyperkalaemia is not a common complication of these drugs but it will occur if there is an associated increased potassium uptake.

Heparin. Large doses of heparin can suppress the synthesis of aldosterone and result in hyperkalaemia.

Renal failure. Chronic renal failure may have an associated hyperkalaemia whereas acute renal shutdown is usually accompanied by hyperkalaemia. In uncomplicated chronic renal insufficiency the remaining nephrons are able to maintain potassium excretion by increasing their workload (increased fractional excretion, page 76) by up to 30-fold, but there comes a stage when this is insufficient due to decreased number of nephrons and potassium is retained causing hyperkalaemia. This occurs when 70-80% of the nephrons are destroyed (serum creatinine >0.35 mmol/L or thereabout). In acute renal shutdown renal function is severely compromised and hyperkalaemia is usual.

Mineralocorticoid deficiency syndromes. Aldosterone increases potassium excretion by increasing the distal tubular cell uptake (see above). Aldosterone deficiency has the reverse effect. These syndromes are discussed in detail in the mineralocorticoid chapter (page 62). Here we will only briefly discuss the syndrome of hyporeninaemic hypoaldosteronism.

Syndrome of hyporeninaemic hypoaldosteronism (SHH). This syndrome is commonly seen in elderly patients where it presents as hyperkalaemia which may be associated with a mild hyperchloraemic metabolic acidosis (page 51). There may be mild renal insufficiency (serum creatinine <0.20 mmol/L) and around 50% of the subjects will have diabetes mellitus, most of the others will have interstitial nephritis. The hyperkalaemia is due to decreased renal potassium excretion as a consequence of hypoaldosteronism.

Evaluation of the renin-aldosterone axis reveals depressed secretion of both hormones -- the exact cause is unknown. A similar biochemical and clinical presentation can be seen in patients on long term prostaglandin inhibitor (e.g., indomethacin) therapy.

Mineralocorticoid resistance syndromes. In these disorders, listed in Table 2.1., the synthesis and secretion of aldosterone is normal but there is end organ resistance. The disorder may be primary (pseudohypoaldosteronism) or secondary to a variety of diseases which affect the kidney (Table 2.1.).

Consequences of hyperkalaemia

The patient's response to hyperkalaemia depends on the rate of rise of the ECF potassium concentration and the level reached. Mild degrees of hyperkalaemia (e.g., <6.0 mmol/L) are usually symptomless, but if there is a rise beyond this figure (particularly if rapid) some or all of the following may occur. The problems of most concern are cardiac arrhythmia and possible arrest.

- listlessness, mental confusion
- muscle weakness
- nausea and vomiting
- paralytic ileus
- parasthesia
- cardiac arrhythmia and arrest
- ECG changes: tall T-waves, wide QRS-complex, wide PR-interval.

Therapy is aimed at decreasing potassium intake (dietary, etc), increasing excretion from the body (use of oral Resonium A, an ion exchange resin which binds potassium, or dialysis) and, in the emergency situation, pushing the potassium into cells with insulin. In the very acute situation calcium, which antagonises the effects of potassium at the tissue level, can be given as IV calcium chloride.

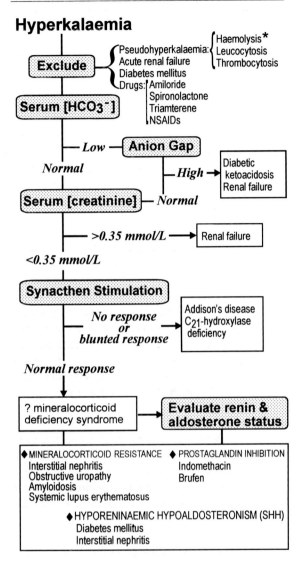

Hyperkalaemia

Exclude {
Pseudohyperkalaemia: { Haemolysis*
Leucocytosis
Thrombocytosis
Acute renal failure
Diabetes mellitus
Drugs: { Amiloride
Spironolactone
Triamterene
NSAIDs

Serum [HCO3⁻]

— *Low* — **Anion Gap**

Normal

— *High* → Diabetic ketoacidosis / Renal failure

Serum [creatinine] — *Normal*

— *>0.35 mmol/L* → Renal failure

<0.35 mmol/L

Synacthen Stimulation

No response or blunted response → Addison's disease / C$_{21}$-hydroxylase deficiency

Normal response

? mineralocorticoid deficiency syndrome → **Evaluate renin & aldosterone status**

◆ MINERALOCORTICOID RESISTANCE ◆ PROSTAGLANDIN INHIBITION
Interstitial nephritis   Indomethacin
Obstructive uropathy   Brufen
Amyloidosis
Systemic lupus erythematosus

◆ HYPORENINAEMIC HYPOALDOSTERONISM (SHH)
Diabetes mellitus
Interstitial nephritis

* Phosphate and LDH may also be increased

Anion Gap = {[Na] + [K]} - {[Cl] + [HCO3]}   RR: 7-17 mEq/L

Figure 2.2. Laboratory evaluation of hyperkalaemia. RR, reference range; LDH, lactate dehydrogenase.

Laboratory evaluation

In most patients presenting with true hyperkalaemia the cause is clinically obvious, e.g., diabetes mellitus, severe renal failure and the like. A logical approach to the evaluation of the patient with hyperkalaemia of obscure origin is outlined in Figure 2.2 which is self-explanatory.

Again it is worth noting that the commonest cause of a high serum potassium is pseudohyperkalaemia and this should be excluded, by analysing a fresh sample if necessary, before pressing on to further tests. Factors to note are haemolysed specimens, time between venesection and cell separation, and the possibility of haematological disorders.

The general approach is to exclude obvious causes such as pseudohyperkalaemia, diabetes mellitus, severe renal failure, and drug-induced hyperkalaemia. Then continue the evaluation on the basis of the plasma bicarbonate and anion gap results as outlined in Figure 2.2. The ACTH (Synacthen) stimulation test is described on page 255 and the evaluation of renin and aldosterone status on page 70.

HYPOKALAEMIA

Hypokalaemia, a plasma [K⁺] less than ~3.5 mmol/L, is the commonest disorder of potassium homeostasis (pseudohyperkalaemia is the commonest plasma potassium abnormality), occurring in around 3 to 6% of all hospitalised patients. The commonest causes of hypokalaemia are diuretic therapy, vomiting, and diarrhoea.

Causes/pathophysiology

Although the commonest mechanism of hypokalaemia is loss from the body, decreased intake plays a significant role because the kidney is not efficient at conserving potassium (~50% of intake appears in the urine within 3 to 4 hours). A useful approach is to consider the causes in terms of decreased intake, transcellular shifts, renal loss and extrarenal loss (Table 2.2.).

Decreased intake. Hypokalaemia due only to a decreased potassium intake is unusual, there being usually an associated increased loss, but it may occur in subjects on potassium-deficient IV therapy, in chronic alcoholics and in anorexia nervosa.

Transcellular shift. Severe hypokalaemia associated with normal total body potassium may occur with a variety of drugs, in barium toxicity (rare), and in hypokalaemic periodic paralysis (uncommon).

Table 2.2. Causes of hypokalaemia.

Decreased intake
  Inappropriate iv therapy
  Anorexia nervosa
  Chronic alcoholism
Transcellular shifts
  Insulin, Vitamin B_{12}
  Salbutamol, Barium toxicity
  Periodic paralysis
Extrarenal loss
  Vomiting
  Diarrhoea
  Laxative abuse
  Villous adenoma of colon
  Urine diversion to gut
Renal loss
  Metabolic alkalosis
  Diuretic therapy
  Mineralocorticoid excess syndromes
  Renal tubular acidosis
  Bartter's syndrome
  Magnesium depletion
  Gentamicin therapy
  Leukaemia

Drugs. Hypokalaemia may complicate insulin therapy in diabetic ketoacidosis if potassium supplements are not given because these patients are potassium deficient. The administration of salbutamol (β_2-agonist), particularly when given as infusions for the prevention of premature labour, can be associated with quite low plasma potassium levels (e.g., <2.5 mmol/L). Newly diagnosed patients with pernicious anaemia, when given vitamin B_{12}, can develop a severe life-threatening hypokalaemia (due to rapid uptake of potassium by newly developing red cells).

Hypokalaemic periodic paralysis. This condition presents with bouts of muscle paralysis associated with hypokalaemia. It is due to increased cellular potassium uptake (cause unknown) which can be initiated by physical stress, large carbohydrate meals, and cold exposure.

Barium toxicity. Several cases of $BaCl_2$ toxicity

have been recorded where severe hypokalaemia has been due to increased cellular potassium uptake.

Renal loss. This is a very important cause for hypokalaemia and is most commonly seen in patients undergoing diuretic therapy.

Diuretic therapy. Therapy with the following groups of diuretics may be associated with hypokalaemia due to excessive renal loss. Although diuretic therapy is a common cause of hypokalaemia in clinical practice, it occurs in less than 5% of patients on therapy.

Carbonic anhydrase inhibitors. These drugs (e.g., acetazolamide) inhibit proximal tubule bicarbonate reabsorption (Figure 2.3) and the increased sodium bicarbonate presented to the distal nephron increases urine flow and hence encourages potassium excretion. This hypokalaemia is associated with a low plasma bicarbonate (metabolic acidosis) rather than the high plasma bicarbonate seen with the other groups of diuretics. These drugs are rarely used as diuretics now but find a use in the treatment of glaucoma.

Thiazide diuretics. These drugs prevent sodium reabsorption in the thick ascending limb of the loop of Henle and the early part of the distal tubule; there is also minimal carbonic anhydrase inhibition (Figure 2.3). The potassium depletion is due to increased renal excretion as a consequence of:

• increased Na^+-K^+ exchange in the distal nephron (increased sodium delivery)
• hyperaldosteronism secondary to minimal hypovolaemia
• increased distal tubule urine flow rate (sodium diuresis)

The hypokalaemia is almost always associated with a high plasma bicarbonate (metabolic alkalosis) which is due to increased renal tubular H^+ secretion resulting from:

1 direct stimulation by thiazide drugs
2 hyperaldosteronism
3 ? potassium depletion *per se*

Loop diuretics. Furosemide and ethacrynic acid,

prevent chloride reabsorption in the thick ascending limb of Henle which in turn prevents the reabsorption of sodium ions. Direct causes of the associated hypokalaemia are similar to those for the thiazide diuretics.

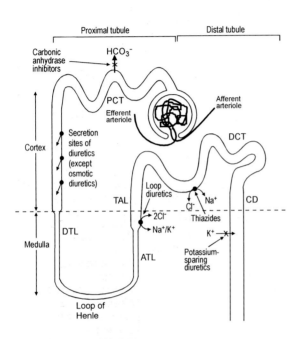

Figure 2.3. Sites of diuretic action in the human nephron. *See text for details.* PCT, proximal convoluted tubules; DTL, descending thin limb; ATL, ascending thin limb; TAL, thick ascending limb of Loop of Henle; DCT, distal convoluted tubule; CD, collecting duct. Redrawn, with permission of W.B. Saunders, from Smith TM. Heart failure. In: Wyngaarden JB and Smith LH (eds), *Cecil Textbook of Medicine, 18th edn.* W.B. Saunders, Philadelphia, 1988.

Extrarenal losses. Both vomiting and diarrhoea are important causes of potassium being lost via extrarenal routes. They may at times be difficult to diagnose as certain patients who induce vomiting or use laxatives surrepticiously may not readily admit to these actions during history-taking.

Vomiting. Prolonged vomiting is nearly always associated with hypokalaemia and in addition the loss of HCl results in metabolic alkalosis (Figure 2.4, and page 44). The potassium is lost from two sources:

- *Vomitus.* Small but significant amounts.
- *Kidney.* Mostly lost in the urine due to increased potassium excretion as a consequence of alkalosis and hyperaldosteronism secondary to hypovolaemia (dehydration due to water loss).

Diarrhoea. Diarrhoeal fluid is rich in bicarbonate (60-80 mmol/L) and potassium (6.0-9.0 mmol/L) and hence the condition results in hypokalaemic metabolic acidosis. Any associated dehydration will result in extra potassium loss *via* the kidney (secondary hyperaldosteronism).

Two similar conditions are laxative abuse and villous adenoma of the colon or rectum.

- *Laxative abuse* results in chronic diarrhoea which may present as hypokalaemia of obscure origin (patient reluctance to admit to self medication).
- Some large bowel *villous adenomas* present with hypokalaemia because of the loss of potassium-rich secretions in the faeces (diarrhoea may not necessarily be a feature).

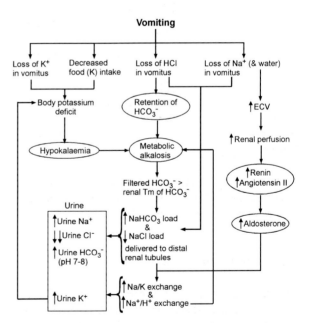

Figure 2.4. Metabolic consequences of vomiting. Tm, maximal tubular reabsorption; ECV, extracellular volume. Redrawn, with permission of W.B. Saunders, from Feldman M. In: Sleisinger MH and Fortran JS (eds), *Gastrointestinal Diseases, 3rd edn.* W.B. Saunders, Philadelphia, 1983.

Renal tubular acidosis (RTA). RTA type 1 always presents with hypokalaemia; in RTA type 2, hypokalaemia generally only occurs after commencement of bicarbonate therapy (page 81).

Urine diversion to large gut. If urine is allowed to collect in the colon, as in ureterosigmoidostomy or vesico-colic fistulae, the urinary chloride is reabsorbed by the gut in exchange for bicarbonate and potassium is secreted into the gut in exchange for ammonium (and sodium) ions, resulting in a hypokalaemic metabolic acidosis. A similar metabolic abnormality occurs with an ileal bladder.

Mineralocorticoid excess syndromes. A characteristic feature of aldosterone excess is hypokalaemia and metabolic alkalosis due to renal loss of potassium and hydrogen ions. These disorders are discussed in detail on page 66.

Miscellaneous causes of hypokalaemia. These include the following:

Gentamicin therapy. Patients on gentamicin therapy may develop occasional hypokalaemia due to renal potassium loss (? inhibition of tubular reabsorption).

Magnesium depletion. Severe depletion may be associated with hypokalaemia which is refractory to potassium therapy until the patient is magnesium-replete (see page 111).

Leukaemia. Occasional hypokalaemia due to renal potassium loss (? toxic effect of lysosomes associated with lysosomuria) is seen in acute myeloid leukaemia.

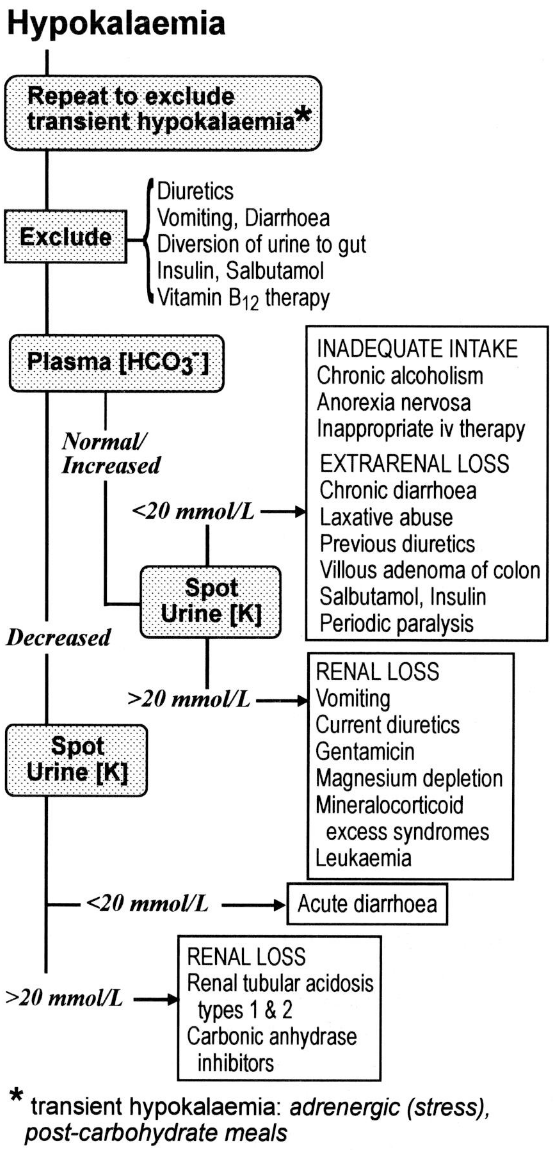

Laboratory evaluation

In clinical practice the commonest causes of hypokalaemia are diuretic therapy, vomiting, diarrhoea, and drug therapy. If after considering these conditions the cause is obscure, the urinary potassium concentration on a spot (untimed) sample should be estimated and the result considered in tandem with the patient's plasma bicarbonate level (Figure 2.5). It is important that the urine sample be collected before giving the subject any potassium therapy as this will invalidate

Hypokalaemia

* transient hypokalaemia: *adrenergic (stress), post-carbohydrate meals*

Figure 2.5. Laboratory evaluation of hypokalaemia.

the result (oral or IV potassium appears in the urine regardless of the clinical condition).

Note: A number of seriously ill patients, e.g., with myocardial infarction, will present with a transient hypokalaemia (i.e., normalises with out therapy). This most likely represents an intracellular shift due to adrenaline stimulation of the cell β-receptors and is seen in stress-associated conditions (stimulation of catecholamine secretion) such as trauma, myocardial infarction and such like.

Consequences of hypokalaemia

The clinical picture is non-specific and depends on the severity of the deficiency; muscle weakness and polyuria (nocturia) are the most characteristic symptoms. The range of signs and symptoms include:

- Muscle weakness: both skeletal and smooth muscle (paralytic ileus). Paralysis of the limbs can occur.
- Loss of tendon reflexes
- Fatigue and apathy
- Tachycardia, cardiac arrhythmia
- Hypotension and postural hypotension
- Polyuria (hypokalaemic nephropathy)
- ECG changes: T-wave depression and occasional inversion, ST depression. In severe cases there may be U waves and widening of the QRS and QT complexes

Patients with hypokalaemia associated with conditions known to cause potassium losses from the body are generally potassium deficient to the tune of 300-350 mmol per 1.0 mmol/L drop in the plasma potassium below 4.0 mmol/L; and will usually require potassium replacement therapy. Potassium can be given orally or intravenously.

The oral preparations are either effervescent KCl tablets with ~14 mmol of K^+ per tablet or slow release preparations with ~8 mmol of K^+ per tablet. Intravenous potassium can be given at the rate of 10 to 20 mmol/hour at a concentration less than 40 mmol/L (to prevent sudden rises in the blood level). The amount of potassium given per day (oral or IV) should be at least 90 mmol because of the ongoing loss in the urine (see above). Close monitoring is essential to prevent the development of hyperkalaemia, particularly with IV therapy.

REFERENCES/FURTHER READING

Bidani A. Electrolyte and acid-base disorders. Med Clinics North Am 1986;70:1013-1036.

DeFronzo RA. Clinical disorders of hyperkalaemia. Ann Rev Med 1982;33:521-554.

Whang R, Whang DD, Ryan MP. Refractory potassium repletion. A consequence of magnesium deficiency. Arch Intern Med 1992;152:40-53.

Williams ME, Rose RM, Epstein M. Hyperkalaemia. Adv Intern Med 1986;31:1409-1412.

Walmsley RN, White GH. Occult causes of hypokalaemia. Clin Chem 1984;30:1406-1408.

Chapter 3

Acid-Base

Acid-base homeostasis depends on the integrated action of the liver, the lungs and the kidney and, to a lesser extent, the gastrointestinal tract, as well as on the efficient working of the physiological buffers in both the extracellular and intracellular compartments. These homeostatic mechanisms are so efficient that the normal extracellular hydrogen ion concentration ($[H^+]$) is maintained at a very low level -- only about 40 nmol/L (pH 7.4) -- with little fluctuations, despite a very large daily flux (net intake of about 70 mmol per day), exceeding the ECF $[H^+]$ by 10^6-fold.

This delicate balance can be, and does become, easily disrupted, as evidenced by the large number of patients presenting with acid-base disorders in critical care practice. Disturbances of acid-base balance occur in a wide range of clinical circumstances and often present as acute medical emergencies for which appropriate urgent intervention is needed and may be life-saving.

We believe that an understanding of the basic physiological and biochemical principles involved in acid-base regulation is crucial to the proper diagnosis and management of patients presenting with such problems. In this chapter, we have provided the background information necessary to appreciate the basis of each clinical disorder, including a germane introductory section on definitions and the concepts of buffering and compensation mechanisms.

DEFINITIONS

Acid: A substance that dissociates in water to produce hydrogen ions (H^+). A strong acid, e.g., hydrochloric acid, dissociates almost completely:

$$HCl \rightarrow H^+ + Cl^-$$

A weak acid, e.g., acetic acid, shows poor dissociation:

$$CH_3COOH \rightleftharpoons H^+ + CH_3COO^-$$

Acidaemia: A raised blood $[H^+]$, greater than 45 nmol/L; or a low blood pH, less than 7.35.

Acidosis: A primary process that generates hydrogen ions. Depending on the buffering and compensatory processes it may, or may not, produce an acidaemia.

Alkali: A substance that dissociates in water to produce hydroxyl ions (OH^-), e.g., sodium hydroxide:

$$NaOH \rightarrow Na^+ + OH^-$$

Alkalaemia: A low blood $[H^+]$, less than 35 nmol/L, or a high blood pH, greater than 7.45.

Alkalosis: A primary disorder that produces excessive hydroxyl ions. It need not always result in alkalaemia.

Base: A substance that can accept hydrogen ions, e.g., Cl^-. A strong base, e.g., CH_3COO^-, has a high affinity for hydrogen ions.

Conjugate base: The dissociation anionic product of an acid, e.g., the bicarbonate ion (HCO_3^-) is the conjugate base of carbonic acid (H_2CO_3):

$$H_2CO_3 \rightleftharpoons H^+ + HCO_3^- \text{ (conjugate base)}$$

Buffer: A mixture of a weak acid and its conjugate base which attenuates a change in $[H^+]$ when a strong acid or base is added, e.g., carbonic acid and bicarbonate. It acts by forming a weaker acid or base.

$HCO_3^- + H^+ \rightarrow H_2CO_3$
(buffer) (strong acid) (weak acid)

$H_2CO_3 + OH^- \rightarrow HCO_3^- + H_2O$
(buffer) (strong base) (weak base)

Blood buffer systems: The three most important buffers in the blood are:

- Bicarbonate system: H_2CO_3/HCO_3^- (~75%)
- Protein system: protein$^+$/protein$^-$ (~20%)
- Phosphate system: $H_2PO_4^-/HPO_4^{2-}$ (~5%)

pH: A measure of the hydrogen ion concentration defined as the logarithm of the reciprocal of the $[H^+]$.
$$pH = \log_{10} 1/[H^+] = -\log_{10}[H^+]$$

pH of a buffer system: This may be calculated from the Henderson-Hasselbalch equation which relates the pH to the concentrations of acid and base.

$$pH = pK + \log_{10} [base]/[acid]$$
(K is overall dissociation constant)

For the bicarbonate system pK is 6.10, thus

$$pH = 6.1 + \log_{10} [HCO_3^-]/[H_2CO_3]$$

This equation shows that the pH of this system is proportional to the ratio of base to acid, i.e.,

$$pH \propto [HCO_3^-]/[H_2CO_3] \qquad \text{Equation (1)}$$

In solution, e.g., in the plasma, the $[H_2CO_3]$ is directly related to the P_{CO_2} (partial pressure of CO_2). The solubility constant of this gas is 0.03, thus

$$P_{CO_2} \text{ (mmHg)} \times 0.03 = [H_2CO_3] \text{ (mmol/L)}$$

Therefore Equation (1) can be recast as:

$$pH \propto [HCO_3^-]/P_{CO_2} \qquad \text{Equation (2)}$$

The hydrogen ion concentration of the bicarbonate buffer system can be calculated, using the Henderson-Hasselbalch equation, as follows:

$$[H^+](nmol/L) = 24 \{P_{CO_2}(mmHg)/[HCO_3^-](mmol/L)\}$$

Respiratory component: The term defines the P_{CO_2} level as this parameter is ultimately controlled by respiration. A high P_{CO_2} (>45 mmHg) is a respiratory acidosis and a low P_{CO_2} (<35 mmHg), a respiratory alkalosis.

Metabolic component: This describes the plasma bicarbonate concentration. Metabolic acidosis is defined by a low plasma $[HCO_3^-]$ (e.g., <23 mmol/L) and metabolic alkalosis, by a high plasma $[HCO_3^-]$ (>33 mmol/L).

Compensation: During acid-base disturbances the body's homeostatic mechanisms try to keep the pH of the body fluids as near normal as possible. As the pH is directly related to the ratio of the $[HCO_3^-]$ to the P_{CO_2}, then during metabolic acidosis (low $[HCO_3^-]$) the pH can be brought back to normal by lowering the P_{CO_2}; i.e., the development of a respiratory alkalosis compensates for the metabolic acidosis. Thus:

Primary lesion	Compensation
metabolic acidosis ($\downarrow[HCO_3^-]$)	respiratory alkalosis ($\downarrow P_{CO_2}$)
metabolic alkalosis ($\uparrow[HCO_3^-]$)	respiratory acidosis ($\uparrow P_{CO_2}$)
respiratory alkalosis ($\downarrow P_{CO_2}$)	metabolic acidosis ($\downarrow[HCO_3^-]$)
respiratory acidosis ($\uparrow P_{CO_2}$)	metabolic alkalosis ($\uparrow[HCO_3^-]$)

NORMAL ACID-BASE HOMEOSTASIS

Hydrogen ions are generated by intermediary metabolism and by the production of carbon dioxide. The majority are re-utilised in other metabolic reactions but hydrogen ions in the form of non-volatile acids and carbon dioxide have to be excreted from the body by the kidneys and the lungs, respectively. Prior to excretion the hydrogen ions are buffered in order to prevent large pH changes which may be deleterious to normal metabolic processes.

HYDROGEN ION METABOLISM

Hydrogen ions are produced in the cells, secreted into the extracellular fluid,, buffered by systems including the bicarbonate system, and then excreted by the kidney.

Hydrogen ion production

The daily turnover is around 150 moles. About 20 moles are due to carbon dioxide production; most of the remaining 130 moles are produced as the result of ATP hydrolysis, respiratory chain reactions, and the reduction of nicotinamide nucleotides, i.e.,

- $ATP^{4-} + H_2O \rightarrow ADP^{3-} + H^+$

- $2Fe^{3+}(cytochrome) + 2H \rightarrow 2Fe^{2+} + 2H^+$

- $NAD^+ + 2HR \rightarrow NADH + 2R^- + H^+$

(No attempt has been made to balance the above equations.)

Under normal circumstances these reactions are reversible and do not result in a net H^+ gain. The hydrogen ions we are concerned with here are those of the *non-volatile,* or *fixed acids,* which are produced at the rate of 40-80 mmol/day, mainly from dietary sources, and have to be excreted by the kidney.

Most of the organic acids formed during the metabolism of fat, carbohydrate, and protein are converted to carbon dioxide and water and do not accumulate in the body. The acids which accumulate and have to be excreted are derived as follows:

- Oxidation of sulphydryl groups (-SH) of sulphur-containing amino acids (cystine, methionine) to H_2SO_4

- Hydrolysis of phosphoesters, phosphoproteins, and phospholipids to H_3PO_4

- Incomplete oxidation of fats and carbohydrates producing small amounts of ketoacids and lactic acid

Thus, dietary protein is the major source of non-volatile acid hydrogen ions; however, this endogenous acid production may be modified, e.g., during fasting and starvation the body fats are the major source of energy and ketoacids (acetoacetic acid, β-hydroxy-butyric acid) account for most of the acid production within the body.

The hydrogen ions, which are produced in the cells, are at first buffered by intracellular mechanisms and then transported, along with their anions, across the cell wall into the ECF. This addition will have resulted in an unacceptable drop in the pH of the ECF. The presence and action of the ECF buffers attenuate the change.

Extracellular buffering

Following secretion from the cells the non-volatile acids are buffered by the ECF buffers including bicarbonate, protein, and phosphate. The most important is the bicarbonate system because it is present in large quantities, can be varied by the lungs via carbon dioxide excretion, and is the only system that can be routinely evaluated in the diagnostic

laboratory. The addition of acid (H^+A^-) to the bicarbonate system results in a fall in the $[HCO_3^-]$ -- referred to as *bicarbonate consumption* -- and a slight increase in the Pco_2.

$$H^+A^- + NaHCO_3 \rightarrow Na^+A^- + H_2CO_3$$
$$H_2CO_3 \rightarrow H_2O + CO_2$$

The final outcome is blood with a low $[HCO_3^-]$, a raised Pco_2, and a low pH, i.e.,

$$pH (\downarrow) \quad \propto \quad \frac{[HCO_3^-] (\downarrow)}{Pco_2 (\uparrow)}$$

As this blood passes through the lungs CO_2 is expired, lowering the Pco_2:

$$pH (\downarrow \rightarrow N) \quad \propto \quad \frac{[HCO_3^-] (\downarrow)}{Pco_2 (\downarrow)}$$

When the blood reaches the kidney hydrogen ions are excreted and bicarbonate ions generated (see below), thus normalising the pH.

Renal H^+ excretion, HCO_3^- generation and reabsorption

The role of the kidney in acid-base homeostasis is three-fold:

1. excretion of H^+ and generation of HCO_3^-
2. excretion of acid anions
3. reabsorption of filtered HCO_3^-

Excretion of H^+ and generation of HCO_3^-. The mechanism whereby the kidney excretes hydrogen ions and generates bicarbonate ions is at present a subject of controversy. There are three prevailing views:

1. the classical textbook view which suggests that all actions occur in the distal nephron
2. a more modern view indicating that the proximal renal tubule is the main site of action
3. a view suggesting that the liver is the main site of action

Here we will consider the classical textbook view (an outline of the other two approaches can be found in the Appendix on page 58).

In the distal nephron, mainly in the collecting ducts, hydrogen ions are excreted in the urine and during this process an equivalent amount of bicarbonate ions is generated and returned to the extracellular fluid. This process involves three closely related mechanisms (Figure 3.1):

- formation of H⁺ (and HCO₃⁻) in the tubular cells
- secretion of H⁺ into the tubular lumen
- excretion of H⁺ in the urine

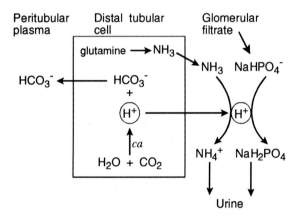

Figure 3.1. Generation of HCO_3^- and excretion of H⁺ by the distal nephron cells. ca, carbonic anhydrase.

Formation of H⁺. The tubular cells contain the enzyme carbonic anhydrase which catalyses the reaction forming hydrogen and bicarbonate ions from water and carbon dioxide.

$$H_2O + CO_2 \rightarrow H_2CO_3 \rightarrow H^+ + HCO_3^-$$

Secretion of H⁺. The luminal membranes of the tubular cells contain specific proton (hydrogen ion) pumps which secrete H⁺ into the lumen in exchange for Na⁺. The reabsorbed Na⁺ are secreted back into the ECF accompanied by the cell-generated HCO_3^-. The amount of bicarbonate generated and returned to the ECF is equivalent to that consumed by the non-volatile acids during buffering.

Excretion of H⁺. The proton pump can maintain a maximal luminal H⁺ gradient of 1:1000, i.e., if the intracellular pH is 7.40 ([H⁺] of 40 nmol/L) then the luminal pH can be decreased to no less than 4.40 ([H⁺] of 40 μmol/L). The kidney, however, has to excrete at least 40 mmol of H⁺ daily. This means that if the urine was pure water, at least 1000 litres would have to be excreted daily. This problem is overcome by the presence of urinary buffers which bind the secreted H⁺ and maintain a low urine concentration of free H⁺.

The two main urinary buffers are *phosphate* and *ammonia* (Figure 3.1). The buffering capacity of the former is limited by the amount of phosphate excreted in the urine daily (20-40 mmol). The urinary ammonia, which is formed in the cells from amino acids, mainly glutamine, is normally excreted at the rate of 20-40 mmol/day and this, in addition to phosphate, is sufficient to rid the body of "normal" amounts of H⁺. If there is a greater H⁺ load to be excreted, as in metabolic acidosis, the ammonia production rate can be increased some 10- to 20-fold.

Whilst other urinary constituents, such as urate and creatinine, can also accept H⁺, they play only a minor role in H⁺ excretion.

Excretion of acid anions. Acid anions, such as SO_4^{2-} and PO_4^{3-}, are filtered by the glomerulus and, providing the GFR is normal, excreted in the urine. In renal impairment the anions may be retained resulting in a high anion gap (see page 40).

Reabsorption of filtered bicarbonate. Eighty to ninety per cent of the filtered HCO_3^- are reabsorbed in the proximal tubule. Most of the remaining 10 to 20% are reabsorbed in the distal nephron with very little escaping in the urine. The mechanism of reabsorption in the proximal tubule (Figure 3.2) is as follows.

Intracellular carbonic anhydrase catalyses the reaction:

$$H_2O + CO_2 \rightarrow H_2CO_3 \rightarrow H^+ + HCO_3^-$$

Subsequently the following occur:

- H⁺ are pumped into the lumen in exchange for Na⁺.

- The reabsorbed Na⁺ are secreted back into the ECF accompanied by the cell-generated HCO_3^-

- In the lumen the H⁺, under the influence of carbonic anhydrase located in the cell brush border, react with luminal (filtered) HCO_3^- to form carbonic acid which degrades to CO_2 and H_2O.

- The generated CO_2 diffuses back into the cell and re-enters the above reaction.

The renal threshold for bicarbonate reabsorption is around 28 to 32 mmol/L. When plasma levels exceed this value bicarbonate appears in the urine.

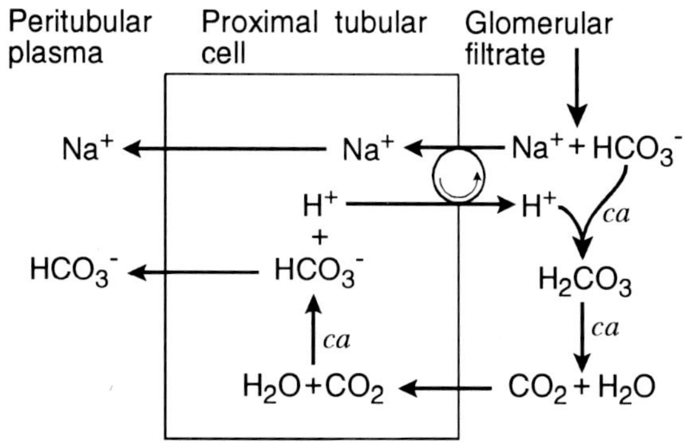

erythrocyte carbonic anhydrase, the CO_2 reacts with water to form H^+ and HCO_3^-. The H^+ are buffered by deoxygenated (reduced) haemoglobin which is less acidic than the oxygenated variety. The HCO_3^- diffuses out into the plasma in exchange for chloride ions, a mechanism called the *chloride* shift. Thus CO_2 is transported to the lung mainly as red cell-generated bicarbonate.

Figure 3.2. Bicarbonate reabsorption by the proximal tubule. ca, carbonic anhydrase.

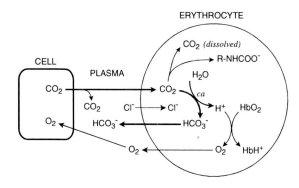

Figure 3.3. Transport of carbon dioxide from cells to erythrocytes. ca, carbonic anhydrase.

CARBON DIOXIDE METABOLISM

Daily, the complete oxidation of fats, carbohydrates, and proteins results in the formation of 15 to 20 moles of carbon dioxide. After diffusing from the cells this CO_2 undergoes a number of reactions in the blood and is then transported to the lungs where it is excreted.

Carbon dioxide transport

Over 90% of the CO_2 generated by intermediary tissue metabolism diffuse out into the blood and enter the red blood cells; the small portion remaining in the plasma is transported in the dissolved state. In the red cells some of the CO_2 remain in the dissolved state, some react with amino acids to form carbamino compounds, but the major portion engages in the following reactions (Figure 3.3).

Within the erythrocytes, under the influence of

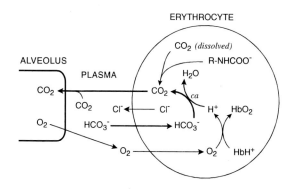

Figure 3.4. Transport of carbon dioxide from erythrocytes to the alveoli.

Carbon dioxide excretion

When the blood enters the lungs the above reactions are reversed (Figure 3.4). Oxygenation of reduced haemoglobin releases the bound hydrogen ions; these ions, under the influence of carbonic anhydrase, react with bicarbonate to form carbonic acid and then carbon dioxide which diffuses out of the cell and into the alveolus. As the red cell bicarbonate level decreases more diffuses in from the plasma in exchange for cellular chloride ions.

THE PLASMA ANION GAP

In plasma, as in any other fluid compartment in the body, the number of electrical charges on the cations equals the number of charges on the anions (Table 3.1), i.e., electrical neutrality is maintained. However, the routine biochemistry laboratory generally only measures the sodium, potassium, chloride, and bicarbonate ions and, by convention, the difference between the sum of the measured cation concentrations ($Na^+ + K^+$) and the sum of the measured anion concentrations ($Cl^- + HCO_3^-$) is called the anion gap (the correct term should be unmeasured anions as there is no anion gap as such). The anion gap is constituted by the charges of the plasma proteins and amino acids, and the organic acid anions (acetoacetate, β-hydroxy-butyrate, etc).

Table 3.1. Major plasma cations and anions (in mEq/L).

Cations		Anions	
Na^+	140	Cl^-	100
K^+	4.0	HCO_3^-	27
*Ca^{2+}	4.5	*Protein⁻	15
*Mg^{2+}	1.5	*PO_4^{3-}	2
		*SO_4^{2-}	1
		*AcidA⁻	5
Total	150		150

* Unmeasured ions, AcidA⁻, Organic acid anions.

Its usefulness lies in the fact that metabolic acidosis can be classified as either a *high anion gap metabolic acidosis* or a *normal anion gap metabolic acidosis*. A high anion gap usually results from abnormal amounts of organic anions such as lactate in lactic acidosis, ketoanions in ketoacidosis, and sulphate, phosphate and other unidentified anions in renal failure. It may infrequently be due to abnormal anions generated by the metabolism of ingested toxins such as salicylates, ethanol, methanol, ethylene glycol, paraldehyde, etc.

For example, in lactic acidosis the addition of hydrogen ions and lactate ions to the plasma results in:

- lowering (consumption) of the plasma bicarbonate
- increase in plasma lactate

Thus the bicarbonate ions are replaced by lactate ions and as the lactate ions are not measured there will be an increase in the anion gap.

On the other hand, if bicarbonate is lost from the body in the form of sodium bicarbonate, as in diarrhoea, it is usually replaced by sodium chloride (diet or therapy origin). In this case bicarbonate is replaced by chloride which is measured in the electrolyte profile and the anion gap does not change; hence normal anion gap metabolic acidosis (also referred to as hyperchloraemic acidosis).

Disturbances of acid-base regulation

There are four simple acid-base disorders -- metabolic acidosis, metabolic alkalosis, respiratory acidosis, and respiratory alkalosis. A subject can also suffer from two simple disorders simultaneously which is termed a mixed acid-base disturbance, e.g., mixed metabolic acidosis and respiratory alkalosis, or even a triple disorder (page 49).

In the routine laboratory a patient's acid-base status is generally evaluated by a 'blood gas' analysis and presented as pH, Pco_2, and $[HCO_3^-]$. These estimations are best thought of in terms of the abbreviated Henderson-Hasselbalch equation:

$$pH \propto \frac{[HCO_3^-]}{Pco_2}$$

- The **pH** evaluates the hydrogen ion concentration: low pH = acidaemia, high pH = alkalaemia.

- The **Pco_2** reflects the respiratory component: high Pco_2 = respiratory acidosis, low Pco_2 = respiratory alkalosis.

- The **$[HCO_3^-]$** indicates the metabolic component: high $[HCO_3^-]$ = metabolic alkalosis, low $[HCO_3^-]$ = metabolic acidosis.

Note: The $[HCO_3^-]$ reported as part of the blood gas

profile is usually a *derived* (calculated) parameter; laboratory instruments (other than the blood gas apparatus) that *measure* the plasma bicarbonate usually present an indirect measurement of this anion in the form of total plasma CO_2 (Tco_2), i.e., it is a measure of the plasma $[HCO_3^-]$ plus the dissolved CO_2. This value differs from the $[HCO_3^-]$ estimated by the blood gas analyser, being usually higher by some 1-2 mmol/L.

Compensation

The concept of compensation is discussed in the section on definitions on page 36. In essence, it is the process whereby the homeostatic mechanisms for acid-base balance are mobilised to return any shifts of the blood pH back towards normal. The pH change caused by a simple acid-base disturbance is attenuated by a secondary acid-base disturbance, e.g., metabolic acidosis (decreased $[HCO_3^-]$) is compensated for by a secondary respiratory alkalosis (decreased Pco_2). There are two important aspects concerning these compensatory processes:

- In the simple acid-base disorders compensation returns the pH towards, but *seldom* to, normal, i.e., in simple disturbances the pH usually remains abnormal. The exception is longstanding respiratory alkalosis and very mild respiratory acidosis where 'complete' compensation may occur.

- In the four simple disorders the compensatory response is fairly predictable, e.g., for a given level of plasma bicarbonate in simple metabolic acidosis the expected Pco_2 can be calculated from the equation shown in the next section. Corresponding equations for calculation of the compensatory responses in the other simple disturbances have also been devised (see appropriate sections).

METABOLIC ACIDOSIS

Simple metabolic acidosis is characterised by a low $[HCO_3^-]$, a low pH and, if compensation has occurred, a low Pco_2.

PRIMARY LESION

The primary lesion is a low plasma $[HCO_3^-]$ due either

to the addition of hydrogen ions to the ECF or loss of bicarbonate from the body.

COMPENSATION

The response to lowering the bicarbonate is shown in Figure 3.5. The low $[HCO_3^-]$ results in a low pH which stimulates the respiratory centre and increases carbon dioxide excretion. This results in a lowered Pco_2 and hence an increase in the pH which returns *towards normal but rarely to normal.* The falling Pco_2 reaches a plateau in 12 to 24 hours and this value can be estimated from the formula below. In uncomplicated simple metabolic acidosis *the Pco_2 usually does not fall below 10 mmHg.*

$$Pco_2 \text{ (mmHg)} = \{1.5 \times [HCO_3^-] \text{ (mmol/L)} + 8\} (\pm 2)$$

CAUSES/PATHOPHYSIOLOGY

A decreased $[HCO_3^-]$ may be due to (a) addition of H^+ to the ECF or (b) loss of HCO_3^- from the body.

Addition of H^+

Increased production
　Ketoacidosis* (page 136)
　Lactic acidosis* (page 139)
　Toxins* (ethanol, methanol, salicylate, ethylene glycol)
　Ingestion/infusions (HCl, NH_4Cl, arginine/lysine HCl)
Decreased renal excretion
　Renal failure* (page 78)
　Obstructive uropathy
　Renal tubular acidosis Type 1(page 81)
　Mineralocorticoid deficiency (page 69)

Loss of HCO_3^-

Extrarenal losses
　Acute diarrhoea (page 218)
　Drainage from pancreatic fistulae
　Diversion of urine to gut (page 33)
Renal losses
　Renal tubular acidosis Type II (page 81)

*These conditions are associated with a high anion gap (see page 40). The others have a normal anion gap (hyperchloraemic metabolic acidosis).

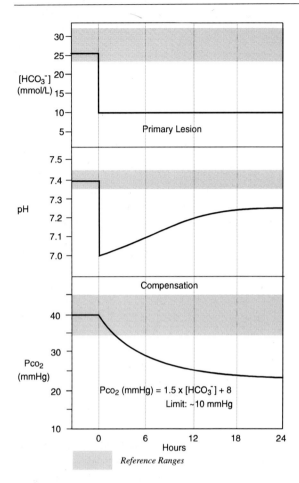

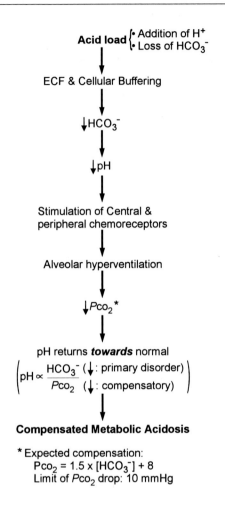

Figure 3.5. The compensatory response to lowering the plasma bicarbonate in simple metabolic acidosis.

Diarrhoea. Severe diarrhoea is associated with a hypokalaemic, hyperchloraemic (normal anion gap) metabolic acidosis which is due to loss of fluid containing high levels of bicarbonate and potassium. The loss of sodium bicarbonate (and water) stimulates renal retention of NaCl (sodium chloride), hence the hyperchloraemia.

Obstructive uropathy. The back pressure of urine in obstructive renal disease results in (a) a decrease in the GFR (raised plasma urea and creatinine levels) and (b) dysfunction of the distal nephron causing retention of potassium (hyperkalaemia) and hydrogen ions (low [HCO_3^-]). An unusual feature is that, although there is a decrease in the GFR, anion retention and a high anion gap tends not to occur to any great extent.

Diversion of urine to gut. When urine comes in contact with intestinal mucosae, as in ileal bladders, vesico-colic fistula, and ureterosigmoidostomy, Cl⁻ are reabsorbed in exchange for HCO_3^- and potassium ions are exchanged with urinary ammonium ions; hence the development of hypokalaemic, hyperchloraemic metabolic acidosis.

CONSEQUENCES

Myocardial function. Acidaemia impairs myocardial contraction which could result in cardiac failure; however, acidaemia also releases catechol-amines which block the pH effect.

Potassium. Hyperkalaemia, due to egress of potassium from cells in exchange for ECF hydrogen ions, may occur in hyperchloraemic metabolic acidosis (page 26) but generally the plasma potassium reflects the causative disorder, e.g., hyperkalaemia in diabetic ketoacidosis, hypokalaemia in renal tubular acidosis and in diarrhoea.

Calcium metabolism. Acidaemia enhances the mobilisation of calcium from bone, decreases the binding of ionised calcium to albumin, and decreases the renal reabsorption of calcium producing hypercalciuria. Thus chronic acidaemia, as in renal tubular acidosis, is associated with a negative calcium balance, and can result in nephrocalcinosis and urolithiasis.

METABOLIC ALKALOSIS

Metabolic alkalosis is characterised by a high pH, a high bicarbonate and, if compensation has occurred, a high Pco_2.

PRIMARY LESION

The causative biochemical lesion is a high $[HCO_3^-]$ which may be due to (a) exogenous ingestion or infusion, or (b) to endogenous production as a consequence of hydrogen ion loss.

COMPENSATION

A high plasma $[HCO_3^-]$ results in a high pH which suppresses respiration and consequently retention of carbon dioxide and a high Pco_2. The high Pco_2 returns the pH *towards normal but rarely to normal* (Figure 3.6). Like metabolic acidosis the compensatory response reaches a maximum in 12 to 24 hours. The approximate level of the Pco_2, for a given bicarbonate concentration can be calculated from:

$$Pco_2 \text{ (mmHg)} = \{0.9 \times [HCO_3^-] \text{ (mmol/L)} + 9\} \ (\pm 2)$$

The rise in the Pco_2 is limited by the fall in the patient's oxygenation status (decreased respiration induces hypoxia, a stimulus for increased respiration) and in simple metabolic alkalosis *it usually does not rise beyond 60 mmHg.*

CAUSES/PATHOPHYSIOLOGY

Persistent metabolic alkalosis requires the simultaneous action of two mechanisms: *generation* of excessive bicarbonate ions and *maintenance* of the high plasma bicarbonate concentration. The necessity for the former is obvious; the latter is needed because the normal kidney is very efficient at excreting excess body bicarbonate, e.g., a normal adult has to ingest some 1000 millimoles of bicarbonate daily before there is any significant rise in the plasma level, and significant metabolic alkalosis occurs at generation levels much less than that figure. Maintenance is solely due to renal bicarbonate retention which in turn can be due to:

- Hypovolaemia, e.g., dehydration
- Severe potassium deficiency
- Mineralocorticoid excess
- High plasma Pco_2

These factors increase renal bicarbonate retention by increasing the proximal tubular reabsorption.

Excessive bicarbonate generation reflects two basic causes:

(1) Increased exogenous bicarbonate, and
(2) Loss of hydrogen ions which results in generation of bicarbonate by the body.

Increased exogenous bicarbonate
  Oral/intravenous bicarbonate
  Antacid therapy, e.g. magnesium carbonate
  Organic acid salts, e.g., lactate, acetate, citrate

Loss of hydrogen ions
  Gastrointestinal tract losses
    Stomach: vomiting, gastric suction
    Bowel: chloride diarrhoea (page 218)
  Kidney losses
    Diuretic therapy
    Mineralocorticoid excess (page 66)

Hydrogen ion loss from the body generates bicarbonate because the eventual source of the H^+ ion

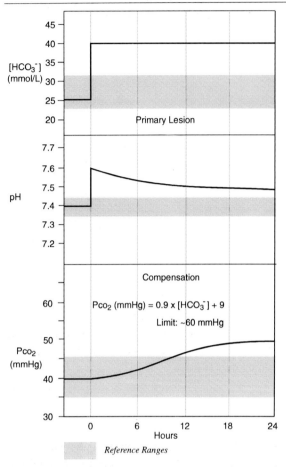

Figure 3.6. Compensatory response to increased plasma bicarbonate in simple metabolic alkalosis.

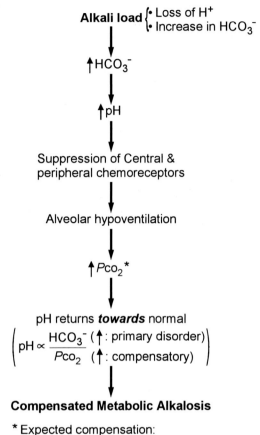

Alkali load { • Loss of H^+
{ • Increase in HCO_3^-

$\uparrow HCO_3^-$

$\uparrow pH$

Suppression of Central & peripheral chemoreceptors

Alveolar hypoventilation

$\uparrow Pco_2$ *

pH returns ***towards*** normal

$\left(pH \propto \dfrac{HCO_3^-}{Pco_2} \begin{array}{l} (\uparrow: \text{primary disorder}) \\ (\uparrow: \text{compensatory}) \end{array} \right)$

Compensated Metabolic Alkalosis

* Expected compensation:
$Pco_2 = 0.9 \times [HCO_3^-] + 9$
Limit of Pco_2 rise: 60 mmHg

---

is carbonic acid and the removal of this ion leaves bicarbonate behind.

$$H_2O + CO_2 \rightarrow H_2CO_3 \rightarrow H^+ + HCO_3^-$$

A similar mechanism occurs with the infusion of organic anions (as salts, not acids) -- the organic anions are eventually taken into the cells and metabolised to carbon dioxide and water, but the ions cross the cell membranes in association with a proton (hydrogen ion) derived from ECF carbonic acid (the bicarbonate is left behind).

Vomiting. Excessive vomiting, from above the pylorus, results in loss of HCl and consequently a rising plasma bicarbonate and a falling plasma chloride level. The hypokalaemia associated with this condition (see page 32, Figure 2.4) is due to some potassium lost in the vomitus and larger amounts lost in the urine. The latter is a consequence of the secondary hyperaldosteronism arising from hypovolaemia (ECV depletion). If the vomiting originates below the pylorus, e.g., gut obstruction, then bicarbonate will be lost in addition to the HCl and the plasma $[HCO_3^-]$ may not deviate far from normal.

Diuretic therapy. The thiazide diuretics and furosemide, but not the potassium-sparing diuretics, may be associated with hypokalaemia (page 31) and metabolic alkalosis. The cause of the metabolic alkalosis is related to increased renal H^+ excretion which may be due to a number of factors, including a

44

direct effect of the diuretic and hyperaldosteronism secondary to diuretic-induced hypovolaemia.

It is important to point out that although diuretic-induced metabolic alkalosis is common, it does not occur in all patients on diuretic therapy (fewer than 5% will develop hypokalaemic metabolic alkalosis and most of these will be oedematous patients who already have some degree of secondary hyperaldosteronism).

CONSEQUENCES

The major effect of alkalaemia is enhanced binding of calcium ions (Ca^{2+}) to protein. The lowered ionised calcium results in increased neuromuscular activity and the characteristic Chvostek and Trousseau signs may occur. Other effects of metabolic alkalaemia are:

- Hypokalaemia due to increased renal potassium excretion and uptake of potassium ions by the cells in exchange for cellular hydrogen ions (page 00)
- Increased renal calcium reabsorption
- Enhanced glycolysis (stimulation of phospho-fructokinase by a high intracellular pH)

RESPIRATORY ACIDOSIS

Respiratory acidosis is characterised by an increased Pco_2 (hypercapnia). It is always due to decreased excretion of CO_2 by the lungs; never to increased CO_2 production in an otherwise normal subject.

PRIMARY LESION

The primary lesion (increased Pco_2) is due to decreased respiratory exchange which may be a consequence of (a) decreased respiration, or (b) decreased respiratory exchange because of local lung disease.

COMPENSATION

The response to hypercapnia is two-fold:

- An acute increase in the plasma [HCO_3^-] during the first 10 minutes (the lower curve, Figure 3.7) followed by,
- A chronic, sustained, rise in the plasma [HCO_3^-]

over the next 2 to 4 days (the upper curve, Figure 3.7), providing the hypercapnia remains.

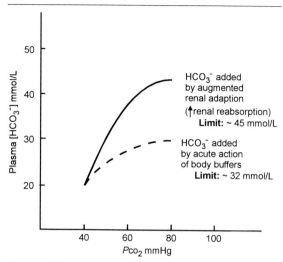

Figure 3.7. Schematic depicting the relative roles of body buffers and renal adaptation to compensate for respiratory acidosis.

Acute phase. Within 10 minutes of the plasma Pco_2 rising there is an increase of some 2 to 4 mmol/L in the plasma [HCO_3^-]. This rise, which results in a plasma [HCO_3^-] at the upper reference limit, is due to the increased CO_2 content forcing the following reaction to the right:

$$H_2O + CO_2 \rightarrow H_2CO_3 \rightarrow H^+ + HCO_3^-$$

This occurs mainly in the red cells where the excess hydrogen ions are buffered by haemoglobin and the bicarbonate remains in solution (see page 39).

Chronic phase. The increased Pco_2 and pH stimulate the kidney to secrete hydrogen ions and during this process bicarbonate is generated (see page 38). The bicarbonate level plateaus out in 2 to 4 days -- *the highest level the bicarbonate reaches in uncomplicated respiratory acidosis is about 45 mmol/L.* The expected bicarbonate value for a given Pco_2 level can be calculated from the following:

$$\text{[HCO}_3^-\text{] (mmol/L)} = \{0.43 \times Pco_2 \text{ (mmHg)} + 7.6\} \pm 2$$

45

Acid-Base

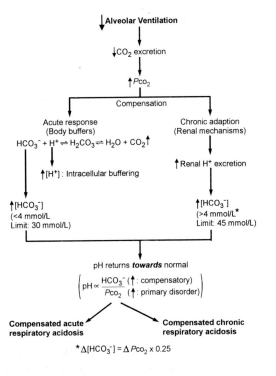

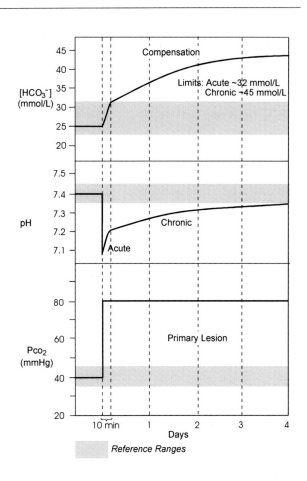

Δ [HCO$_3^-$] and Δ Pco$_2$ = change in [HCO$_3^-$] and Pco$_2$, respectively, from an arbitrary normal value, taken as 25 mmol/L and 40 mm Hg, respectively.

Figure 3.8. Simple respiratory acidosis and the two-phase compensation involving body buffers and renal adaptation.

CAUSES/PATHOPHYSIOLOGY

Hypercapnia, which is tantamount to alveolar hypoventilation, may be due to intrathoracic disease, neuromuscular or chest wall disease, or central depression of respiration.

Thoracic disease

Restrictive defects
hydrothorax, pneumothorax, flail chest
Obstructive disease
bronchitis, emphysema, pneumonia, infiltrations, oedema, foreign body obstruction

Neuromuscular disease
poliomyelitis, Guillain-Barré syndrome, multiple sclerosis, myopathies

Central depression
trauma, cerebrovascular accidents, CNS infections, CNS tumours, drug overdose.

CONSEQUENCES

Brain: Hypercapnia induces cerebral vasodilation and increased blood flow which can increase the intracerebral pressure producing drowsiness, headaches, stupor, and coma.

Potassium: Theoretically acidaemia could result in the release of potassium from the cells (exchange for H^+) but this is not a consistent feature of respiratory acidosis.

Respiratory Alkalosis

This disorder is characterised by hypocapnia (low Pco_2) due to increased ventilation.

PRIMARY LESION

The primary lesion is a low blood Pco_2 due to increased ventilation as a consequence of either (a) central stimulation of the respiratory centre, or (b) reflex stimulation from lung pathology.

COMPENSATION

The compensatory response to a low Pco_2 is a decrease in plasma $[HCO_3^-]$ which occurs in two phases, acute and chronic (Figure 3.9).

Acute phase. Within 10 minutes of the Pco_2 falling there is a drop of some 2 to 4 mmol/L in the plasma $[HCO_3^-]$ due to the following reaction proceeding to the left:

$$H_2O + CO_2 \leftarrow H_2CO_3 \leftarrow H^+ + HCO_3^-$$

As for the reaction in respiratory acidosis (see above), this occurs mainly in the red cells. *Plasma [HCO₃⁻] can fall to 18 mmol/L but rarely below this level.*

Chronic phase. Following the acute drop in $[HCO_3^-]$ there is a further sustained drop due to retention of hydrogen ions by the kidney (normal HCO_3^- regeneration proceeds at a lower than normal rate). If the condition continues for seven days or more the $[HCO_3^-]$ may drop sufficiently for the pH to return to the normal range, i.e., complete compensation may occur. *The limit to which the plasma [HCO₃⁻] can go down to in uncomplicated respiratory alkalosis is 12 to 14 mmol/L.*

CAUSES/PATHOPHYSIOLOGY

Hyperventilation and increased CO_2 excretion can be due to central (CNS) or pulmonary mechanisms. It is never due to decreased CO_2 production.

Central stimulation
Anxiety/hysteria
Pregnancy (stimulation by progesterone)
Hypoxaemia
Hepatic encephalopathy
Gram-negative septicaemia
Salicylate overdose
Infection, trauma
Tumour

Pulmonary pathology
Embolism
Congestive cardiac failure (oedema)
Asthma, pneumonia

CONSEQUENCES

Calcium metabolism. The main clinical feature of respiratory alkalosis is tetany (carpopedal spasm) due to a lowering of the plasma ionised calcium level (alkalaemia causes increased binding of calcium ions to protein).

Potassium. Initially there may be a mild hypokalaemia due to increased cellular uptake (exchange with cellular H^+) but generally the plasma potassium remains normal.

Phosphate. Transient severe hypophosphataemia (e.g., <0.4 mmol/L) is not uncommon. This is due to alkalaemia-induced cellular phosphate uptake (stimulation of phosphofructokinase).

Glucose metabolism. A low intracellular $[H^+]$ stimulates phosphofructokinase activity and hence glycolysis. This produces increased lactate production and may result in a 1 to 2 mmol/L increase in the plasma lactate concentration.

Brain. Hypocapnia induces cerebral vasoconstriction which may result in light-headedness.

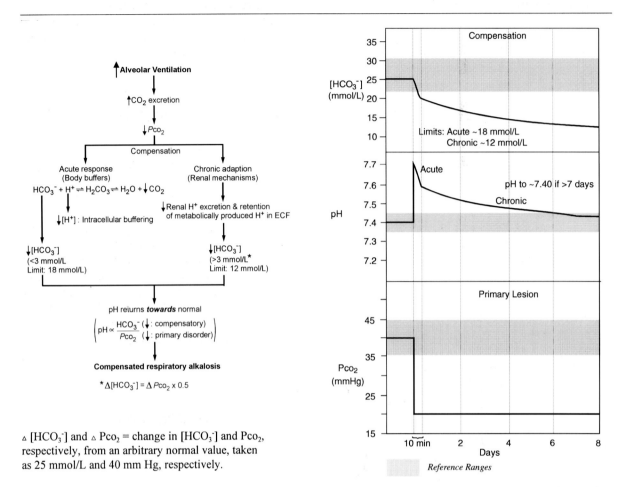

$\triangle$ [HCO$_3^-$] and $\triangle$ Pco$_2$ = change in [HCO$_3^-$] and Pco$_2$, respectively, from an arbitrary normal value, taken as 25 mmol/L and 40 mm Hg, respectively.

Figure 3.9. Perturbations caused by primary respiratory alkalosis and the effects of the acute and chronic compensatory mechanisms.

MIXED ACID-BASE DISTURBANCES

In hospital practice about 40% of the blood gas reports reveal a mixed disorder, i.e., two or more simple disturbances occurring together. Some of the more common combinations are listed in the sections below.

Characteristically they present in one of two ways:

- a severe acidaemia or alkalaemia

- a normal, or near normal, pH associated with abnormal levels of Pco$_2$ and [HCO$_3^-$] (suggesting complete compensation of simple disorder)

Metabolic and respiratory acidosis

Blood gases

pH	-	usually very low (e.g. <7.00)
Pco$_2$	-	increased (respiratory acidosis)
[HCO$_3^-$]	-	decreased (metabolic acidosis)

CAUSES

- cardiopulmonary arrest
- respiratory failure with hypoxia

In these two disorders there is inadequate oxygen presented to the tissues which results in anaerobic glycolysis and lactic acidosis (page 139).

48

Metabolic and respiratory alkalosis

Blood gases

pH	-	usually very high (e.g., >7.60)
Pco_2	-	decreased (respiratory alkalosis)
$[HCO_3^-]$	-	increased (metabolic alkalosis)

CAUSES

- vomiting and congestive cardiac failure
- diuretic therapy and hepatic failure
- diuretic therapy and pneumonia

Vomiting and diuretic therapy are causes of metabolic alkalosis; cardiac and hepatic failure and pneumonia are causes of respiratory alkalosis.

Metabolic alkalosis and respiratory acidosis

Blood gases

pH	-	normal or near normal
Pco_2	-	increased (usually >60 mmHg)
$[HCO_3^-]$	-	increased (usually >45 mmol/L)

CAUSES

- diuretic therapy and chronic obstructive lung disease
- vomiting and chronic obstructive lung disease

Metabolic acidosis and respiratory alkalosis

Blood gases

pH	-	normal or near normal
Pco_2	-	decreased (respiratory alkalosis)
$[HCO_3^-]$	-	decreased (metabolic acidosis)

CAUSES

- salicylate overdose
- septic shock
- renal failure and sepsis
- renal failure and congestive cardiac failure

Salicylate stimulates the respiratory centre (respiratory alkalosis) and interferes with intermediary metabolism to produce an organic acid acidosis. In septic shock the bacteraemia, if Gram-negative, stimulates the respiratory centre and inadequate tissue perfusion (shock) results in local anoxia and lactic acidosis.

Metabolic acidosis and alkalosis

Blood gases

pH	-	variable, but near normal
Pco_2	-	variable, often near normal
$[HCO_3^-]$	-	variable, often near normal

The characteristic feature is a normal, or near normal, plasma $[HCO_3^-]$ associated with a very high anion gap. The high anion gap represents a metabolic acidosis which would have decreased the plasma $[HCO_3^-]$ by an equivalent amount; and if the $[HCO_3^-]$ was originally high (metabolic alkalosis) then the fall caused by the addition of organic acid ions could produce a normal, or near normal, plasma $[HCO_3^-]$.

CAUSES

- diuretic therapy and ketoacidosis
- vomiting and renal failure
- vomiting and severe dehydration (lactic acidosis)
- vomiting and ketoacidosis

Triple acid-base disturbance

This unusual disorder represents a mixed metabolic acidosis and metabolic alkalosis associated with a third disorder which can be either respiratory acidosis or respiratory alkalosis. Again the characteristic feature is a normal, or near normal, bicarbonate associated with a high anion gap.

Blood gases

pH	-	increased or decreased
Pco_2	-	increased or decreased
$[HCO_3^-]$	-	normal or near normal

Note: The key to the diagnosis of mixed disorders is the application of the compensation formulae mentioned above, i.e., if the calculated value of compensation is significantly more or less than the measured value then a mixed disorder is probable.

Table 3.2. Common causes of mixed acid-base disturbances.

Metabolic acidosis + respiratory acidosis
  cardiopulmonary arrest
  respiratory failure with hypoxia
  severe pulmonary oedema

Metabolic alkalosis + respiratory alkalosis
  vomiting and congestive cardiac failure
  diuretic therapy and hepatic failure or pneumonia

Metabolic alkalosis + respiratory acidosis
  diuretic therapy + chronic obstructive lung disease
  vomiting and chronic obstructive lung disease

Metabolic acidosis + respiratory alkalosis
  salicylate toxicity
  septic shock
  renal failure and sepsis
  renal failure and congestive cardiac failure
  diabetic ketoacidosis and pneumonia

Metabolic alkalosis + metabolic acidosis
  diuretic therapy and ketoacidosis
  vomiting and renal failure

Triple acid-base disturbance
  mixed metabolic acidosis and metabolic alkalosis
  PLUS either respiratory acidosis or alkalosis

EVALUATION OF ACID-BASE DISORDERS

From a laboratory point of view acid-base disturbances present as an abnormality in one or more of the following:

- Blood gas results
- Serum anion gap
- Serum bicarbonate

It is of course possible, but unusual, to have a severe acid-base disorder in a subject who has normal values for all of the above parameters. Such may occur if there is a mixed metabolic acidosis and metabolic alkalosis (page 49) where the metabolic acidosis is of a normal anion gap variety, e.g., severe vomiting (increases the plasma $[HCO_3^-]$) in a patient with untreated renal tubular acidosis (decreases the plasma $[HCO_3^-]$ without increasing the anion gap, see page 82). Obviously such occurrences are rare but these possibilities emphasise the importance of considering closely the patient's clinical picture in all cases of suspected acid-base disturbance.

The clinical spectrum of acid-base disturbances is dealt with adequately in other texts and this section will only deal with the laboratory aspects of acid-base evaluation.

BLOOD GASES

Some 40% of patients with acid-base disturbances will have a mixed disorder and these will be missed unless the blood gas results are evaluated in a logical manner. The key to diagnosis is to consider the parameters in the light of the known compensatory responses (discussed earlier). A simple approach is along the following lines:

1. Determine the biochemical diagnosis
2. Evaluate the compensatory response

Determine biochemical diagnosis

Evaluate each of the three analytes to produce a provisional diagnosis.

pH	- ↑	=	alkalaemia, primary lesion likely to be an alkalosis
	- ↓	=	acidaemia, primary lesion likely to be an acidosis
Pco_2	- ↓	=	respiratory alkalosis
	- ↑	=	respiratory acidosis
$[HCO_3^-]$	- ↓	=	metabolic acidosis
	- ↑	=	metabolic alkalosis

At this point a provisional diagnosis should be made, e.g., acidaemia with a metabolic acidosis and a respiratory alkalosis. The next step is to determine if the disorder is simple or mixed; this can be resolved by evaluating the compensatory responses.

Evaluate compensatory responses

The compensatory responses can be evaluated by applying the formulae mentioned above as in the case of the simple acid-base disturbances. Generally, although a useful intellectual exercise, this is not necessary in the majority of cases. The most important clues come from consideration of the pH.

1. A low pH indicates acidaemia and in simple disturbances the other two analytes tend to proceed in the same direction: In simple metabolic acidosis the expected results are low levels for both [HCO_3] (primary lesion) and Pco_2 (compensation by respiratory alkalosis). In simple respiratory acidosis the reverse is expected -- high Pco_2 (primary lesion) and high [HCO_3^-] (compensatory response). If the [HCO_3^-] and the Pco_2 proceed in opposite directions, contrary to what is expected -- a high Pco_2 and a low [HCO_3^-] -- then the patient has a mixed respiratory and metabolic acidosis, in which case the pH tend to be very low.

2. Similarly, a [HCO_3^-] and a Pco_2 proceeding in opposite directions (low Pco_2 with a high [HCO_3^-]) with a markedly high pH (alkalaemia), indicates a mixed metabolic and respiratory alkalosis.

3. If the pH is normal, or near normal, suspect a mixed disorder:

    (a) if both [HCO_3^-] and Pco_2 are decreased consider mixed respiratory alkalosis and metabolic acidosis (page 50). This is based on the premise that simple disorders do not compensate completely (producing a normal pH); however, longstanding chronic respiratory alkalosis may show complete compensation (Figure 3.10) and should be considered -- in this case the diagnosis is made on the basis of the clinical picture.

    (b) if both [HCO_3^-] and Pco_2 are increased consider mixed respiratory acidosis and metabolic alkalosis (page 50). The exception to this rule is mild respiratory acidosis with a Pco_2 less than 60 mmHg which may exhibit complete compensation resulting in a normal pH.

Evaluation of a low bicarbonate

A low bicarbonate is, by definition, a metabolic acidosis. It may be a primary disorder or secondary to respiratory alkalosis; hence the necessity for blood gas determination for proper diagnosis although the history will give a good indication of the probable cause. An approach to evaluation of metabolic acidosis is outlined in Figure 3.10.

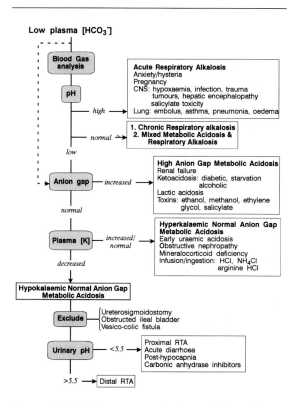

Figure 3.10. Laboratory evaluation of a low plasma bicarbonate. RTA, renal tubular acidosis; HCl, hydrochloric acid; NH_4Cl, ammonium chloride.

1   Determine the anion gap which casts the causes into two groups (high and normal anion gap metabolic acidosis, see Figure 3.10). If the anion gap is *high,* further investigations may involve the determination of plasma creatinine (renal failure), plasma glucose (diabetes mellitus, alcoholic keto-sis), and plasma lactate (lactic acidosis). If it is *normal,* review the plasma potassium concentration [see step (2)].

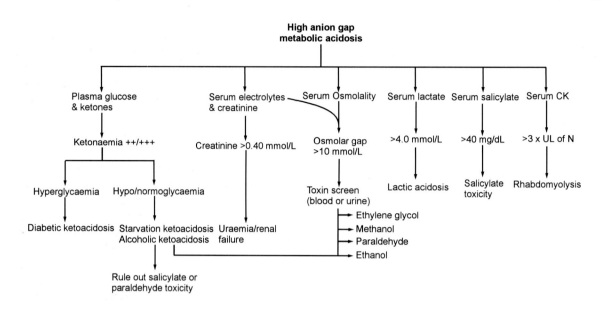

Figure 3.11. Laboratory evaluation of high anion gap metabolic acidosis.

In most cases of metabolic acidosis, the information derived from the blood gas estimation and calculation of the anion gap, coupled with the clinical findings, is usually sufficient for diagnosis and treatment. Further investigations are only necessary if the diagnosis is unclear. These may include estima-tions of plasma creatinine, glucose, lactate, ketoacids, salicylates, etc. (Figure 3.11). If the history is unavailable or inadequate, it may be necessary to perform all the above tests, including a drug screen, before the diagnosis becomes evident.

2   Evaluation of **plasma potassium** in the patient with a normal anion gap metabolic acidosis:

(a) In the case of *hyperkalaemia,* consider:

- Early uraemic acidosis
- Mineralocorticoid deficiency (page 69)
- Obstructive uropathy (page 42)
- Infusion/ingestion of HCl or NH_4Cl

(b) If there is *hypokalaemia* consider:

- Diarrhoea (page 218)
- Renal tubular acidosis (page 81)

- Carbonic anhydrase inhibitor drugs
- Diversion of urine into the gut (page 33)

Evaluation of a high bicarbonate

A high bicarbonate indicates metabolic alkalosis which may be primary or secondary and which may require a blood gas estimation for the correct diagnosis (Figure 3.12). The commonest causes of simple metabolic alkalosis are:

- Diuretic therapy
- Vomiting
- Mineralocorticoid excess syndromes (page 66).

In most cases the diagnosis will be evident from the clinical picture but surreptitious vomiting and diuretic administration are not uncommon and these possibilities can be evaluated by determining *the urinary potassium and chloride* concentrations on a spot (untimed) urine sample (Figure 3.12). A urinary chloride value less than 10 mmol/L is characteristic of vomiting.

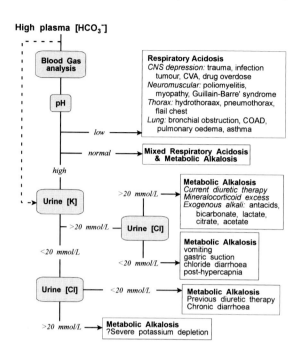

High plasma [HCO₃⁻]

Respiratory Acidosis
CNS depression: trauma, infection
tumour, CVA, drug overdose
Neuromuscular: poliomyelitis,
myopathy, Guillain-Barre' syndrome
Thorax: hydrothoraax, pneumothorax,
flail chest
Lung: bronchial obstruction, COAD,
pulmonary oedema, asthma

Mixed Respiratory Acidosis & Metabolic Alkalosis

Metabolic Alkalosis
Current diuretic therapy
Mineralocorticoid excess
Exogenous alkali: antacids,
bicarbonate, lactate,
citrate, acetate

Metabolic Alkalosis
vomiting
gastric suction
chloride diarrhoea
post-hypercapnia

Metabolic Alkalosis
Previous diuretic therapy
Chronic diarrhoea

Metabolic Alkalosis
?Severe potassium depletion

Figure 3.12. Laboratory evaluation of a high plasma bicarbonate. COAD, chronic obstructive airway disease.

OXYGEN METABOLISM

The cells have no capability to store oxygen, yet all cells require it as an essential metabolic fuel. Without constant delivery, tissue hypoxia and anaerobic metabolism ensue. Tissue hypoxia is defined as inadequate critical oxygen tension to meet the needs of the cell. It is not synonymous with, but closely related to, arterial hypoxaemia which is decreased Po_2 in the arterial blood.

Blood requires an oxygen carrier because of the limited solubility of oxygen. At a Po_2 of 100 mmHg, one litre of plasma will contain only about 3.03 mL of *dissolved* oxygen (0.136 mmol/L). At rest the cardiac output is ~5 L/min giving a delivery of *dissolved* oxygen to the tissues of ~15 mL/min -- a grossly inadequate amount considering that tissue requirements for oxygen are ~250 mL/min at rest and ~4L/min during exercise. This problem is overcome by haemoglobin which enables the blood to carry up to 200 mL of oxygen per litre.

Haemoglobin and oxygen reactions

Haemoglobin is a protein (MW ~67 000) comprised of four interlinked polypeptide chains, each attached to a protoporphyrin group containing a ferrous iron atom. Oxygen binds to the iron complex and each haemoglobin molecule is capable of binding four molecules of oxygen.

$$Hb + 4O_2 \rightleftarrows Hb(O_2)_4$$

One gram of haemoglobin, when fully saturated, can bind 1.34 mL of oxygen. Therefore one litre of blood, with a haemoglobin concentration of 150 g/L and at 98% saturation, will combine with ~196 mL of oxygen (8.8 mmol/L). The inclusion of the dissolved oxygen give a total carriage capacity of ~ 200 mL/L.

The relationship between arterial and tissue oxygenation is explained in large part by the relationship between haemoglobin and oxygen because, to a large extent, oxygen delivery to the tissues depends on the ease with which haemoglobin gives up its oxygen once it reaches the tissues. The relationship between oxygen and haemoglobin is non-linear.

A graphic plot of the percentage oxygen saturation of haemoglobin against the partial pressure of oxygen (Po_2) to which it is exposed gives an S-shaped curve (the haemoglobin-oxygen dissociation curve) which describes the affinity of haemoglobin for oxygen.

Haemoglobin-Oxygen Dissociation Curve

This curve is shown graphically in Figure 3.13. Features to note are:

- At normal alveolar Po_2 (~100 mmHg) haemoglobin is ~98% saturated with oxygen.

- Half saturation (called P_{50}) occurs at a Po_2 of about 27 mmHg at pH 7.4 (Curve B).

- The steep part of the curve lies in the range of the oxygen tensions prevailing in the extrapulmonary tissues of the body (Po_2 levels down to 20-30 mmHg).

- If the curve is *shifted to the left* (Curve A, e.g, at high pH), less oxygen is released due to increased affinity and a higher % saturation for a given Po_2 is obtained.

- If the curve is *shifted to the right* (e.g., at low pH, Curve C), more oxygen is released (decreased affinity) resulting in a lower % saturation for a given Po_2.

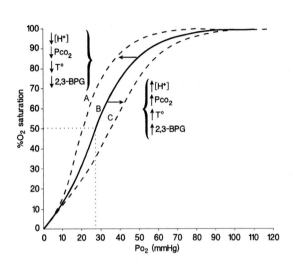

Figure 3.13. The haemoglobin-oxygen dissociation curve.

The extent that oxygen combines with haemoglobin depends on two elements:

(1) the partial pressure of oxygen (Po_2), also known as the oxygen tension, and

(2) factors which displace the curve to the right or left
  (a) hydrogen ion concentration
  (b) partial pressure of carbon dioxide
  (c) temperature
  (d) red cell levels of 2,3-bisphosphoglycerate (2,3-diphosphoglycerate, 2,3-DPG).

Po_2 and haemoglobin saturation

An inspection of the curve in Figure 3.14 shows a steep slope between a Po_2 of 10 and 60 mmHg and a plateau between 70 and 100 mmHg. The plateau provides a safety factor so that significant falls in the Po_2, e.g., at high altitudes or with pulmonary disease, will be associated with only small falls in the oxygen-

carrying capacity of haemoglobin. A drop in the Po_2 from 100 to 60 mmHg will be associated with a decrease in oxygen saturation from ~95% to 90%.

Oxygen is delivered by a linked chain of transfers from the atmosphere to the alveoli, to the blood, and then to the tissues and cells of the body. It diffuses from areas of higher partial pressure to areas of lower partial pressure. The Po_2 at sea level is equal to the barometric pressure of 760 mm Hg multiplied by the fraction of oxygen in dry air (20.93%) which equals 159 mm Hg. As the inspired air is warmed and humidified in the upper airways, it gets diluted by water vapour causing the Po_2 of tracheal /bronchial air to fall to ~149 mm Hg (Figure 3.14). The inspired air is further diluted by carbon dioxide in the lower airways and alveoli -- thus Po_2 of alveolar air is ~100 mmHg. Likewise, arterial blood entering the capillaries has a Po_2 of ~100 mmHg and an oxygen saturation of ~98%.

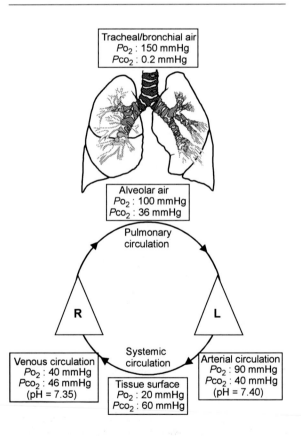

Figure 3.14. Average gas content in the lungs, the pulmonary and systemic circulation and the tissues. R and L represents the right atrium and ventricle and the left atrium and ventricle, respectively.

At the tissue level the Po_2 is low (20-40 mmHg) and this induces removal of oxygen from haemoglobin. At a Po_2 of 40 mmHg the haemoglobin will still be 70-80% saturated and this allows for the release of more oxygen should it be required, e.g., during exercise muscle Po_2 may drop to 10 mmHg. The Po_2 of venous blood returning to the lungs will depend on the amount of oxygen extracted by the tissues but, in the resting condition, is around 40-45 mmHg (75-80% saturated).

Hydrogen ion concentration and haemoglobin saturation. A low pH (acidaemia) shifts the curve to the right (enhances oxygen delivery) and a high pH (alkalaemia) shifts it to the left (decreases oxygen delivery). This effect of pH on haemoglobin oxygen saturation is known as the Bohr effect.

$$HHb + O_2 \rightleftarrows HbO_2 + H^+$$

Thus:
(a) reduced haemoglobin (deoxyhaemoglobin) is more basic than oxyhaemoglobin, and
(b) acidity stimulates oxygen release.

The physiological significance of the hydrogen ion effect is two-fold:

- Metabolically active tissues produce CO_2 (and ultimately acid, see below) and perhaps lactic acid resulting in a low pH; this encourages local oxygen release.

- Patients with poor tissue perfusion are usually acidaemic (e.g, lactic acidosis develops), encouraging local oxygen release. Treatment with bicarbonate would increase the pH and lessen the availability of oxygen. Thus it is probably wise to attend to the patient's circulatory status before administering bicarbonate.

Pco2 and haemoglobin saturation. A high Pco_2 shifts the curve to the right whilst a low Pco_2 shifts it to the left. This is probably a reflection of the Bohr effect as a high Pco_2 results in acidaemia (respiratory acidosis). The physiological implications are obvious: in the tissues where the Pco_2 is high, it favourably increases release of oxygen whilst in the lungs where the Pco_2 is lowered, it encourages the uptake of oxygen by haemoglobin.

Temperature and haemoglobin saturation. As shown in Figure 3.13 a high temperature displaces the curve to the right and a low temperature to the left. The implications are similar to those for pH, i.e., metabolically active tissue will have an elevated temperature and this encourages oxygen release from haemoglobin.

2,3-bisphosphoglycerate (2,3-BPG) and haemoglobin saturation. 2,3-BPG, previously called 2,3-diphosphoglycerate (2,3-DPG, DPG), is produced in the red cell by a glycolytic shunt pathway and functions as the most important controller of oxygen release from haemoglobin.

All cells contain small amounts of 2,3-BPG but red cells have a relatively high level (3-5 mmol/L). 2,3-BPG binds strongly to deoxygenated haemoglobin, preventing re-oxygenation, and less strongly to oxygenated haemoglobin. Thus 2,3-BPG shifts the saturation curve to the right favouring the release of oxygen, e.g., a 24% increase in 2,3-BPG shifts the half-saturation point up by 3 mmHg giving a 22% increase in oxygen release.

The red cell concentration of 2,3-BPG is increased in hypoxic conditions such as chronic lung disease, congenital heart disease, severe anaemia, and high altitude living. Decreased levels occur in stored blood (blood banking), diabetes mellitus, and phosphate-depleted conditions. Although high levels of 2,3-BPG decrease the binding of oxygen to haemoglobin the high oxygen tension in the lungs is sufficient to overcome this inhibition and full oxygenation occurs at this level.

ABNORMALITIES OF THE Po2

In the normal subject the arterial Po_2 (Pao_2) is around 80-110 mmHg. Abnormalities may be due to:

(1) reduction (or increase) in the inspired Po_2 (PIo_2)

(2) hypoventilation

(3) lung disease

A useful procedure in the evaluation of patients with respiratory problems is the application of the alveolar gas equation and estimation of the alveolar-arterial oxygen gradient. The equation is simplified as:

$$PAo_2 = PIo_2 - Paco_2/R$$

Where, PAo_2 = alveolar Po_2; PIo_2 = Po_2 of inspired air; $Paco_2$ = arterial Pco_2, R = respiratory quotient (=0.8).

The PIo_2 is calculated as follows:

PIo_2 = 0.2093 (fraction of O_2 in air at sea level) x {barometric pressure (760 mmHg) - water vapour pressure (47 mmHg)}

Thus at sea level the PIo_2 is 150 mmHg
  {i.e., 0.2093 x (760 - 47)}

Therefore:
  $$PAo_2 = 150 - 1.25 \times Paco_2$$

If the patient is on 40% oxygen then the calculation is

$$PAo_2 = 0.4(760 - 47) - 1.25 Paco_2$$

The alveolar-arterial oxygen gradient
  = $PAo_2 - Pao_2$ (arterial Po_2)

Normally this is less than 15-20 mmHg but it increases with age (e.g., up to 30 mmHg).

Calculation of the alveolar-arterial oxygen gradient allows evaluation of the cause of a low arterial Po_2. In pure hypoventilation (no lung disease) the arterial Pco_2 rises and the arterial Po_2 falls -- the low Po_2 is due to the high Pco_2 -- but the gradient remains normal (e.g, <15 mmHg, see below). In intrinsic lung disease (reduced diffusion of oxygen) the gradient is wide (e.g, >30 mmHg).

Reduction in inspired Po_2 and hypoventilation

These two conditions can result in a lowered arterial Po_2 but if there is no lung disease the alveolar-arterial oxygen gradient will remain normal, i.e., both the alveolar and arterial Po_2 will fall in parallel.

Lung disease. Decreased arterial Po_2 associated with a wide alveolar-arterial oxygen gradient can occur in :

  (a) diffusion defects

  (b) ventilation perfusion inequality
  (c) shunts

Diffusion defects: Such occur in diffuse interstitial lung fibrosis and fluid-filled alveoli (oedema, pneumonia) where oxygen has difficulty in diffusing across into the capillaries. However, it is now considered that hypoxaemia of lung disease is due more to ventilation-diffusion inequality than to diffusion defects.

Ventilation-perfusion inequality: Pulmonary gas exchange depends on a balance between alveolar ventilation (V) and capillary blood flow or perfusion (Q) -- a ventilation-perfusion ratio (V/Q) of 1.0 is considered ideal. Alveolar ventilation is about 4 litres of air per minute. Cardiac output and resulting tissue perfusion is about 5 litres of blood per minute.

In diseased lungs (e.g, emphysema, asthma) the ratio falls in areas throughout the lung and this results in hypoxaemia. For example, hypoventilation of a lung unit may result in a ratio of 0.1 and blood leaving this unit will be poorly oxygenated. There may be a compensatory increase in ventilation and perfusion of surviving lung units, but blood leaving these areas with a high V/Q will not contain more oxygen than that leaving areas with a normal V/Q ratios because of the slope of the O_2 dissociation curve (saturation will not go beyond ~98%).

The situation with CO_2 is different. A low V/Q will result in retention of CO_2 and a high Pco_2 but this can be compensated by increased ventilation in normal lung units -- the CO_2 dissociation curve is linear and increased ventilation can lower the Pco_2 considerably, e.g., to ~7 mmHg. Thus the mixture of blood with high and low Pco_2 can result in an overall normal Pco_2.

Shunts: The shunting of blood through non-gas exchanging lung units (V/Q ratio = 0) will result in lowering of the Po_2 of the mixed venous blood. This may arise when blood passes through the capillaries supplying alveoli that are atelectatic, or filled with oedema fluid, or are filled with inflammatory exudate. It will also occur in a right to left heart shunt.

Low Po_2 associated with a low Pco_2

In lung disease a low Po_2 is usually associated with a high Pco_2, i.e., oxygen cannot get into the blood and carbon dioxide cannot get out. However one often sees a low P_{O_2} associated with a low P_{CO_2}. This is due to the fact that the CO_2 dissociation curve is linear whilst that of oxygen is sigmoid; thus, hyperventilation can lower the arterial P_{CO_2} to very low levels (e.g, to <10 mmHg) but cannot increase the P_{O_2} above ~100-110 mmHg (the level in breathing air). Consider a defect where a large number of alveoli with a normal blood supply are not ventilated. The blood from the diseased lung will have a low P_{O_2} (e.g., <30 mmHg) and a moderately increased P_{CO_2} (e.g., 44-52 mmHg). If the patient is hyperventilating (anoxic drive) then the blood from the normal portion of lung will have a low P_{CO_2} (e.g., 7 mmHg) but a normal P_{O_2} (~100 mmHg). Mixing of these two samples of blood could therefore result in a low P_{O_2} associated with a normal or low P_{CO_2}.

Tissue oxygenation

The oxygen content of blood obviously depends in the first instance on the P_{O_2}. At a given P_{O_2} the oxygen content will be reduced if there is a reduction of the haem binding sites (in anaemia, methaemoglobin-aemia, carboxyhaemoglobinaemia) or if the dissociation curve is shifted to the right. However, the tissue P_{O_2} depends largely on the cardiac output and local blood flow; thus patients with hypoxaemia who have a good cardiac output can tolerate fairly low levels of arterial P_{O_2}. Furthermore, such patients will have an increased red cell 2,3-BPG level which will encourage oxygen release at the tissue level. A marker of the tissue oxygen supply is the blood lactate level but this is relatively crude and hyperlactataemia usually represents a gross defect.

OXYGEN TOXICITY

Molecular oxygen produces toxic compounds such as superoxide, hydrogen peroxide, hydroxyl radicals, and hydroperoxyl radicals, which are very active oxidants and have the potential to destroy cell components such as unsaturated lipids, proteins, and DNA. Superoxide ($O_2^{\cdot}$) is a charged free radical originating from molecular oxygen acquiring a single electron ($O_2 + e^- \rightarrow O_2^{\cdot}$). Hydroxyl radicals arise from the interaction of superoxide with hydrogen peroxide ($H_2O_2 + O_2^{\cdot} \rightarrow O_2 + OH^- + OH\cdot$). Hydroperoxyl radicals arise from protonation of superoxide ($O_2^{\cdot} + H^+ \rightarrow HO_2^{\cdot}$).

The tissues (and tissue components) at risk in oxygen toxicity include:

- *Red cells:* membrane damage resulting in haemolysis
- *Haemoglobin:* oxidation of iron atoms producing methaemoglobin
- *Lung:* damage to alveolar walls
- *Retina:* development of retrolental fibroplasia
- *Brain:* damage to cell membranes

The neonate, for example, risks oxygen toxicity if ventilated with pure oxygen; this could lead to damage of the lungs and development of retrolental fibroplasia.

The cells are protected from oxidative destruction by a number of mechanisms including:

Superoxide dismutase: An enzyme present in most cells which converts superoxide to hydrogen peroxide. The hydrogen peroxide is then removed by catalase.
$$2O_2^{\cdot} + 2H^+ \rightarrow H_2O_2 + O_2$$

Catalase: Converts hydrogen peroxide to water and oxygen
$$H_2O_2 \rightarrow O_2 + H_2O$$

Glutathione peroxidase: Converts hydrogen peroxide to water
$$H_2O_2 + 2GSH \rightarrow GSSG + 2H_2O$$

Glutathione reductase: The reduction of oxidised glutathione back to reduced glutathione is mediated by the enzyme glutathione reductase. This reductase requires NADPH which is produced by the *glucose 6-phosphate dehydrogenase* reaction. Deficiency of the enzyme glucose 6-phosphate dehydrogenase will result in decreased production of reduced glutathione and thus the potential for red cell damage.

Antioxidants: A number of naturally occurring compounds such as vitamin E and β-carotene have the ability to react with free radicals without generating further free radicals.

REFERENCES AND FURTHER READING (on page 61)

APPENDIX

RENAL H⁺ EXCRETION

Recent experimental evidence has indicated that the traditional view of renal hydrogen ion excretion and bicarbonate generation may be incorrect. Two different approaches are outlined below.

THE MODERN VIEW

The method of hydrogen ion disposal by the distal renal tubules outlined on page 00 is the traditional textbook view. Recent investigations, however, have shown that this is erroneous because of two factors:

- The pK of the reaction $NH_3 + H^+ \rightleftharpoons NH_4^+$ is 9.03 at physiological pH (~7.40) and thus the products of glutamine produced by the glutaminase reaction are glutamate and NH_4^+ not glutamic acid and NH_3, Thus formation and excretion of ammonia by the kidney will not result in the net excretion of a hydrogen ion.

- In the kidney the glutaminase reaction and the formation of ammonium ions occurs mainly in the *proximal tubular cells*, not the cells of the distal nephron.

The following short discussion takes these two factors into account and provides a more up-to-date view of renal hydrogen ion excretion. Those readers interested in pursuing the subject further should consult the reviews by the following authors: Halperin M.L. and Jungas R.L. (1983), Halperin M.L. et al (1987), Halperin M.L. (1989).

In the proximal renal tubular cells one molecule of glutamine is metabolised to two molecules each of NH_4^+ (ammonium ion) and HCO_3^- (bicarbonate ion). The NH_4^+ is excreted in the urine and the HCO_3^- returns to the blood. Thus for each NH_4^+ excreted in the urine a HCO_3^- is generated (Figure 3.16). There are three important aspects to these mechanisms:

1. formation of two NH_4^+ by conversion of glutamine to 2-oxoglutarate

2. generation of two HCO_3^- by metabolism of 2-oxoglutarate

3. secretion of NH_4^+ into the renal tubule and excretion in the urine

Formation of NH_4^+. Glutamine is transported into the mitochondria where two enzymes, glutaminase and glutamate dehydroge-nase, convert it to 2-oxoglutarate and two molecules of NH_4^-

glutamine ----------------> NH_4^+ + glutamate
　　　　　glutaminase

glutamate --------------------> NH_4^+ + 2-oxoglutarate
　　　glutamate dehydrogenase

As stated above ammonia is formed from glutamine as the ammonium ion and excretion of this ion by the kidney will not result in a net loss of hydrogen ion. However, if we consider the further metabolism of 2-oxoglutarate we will see that two molecules of bicarbonate are generated and that excretion of ammonium ions will result in a net loss of hydrogen ions from the body.

Generation of HCO_3^-. 2-oxoglutarate contains two carboxylate anions ($-COO^-$). Metabolism of these anions to non-ionic structures results in consumption of H^+. This can occur by either *decarboxylation* (formation of CO_2):

$$R\text{-}COO^- + H^+ \rightarrow R\text{-}H + CO_2$$

or by *reduction to an aldehyde group* ($-CHO$), i.e.,

$$R\text{-}COO^- + H^+ + 2H \rightarrow R\text{-}CHO + H_2O$$

Note. From the ubiquitous reaction between water and carbon dioxide, consumption or removal of a hydrogen ion is tantamount to production of a bicarbonate ion, which is left behind, i.e.,

$$CO_2 + H_2O \rightleftharpoons H^+ + HCO_3^-$$

In the kidney the 2-oxoglutarate generated from glutamine can be further metabolised along either of two pathways, gluconeogenesis or oxidation in the TCA cycle, both of which involve destruction of the carboxylate ions and the consumption of H^+.

Gluconeogenesis: In the mitochondria 2-oxoglutarate is converted to malate (2-oxoglutarate →

succinyl-CoA → succinate → fumarate → malate). The malate exits to the cytosol where it is converted to oxaloacetate which then proceeds via gluconeogenesis to glucose. The two hydrogen ion consuming reactions in this process are:

1 conversion of oxaloacetate to phosphoenol-pyruvate by phosphoenolpyruvate carboxykinase (PPCK)

$$oxaloacetate + H^+ \rightarrow CO_2 + phosphoenolpyruvate$$

2 reduction of 1,3-bisphosphoglycerate to glyceraldehyde 3-phosphate by glyceraldehyde 3-phosphate dehydrogenase (G3PDH).

$$1,3\text{-bisphosphoglycerate} + H^+ \rightarrow$$
$$glyceraldehyde\ 3\text{-phosphate} + Pi$$

Thus, the conversion of 2-oxoglutarate to glucose utilises hydrogen ions (or generates bicarbonate).

$$2\text{-oxoglutarate} + 2H^+ \rightarrow 1/2glucose$$

Oxidation of 2-oxoglutarate in the TCA cycle:
In this process 2-oxoglutarate is converted to acetyl-CoA which enters the TCA cycle. There are a number of reactions involved both inside and outside the mitochondria:

(1) conversion of 2-oxoglutarate to malate (mitochondrial)

(2) exit of malate from the mitochondria and conversion to pyruvate in the cytosol. This is a hydrogen consuming reaction (decarboxylation) catalysed by the *malic enzyme*.

$$malate + H^+ \rightarrow pyruvate + CO_2$$

(3) entry of pyruvate into mitochondria and conversion to acetyl-CoA

(4) entry of acetyl-CoA into TCA cycle as citrate by condensation with oxaloacetate

(5) destruction of one of the three carboxylate ions of citrate by *isocitrate dehydrogenase*

$$citrate + H^+ \rightarrow 2\text{-oxoglutarate} + CO_2$$
$$(3COO^-) \qquad\qquad (2COO^-)$$

Thus the overall reaction is:

$$2\text{-oxoglutarate} + 4O_2 + 2H^+ \rightarrow 5CO_2 + 3H_2O$$

Again, as for gluconeogenesis, two hydrogen ions are consumed (or two bicarbonate ions generated).

Excretion of NH_4^+. The formation of NH_4^+ in the proximal tubule generates HCO_3^- but there will only be a net gain in bicarbonate if the ammonium ion is excreted from the body, i.e., if it is retained it will be metabolised to urea, a process producing hydrogen ions (thus neutralising the generated bicarbonate):

$$CO_2 + 2NH_4^+ \rightarrow urea + 2H_2O + 2H^+$$

The exact mechanism of ammonium ion excretion is unclear but two points emerge: (a) secretion by the proximal tubule results in Na^+ reabsorption, (b) reactions in the loop of Henle probably result in reclamation of some of the filtered HCO_3^-.

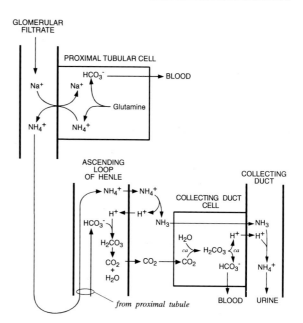

Figure 3.15. Ammonium and hydrogen ion metabolism in the proximal and distal nephrons.

Proximal tubule: In the proximal cells NH_4^+ is

secreted into the lumen via the Na^+/H^+ antiporter in exchange for luminal Na^+ (Figure 3.15); thus sodium conservation. Under normal circumstances about 40 mmol of ammonia are excreted daily, this can rise to ~400 mmol during severe acidosis.

Loop of Henle and collecting ducts: In the thick ascending limb NH_4^+ is reabsorbed, probably by the $Na^+-K^+/2Cl^-$ cotransporter. In this area of the nephron the ammonium ion may be involved in bicarbonate recycling. About 85% of the filtered bicarbonate is reabsorbed in the proximal tubule and the remainder (some 600 mmol/day) distally. Some of the bicarbonate escaping proximal reabsorption may be reclaimed by the following mechanism (Figure 3.15).

The absorbed NH_4^+ dissociates to H^+ and NH_3. The H^+ is secreted back into the tubular lumen to form H_2CO_3 with luminal HCO_3^-. CO_2, generated from luminal H_2CO_3, diffuses across to the collecting duct tubule (along with NH_3) and under the influence of carbonic anhydrase forms H^+ and HCO_3^-. The HCO_3^- is returned to the blood (recycled) and the H^+ is secreted into the tubular lumen. The NH_3 (formed from the NH_4^+ reabsorbed in the loop of Henle) diffuses across the cell and into the collecting duct lumen where it buffers the secreted H^+ and is excreted in the urine as NH_4^+ (Figure 3.15).

Therefore the generation and excretion of ammonium ions results in:

(1) generation of bicarbonate
(2) conservation of sodium
(3) conservation of bicarbonate

Thus, although the excretion of NH_4^+ does not really result in the excretion of hydrogen ions by the kidney it does reflect the rate of hydrogen ion disposal by the kidney. The above mechanism also differs from the traditional view in that it suggests that bicarbonate is regenerated in the proximal, not the distal, tubule.

AN ALTERNATIVE VIEW

This view (Figure 3.16), championed by Atkinson and Bourke (1984, 1987), is based on two premises:

(1) catabolism of amino acids produces bicarbonate and ammonium ions, e.g., for alanine

$$CH_3\text{-}CH(NH_3^+)\text{-}COO^- + 3O_2 \rightarrow 2CO_2 + HCO_3^- + NH_4^+ + H_2O$$

(2) ureagenesis consumes bicarbonate

$$2NH_4^+ + HCO_3^- \rightarrow urea + CO_2 + 3H_2O$$

Thus, they argue, protein catabolism produces a bicarbonate load and the bicarbonate level is controlled by the rate of ureagenesis. They go on to suggest that:

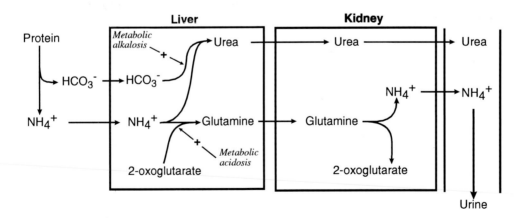

Figure 3.16. Bicarbonate and ammonia metabolism in the liver and kidney and the effects of acidosis and alkalosis. *See text for details.*

(a) In metabolic acidosis (low bicarbonate) ureagenesis is inhibited (decreased utilisation of bicarbonate) and the excretion of ammonium ions by the kidney is increased, i.e., ammonia not converted to urea

(b) In metabolic alkalosis ureagenesis is stimulated (consumption of bicarbonate) and the rate of renal ammonium excretion is suppressed, i.e., ammonia converted to urea

The experimental evidence for this view is strengthened by the fact that urea production is decreased in acidaemia and increased in alkalaemic. This mechanism, however, is disputed by Halperin et al (1987) and the reader is directed to this review and those cited above for further information.

REFERENCES/FURTHER READING

Albert MS, Dell RB, Winter RB. Quantitative displacement of acid-base equilibrium in metabolic acidosis. Ann Intern Med 1967;66:312-322.

Bia M, Thier SO. Mixed acid-base disturbances: a clinical approach. Med Clinics North Am 1981;65: 347-361.

Brackett NC, Cohen JJ, Schwartz WB. Carbon dioxide tritration curve of normal man. N Engl J Med 1965;272:6-12.

Brenner BM, Rector FC Jr. (eds): *The Kidney, 4th edn.* Philadelphia: WB Saunders, 1990.

Emmett MD, Nairns RG. Clinical use of the anion gap. Medicine 1977;56:38-54.

Fulop M. Hypercapnia in metabolic alkalosis. NY State J Med 1976;76:19-23.

Walmsley RN, White GH. Mixed acid-base disorders. Clin Chem 1985;31:321-325.

Walmsley RN, White GH. Normal 'anion gap' (hyperchloraemic) acidosis. Clin Chem 1985;31:309-313.

ADDITIONAL REFERENCES (APPENDIX)

Atkinson DE and Bourke E. The role of ureagenesis in pH homeostasis. TIBS 1984;9:297-300.

Atkinson DE and Bourke E. Metabolic aspects of the regulation of systemic pH. Am J Physiol 1987;252 (Renal fluid electrolyte physiology, 21):F987-F965.

Halperin ML. and Jungas RL. Metabolic production and renal disposal of hydrogen ions. Kidney Internl 1983;24:709-713.

Halperin ML, Jungas RL, Cheema-Dhadi S, Brosnan JT. Disposal of the daily acid load: an integral function of the liver, lungs, and kidney. TIBS 1987; 12:197-199.

Halperin ML How much 'new' bicarbonate is formed in the distal nephron in the process of net acid excretion? Kidney Internl 1989;35:1277-1281.

Chapter 4

Mineralocorticoids

The mineralocorticoids are C_{21} steroids which originate in the zona glomerulosa of the adrenal cortex and influence potassium, sodium, and hydrogen ion homeostasis. The major and most important of these steroids is aldosterone but a precursor, 11-deoxy-corticosterone, also has significant mineralocorticoid activity (~6% of that of aldosterone). Corticosterone, another intermediate product, and cortisol, the principal glucocorticoid, have minimal mineralo-corticoid activity (<1% of that of aldosterone). The major synthetic mineralocorticoid used in therapy is fludrocortisone (~80% of aldosterone potency).

Normal physiology

Aldosterone is synthesised in the adrenal cortex and transported in the blood attached to albumin and specific binding proteins. It influences potassium and sodium homeostasis and is inactivated by the liver and excreted in the urine.

ALDOSTERONE ACTION

The overall effect of aldosterone is sodium uptake and secretion of potassium and hydrogen ions by the epithelial cells of the distal nephron, large gut, sweat glands, salivary glands, and mammary glands.

The most important site of action is the distal nephron where it increases sodium reabsorption from the lumen and increases potassium and hydrogen ion secretion producing sodium retention, and potassium and hydrogen excretion. The exact mechanism is unclear but it appears to increase cellular K^+ uptake from the ECF producing a high cellular potassium concentration ($[K^+]$) and actively induce Na^+ reabsorption from the luminal fluid producing a luminal negative potential. The high cellular $[K^+]$ and luminal negativity 'encourages' K^+ secretion into the tubular lumen (see page 26).

The effect of aldosterone on distal H^+ secretion appears to be mediated by increasing the number of proton pumps rather than increasing the activity of individual pumps. For example, in aldosterone deficiency the amount of H^+ secreted is decreased but

the cell to luminal gradient is unchanged and a urinary pH as low as 4.50 can be attained.

Prolonged *aldosterone excess* is associated with:

(a) increased renal sodium reabsorption and body sodium excess which will induce water retention
(b) increased renal potassium excretion, potassium depletion, and hypokalaemia
(c) increased renal hydrogen excretion and renal bicarbonate generation, and metabolic alkalosis (high plasma $[HCO_3^-]$)

Prolonged aldosterone deficiency will produce:

(a) renal sodium loss and sodium depletion
(b) renal potassium retention and hyperkalaemia
(c) renal H^+ retention and metabolic acidosis (low plasma $[HCO_3^-]$)

ALDOSTERONE SYNTHESIS

The following section deals with cortisol synthesis as well as that of aldosterone. The starting point (Figure 4.1) is cholesterol which is converted to aldosterone, cortisol, or C_{19} steroids (e.g., dehydroepiandrosterone, DHEA) by five apoenzymes. (Refer to Table 4.1 for details and abbreviations.) Four of the five enzymes are members of the cytochrome P450 group of mixed function oxidases, several have more than one enzyme activity, two are located in the mitochondria, and three are located in the endoplasmic reticulum.

It is convenient to discuss steroidogenesis (Figure 4.1) in five parts:

(1) conversion of cholesterol to pregnenolone,
(2) pregnenolone metabolism,
(3) progesterone metabolism and aldosterone production,
(4) cortisol formation, and
(5) C_{19}-steroid synthesis.

Cholesterol to pregnenolone: The rate limiting step in cortisol synthesis (enzyme involved: P450$_{SCC}$) is the *side-chain cleavage* of cholesterol to form pregneno-

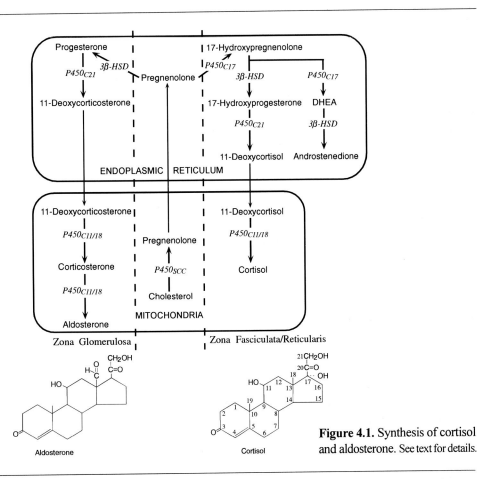

Figure 4.1. Synthesis of cortisol and aldosterone. See text for details.

Enzyme	Location	Activity
$P450_{SCC}$	mitochondrial	cholesterol side chain cleavage enzyme
$P450_{C17}$	endoplasmic reticulum	17-hydroxylase and 17,20-desmolase activity
$P450_{C21}$	endoplasmic reticulum	21-hydroxylase activity
$P450_{C11/18}$	mitochondrial	11β-hydroxylase, 18-hydroxylase activity
3β-HSD	endoplasmic reticulum	3β-hydroxysteroid dehydrogenase and Δ^5-3-ketosteroid isomerase (not a P450 cytochrome complex)

Table 4.1. Enzymes involved in adrenal steroido-genesis.

lone, which is transported to the endoplasmic reticulum. The cholesterol is derived largely from low density lipoproteins (LDL). The cellular uptake of cholesterol and side-chain cleavage are both stimulated by pituitary-derived adrenocorticotrophic hormone (ACTH).

Pregnenolone metabolism: In the zona glomerulosa 3 β-HSD predominates and progesterone is formed. In the zona fasciculata and zona reticularis $P450_{C17}$ predominates with the formation of 17-hydroxy-pregnenolone.

Progesterone metabolism: Progesterone is converted by $P450_{C21}$ (hydroxylation at C_{21} of the steroid nucleus) to 11-deoxycorticosterone (11DOC) which is transferred back to the mitochondria where the activities of a single enzyme complex ($P450_{C11/18}$) convert it through corticosterone (hydroxylation at

C_{11}) to aldosterone (hydroxylation at C_{18} and formation of an aldehyde group on C_{18}).

Cortisol formation: In the endoplasmic reticulum 17-hydroxypregnenolone is converted to 17-hydroxyprogesterone (3β-HSD) and then to 11-deoxycortisol by hydroxylation at C_{21} (P450$_{C21}$). The 11-deoxy-cortisol is then moved inside the mitochondria where hydroxylation of C_{11} occurs (P450$_{C11/18}$), producing cortisol. There is some evidence to suggest that there are two forms of the P450$_{C11/18}$ complex: one in the zona glomerulosa for aldosterone synthesis and the other in the zona fasciculata/reticularis for cortisol synthesis.

C₁₉-steroid synthesis: The 17,20-desmolase activity of the P450$_{C17}$ complex converts 17-hydroxypregnenolone to dehydroepiandrosterone (DHEA) which is then converted to androstenedione by 3β-HSD. Androstenedione is a precursor of both testosterone and oestrogens. DHEA, which is converted to its sulphate conjugate (DHEA-S) by sulphotransferase, is the main steroid produced by the foetal adrenal.

CONTROL OF SYNTHESIS AND SECRETION

Cortisol

Cortisol synthesis and secretion are controlled (stimulated) by pituitary-derived ACTH which is in turn controlled by corticotrophin releasing factor and by feedback inhibition by cortisol (page 249).

Aldosterone

The rate of aldosterone synthesis and secretion is influenced by ACTH, angiotensin II, and potassium.

ACTH: Aldosterone, like cortisol, exhibits a circadian rhythm and pharmacological doses of ACTH increases its secretion rate. However, the action of ACTH on aldosterone secretion is probably of little physiological importance considering that:

- Hypopituitarism (ACTH deficiency) is not associated with decreased aldosterone synthesis or secretion.

- The high circulating levels of ACTH in Cushing's disease do not result in increased aldosterone secretion.

Angiotensin II: Angiotensin II, a product of the renin-angiotensin system (see below), stimulates aldosterone synthesis and secretion. This is the most important control mechanism of aldosterone secretion.

Potassium: Aldosterone synthesis is very sensitive to changes in the circulating potassium level: hyperkalaemia stimulates, and hypokalaemia inhibits, synthesis and secretion. An increase in the plasma potassium concentration of as little as 0.1 mmol/L will increase aldosterone secretion. This is a direct effect at the adrenal level.

THE RENIN-ANGIOTENSIN SYSTEM

Renin, an enzyme synthesised in the kidney by the juxtaglomerular apparatus, regulates aldosterone secretion through the action of angiotensin II (Figure 4.2). Renin is synthesised in, and released from, the juxtaglomerular apparatus, a group of cells comprising the juxtaglomerular cells of the afferent glomerular arteriole and the macula densa cells of the distal tubule. Renin converts a renin substrate (angiotensinogen), a glycoprotein synthesised by the liver, to a decapeptide angiotensin I. This substance is converted, mainly in the lung, by angiotensin converting enzyme (ACE) to an octapeptide, angiotensin II. Angiotensin II has four main actions:

(1) arteriolar vasoconstriction
(2) aldosterone release
(3) inhibition of renin release (short feedback loop)
(4) stimulation of liver synthesis of renin substrate

Renin

Renin release is controlled by several factors:

(1) renal perfusion pressure
(2) sodium concentration at the macula densa
(3) sympathetic nervous system
(4) angiotensin II

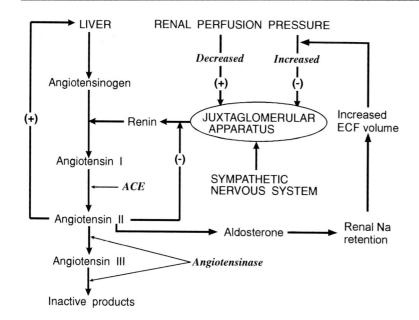

ACE, angiotensin converting enzyme. The plus and minus signs indicate stimulation and inhibition, respectively.

Figure 4.2. The renin-angiotensin-aldosterone system. See text for details.

Renal perfusion pressure: A fall in renal perfusion (blood) pressure produces renin release; thus shock, haemorrhage, dehydration, renal artery stenosis, etc, will increase renin secretion. Increased secretion also occurs when the subject moves from the supine to the upright position, as a result of decreased venous return and cardiac output due to gravitational pooling of blood in the extremities. Renin release is reduced by a raised renal perfusion pressure, e.g., ECF volume expansion. These pressure changes are thought to be detected by the juxtaglomerular cells of the afferent arterioles.

Sodium concentration at the macula densa: It was originally thought that a decreased sodium concentration in the fluid perfusing the distal renal tubule increased renin secretion. However, it has recently been suggested that the macula densa responds rather to the rate of chloride reabsorption in the ascending loop of Henle.

Sympathetic nervous system: The sympathetic nervous system activates renin release through β-adrenergic receptors. This mechanism is thought to be important for the increased renin release associated with postural changes, and with minor

decreases in the extracellular fluid volume. Infusions of catecholamines will also increase renin release.

Angiotensins II and III: These two metabolites inhibit renin release -- they act directly on the juxtaglomerular cells -- and thus constitute a short negative feedback mechanism.

Plasma volume and aldosterone

From the above discussion it can be seen that there is an intimate relationship between plasma volume, renin, and aldosterone. For example, if plasma volume falls (dehydration, ECV depletion), the following sequence of events occurs:

↓ plasma volume › ↑ renin › ↑ angiotensin II ›
    (a) vasoconstriction
    (b) ↑ aldosterone

↑ aldosterone › ↑ renal sodium reabsorption ›
↑ extracellular [Na] → ↑ osmolality →
    (a) thirst
    (b) ↑ ADH release

↑ ADH + thirst → positive water balance →
↑ plasma volume → ↓ renin secretion

ALDOSTERONE METABOLISM

Normally, about 50-250 μg (0.14-0.17 μmol) of aldosterone are produced daily. It circulates in the plasma weakly bound to albumin and more tightly bound to transcortin and a specific binding protein, aldosterone-binding globulin. The principal site of catabolism is the liver, where over 90% of aldosterone is cleared from the blood during a single passage. Here it is inactivated by reduction to the tetrahydro derivatives and then conjugated to glucuronic acid (at the C_3 position) and excreted in the urine. The normal plasma level of aldosterone is around 0.03-0.55 nmol/L.

Mineralocorticoid excess syndromes

The *sine qua non* of all the mineralocorticoid excess syndromes (MES) is hypokalaemia and increased renal potassium excretion. Patients with MES usually present with hypokalaemia and metabolic alkalosis; in addition the primary MES disorders are associated with sodium and water excess which may lead to hypertension.

CAUSES/PATHOPHYSIOLOGY

The MES can be secondary to increased plasma renin activity or they may be primary adrenal disorders associated with depressed plasma renin levels (Table 4.2). The essential difference between the two is the subject's intravascular volume which is decreased in the secondary and increased in the primary disorders.

Primary hyperaldosteronism

Conn's syndrome, due to chronic autonomous aldosterone secretion by an adrenal adenoma or bilateral hyperplasia, characteristically presents with hypertension, hypokalaemic metabolic alkalosis and renal potassium wasting. All of these features can be assigned to excessive aldosterone activity, including the hypertension which relates to fluid retention secondary to sodium retention. Aldosterone secreted autonomously from an adrenal adenoma is not

subject to the normal negative feedback control exerted by suppressed renin production due to aldosterone-mediated ECV expansion. (Figure 4.3). The diagnosis depends on the demonstration of hyperaldosteronism associated with low plasma renin activity. It is a rare cause of hypertension (<0.5%).

Table 4.2. Causes of mineralocorticoid excess.

Primary (low plasma renin activity)
Hyperaldosteronism (Conn's syndrome)
    Adrenal adenoma, Adrenal hyperplasia
Other steroid excess
    Enzyme deficiency: 11β-hydroxylase,
        17α-hydroxylase
    Cushing's syndrome (page 257)
    Ectopic ACTH syndrome (page 258)

Secondary (high plasma renin activity)
Physiological
    Volume depletion: dehydration, diuretic therapy,
        haemorrhage, etc
Oedema-associated
    Cardiac failure, nephrotic syndrome, cirrhosis
Hypertension-associated (page 294)
    Renovascular disorders, malignant hypertension,
    Renin-secreting tumour, oestrogen therapy
Drugs/exogenous steroids
    Steroid/carbenoxolone therapy, licorice ingestion
Pseudohyperaldosteonism (Liddle's syndrome)

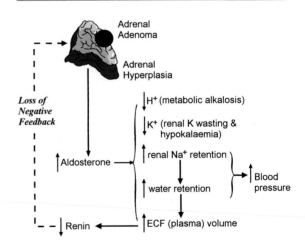

Figure 4.3. Pathophysiology of primary hyperaldosteronism.

Adrenal enzyme defects

The adrenal enzyme defects resulting in mineralo-corticoid excess also result in deficient cortisol secretion. The latter stimulates pituitary ACTH release; chronic stimulation of the adrenal with this hormone causes adrenal hyperplasia. These syndromes are present from birth and hence the designation congenital adrenal hyperplasia (CAH). The C_{11} defect is the commonest of these conditions but they are all rare.

17α-hydroxylase: Deficiency of this enzyme reduces cortisol production (decreased conversion of progesterone to 17-hydroxyprogesterone) which in turn increases ACTH production (page 249). Prolonged adrenal stimulation by ACTH will activate the aldosterone pathway increasing production of corticosterone and 11-deoxycorticosterone (11-DOC), with resultant increased mineralocorticoid activity. The production of aldosterone itself is often suppressed probably because the increased mineralo-corticoid activity of 11-DOC induces hypokalaemia which inhibits its conversion to aldosterone.

11β-hydroxylase: Impaired conversion of 11-DOC to corticosterone results in the accumulation of the 11-deoxysteroid. Cortisol production is also impaired resulting in increased ACTH secretion and adrenal hyperplasia.

Secondary hyperaldosteronism

This describes increased aldosterone production secondary to increased renin secretion which distinguishes it biochemically from primary hyper-aldosteronism. The initiating disorder is usually hypovolaemia (low blood volume resulting in poor renal perfusion), e.g., dehydration, diuretic therapy, Bartter's syndrome (page 82), haemorrhage, etc. It also occurs in the oedematous situations (with low effective arterial blood volume, page 11), renovascular disease (page 292), and in the rare renin-secreting tumour.

Drugs

Drugs that may be associated with clinical mineralo-corticoid excess are steroids (e.g., cortisol in large doses, fludrocortisone) and the glycyrrhizinic acid derivatives (licorice and carbenoxolone).

Glycyrrhizinic acid. The aldosterone receptor cannot distinguish between cortisol and aldosterone and reacts to both equally. However, aldosterone-sensitive tissues contain the enzyme 11β-hydroxy-steroid dehydrogenase (11β-HSD) which converts cortisol to the inactive cortisone, thus impeding the action of cortisol on the receptor. The glycyrrhizinic acid derivatives inhibit 11β-HSD activity and allow cortisol access to the receptors in aldosterone-sensitive tissues.

Pseudohyperaldosteronism

This rare familial disorder (Liddle's syndrome) is characterised by hypertension and hypokalaemic metabolic alkalosis associated with low circulating aldosterone levels. The nature of the defect is unknown but is thought to be a renal transport problem because it does not respond to spirono-lactone which blocks the action of aldosterone, but responds to the diuretic triamterene which causes natriuresis and potassium retention by a mechanism not involving aldosterone.

CONSEQUENCES

The classical features of mineralocorticoid excess are hypokalaemia and metabolic alkalosis. Hypertension is a feature of the primary syndromes whilst the secondary syndromes are often consequent to hypovolaemia.

Salt and water metabolism. In primary hyperaldosteronism the retention of sodium results in an expanded ECF volume. However, this is not progressive and the patient does not become oedematous because subsequently the positive sodium (and water) balance reverts to normal. This has been termed the 'escape' phenomenon (the mechanism is unclear but may be related to atrial natriuretic peptide stimulating renal sodium excretion). Although oedema does not occur, hypertension, due to increased blood volume, does.

Potassium metabolism. Increased potassium

excretion, which occurs in both primary and secondary disorders, results in hypokalaemia and potassium depletion. Severe depletion may produce hypokalaemic nephropathy which is manifested clinically by polyuria and nocturia.

Acid-base metabolism. Aldosterone-induced renal H^+ excretion and HCO_3^- generation produces metabolic alkalosis. Although this is very common in the secondary disorders it is not always present in the primary disorders. A possible reason is that hypovolaemia stimulates renal bicarbonate retention whereas hypervolaemia increases its excretion.

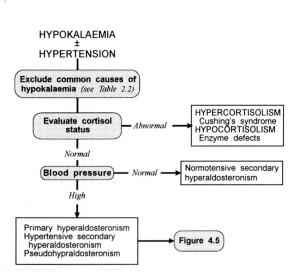

Figure 4.4. Laboratory evaluation of suspected hyperaldosteronism.

LABORATORY EVALUATION

The laboratory evaluation of the patient with suspected mineralocorticoid excess (hypertension or hypokalaemia or both) is outlined in Figures 4.4 and 4.5. The logical procedure is:

1   Exclude common causes of hypokalaemia, vomiting, diuretics, diarrhoea, etc.

2   Check the potassium concentration of a spot urine -- if less than 20 mmol/L, seek an

extrarenal cause; if greater than 20 mmol/L, proceed to the evaluation of cortisol (page 259) and renin/ aldosterone status.

3   In cases of suspected adrenal adenoma, diagnostic imaging techniques such as computerised axial tomography (CT scanning) can be useful providing the lesion ia above 0.5 cm in diameter.

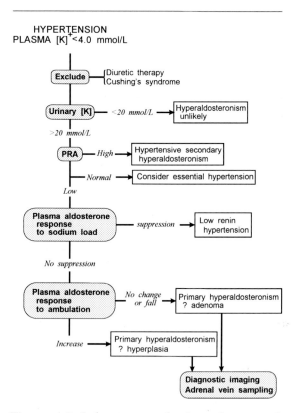

Figure 4.5. Laboratory evaluation of suspected primary hyperaldosteronism.

Evaluation of renin and aldosterone status

1. Determine renin response to ambulation. Determine renin activity on a blood sample (a) before patient gets out of bed in the morning and (b) after 2 to 4 hours ambulation. In the normal subject the plasma renin should be within normal limits and increase at least two-fold on ambulation. In primary hyperaldosteronism the renin level is suppressed and does not increase on ambulation.

2. Aldosterone response to saline load.
Administering a sodium (saline) load to a normal subject should cause a suppression of the plasma aldosterone to values less than 10 ng/100 mL. The simplest and quickest sodium loading protocol is to infuse 2 litres of saline over 4 hours and taking pre- and post-load blood samples for aldosterone estimation.

3. Adrenal venous sampling. Samples of adrenal venous blood, obtained under radiological guidance, can be used to determine the site of an adenoma or to provide differential diagnosis of bilateral hyperplasia.

Mineralocorticoid deficiency syndromes

The mineralocorticoid deficiency syndromes (MDS) characteristically present with:

- hyperkalaemia
- hyperchloraemic metabolic acidosis
- renal salt wasting, with or without hypo-natraemia and evidence of hypovolaemia

The constant feature is hyperkalaemia whilst the other electrolyte abnormalities may not be present or obvious. The complex of hyperkalaemic, hyperchloraemic metabolic acidosis due to mineralocorticoid deficiency is often referred to as renal tubular acidosis type 4.

CAUSES/PATHOPHYSIOLOGY

The mineralocorticoid deficiency syndrome may be due to:

(1) general adrenocortical disease (cortisol and aldosterone deficiency),
(2) specific aldosterone deficiency,
(3) renal tubular resistance to aldosterone, and
(4) potassium-sparing diuretics.

Enzyme defects

21β-hydroxylase deficiency is the commonest type of adrenal enzyme defect. Both cortisol and aldo-

Table 4.3. Causes of mineralocorticoid deficiency.

Cortisol & aldosterone deficiency
Addison's disease (page 252)
Enzyme defect (21β-hydroxylase)

Selective aldosterone deficiency
Syndrome of hyporeninaemic hypoaldosteronism
Drugs: indomethacin, captopril, heparin
Enzyme defect: corticosterone methyl oxidase

Tubular resistance
Renal disease: interstitial nephritis, SLE,
 obstructive uropathy
Renal transplant
Sickle cell disease
Pseudohypoaldosteronism

Potassium-sparing diuretics
spironolactone, amiloride, triamterene (page 28)

sterone synthesis are defective resulting in:

- Loss of negative feedback by cortisol with increased ACTH secretion resulting in (a) bilateral adrenal hyperplasia and (b) increased adrenal androgen synthesis.

- Renal sodium wasting and hyperkalaemia (aldosterone deficiency).

Syndrome of hyporeninaemic hypoaldosteronism (SHH)

SHH is an unusual, but fairly common, cause of hyperkalaemia due to the deficient secretion of renin and aldosterone. The mechanism of the disorder is unclear but certain characteristics are associated with it.

- It occurs most commonly in subjects over the age of 60-years.
- 50% of cases have diabetes mellitus.
- 50% of subjects have mild renal insufficiency (plasma creatinine <0.20 mmol/L).
- 50% present with hyperchloraemic metabolic acidosis.

- Renal salt-wasting is not a common feature.
- Plasma renin and aldosterone levels are low and do not respond to the stimulus provided by ambulation.

Drugs & selective aldosterone deficiency

Prostaglandin synthetase inhibitors. Drugs that inhibit prostaglandin production, such as indomethacin and ibuprofen, can result in hyperkalaemia because prostaglandins are necessary for the normal secretion of renin and aldosterone. This condition has similar biochemical features to the SHH syndrome.

Heparin. Chronic heparin administration can selectively suppress aldosterone production in the adrenal gland.

Captopril. Angiotensin converting enzyme (ACE) inhibitors depress the production of aldosterone by suppressing the conversion of angiotensin I to angiotensin II. Their administration is associated with high plasma renin levels and low aldosterone levels.

LABORATORY EVALUATION

The characteristic, and constant, presenting feature of the MDS is hyperkalaemia and the evaluation of this abnormality is dealt with on page 30. After excluding the common causes of hyperkalaemia such as pseudohyperkalaemia, renal failure, diabetic keto-acidosis, use of potassium-sparing diuretics, etc, and the possibility of a mineralocorticoid deficiency exists, the next action (Figure 4.6) is to exclude general adrenal disease with the short Synacthen test (page 255). If this test proves normal then the renin and aldosterone response to ambulation should be evaluated.

CONSEQUENCES

The clinical and biochemical features of the MDS depend on the aetiology and status of the other adrenal steroids. Mineralocorticoid deficiency *per se* is manifested by abnormalities of potassium, acid-base, and salt and water metabolism.

Potassium. Decreased renal potassium secretion and hyperkalaemia may be the only abnormality present.

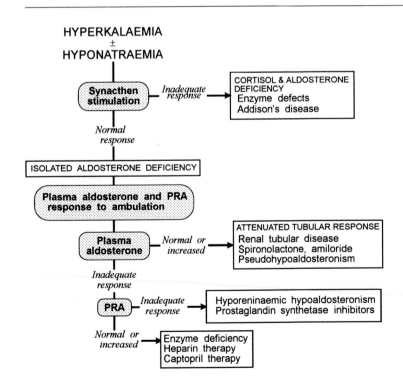

PRA, plasma renin activity

Figure 4.6. The laboratory evaluation of suspected hypoaldosteronism.

Acid-base. Often, but not always, a hyperchloraemic metabolic acidosis (page 51) may occur.

Salt and water. The renal sodium wasting can result in hypovolaemia, hyponatraemia, and hypo-osmolality (see Addison's disease, page 252). This does not occur in all cases, for example, in the SHH syndrome the circulating aldosterone appears to be sufficient to prevent salt wasting but insufficient to prevent renal potassium retention.

REFERENCES/FURTHER READING

Axelrod L. Case records of the Massachusetts General Hospital. N Engl J Med 1992;326:1617-1623.

Batlle DC, Kurtzman NA. Syndromes of aldosterone deficiency and excess. Med Clinics North Am 1983; 67:879-902.

Edwards CW, Burt D, Stewart PM. The specificity of the human mineralocorticoid receptor: clinical clues to a biological conundrum. J Steroid Biochem 1989; 32:213-216.

Gordon RD, Klemm SA, Tunny TJ, Stowasser M. Primary aldosteronism: hypertension with a genetic basis. Lancet 1992;340:159-161.

Young WF, Klee GG. Primary aldosteronism: diagnostic evaluation. Endocrinol Metabol Clinics North Am 1988;17:367-395.

Chapter 5

The Kidney and Renal Disease

In laboratory medicine the commonest presentation of renal disease is an elevated plasma creatinine or urea or both. Given that renal disease is not only common in its own right but also a frequent complication of high prevalence diseases such as diabetes mellitus and hypertension, it is not unusual to find numerous patients with plasma creatinine and urea abnormalities in general medical practice. If we add to this the fact that after the age of 35 years kidney function progressively deteriorates, then the importance of some knowledge of normal renal function and diseases of the kidney becomes apparent.

Normal physiology

The major function of the kidney is to maintain the volume and composition of the extracellular fluid and, indirectly, the intracellular fluid. This is performed by filtration of the blood by the glomerulus and processing of this fluid by the tubules (Figure 5.1). This process involves:

- reabsorption of essential metabolites, e.g., glucose, amino acids
- excretion of waste products, e.g., urea, urate
- maintenance of water, electrolyte, acid-base, calcium, magnesium and phosphate balance.

Other functions of the kidney involve vitamin D metabolism (page 90), synthesis and secretion of renin (page 64), and erythrocyte production (synthesis of erythropoietin).

GLOMERULAR FILTRATION

The kidneys receive about 20% of the cardiac output or about 1200 mL of blood a minute (~600 mL of plasma a minute) and from this about 120 mL of filtrate passes through the glomerulus to the proximal tubule. The filtrate is equivalent to cell and protein-free blood (a small amount of low molecular weight proteins appears in the filtrate but most of this is reabsorbed in the tubule), e.g., its albumin content is around 100-300 mg/L compared to plasma albumin concentration of 35-55 g/L.

Factors that influence the rate of filtration are:

- renal blood flow and pressure in the afferent arterioles
- number of functional glomeruli
- permeability of the glomeruli
- blood colloidal osmotic pressure
- back pressure in the tubules
- pressure in the afferent glomeruli

The glomerular filtration rate (GFR) in young adult males is around 130 mL/min/1.73 m^2 body surface area ($\pm 15\%$). After the age of 35 years, due to age-related nephron 'drop-out', the rate falls ~10% per decade. There is an increase of 30 to 50% before the end of the first trimester of pregnancy. A high protein diet will increase the GFR slightly and there is a small decrease during protein restriction.

The approximate daily amounts of water and plasma analytes filtered by the glomeruli and the resulting urine composition are illustrated in Figure 5.1.

RENAL TUBULAR FUNCTION

The renal tubules are responsible for processing the glomerular filtrate and dealing with waste product excretion, retention of essential metabolites, and water, electrolyte, and acid-base homeostasis. These are complex processes and will only be dealt with briefly. Further information is available in this text in the sections on the particular analytes (page numbers supplied) but for comprehensive information the reader is directed to the text by Brenner and Rector (1990) which is referenced at the end of the chapter.

Proximal tubule

Most of the essential metabolites (glucose, amino acids, etc), sodium, chloride, potassium, bicarbonate, calcium, phosphate, and water are reabsorbed in the proximal tubule. The appproximate amounts are listed in Figure 5.1.

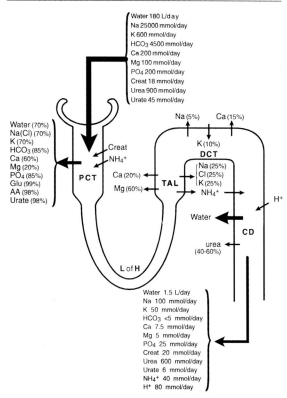

Figure 5.1. The nephron: normal function. See text for details. AA, amino acids; Glu, glucose; PCT, proximal convoluted tubules; L of H, loop of Henle; TAL, thick ascending limb; DCT, distal convoluted tubule; CD, collecting duct.

Glucose. Nearly all of the filtered glucose is reabsorbed. However, if the plasma glucose level exceeds 10 mmol/L (normal renal threshold), significant amounts will appear in the urine.

Amino acids. Almost all (~98%) of the filtered amino acids are reabsorbed. There are specific transport mechanisms for the particular groups.

Sodium and chloride. Sodium ions are actively reabsorbed (about 70 to 80%); chloride ions follow passively along the created electrochemical gradient.

Potassium. There is active transport of 70 to 80% of filtered potassium ions in this part of the nephron via a process independant of sodium and chloride reabsorption.

Calcium. Calcium ions are actively reabsorbed in association with sodium ions. (PTH has no effect on calcium reabsorption in this part of the tubule).

Magnesium. The mechanism for proximal handling of magnesium ions is not known -- they are probably passively reabsorbed.

Bicarbonate. 80 to 90% of the filtered bicarbonate is reabsorbed in the proximal tubule, the process being dependant on carbonic anhydrase activity and hydrogen ion secretion. This is discussed on page 38 in the acid-base section.

Phosphate. The active reabsorption of phosphate is influenced by PTH levels (increased PTH decreases reabsorption).

Water. There is passive reabsorption, along with sodium. The luminal fluid presented to the descending limb of the loop of Henle has the same tonicity as that of the filtrate.

Loop of Henle

Descending limb. As the loop of Henle descends into the renal medulla the high tonicity of the interstitial tissue causes sodium ions and water to move out of the lumen into the interstitial tissue (see countercurrent multiplier, page 5).

Ascending limb. In the thick ascending limb the active reabsorption of chloride ions is followed by the reabsorption of 20-25% of the filtered sodium and potassium ions. As this portion of the nephron is impermeable to water the luminal fluid becomes diluted (fluid osmolality 50-100 mmol/kg). Twenty to 25% of the filtered calcium is reabsorbed here as well as some 50-60% of the filtered magnesium.

Distal tubule

The distal tubule, in conjunction with the collecting ducts, is an important regulator of sodium, potassium, and hydrogen ion homeostasis.

Sodium. An additional 5 to 10% of the filtered sodium is reabsorbed in this area. This occurs through out the whole distal tubule but mostly in the proximal portion. Sodium ions are actively reabsorbed through specific sodium channels under the influence of aldosterone. This sodium ion movement creates a negative charge on the luminal aspect of the tubular cell which is important for the secretion of hydrogen and potassium ions.

Potassium. The major portion of the filtered potassium (>95%) is reabsorbed in the nephron proximal to the distal tubule. In the distal tubule and collecting ducts potassium ions are secreted into the tubular lumen accounting for the major portion appearing in the urine. The rate of secretion depends on the potassium concentration in the distal tubular cell (which is influenced by aldosterone), the magnitude of the luminal negative charge, and the rate of urine flow past the distal tubule (see page 27).

Hydrogen ions. The distal nephron and the collecting ducts are the sites of hydrogen ion excretion. This is covered in the acid-base chapter on page 38.

Calcium. About 10% of the filtered calcium is reabsorbed in the distal tubule under PTH control.

Magnesium. 2-5% of the filtered magnesium is passively reabsorbed in the distal tubule and collecting ducts.

Collecting ducts

The function of the collecting ducts is similar to that of the distal tubule and it is here that the 'fine tuning' of sodium and potassium homeostasis occurs. However, the major activity of this portion of the nephron is water reabsorption and concentration of the urine. Normally this portion of the nephron is impermeable to water but the addition of arginine vasopressin (AVP) imparts permeability and allows the reabsorption of water. The fluid entering the collecting ducts has an osmolality of 50 to 100 mmol/kg because of the diluting effect of the thick ascending limb of the loop of Henle.

If AVP is absent then the urine reaching the bladder will be copious and have a low concentration.

On the other hand, in the presence of AVP water is reabsorbed from the urine resulting in a decreased output of urine with a high concentration. This is made possible by a tonicity gradient due to the high solute content of the interstitial tissue (created by the countercurrent and counterexchange mechanisms, see pages 5, 6).

UREA METABOLISM

Urea is produced in the liver as the end product of amino acid metabolism. They are normally catabolised by transamination and deamination which produces ammonia, a toxin. Detoxification of ammonia occurs in the urea cycle where two molecules are joined to a molecule of carbon dioxide to form urea. The rate of production, normally around 25 to 35 g/day (400-600 mmol), varies with the amount of ingested protein (100 g of proteins produces ~30 g of urea) and the integrity of the liver (severe liver dysfunction can result in low production and low plasma levels).

Urea is freely filtered by the glomerulus and passes freely through the nephron until it reaches the collecting ducts. Here a portion, depending on urine flow rate, is reabsorbed. At high flow rates (>2.0 mL/min) about 40% is reabsorbed whereas at low flow rates (~0.5 mL/min) around 60% is reabsorbed. Most of the reabsorbed urea finds its way back into the nephron lumen by diffusing into the descending limb of the loop of Henle. The reabsorbed urea plays an important role in the countercurrent mechanism which determines the interstitial tonicity.

The plasma urea level reflects the balance between production and excretion:

- ***Increased production*** occurs with high protein intakes, and in association with the anti-anabolic effects of tetracyclines, glucocorticoids, trauma, and serious illness; all of which may produce a high plasma level.

- ***Decreased excretion*** is associated with a lowered GFR. If the lowered GFR is due to decreased renal blood flow (e.g., dehydration) in an otherwise normal kidney there is an early rise in the plasma urea (cf to creatinine) due to the increased tubular reabsorption related to the low urine flow rate. Hence it is not unusual to find subjects with normal plasma creatinine levels associated with high plasma urea levels (see prerenal uraemia, page 78).

The plasma urea level is a poor indicator of the GFR because:

- Decreased production (low protein intake) can lower the plasma urea sufficiently to enable a normal plasma level to be associated with severe renal insufficiency.

- The GFR has to drop some 40-60% before the plasma urea begins to rise.

- Increased production (e.g., high protein intake) in the face of minor degrees of decreased renal function can result in disproportionately high plasma levels.

NOTE: As stated above the GFR drops with age so that, for example, a 70-year-old subject could only have 60% of renal function remaining. Under normal circumstances the plasma urea value can be within the normal reference range but if he develops mild dehydration with a further drop of 5-10% in the GFR then the plasma urea value will increase dramatically.

CREATININE METABOLISM

Creatinine is derived from the high energy phosphate compound, phosphocreatine, which maintains the muscle ATP level. This compound loses its phosphate and cyclises irreversibly to form 10 to 25 mmol daily of the waste product, creatinine, which is excreted in the urine. The filtered creatinine passes straight through the nephron without being reabsorbed by the tubules. A small amount, which increases during renal failure, is added to the urine by tubular secretion. The plasma level depends on two factors:

- *Rate of production:* This is related to muscle mass, i.e., large masses are associated with large production rates and high plasma levels (and *vice versa*). Thus children and elderly women will have lower plasma levels (e.g., <0.06 mmol/L) than big-size, manual working males (e.g., <0.13 mmol/L).

- *Rate of excretion:* This is wholly dependant on the GFR, i.e., a low GFR causes retention and high plasma levels.

Although plasma values directly reflect the subject's GFR it is not always a good indicator of this parameter because:

- The plasma level is dependant on muscle mass.

- Creatinine secretion by the proximal tubule increases as the GFR decreases. Some drugs, e.g., cimetidine, interfere with this secretion.

- A number of substances interfere with the (Jaffé reaction) assay, e.g., acetoacetate, cephalosporins.

- Roasted meats contain significant amounts of creatinine and ingestion of these can raise the plasma level temporarily.

However, for clinical purposes, it can be used as a simple and fairly reliable indicator of the GFR, and a number of equations have been developed to determine the GFR from the plasma value (see below).

CONCEPT OF CLEARANCE

The renal clearance of a substance is the amount of blood (or plasma) completely cleared (theoretically) of that material, by the kidney, in a given time. It is calculated from the following formula:

$$\text{Clearance of x (mL/min)} = \frac{UV}{P}$$

U = urinary concentration of x (mmol/L), V = urine volume per minute, P = plasma concentration of x (mmol/L).

If a substance filtered by the glomerulus passes straight through the nephron without being decreased by reabsorption or increased by tubular secretion then its clearance will equal the GFR (inulin is such a substance). Some substances, such as ρ-aminohippuric acid, are completely removed from the blood during one passage through the kidney; their renal clearance will estimate the renal blood flow.

Creatinine clearance

In routine medicine the GFR is usually estimated by the creatinine clearance but such values will be slightly higher than those obtained by inulin clearance because of the portion secreted by the tubules. This secretion becomes more of a problem in late renal failure because it increases in magnitude; in fact up to 30% of the urinary creatinine may be derived from this mechanism in severe renal failure, thus overestimating the GFR. The main problem with estimating the creatinine clearance is the timing and completeness of the urine collection, which are crucial to the estimation. It has been shown that clearances estimated on the same subject on repeated 24-hour collections can vary by up to 25%.

A number of equations have been derived to estimate the creatinine clearance from the plasma creatinine value. One such (Crockcroft and Gault, 1976) is:

$$\text{clearance (mL/min)} = \frac{(140 - \text{age in years}) \times Wt\,(kg)}{814 \times \text{plasma [creat] (mmol/L)}}$$

This gives a reasonably good correlation with measured values provided that (a) the plasma creatinine value is not within the normal range, (b) the renal failure is not severe, and (c) there is no inhibition of tubular secretion of creatinine by medications.

Urea clearance

Urea clearance values are less than those obtained for creatinine because of the urea reabsorption in the collecting ducts; they will also vary according to the urine output. The one advantage urea clearance has over creatinine clearance is the ease and precision of the urea measurement in the laboratory (no corresponding interferences as occurs with the creatinine assay, see above); however, despite this, this parameter of renal function is rarely used today.

FRACTIONAL EXCRETION

The renal fractional excretion ($FE\chi$) of a substance is that per centage of the total amount filtered by the glomerulus which is finally excreted in the urine.

$$FE\chi(\%) = \frac{U\chi \times Pcr}{Ucr \times P\chi} \times 100$$

$U\chi$=urine concentration of χ,$P\chi$=plasma concentration of χ, Pcr=plasma creatinine concentration,Ucr=urine creatinine concentration (all in mmol/L).

The test requires only a spot, or untimed, urine sample and a blood sample taken at the same time. It is used essentially as a measure of the renal handling of the particular analyte and gives some indication of tubular activity and function. Particularly useful is the fractional excretion of sodium in oliguric patients (page 80).

Renal dysfunction

Although the number of diseases that can involve the kidney are numerous the biochemical presentations are limited to a small number of syndrome-like complexes such as chronic renal failure, acute renal failure, and tubular syndromes; these will be briefly discussed.

Chronic renal failure (CRF)

Chronic renal failure is defined as progressive azotaemia (increasing plasma urea and creatinine levels) occurring over a period of weeks and months.

CAUSES

Any acute kidney disease can progress to endstage renal failure over periods ranging from months to several years but the commonest causes are:

- Glomerulonephritis
- Polycystic kidney disease
- Diabetic nephropathy
- Chronic pyelonephritis
- Hypertensive renal disease
- Analgesic nephropathy
- Urinary tract abnormalities, e.g., obstruction

PATHOPHYSIOLOGY

As functional nephrons 'drop out', characteristic and predictable abnormalities of fluid and electrolyte homeostasis occur because the kidney is unable to maintain the normal physiological environment. Most of these abnormalities only become manifest when the GFR has fallen by 60 to 70% (Table 5.1), but early in the process the characteristic presenting feature is an inability to concentrate the urine resulting in nocturia or enuresis.

The only abnormality in the plasma early in the process may be an increase in the plasma levels of urea and creatinine (which do not occur until 50-70%

of the nephrons are destroyed). As the disease progresses, reflected by a further fall in the GFR, other analytes such as potassium, hydrogen ions, phosphate, and urate appear in the blood in increasing amounts.

Table 5.1. Plasma levels of various analytes in progressive renal failure.

Creatinine clearance	Analyte increased
60-120 (mL/min)	Nil
30-60	Creatinine, Urea
20-30	K^+, H^+ ($\downarrow[HCO_3^-]$)
10-20	Urate, PO_4

Sodium homeostasis

Patients with CRF are able to maintain sodium balance despite a massive loss of nephrons. This reflects the hypertrophy and increased workload of the remaining nephrons as evidenced by an increase in the fractional excretion of sodium. This is normally less than 1% but in renal insufficiency it can increase up to 25%, a 20- to 30-fold increase. When the FE_{Na} reaches its limit further deterioration of renal function will result in sodium and water retention and lead to hypertension. At this stage salt intake should be restricted. In some patients, particularly those with tubulointerstitial disease, e.g., pyelonephritis, sodium wasting may occur resulting in a negative sodium balance (salt-losing nephritis).

Water homeostasis

As CRF progresses and there is damage to the tubules and collecting ducts, the kidney's ability to concentrate and dilute urine is lost. The concentrating ability is lost before the diluting ability and may be the first indicator of renal insufficiency. In the later stages of the disease, despite a varying fluid intake, the urine osmolality becomes fixed around 300 mmol/kg (isosthenuria).

Potassium homeostasis

Patients with progressive renal disease remain in potassium balance and maintain a normal plasma potassium for a long period due to:

- *Increased renal FE_K:* The normal FE_K is around 10-20% and it can increase up to 300% in renal insufficiency. When the GFR falls to less than 20 to 30 mL/min the FE_K is usually maximal and thereafter plasma $[K^+]$ begins to rise.

- *Increased colonic secretion:* Normally about 10% of ingested potassium appears in the stools. In CRF this can increase t o 30 to 40%. The mechanism is probably related to increased colonic secretion subsequent to increased aldosterone secretion induced by hyperkalaemia.

Acid-base homeostasis

In the later stages of CRF (e.g., when the GFR is <20 mL/min) the patient characteristically develops a high anion gap metabolic acidosis (page 41). As renal failure progresses the remaining normal nephrons, though able to normally excrete H^+ and develop a hydrogen ion gradient across the tubular cell membrane (urine pH to <5.5), are unable to secrete sufficient H^+ (80-100 mmol/day) to maintain normal acid-base balance, and thus the plasma $[HCO_3^-]$ falls. In uncomplicated renal failure this develops when the GFR falls below ~20 mL/min.

The high anion gap represents the retention, by the failing glomerulus, of anions such as phosphate, sulfate, and organic acid anions. If the renal disease affects the tubules to a greater extent than the glomerulus, as occurs in pyelonephritis and analgesic nephropathy, the H^+ may be retained in the absence of significant glomerular retention of anions and a hyperchloraemic (normal anion gap) metabolic acidosis occurs (page 41).

An interesting feature of severe CRF is that, despite a retention of some 10 to 20 mmol of H^+ daily, the plasma $[HCO_3^-]$ remains fixed at around 12 to 14 mmol/L. This is due to buffering of the retained H^+ by the calcium carbonate of bone. The trade-off here is loss of bone calcium which contributes to the condition of uraemic osteodystrophy.

Calcium and phosphate homeostasis

Advanced CRF is associated with phosphate retention and negative calcium balance which results in hyperphosphataemia, hypocalcaemia, and bone disease (uraemic osteodystrophy).

The plasma phosphate level remains within normal limits until the GFR falls to below ~20 mL/min. The suggested mechanism is:

↓GFR
→ ↑plasma [PO_4]
→ ↓ plasma [Ca^{2+}] (precipitated as calcium phosphate)
→ ↑PTH secretion
→ ↑PO_4 excretion
→ normal plasma [PO_4].

Eventually there will be insufficient nephrons to maintain phosphate excretion and the plasma level rises.

Early in CRF the plasma ionised calcium (Ca^{2+}) level falls due to phosphate retention (precipitation as insoluble calcium phosphate *in vivo* and in the gut) and decreased absorption from the gut as a consequence of disturbance of vitamin D metabolism (decreased production of 1,25-dihydroxyvitamin D, page 90). The low [Ca^{2+}] stimulates PTH secretion which, in addition to its effect on phosphate metabolism, increases the removal of calcium from bone. The end result is a low total plasma [Ca] (usually 1.7 to 1.8 mmol/L), and a negative calcium balance resulting in bone demineralisation.

Magnesium homeostasis

Magnesium, like the other analytes discussed above, remains in balance (because of increased fractional excretion) until severe CRF develops and then its level begins to rise in the plasma. This occurs when the GFR falls to below ~20 mL/min (plasma levels rise earlier if magnesium intake is increased, e.g., ingestion of magnesium-containing antacids).

Metabolic and endocrine disturbances

In severe renal insufficiency (e.g., plasma creatinine >0.8 mmol/L) glucose intolerance is not uncommon (? toxic inhibition of insulin action) and in some cases hypoglycaemia occurs (? decreased renal clearance of insulin). Prolactin levels are often elevated, presumably due to decreased renal clearance, and in men decreased circulating testosterone levels are usual (cause unclear). Erythropoietin production is suppressed and severe anaemia ensues.

Acute renal failure

Acute renal failure is characterised by a sudden increase in the plasma urea or creatinine or both occurring over hours or days. It is usually accompanied by oliguria; but often there is anuria (<400 mL/day), and occasionally diuresis but this is uncommon and seen only in some cases of acute tubular necrosis.

If we bear in mind that three general conditions are necessary for normal renal function, i.e., adequate blood flow to the glomerulus, normally functioning parenchy-ma, and patent urinary tracts for free passage of urine from the body, then we can divide the causes of acute renal failure into:

- *Prerenal uraemia:* inadequate blood flow to an otherwise normally functioning kidney
- *Renal uraemia:* adequate blood flow but diseased or dysfunctional parenchyma
- *Postrenal uraemia:* obstruction to urine outflow.

Prerenal uraemia (PRU)

The basic problem in this condition is a decreased GFR in an otherwise normal urorenal system. The decrease is usually due to hypovolaemia resulting in decreased renal blood flow but there are a number of other causes (Table 5.2) including congestive cardiac failure.

Table 5.2. Causes of prerenal uraemia.

Extracellular volume (ECV) depletion
Haemorrhage: external, into gut, into tissues
Burns
Gut loss: vomiting, diarrhoea
Renal loss (salt-losing conditions):
    diuretic therapy, osmotic diuresis,
    Addison's disease, salt-losing nephritis

Normal/increased ECV with ineffective blood volume
Shock
Cardiac failure
Nephrotic syndrome
Hepatorenal syndrome
Third space loss: pancreatitis, ascites, crush injury

The physiological response to hypovolaemia and the resulting biochemical manifestations are:

Hypovolaemia →

1. Increased renal Na$^+$ reabsorption →

    (a) decreased urinary 'spot' [Na] (<10 mmol/L)
    (b) FE$_{Na}$ less than 1%

2. Increased AVP secretion →

    (a) decreased urinary output
    (b) concentrated urine:
        urine:plasma osmolality >1
        urine:plasma creatinine >20
        urine:plasma urea >20

3. Decreased GFR → Increased plasma urea and creatinine levels. The urea value is usually relatively higher than the creatinine value, e.g., urea:creatinine ratio >50 (mmol/L:mmol/L).

The importance of this disorder is that if it is not treated promptly, it may lead to the development of acute tubular necrosis (see below).

CAUSES

Most of the described causes are listed in Table 5.3, but there are five common groups.

Renal hypoperfusion. Hypoperfusion is the commonest cause of acute renal failure and can result in parenchymal dysfunction ranging from prerenal uraemia to acute tubular necrosis.

Acute tubular necrosis. This is reversible in most patients, with the oliguric phase lasting from a few days to 4-6 weeks.

Drug toxicity. Drugs commonly associated with acute renal failure are: non-steroidal anti-inflammatory drugs (e.g., ibuprofen), angiotensin-converting enzyme inhibitors, aminoglycosides (e.g., gentamicin, neomycin, streptomycin), amphotericin B, and cyclosporins.

Myoglobuinuria. This may occur during crush injury or the severe rhabdomyolysis associated wth disorders such as alcohol abuse. Myoglobin is toxic to the tubules.

Transfusion reactions. Severe intravascular haemolysis is a well known cause of acute renal failure.

Table 5.3. Causes of acute renal failure (renal).

Acute tubular necrosis
    Post-ischaemic
    Nephrotoxic
Acute interstitial nephritis
    Drug hypersensitivity
    Infection
Gram-negative sepsis
Postpartum haemorrhage
Renal artery occlusion (bilateral)
Acute glomerulonephritis

PATHOPHYSIOLOGY

The exact mechanism of the oliguric phase is unclear but three suggestions have been put forward.

- Redistribution of intrarenal blood flow where blood is shunted from the cortex to the medulla.
- Obstruction of the tubular lumen by cellular debris.
- Diffusion of urine back to blood via damaged tubules.

The characteristic biochemical features are:

(1) high anion gap metabolic acidosis,
(2) hyperkalaemia,
(3) raised plasma urea and creatinine levels,
(4) hypocalcaemia and hyperphosphataemia,
(5) high urinary sodium concentration.

Features of the oliguric phase can be explained in terms of a *decreased GFR* and *tubular damage* (Figure 5.2).

(1) *Decreased GFR* →

    (a) low urine output (oliguria)
    (b) retention of waste products (high plasma urea, creatinine, and anion gap).
    (c) retention of phosphate → hyperphosphataemia and hypocalcaemia (precipitation as insoluble calcium phosphate)

(2) *Tubular dysfunction* →

  (a) decreased renal Na^+ reabsorption (urinary [Na]
      >20 mmol/L, FE_{Na} >1%)
  (b) retention of H^+ and K^+ → hyperkalaemia and
      metabolic acidosis
  (c) resistance to AVP (dilute urine with
      urine:plasma osmolality ~1)

Thus the biochemical features are similar to those of
severe chronic renal failure, the only difference is the
time it took to develop the lesion. Table 5.4 shows the
biochemical features which may be useful in the
differentiation of this condition from prerenal uraemia.
The most important parameter is the urinary sediment:
in ATN there is blood staining, cellular debris, casts,
red blood cells, and amorphous material; in PRU the
urine is generally clean.

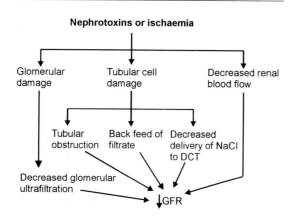

Figure 5.2. Pathophysiology of oliguria in acute renal
failure. DCT, distal convoluted tubule.

Table 5.4. Differentiation of PRU from ATN.

Index	PRU	ATN
UNa mmol/L	<10	>20
FE_{Na} %	<1	>3
UCl mmol/L	<10	>20
FE_{Cl} %	<1	>3
U:P Osmo	>3	~1
Sediment	clear	RBCs, casts, cell debris

UNa (UCl), spot urine sodium (chloride) concentration;
FE_{Na}, (FE_{Cl}), fractional excretion of sodium (chloride); U:P
Osmo, ratio of urine to plasma osmolality.

Renal tubular disorders

Renal tubular disorders may involve abnormalities of
a number of functions (e.g., Fanconi syndrome) or of
a single function (e.g., hydrogen ion secretion defect).
Disorders of almost every function have been
described but in this section we will only consider the
more common ones.

Classification

Multiple functions affected
  Fanconi syndrome

Single function defect
Proximal nephron:
  Renal glycosuria
  Aminoaciduria
  Proximal renal tubular acidosis
  Familial hypophosphataemia (page 107)
Distal nephron:
  Distal renal tubular acidosis
  Nephrogenic diabetes insipidus (page 21)
  Bartter's syndrome
  Pseudohypoaldosteronism (page 69)
  Pseudohypoparathyroidism (page 97)

Fanconi syndrome

This disorder, which usually presents as failure to
thrive, or as rickets in children, is characterised by
glycosuria, aminoaciduria, and phosphaturia (proximal
tubule reabsorption defect). In addition, there may be
proximal renal tubular acidosis due to impaired
proximal bicarbonate reabsorption and an impaired
concentrating ability.

  The cause may be idiopathic (primary), or acquired
due to heavy metal poisoning (e.g., lead), drugs (e.g.,
old tetracyclines), amyloidosis, and multiple myeloma.
In addition, it is a feature of a number of inborn errors
of metabolism, including Wilson's disease, galactosaemia, glycogen storage disease, and cystinosis.

Renal glycosuria

This benign disorder is due to a defect in the proximal
tubular transport of glucose. Normally almost all of
the glucose presented to the proximal tubule is
reabsorbed and no significant amounts appear in the

urine; however, if the plasma glucose rises above ~10 mmol/L the threshold for reabsorption is exceeded and glycosuria ensues. In renal glycosuria the renal threshold is much lower and glycosuria is associated with plasma glucose values as low as 5.5 mmol/L. It is an uncommon and harmless disorder which may be confused with the glycosuria of diabetes mellitus.

Aminoacidurias

Filtered amino acids are almost completely (~99%) reabsorbed by specific transport mechanisms located in the proximal tubule. They can appear in the urine if the transport mechanisms are overwhelmed by massive amounts (overflow) or if the transport mechanisms are defective (transport defects).

Overflow. This is the underlying problem in those disorders associated with very high plasma amino acid levels and may be generalised, as in severe liver disease, or it may be restricted to a specific amino acid, as in some of the inborn errors of metabolism (page 300), e.g., phenylalanine in phenylketonuria.

Transport. Tubular transport defects may be generalised, as in the Fanconi syndrome or specific, as in cystinuria and the Hartnup syndrome. Proximal tubular amino acid transport occurs in groups, the four most important being:

- *Dibasic group:* cystine, ornithine, arginine, and lysine (cystinuria)
- *Hartnup group:* monoamine-monocarboxylic acids excluding iminoacids and glycine (Hartnup disease)
- *Iminoacids and glycine* (iminoglycinuria)
- *Dicarboxylic acids* (glutamic and aspartic acid)

Cystinuria. This is due to a defect in the transport of the dibasic group of acids (cystine, ornithine, arginine, lysine). Cystine and varying combinations of the other three acids appear in the urine and there may be cystine stone formation; otherwise the condition is harmless. The transport defect is also present in the gut but the four amino acids are able to shortcircuit this deficiency by being absorbed as components of small peptides.

Hartnup disease. In this disorder there is a defect in the transport of the neutral amino acids (monoamine, monocarboxylic amino acids, including tryptophan), in both the gut and the proximal renal tubule. Other than the characteristic aminoaciduria, the prominent features are a pellagra-like rash and ataxia which are probably related to tryptophan deficiency (tryptophan is the precursor of nicotinic acid, vitamin B_2).

Renal tubular acidosis

Renal tubular acidosis (RTA) is defined as a metabolic acidosis due to renal tubular dysfunction which occurs in the absence of significant glomerular dysfunction, e.g., plasma creatinine < 0.20 mmol/L. It is of the normal anion gap (hyperchloraemic) variety, presenting as one of three distinct types: *type 1* or distal, *type 2* or proximal, and *type 4* which is associated with the mineralocorticoid deficiency syndromes (page 00). In addition, there may be combinations of types 1 and 2, for example, the term type 3, which is no longer in use, was used to describe type 1 disease associated with significant bicarbonate wasting (type 2).

Type 1 (distal) RTA

This is due to an inability of the distal nephron to secrete and excrete hydrogen ions (see page 00). This results in:

- An inability to lower the urinary pH to below 5.50.
- Retention of hydrogen ions resulting in metabolic acidosis (low plasma [HCO_3^-]).
- Renal potassium wasting (mechanism unclear).

Patients present with:

- Hyperchloraemic metabolic acidosis
- Hypokalaemia
- Urine pH >5.5 during acidaemia (normally 4.5-5.0)
- Hypercalciuria -- chronic acidaemia results in bone dissolution and increased renal calcium excretion; renal stones are thus a common complication.

It may present as a primary (idiopathic) disorder or, more usually, secondary to autoimmune disorders (Sjögren's syndrome, chronic active hepatitis, dysgammaglobulinaemias), nephrocalcinosis, toxins/

drugs (amphotericin B, toluene), and renal disease (pyelonephritis, obstructive uropathy, renal transplant). Treatment is with oral bicarbonate, the amount required being 1-3 mmol/kg/day which is equivalent to the amount of hydrogen ions excreted daily by the kidney in the normal subject.

Type 2 (proximal) RTA

Here there is an inability of the proximal renal tubule to reabsorb bicarbonate (page 38), resulting in significant bicarbonaturia and a low plasma [HCO_3^-]. A similar situation occurs in patients treated with the carbonic anhydrase inhibitor, acetazolamide. It is a self-limiting disorder in that the tubular defect is not absolute and when the filtered bicarbonate falls to levels that can be reabsorbed the plasma [HCO_3^-] stabilises. The distal nephron is unaffected and hence the patient can lower his urinary pH to below 5.50. Hypokalaemia may occur but usually not until the patient is treated with bicarbonate.

It may be part of the Fanconi syndrome, it may present as an isolated defect, or it may be secondary to disorders such as cystinosis, Wilson's disease, Lowe's syndrome, primary hyperparathyroidism, and renal transplant. Treatment with bicarbonate is difficult because it is rapidly excreted in the urine (requirements in excess of 20 mmol/kg/day may be needed) and is often associated with potassium wasting.

LABORATORY EVALUATION

The renal acidoses include:

- Uraemic acidosis
- Type 1 RTA
- Type 2 RTA
- Type 4 RTA (mineralocorticoid deficiency)

The *minimal laboratory investigations* necessary for the evaluation of suspected RTA are (Table 5.5):

- Plasma electrolytes and creatinine
- Urinary pH during acidaemia (a pH on an early morning urine sample is a useful screening test, a value in excess of 6.0 suggests type 1 RTA).

The *definitive* diagnosis may require an *ammonium chloride challenge*. In this test the patient is given 0.1 g of ammonium chloride per kg body weight at 0800 h and urine is collected hourly for at leat 8 hours and

the hydrogen ion (titratable acidity) and ammonium excretion rates are measured. The normal response is:

- pH falls to below 5.50
- titratable acidity (H^+ excretion): >25 mmol/min
- ammonia excretion: >35 mmol/min.

Table 5.5. Some diagnostic features of the renal acidoses.

	Uraemic acidosis	Type 1 RTA	Type 2 RTA	Type 4 RTA
Plasma				
[Cr] mmol/L	>0.20	<0.20	<0.20	<0.20
AG mEq/L	high	normal	normal	normal
[K] mmol/L	N-I	D	N-D	I
Urine during acidaemia				
pH	<5.50	>5.50	<5.50	<5.50
H^+ excretion (mmol/min)	<25	<25	>25	<25
NH_3 excretion (mmol/min)	<35	<35	>35	<35

[Cr], creatinine concentration, N=normal, D=decreased, I=increased, AG=anion gap.

Bartter's syndrome

This is an autosomal recessive disorder which presents with severe hypokalaemia, metabolic alkalosis, high renin and aldosterone secretion and hyperplasia of the juxtaglomerular apparatus. The cause is unclear but may be due to defective chloride reabsorption in the thick ascending limb of the loop of Henle, i.e.,

- The decreased chloride absorption results in sodium depletion, water depletion, and hypovolaemia.

- The hypovolaemia stimulates renin secretion, chronic secondary hyperaldosteronism and consequent hypokalaemia and juxtaglomerular hyperplasia.

Proteinuria

The glomerular basement membrane (and its associated structures), due to its anatomical arrangement and negative charge is poorly permeable to plasma proteins (most plasma proteins are also negatively charged), allowing only small amounts through with the ultrafiltrate (100-300 mg/L). Most of the small amounts of albumin, low molecular weight proteins and peptides (enzymes, hormones, immunoglobulins) that escape the glomerulus are reabsorbed and metabolised by the renal tubules (Figure 5.3). The final amount excreted in the urine by the normal subject is less than 150 mg/day consisting of *filtered proteins* (60%) including albumin (25-35 mg/day), plasma-derived immunoglobulins, β_2-, α_1-, and α_2-microglobulins, and *uroepithelial-secreted proteins* (40%) such as secretory IgA and the Tamm-Horsfall protein.

Proteinuria, defined as a urinary protein excretion rate in excess of 150 mg/day may be due to one, or more, of four mechanisms:

- Glomerular disease (glomerular proteinuria)
- Tubular disease (tubular proteinuria)
- Overflow from a high plasma level of low molecular weight proteins (overflow proteinuria)
- Secretion by the uroepithelium (secretory proteinuria)

Glomerular proteinuria

Increased glomerular filtration of plasma proteins occurs when the filtration barrier is altered by disease (pathological) or when haemodynamic factors result in an increased filtration fraction (benign).

Pathological glomerular proteinuria. Any form of glomerular disease may cause increased glomerular membrane permeability to proteins and when the amount filtered exceeds the reabsorptive capacity of the tubules, proteinuria occurs (Figure 5.3). In the glomerular disease termed *minimal change disease* the albuminuria reflects a change in the charge on the basement membrane whereas in *proliferative* and *membranous disease* there is probably a defect in the sieving properties which allows filtration of larger proteins such as the γ-globulins (immunoglobulins). Glomerular proteinuria usually exceeds 1-2 g/day and

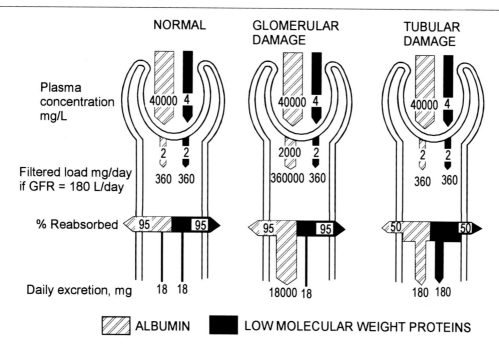

Figure 5.3. Schematic diagram illustrating the normal mechanism of protein excretion and two faulty mechanisms resulting in glomerular and tubular proteinuria. Adapted from Maack TM, Sherman RL. Proteinuria. Am J Med 1974;56:71, with permission.

values up to 10-20 g/day are characteristic of the nephrotic syndrome.

Benign glomerular proteinuria. Haemodynamic alterations may result in an increased filtration fraction which can be associated with significant proteinuria. Such occurs in cardiac failure, hypertension, stress, fever, severe exercise. The proteinuria is usually less than 1g/day and disappears when the primary problem is relieved.

Orthostatic proteinuria. This benign disorder is associated with posture. Proteinuria of up to 1g/day occurs in the upright posture but disappears on prolonged recumbency (e.g., asleep overnight). It is found in adolescents and young adults and is thought to be due to an exaggerated renin or catecholamine release on standing, resulting in an increased filtration fraction.

Tubular proteinuria

The small proteins such as β_2-, α_1-, and α_2-microglobulins and large peptides such as parathyroid hormone and insulin are almost completely (~99.9%) reabsorbed by the tubules but tubular injury (even minimal) inhibits this uptake resulting in a proteinuria of around 1-2 mg/day (Figure 5.3). The better studied of these proteins is β_2-microglobulin which serves as a good marker of tubular dysfunction in conditions such as heavy metal poisoning, the Fanconi syndrome, chronic hypokalaemia, and the like. Measurement of renal excretion rates is of little diagnostic value in renal disease associated primarily with glomerular dysfunction.

Overflow proteinuria

Small molecular weight proteins such as haemoglobin, myoglobin, and immunoglobulin light chains are filtered in very small amounts and reabsorbed by the tubules; hence very little appears in the urine in the normal subject. However, when the plasma levels are grossly elevated the filtration rate exceeds the reabsorption rate and they appear in the urine.

Such occurs during intravascular haemolysis (haemoglobinuria), crush injury and rhabdomyolysis (myoglobinuria), and in the paraproteinaemias such as myeloma when light chains are excreted (Bence-Jones proteinuria).

Secretory proteinuria

Inflammatory processes of the urinary tract cause increased secretion of uroepithelial mucoproteins and secretory IgA. However, they are not present in large quantities and special techniques are required to demonstrate them.

Nephrotic syndrome

This describes a condition due to glomerular damage which is characterised by:

- *Proteinuria (glomerular proteinuria).* Varies from 1-2 g/day up to 20-30 g/day, consisting mainly of albumin but other plasma proteins may be also present, e.g., immunoglobulins, transferrin.

- *Hypoalbuminaemia.* Due to renal albumin loss.

- *Hypercholesterolaemia* (see page 208).

- *Oedema.* Due to renal sodium and water retention (see page 11).

- *Secondary hyperaldosteronism.* Due to low effective arterial blood volume as a consequence of hypoalbuminaemia. It may result in hypokalaemic metabolic alkalosis (page 43).

- Plasma creatinine and urea levels are usually normal unless the disorder has progressed to chronic renal failure.

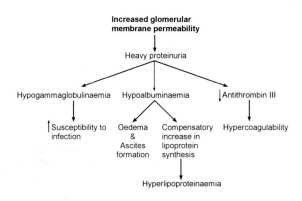

Figure 5.4. Pathophysiology of the nephrotic syndrome.

It may be a primary disorder (e.g., in children) or secondary to a wide variety of diseases: diabetes mellitus, drug toxicity (e.g., gold, penicillinamine), infections (e.g., hepatitis B, malaria), connective tissue diseases (e.g., systemic lupus erythematosus), and heavy metal toxicity (e.g., mercury).

CLINICAL AND LABORATORY EVALUATION OF PROTEINURIA

Clinically there are two groups of subjects, those with *proteinuria associated with renal disease* and those with *isolated proteinuria.*

Proteinuria and renal disease

Many types of renal disease are associated with proteinuria, e.g., glomerulonephritis, nephrotic syndrome, tubulo-interstitial disease, primary tubular disease. Thus, once proteinuria is documented further tests should include plasma electrolytes, creatinine and urea, and albumin. In addition, a 24-hour urinary protein excretion rate and a creatinine clearance should be performed.

Isolated proteinuria

Proteinuria found in an otherwise normal and asymptomatic subject is not uncommon, with a prevalence of between 0.5% to 10%, depending on the population studied and the definition of proteinuria. The proteinuria is usually less than 1 g/day. There are a number of classifications but the following is a useful clinical guide: *benign isolated proteinuria* and *persistent isolated proteinuria.*

Benign isolated proteinuria. As the name suggests these disorders are benign; they may present as:

● *Functional proteinuria:* secondary to fever, exercise, cardiac failure, etc.

● *Transient proteinuria:* often seen in young adults; as the term implies the proteinuria disappears on re-testing.

● *Intermittent proteinuria:* occurs in young adults and defined as proteinuria found in at least half of samples from multiple testings; follow up generally reveals no apparent cause.

● *Orthostatic proteinuria:* see above.

Persistent isolated proteinuria. This is said to be found in 5-10% of young adults presenting with isolated proteinuria. The proteinuria is present in all urine samples tested. Compared with the benign group these subjects, as a group, have increased morbidity and mortality and the risk of developing renal disease is high (~50%). If the proteinuria exceeds 0.5 g/day a renal biopsy is usually recommended.

Nephrolithiasis

Renal stone disease occurs in around 1:1000 men and 1:3000 women. It is usually unilateral but recurs in some 60% of cases, particularly those with hyper-oxaluria, cystinuria, chronic pyelonephritis, and those with a persistently alkaline urine, e.g., distal renal tubular acidosis. About 70-75% of the stones contain calcium oxalate or calcium phosphate, 10% are composed of triple phosphate (magnesium ammonium phosphate or struvite), 10% are uric acid stones; cystine and xanthine stone make up less than 1%.

CAUSES

The precipitation of solutes in the urine and stone formation can be due to:

Lack of inhibitors: Amongst the inhibitors that prevent solute precipitation are inorganic pyrophosphate, citrate, magnesium, some glycoproteins, and acid mucopolysaccharides. For example, distal renal tubular acidosis is associated with hypocitraturia and with recurrent stone formation.

Supersaturation of the urine by the offending solute due to:

● *Increased excretion of crystalloid:* hypercalciuria, cystinuria, xanthinuria, hyperoxaluria

● *Decreased urinary volume,* e.g., living in the tropics

Absorptive Hypercalciuria

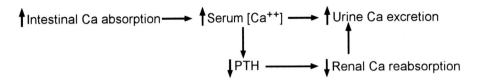

Renal Hypercalciuria

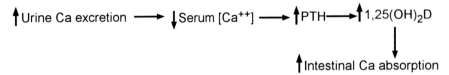

Resorptive Hypercalciuria

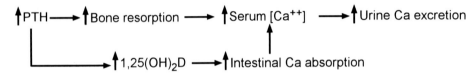

Figure 5.5. Pathophysiology of various types of hypercalciuria associated with calcium stone formation. Modified after Pak CYC. Kidney stones. In Foster DW, Wilson JE (eds): *Williams Textbook of Endocrinology, 8th Edn..* W.B. Saunders, Philadelphia, 1994.

• *Urinary stagnation,* e.g., obstruction of the urorenal tract

• *Urinary pH changes,* e.g., calcium salts tend to precipitate at alkaline pH; uric acid at low pH (<5.5)

• *Infections,* e.g., urea-splitting bacteria produce ammonia and an alkaline pH; clumps of bacteria may provide a nidus for precipitation.

Calcium stones. Most calcium stones are composed of calcium oxalate (a lesser number are of calcium phosphate) and 80 to 90% are idiopathic (no discoverable cause). Some are associated with increased oxalate secretion (see below) and 10 to 15% are associated with hypercalciuria.

Hypercalciuria may be associated with hypercalcaemia (page 93), particularly those associated with primary hyperparathyroidism, or normocalcaemia (*normocalcaemic hypercalciuria*) -- idiopathic or associated with: renal tubular acidosis, carbonic anhydrase inhibitors, immobilisation, hyperthyroidism, Paget's disease, medullary sponge kidney. Depending on the cause (see Figure 5.5), hypercalciuria may be:

• absorptive, due to increased intestinal calcium absorption
• renal, due to decreased tubular calcium reabsorption, with secondary enhanced intestinal absorption of calcium
• resorptive, due to increased mobilization of skeletal (bone) calcium

Triple phosphate stones. The magnesium ammonium phosphate stones develop in relation to urinary tract infection where urea-splitting organisms increase the urinary pH by the release of ammonia.

Uric acid stones. These are associated with

increased urate secretion (page 115) and an acid urine (pH <5.5). The commonest cause is gout (35 to 40% of gouty patients form stones).

Oxalate stones. Oxalate is a common constituent of calcium stones and pure oxalate stones are rare. Hyperoxaluria occurs in the very rare primary hyperoxaluria and in gut diseases such as inflammatory disease of the terminal ileum, jejunoileal bypass surgery, small bowel resections where there is increased absorption of dietary oxalate.

Cystine stones. These are uncommon and associated with cystinuria (see page 300).

Xanthine stones. Very rare and usually indicate xanthine oxidase deficiency (page 121).

LABORATORY EVALUATION

A careful clinical work-up is important with particular reference to any history of urinary tract infections, gout, intestinal surgery, high calcium intakes, etc. Calcium-containing stones and cystine stones are radio-opaque whereas urate stones are radiolucent and may require an IVP or ultrasound for their recognition.

From the laboratory point of view any available stones should be analysed which will give a hint about the analyte to follow-up. In the absence of stone analysis a 24-hour urine should be obtained for estimation of calcium, oxalate, and urate, and serum levels of calcium and urate should be estimated. Other more specific examinations may include urinary pH (renal tubular acidosis and urinary infection) and specific gravity (increased SG suggests supersaturation).

Microscopy and a bacterial culture should be carried out to exclude urinary tract infection, and evaluation of urine for cystine and xanthine to exclude cystinuria and xanthinuria. If hyperparathyroidism is suspected plasma PTH should be measured.

REFERENCES/FURTHER READING

Batlle DC. Renal tubular acidosis. Med Clinics North Am 1983;67:859-878.

Berry CA and Rector FC Jr. Renal transport of glucose, amino acids, sodium, chloride, and water. *In:* Brenner BM and Rector FC Jr (eds), *The Kidney, 4th edn*, Philadelphia: WB Saunders, 1990, pp 215-282.

Cockcroft DW and Gault MH. Prediction of creatinine clearance from serum creatinine. Nephron 1976;16:31-41.

Coe FL, Parks JH, Asplin JR. The pathogenesis and treatment of kidney stones. N Engl J Med 1992; 327:1141-1152.

Larson TS. Evaluation of proteinuria. Mayo Clin Proc 1994;69(12):1154-8.

Massry SG and Glassock RJ (eds). *Textbook of Nephrology, 2nd edn,* Baltimore: Williams and Wilkins, 1989.

Robertson GL. Differential diagnosis of polyuria. Ann Rev Med 1988:39:425-442.

Samuell CT, Kasidas GP. Biochemical investigations in renal stone formers. Ann Clin Biochem 1995;32: 112-122.

Warnock DG. Uremic acidosis. Kidney 1988;34:278-287.

Chapter 6

Calcium

Calcium is a major constituent of bone and hence an important structural element in the body. Besides its pivotal function in bone mineralisation, it also plays an essential role in neuromuscular excitability and blood clotting. The activation of cells by hormones and many intracellular processes, including enzyme activation, are controlled by intracellular calcium.

Normal homeostasis

The total body calcium content is about 25 to 35 moles -- over 99% is in the skeleton, less than 0.5% occurs in the soft tissues and less than 0.1% resides in the ECF.

INTAKE

The average oral intake is around 10-20 mmol/day; 20-40% of this is absorbed by the gut (Figure 6.1) depending on:

- Availability of ionised calcium (Ca^{2+}). This is decreased by substances such as phytates and oxalates which bind the ionised calcium and by an alkaline pH which precipitates insoluble calcium complexes. An acid medium promotes absorption by increasing ionisation.

- Availability of the active vitamin D metabolite, 1,25-dihydroxycholecalciferol (1,25-DHCC, see below).

It is absorbed in the small bowel by both passive diffusion and active transport, the amount absorbed being determined largely by the cellular concentration of a specific calcium binding protein that is regulated by the plasma activity of 1,25-DHCC. The rate of absorption is increased during periods of high demand, e.g., pregnancy and lactation.

The intestinal secretions and bile contain calcium which adds to the load; hence if substances which form insoluble complexes with calcium are present in the gut, it is possible for the faecal calcium to exceed the oral intake, but under normal circumstances faecal excretion is not an important excretion route.

PLASMA CALCIUM

The total plasma calcium concentration is around 2.15-2.55 mmol/L and consists of three fractions:

- Protein bound: 40-45% mainly to albumin
- Ionised: 45-50%
- Complexed: 5-10% (as citrate, phosphates, and bicarbonate)

The ionised portion (Ca^{2+}) is the biologically active fraction and is maintained at a fairly constant level (1.05-1.35 mmol/L) by an intricate control system involving parathyroid hormone (PTH). It is sensitive to pH changes, with alkalaemia lowering the level by increasing the protein bound fraction; acidaemia results in the reverse situation. A decrease in the plasma ionised calcium level increases neuromuscular excitability and stimulates PTH synthesis and secretion (see below).

One gram of albumin binds approximately 0.25 mmol of calcium and thus a fall in the plasma albumin level of 10 g/L will be associated with a total calcium fall of around 0.25 mmol/L (the level of ionised calcium will not decrease as it is kept constant by the action of PTH).

BONE FLUX

Bone undergoes continuous resorption and remodelling and thus calcium is in a constant state of flux between bone and the available calcium pool (Figure 6.1). Under normal conditions about 10 mmol of calcium is resorbed from and laid down in bone each day.

OUTPUT

The major calcium excretion route is via the kidneys where, depending on the intake, some 2.5 to 7.5 mmol of calcium are excreted daily. Approximately 250 mmol/24 h of calcium are filtered by the glomerulus but most of this is reabsorbed by the renal tubules with only about 1-5% appearing in the urine.

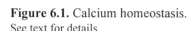

Figure 6.1. Calcium homeostasis.
See text for details.

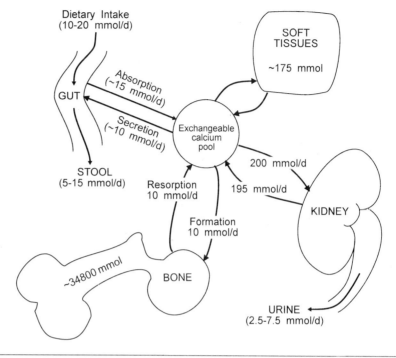

Tubular reabsorption. Calcium reabsorption occurs along the whole length of the nephron and is mainly under the control of PTH which influences calcium absorption in the distal nephron.

- *Proximal tubule*: ~65% reabsorbed
- *Ascending limb of loop of Henle*: ~20% reabsorbed (in thick portion)
- *Distal convoluted tubule and collecting duct*: ~15% reabsorbed (influenced by PTH)

In the proximal tubule calcium reabsorption appears to be tightly coupled to sodium reabsorption, for example during hypovolaemia, which is associated with increased sodium reabsorption in this part of the nephron, the reabsorption of calcium is increased; and during volume expansion with saline infusion the proximal reabsorption of calcium is decreased.

Tubular calcium reabsorption is energy dependant and, in most sections, an obligatory process with no known control; the exception is the distal nephron where PTH exerts some control. Increased PTH activity increases reabsorption and decreased activity results in increased renal calcium excretion.

CONTROL OF HOMEOSTASIS

The two major controllers of calcium homeostasis are *parathyroid hormone* (PTH) and *vitamin D*. Other factors that are known to influence calcium metabolism but play a minor, if any, role in the normal subject are: *calcitonin, thyroid hormones, adrenal steroids, prostaglandins, osteoclast activating factor, PTH-related protein.*

Parathyroid hormone (PTH)

PTH, which is secreted in response to a decrease in the plasma ionised calcium level, influences calcium homeostasis by: (a) directly effecting calcium and phosphate reabsorption by the kidney, (b) influencing bone mineralisation and calcium flux from bone, and (c) stimulating 1,25-dihydroxycholecalciferol (1,25-DHCC) synthesis by the kidney.

Structure and metabolism. PTH is a polypeptide of 84 amino acid residues synthesised and secreted by the parathyroid glands (Figure 6.2). The initial product is a preprohormone of 115 amino acids; this is processed to a prohormone of 90 residues and finally to the native hormone of 84 residues which is stored in secretory granules and released into the plasma. In the circulation the half-life of the intact hormone is around 5 minutes as it is rapidly degraded to carboxy-terminal and amino-terminal fragments by the liver and kidney (cleavage between amino acids 33 and 37). The carboxy-terminal fragments are biologically inactive, have a plasma half-life of 30 minutes, and are cleared by glomerular filtration. Biologically active amino-terminal fragments are probably also secreted by the parathyroid glands but the plasma level of these fragments is always lower than that of the intact hormone, suggesting that they may not be physiologically important (the biological activity of PTH resides in amino acids 2 to 6 of the amino portion of the hormone).

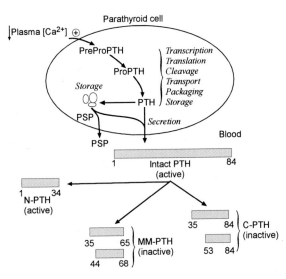

Figure 6.2. Metabolism of parathyroid hormone. PSP, parathyroid secretory protein; N-PTH, amino-terminal PTH fragment; MM-PTH, mid molecule fragment; C-PTH, carboxy-terminal fragment.

Action. PTH acts on bone and the kidney and in addition plays an important role in vitamin D metabolism.

- *Bone:* stimulates osteoclast activity causing release of calcium and phosphate (1,25-DHCC has a complementary role in this activity)

- *Kidney:* (1) increases calcium reabsorption by the distal nephron through the adenyl cyclase-cyclic AMP mechanism, (2) decreases phosphate reabsorption by the proximal tubule, (3) increases 1,25-DHCC production and subsequently increases the absorption of calcium in the gut.

- *Vitamin D:* stimulates renal 1α-hydroxylase activity which increases the production of 1,25-DHCC (see below).

The overall effect is to increase the plasma ionised calcium and decrease the plasma phosphate (due to increased renal phosphate excretion). Prolonged excess of PTH will be associated with hypercalcaemia, hypophosphataemia, and increased plasma ALP activity (stimulation of osteoblasts); PTH deficiency (hypoparathyroidism) will be associated with hypocalcaemia and hyperphosphataemia.

Control of secretion. The rate of secretion is inversely related to the plasma ionised calcium concentration; changes of as little as 1% in the ionised calcium level will stimulate or suppress PTH release. Hypomagnesaemia, and to a lesser extent, hyper-magnesaemia, inhibit PTH secretion.

Vitamin D

Vitamin D, through its polar metabolite 1,25-dihydroxycholecalciferol (1,25-DHCC), influences intestinal calcium absorption and bone calcium flux.

Metabolism (Figure 6.3). Vitamin D occurs in two forms: (1) cholecalciferol (vitamin D_3) which is formed in the skin by the action of ultraviolet light on the epidermal steroid compound 7-dehydrocholesterol, (2) ergocalciferol (vitamin D_2), derived from plant products and irradiated yeast and bread (usually added to foods). Normally the dietary component is a less important source of vitamin D than the skin-derived compound.

Vitamin D is taken up by the blood and transported attached to a specific binding protein, D-binding protein (DBP), to the liver where it is hydroxylated (25-hydroxylase) to 25-hydroxycholecalciferol (25-HCC). This metabolite is then transported (attached to DBP) to the kidney where it is converted to the active metabolite 1,25-DHCC by the enzyme 1-α-hydroxylase. This enzyme is stringently regulated:

90

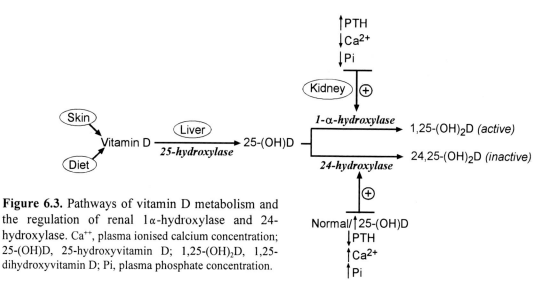

Figure 6.3. Pathways of vitamin D metabolism and the regulation of renal 1α-hydroxylase and 24-hydroxylase. Ca^{++}, plasma ionised calcium concentration; 25-(OH)D, 25-hydroxyvitamin D; 1,25-(OH)$_2$D, 1,25-dihydroxyvitamin D; Pi, plasma phosphate concentration.

- Activity stimulated by: (a) hypophosphataemia
  (b) PTH
  (c) hypocalcaemia

- Activity suppressed by: (a) hyperphosphataemia
  (b) 1,25-DHCC
  (short feedback)
  (c) hypercalcaemia

In states of calcium sufficiency another kidney enzyme (24-hydoxylase) becomes active and converts the precursor to the less active metabolite 24,25-DHCC. The 1α-hydroxylase may also occur in extrarenal tissues, e.g., granulomatous tissues such as in sarcoidosis and some lymphoma cells (see below).

1,25-DHCC is transported in the blood attached to DBP to its main target tissues, the gut, bone, and kidney where it operates through a mechanism similar to that of the steroid hormones (it binds to intracellular receptors and regulates gene transcription).

Action. Vitamin D influences calcium metabolism by its action on the small intestine, bone, and kidney.

Small intestine: 1,25-DHCC increases the absorption of calcium mainly by stimulating the synthesis of a calcium-binding protein which facilitates the uptake of calcium across the brush border of the intestinal mucosal cell. It also increases phosphate uptake.

Bone: Both calcium and phosphate are mobilised from bone by 1,25-DHCC-mediated stimulation of osteoclast activity.

Kidney: 1,25-DHCC increases the renal retention of both calcium and phosphate (? direct action on tubules).

- Vitamin D excess is associated with hypercalcaemia (increased renal and gut absorption, and bone mobilisation) and hyperphosphataemia (increased gut absorption and increased renal reabsorption due mainly to hypercalcaemia-induced PTH suppression).

- Vitamin D deficiency is associated with (a) decreased calcium absorption which will result in hypocalcaemia, and (b) increased PTH activity (stimulated by low plasma ionised calcium) which results in increased osteoclast activity (elevated serum alkaline phosphatase), and hypophosphataemia (decreased renal phosphate reabsorption).

In addition to the above actions there is now evidence that vitamin D plays a role (? importance) in cell proliferation, immune mechanism, and neurological function.

Miscellaneous factors

Calcitonin, thyroid hormones, steroids, prostaglandins, and osteoclast activating factor are compounds that are known to influence calcium metabolism when present in excessive (supra-physiological) amounts; Their role in normal calcium homeostasis in the normal subject is doubtful and may be of little import.

Calcitonin. This is 32-amino acid polypeptide secreted by the parafollicular (C) cells of the thyroid gland. In high doses, in patients with increased bone turnover (e.g., Paget's disease), it inhibits osteoclastic bone reabsorption and increases the renal excretion of calcium and it can lower the plasma calcium level in such patients with hypercalcaemia due to increased bone turnover. Its role in calcium homeostasis is probably of little importance because high plasma levels, as seen in medullary tumours of the thyroid, are usually not associated with hypocalcaemia, and the low values which are associated with total removal of the thyroid are not associated with hypercalcaemia.

Thyroid hormones. These hormones increase the rate of calcium removal from bone, e.g., severe hyperthyroidism may be associated with mild hypercalcaemia and an increased renal calcium excretion rate producing a negative calcium balance.

Adrenal steroids. Addison's disease is occasionally associated with hypercalcaemia but this is more likely due to haemoconcentration and increased renal calcium reabsorption (consequence of hypovolaemia) rather than to any direct effect of cortisol deficiency.

Prostaglandins. Prostaglandins stimulate bone reabsorption *in vitro* and infusions in experimental animals can result in hypercalcaemia. In some cases of malignant hypercalcaemia inhibition of prostaglandin synthesis by indomethacin can lower the serum calcium level. These factors suggest that in unusual circumstances prostaglandins have an effect on calcium metabolism; their importance in the normal subject is doubtful.

Osteoclast activating factor (OAF). The OAFs are a group of compounds produced by proliferating lymphocytes which are capable of stimulating local bone resorption. A role in normal calcium homeostasis is unlikely.

REGULATION OF PLASMA CALCIUM

Normally the plasma total calcium concentration is kept within narrow limits (2.15-2.55 mmol/L) by the following processes:

A *fall* in $[Ca^{2+}]$ $\rightarrow$ ↑PTH secretion which $\rightarrow$

   (a) release of calcium from bone
   (b) increased renal calcium reabsorption
   (c) increased 1,25-DHCC production →increased
       gut absorption of calcium

(a) + (b) + (c) → ↑plasma $[Ca^{2+}]$ →suppression of PTH

A *rise* in $[Ca^{2+}]$ $\rightarrow$ ↓PTH secretion which $\rightarrow$

   (a) decreased bone reabsorption
   (b) decreased renal calcium reabsorption
   (c) decreased 1,25-DHCC production $\rightarrow$
       decreased gut absorption of calcium

(a) + (b) + (c) → ↓plasma $[Ca^{2+}]$ → stimulation of PTH

Disorders of calcium homeostasis

Hypercalcaemia

The definition of hypercalcaemia depends on the reference range provided by the laboratory and the precision of the analytical method; with a reference range of 2.15-2.55 mmol/L a value in excess of 2.60 mmol/L should be considered to be sufficiently abnormal to warrant further evaluation.

The disorder is common with about 1% of the general population and 4% of the hospital population presenting with a total serum calcium in excess of 2.60 mmol/L. However, it is important to note that on analysis of a further blood sample many of these "hypercalcaemics" will produce a second value which is within the reference range. This phenomenon, sometimes referred to as "regression towards the mean", reflects biological variation and collection and analytical errors. Hence all subjects presenting with hypercalcaemia should have the level confirmed by analysis of a second blood sample.

CAUSES/PATHOPHYSIOLOGY

The common causes of hypercalcaemia are listed in Table 6.1. In hospitalised patients the commonest cause is malignancy whilst in the general population the commonest cause is primary hyperparathyroidism. These two disorders plus hypercalcaemia due to vitamin D excess cover 95-98% of the causes of hypercalcaemia seen in clinical practice.

Primary hyperparathyroidism

Primary hyperparathyroidism, due to hypersecretion of PTH, is the commonest cause of hypercalcaemia after malignancy with a prevalence of 25 per 10,000 in the general population. It has a female:male preponderance of 3:1 with a prevalence among women over the age of 65-years some 10-times that of the general population. The commonest cause is a solitary adenoma (80-90% of cases); chief cell hyperplasia involving all glands occurs in about 15% of cases whilst carcinoma is rare (less than 2%). It can also present as a familial disease and as part of the multiple endocrine adenosis syndrome (page 287).

Most subjects with the disease are asymptomatic, being identified only when their plasma calcium level is estimated as part of an investigation process for another disorder, or during "screening". However, loss of calcium from bone can result in overt bone disease such as osteoporosis or the more dramatic localised osteitis fibrosa cystica; in addition, hypercalcaemia and hypercalciuria can result in nephrocalcinosis, nephrolitihiasis, and renal failure.

Biochemical features. Some or all of the following may occur:

Hypercalcaemia: Hypercalcaemia is almost always present in primary hyperparathyroidism although it may be intermittent in patients with early or mild disease. PTH causes release of calcium from bone and

Table 6.1. Causes of hypercalcaemia.

Malignancy
 Solid tumours
 Breast, bronchus, cervix, ovary kidney
 Haematological
 Multiple myeloma, leukaemia, Hodgkin's disease, non-Hodgkin's lymphoma

Hyperparathyroidism
 Primary, tertiary, Multiple endocrine adenosis

Non-malignant/non-hyperparathyroidism
 Vitamin D excess syndromes
 Overdose, sarcoidosis, granulomas
 Iatrogenic
 IV calcium infusion
 Increased bone reabsorption
 Thyrotoxicosis, immobilisation, vitamin A excess
 Renal failure
 Post-dialysis, post-acute renal failure
 Decreased renal excretion
 Familial benign hypercalcaemia, thiazide diuretics, lithium therapy
 Miscellaneous
 Milk-alkali syndrome, Addison's disease, acromegaly, phaeochromocytoma

increased renal calcium reabsorption. The latter is probably the most important factor maintaining the high plasma calcium level.

Hypophosphataemia: PTH induces increased renal phosphate excretion which can result in hypophosphataemia. This is usually a late development and is seen in only about 50% of cases these days because of early diagnosis due to screening. If renal failure intervenes hyperphosphataemia will occur.

High plasma alkaline phosphatase activity: This reflects the increased bone turnover and, like hypophosphataemia, is not seen in all cases. The activity is moderate and usually not exceeding 350 U/L.

Hypercalciuria: This can be demonstrated in 25-50% of cases. PTH induces increased renal tubular calcium reabsorption; hence the degree of urinary calcium excretion is less than in other causes of hypercalcaemia.

High plasma PTH levels: The plasma level of the intact hormone is generally above the upper reference limit but normal values do not exclude the diagnosis, for example, a value within the normal range but above the mean level is inappropriately high in the presence of hypercalcaemia (hypercalcaemia due to non-parathyroid causes will generally suppress the plasma PTH level to below, or near, the lower reference limit). Extremely high values have been described in carcinoma of the parathyroid glands.

Malignant disease

In hospitalised patients malignancy is the commonest cause of hypercalcaemia (~40% of all causes) and it is found in up to 20% of subjects with malignant neoplasm. In most instances it is a late complication of the disease, presenting in a patient known to have cancer. The presentation is usually abrupt with the serum calcium values often reaching very high levels, e.g., >3.5 mmol/L. In some cases the tumour may not be overt, with hypercalcaemia being the presenting feature. Carcinomas of the bronchus, breast, and kidney and haematological malignancies (myeloma, leukaemia, lymphoma, Hodgkin's disease) are the common tumour types which may be associated with hypercalcaemia.

Recent evidence suggests that up to 10% of patients with malignant-related hypercalcaemia have primary hyperparathyroidism, which is not surprising considering the prevalence of malignancy and hyperparathyroidism in the community.

Pathophysiology

From the clinical and biochemical aspects there are three main types of malignant hypercalcaemia:

(1) Tumours with bone metastases. In about 40% of cases there is excessive bone resorption due to direct invasion by metastatic tumour. In some cases, e.g., breast cancer, there may be direct phagocytosis of bone, but in most cases there is most likely local secretion of osteoclast-activating factors. In multiple myeloma interleukin-1 has been identified as the active factor.

(2) Tumours without bone metastases. In

this group of patients (30-40%) the term *humoral hypercalcaemia of malignancy* has been applied. It occurs in the squamous cell carcinomas (lung, oesophagus), and carcinomas of the kidney, ovary, and pancreas. The factor responsible is parathyroid hormone-related protein which is elaborated by the tumour.

Parathyroid hormone-related protein (PTHrP) is a peptide of 141 amino acid residues with the N-terminal 1-13 residues showing some homology with PTH. It binds to the PTH receptors in bone and kidney, producing the same biological effects as PTH. The messenger RNA that encodes for PTHrP has been located in various foetal tissues suggesting possible roles in cell differentiation and in foetal calcium homeostasis.

Subjects with this type of malignant hypercalcaemia have the biochemical features of primary hyperparathyroidism (hypercalcaemia, hypophosphataemia, raised alkaline phosphatase) but with a low serum PTH level.

(3) Lymphoma-related hypercalcaemia. Subjects with lymphoma may develop hypercalcaemia due to increased circulating levels of 1,25-DHCC. In this situation the tumour cells possess 1α-hydroxylase activity which converts 25-HCC to 1,25-DHCC, causing vitamin D intoxication.

Biochemical features

The hypercalcaemia is usually of abrupt onset and rises rapidly to very high values (levels in excess of 4.0 mmol/L are not uncommon). The serum phosphate level is variable. Hyperphosphataemia is seen in subjects with the metastatic variety of hypercalcaemia, in the lymphomas with vitamin D excess, and if there is renal failure. Hypophosphataemia is characteristic of the humoral hypercalcaemia of malignancy. The serum alkaline phosphatase level is generally elevated and the urinary calcium excretion rate is high.

Vitamin D excess

This is the third commonest cause of hypercalcaemia and it is becoming more prevalent with the use of vitamin D preparations in the treatment of osteoporosis. The hypercalcaemia is due to increased gut absorption; this suppresses PTH secretion which in turn inhibits renal phosphate excretion resulting in hyperphosphataemia. The serum alkaline phosphatase is characteristically normal. The vitamin D excess syndrome can also occur in lymphomas (see above) and in a number of granulomatous diseases such as sarcoidosis, tuberculosis, and histoplasmosis, all of which include monocytic cells containing the 1α-hydroxylase enzyme.

Familial benign hypercalcaemia

This condition, previously called familial hypo-calciuric hypercalcaemia, is an autosomal dominant disorder that presents with asymptomatic, non-progressive hypercalcaemia, usually before the age of 10 years. It is characterised by mild hypercalcaemia (usually <3.00 mmol/L), hypermagnesaemia, normal or slightly elevated PTH levels, and relative hypocalci-uria. The cause is unclear but appears to be related to increased renal tubular calcium reabsorption. Recent work suggests that the disorder is due to a mutation of the ionised calcium receptor gene.

Diagnosis depends on demonstration of (a) the familial connection (persistent hypercalcaemia in parents and siblings) and (b) low renal calcium excretion rate (see below).

Thyrotoxicosis

Thyroid hormones increase the rate of bone turnover and thereby increase the mobilisation of bone calcium. This may occasionally result in hypercalcaemia of a modest degree. The plasma calcium value reverts to normal after the thyroid problem has been resolved.

Lithium therapy

Chronic lithium therapy may be associated with hypothyroidism (inhibition of TSH action), diabetes insipidus (interference with AVP activity) and hypercalcaemia. The cause of the latter is unclear but increased secretion of PTH and decreased renal calcium excretion has been demonstrated. The suggested cause for the increased PTH secretion is lithium-induced desensitisation of the parathyroid glands to Ca^{2+} (i.e., a higher than normal plasma level of Ca^{2+} is required to suppress PTH release).

Immobilisation

Since the bone calcium is in constant flux due to

muscle stresses then immobilisation will result in calcium resorption in excess of calcium deposition. Hypercalciuria and a negative calcium balance occur in all subjects who are immobilised for long periods. If the subject has increased bone turnover, such as growing children and adults with Paget's disease, hypercalcaemia may occur.

Milk-alkali syndrome

This rare and unusual disorder is seen in some patients who ingest large amounts of milk (calcium and vitamin D) and alkalies (e.g., $CaCO_3$) -- a past treatment for peptic ulcers. They present with hypercalcaemia (increased dietary calcium and vitamin D), metabolic alkalosis (alkali ingestion), and renal failure (hypercalcaemia and hypercalciuria). The alkalaemia increases renal calcium reabsorption and further aggravates the hypercalcaemia.

Vitamin A toxicity

Excessive consumption of vitamin A can result in increased bone resorption and hypercalcaemia which may be associated with nephrocalcinosis and renal failure.

Thiazide diuretics

There have been a number of reports of mild hypercalcaemia associated with long-term thiazide diuretic therapy. The cause is unclear but suggestions include increased renal calcium reabsorption (? hypovolaemia-related), thiazide-induced PTH release, and increased calcium absorption by the gut. Patients with pre-existing metabolic bone disease are likely to exhibit this problem and thiazides can worsen the hypercalcaemia of primary hyperparathyroidism.

CONSEQUENCES OF HYPERCALCAEMIA

The clinical features of hypercalcaemia relate to the plasma ionised calcium and are fairly non-specific. At total calcium values in excess of 3.00 mmol/L there may be anorexia, nausea, vomiting, constipation, and muscle weakness. When the value exceeds 4.00 mmol/L stupor and coma may occur. Polyuria is a common symptom due to calcium interference with the action of ADH on the collecting ducts.

Deposition of calcium salts in tissues may lead to conjunctival deposits, band keratopathy, and nephrocalcinosis (renal failure). If there is chronic hypercalciuria renal calculi may form.

Hypercalcaemia may predispose to acute pancreatitis, duodenal ulcers, and hypertension.

CLINICAL AND LABORATORY EVALUATION

The cause of hypercalcaemia in most cases can be determined from the clinical picture, the degree of hypercalcaemia, the serum PTH level, and the evaluation of the urinary calcium excretion rate (Figure 6.4). In obscure cases specialised investigations such as serum vitamin D estimations and bone scans may be required.

Clinical picture. Important points to consider are:

- *Age and sex* (primary hyperparathyroidism is common in women over the age of 60 years, familial benign hypercalcaemia usually presents in childhood)
- *Presence or absence of malignancy*
- *Bone pain* (malignancy, primary hyperparathyroidism)
- *Drug history* (particularly vitamin D preparations, lithium, thiazides)
- *Kidney stones* (common in hyperparathyroidism but not in malignancy)
- *Family history* (familial benign hypercalcaemia)

Degree of hypercalcaemia. Primary hyperparathyroidism and familial benign hypercalcaemia are usually associated with modest hypercalcaemia (e.g.,<3.00 mmol/L), whereas malignancy and, occasionally, vitamin D intoxication can be associated with very high plasma calcium levels (e.g., >3.5 mmol/L). It is important that the calcium level is evaluated in the light of the serum albumin level and if the albumin value is very high or very low appropriate adjustments should be made, e.g.,

For each 1g/L the albumin is above (or below) 40 g/L subtract (or add if albumin is lower) 0.02 mmol/L from the measured total calcium value. (An albumin of 40 g/L is the midpoint of its reference interval.)

Ideally, in suspected cases of disordered calcium

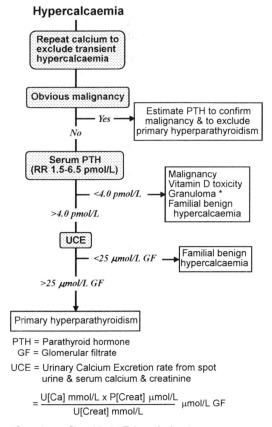

PTH = Parathyroid hormone
GF = Glomerular filtrate
UCE = Urinary Calcium Excretion rate from spot urine & serum calcium & creatinine

$$= \frac{U[Ca] \text{ mmol/L} \times P[Creat] \text{ }\mu mol/L}{U[Creat] \text{ mmol/L}} \text{ }\mu mol/L \text{ GF}$$

*Granuloma: Sarcoidosis, Tuberculosis, etc

Figure 6.4. Evaluation of hypercalcaemia.

homeostasis the serum ionised calcium should be estimated, not the serum total calcium. However, this measurement is not generally available in all routine laboratories and there are a number of technical difficulties with the method which make interpretation difficult and often unreliable.

Serum PTH. Measurement of the intact molecule using a two-site immunoradiometric assay gives the greatest sensitivity and specificity. Other radioimmunoassays measuring carboxy-terminal and other fragments are unreliable and difficult to interpret. A high PTH in association with hypercalcaemia is characteristic of primary hyperparathyroidism; PTH values below and at the lower end of the reference range are characteristic of non-parathyroid causes. An important point to bear in mind is that in primary hyperparathyroidism the PTH level may be within the reference values but still be inappropriately high. For example in the Author's laboratory normal subjects given a calcium load have a serum PTH ranging from undetectable to 3.0 pmol/L (RR: 1.5-6.5 pmol/L) and we use a cut-off value of 4.0 pmol/L (i.e., a PTH value in excess of 4.0 pmol/L is inappropriately high if there is an associated hypercalcaemia. Patients with hypercalcaemia due to malignancy and vitamin D toxicity have PTH values less than 3.0 pmol/L. (NOTE: malignancy and primary hyperparathyroidism can occur in the same patient).

Urinary calcium excretion. There are a number of ways of estimating the urinary calcium excretion, e.g., 24-hour excretion rate, calcium: creatinine clearance ratio, but the most useful is the urinary calcium excretion rate (UCE) which can be performed on a spot urine sample; it is calculated as follows.

$$\frac{Uca\ mmol/L \times Pcr\ \mu mol/L}{Ucr\ mmol/L} = \mu mol/L$$

Uca, urine calcium; Pcr, plasma creatinine; Ucr, urine creatinine

UCE values less than 25 μmol/L glomerular filtrate are deemed low and are characteristic of familial benign hypercalcaemia; values in excess of 25 μmol/L glomerular filtrate occur in hypercalcaemia due to primary hyperparathyroidism and malignancy.

Miscellaneous tests. The following may be useful selectively:

Serum phosphate: Hypophosphataemia is characteristic of primary hyperparathyroidism and humoral hypercalcaemia of malignancy, hyperphosphataemia occurs in vitamin D excess and some malignancies (and if there is severe renal impairment).

Serum alkaline phosphatase: Elevated values are associated with malignancy and primary hyperparathyroidism, normal values occur in vitamin D toxicity and familial benign hypercalcaemia (up to 50% of cases of primary hyperparathyroidism have normal values).

Total protein: a high serum total protein due to increased globulin levels is characteristic of multiple myeloma.

Vitamin D studies: if vitamin D toxicity is suspected a serum 25-HCC estimation may be useful.

Hypocalcaemia

Hypocalcaemia is defined as a plasma calcium level below the lower limit of the reference range, e.g., <2.15 mmol/L. Mild degrees of hypocalcaemia, e.g., 1.90-2.10 mmol/L, are common, usually transient and probably of no importance; however, they should not be disregarded and the appropriate response is to re-assay using a fresh blood sample.

CAUSES/PATHOPHYSIOLOGY

A list of the causes of hypocalcaemia is given in Table 6.2. The commonest cause is hypoalbuminaemia and thus all patients who record a low plasma total calcium level should have their plasma albumin estimated. If the albumin is below the stated reference range a correction should be attempted to determine the contribution due to the low albumin, e.g,

Corrected calcium (mmol/L) =
measured calcium (mmol/L) + 0.02(40 - [Alb] g/L)

The next commonest causes are renal failure and acute pancreatitis. These three conditions usually only result in mild hypocalcaemia (e.g., 1.80-2.00 mmol/L); conditions such as hypoparathyroidism and the vitamin D deficiency syndromes usually produce a plasma calcium value below 1.80 mmol/L but are fairly rare causes of hypocalcaemia.

Factitious hypocalcaemia

Ethylenediamine tetra-acetic acid (EDTA), an anti-coagulant used for the collection of haematological blood specimens, acts by chelating calcium ions. Thus if these specimens are used for plasma calcium analysis very low values (<0.50 mmol/L) will be obtained. The common cause of contamination is when blood specimens for biochemistry are 'topped-up' from the EDTA-containing specimen meant for the haematological laboratory.

Table 6.2. Causes of hypocalcaemia.

Hypoalbuminaemia
Factitious
 EDTA contamination, citrated blood
Decreased intake
 Vitamin D deficiency (Table 6.3)
 Malabsorption
 Inadequate parenteral nutrition
Decreased flux from bone
 PTH deficiency: hypoparathyroidism, hypo-
  magnesaemia
 Bone resistance to PTH: uraemia, hypo-
  magnesaemia, pseudohypoparathyroidism
Increased bone uptake
 Hungry bone syndrome
 Vitamin D therapy for osteomalacia
Extra-skeletal sequestration
 Acute pancreatitis
 Hyperphosphataemia
Renal failure (multifactorial)
Drug therapy
 EDTA, calcitonin, mithramycin, phosphates

Vitamin D deficiency syndromes

Vitamin D deficiency, in addition to producing hypocalcaemia, hypophosphataemia and hyper-phosphatasaemia, causes rickets in children and osteomalacia in adults. The biochemical features are due to decreased calcium absorption by the gut, i.e.,

↓ vitamin D → calcium absorption
→ hypocalcaemia → ↑PTH secretion →

(a) ↑renal phosphate excretion → hypophosphataemia
(b) ↑osteoblastic activity → hyperphosphatasaemia

The commoner causes of the vitamin D deficiency syndromes are listed in Table 6.3.

Hypoparathyroidism

In hypoparathyroidism there is deficient PTH activity which results in moderate to severe hypocalcaemia (1.40-1.70 mmol/L) and hyperphosphataemia

(increased tubular phosphate reabsorption). The plasma alkaline phosphatase is usually normal. The hypocalcaemia is due to decreased renal calcium reabsorption, decreased calcium release from bone, and decreased calcium absorption from the gut (decreased 1,25-DHCC due to suppressed 1α-hydroxylase activity). The causes include:

- Congenital
- Idiopathic
- Ablation (surgery, irradiation)
- Magnesium deficiency (suppression of PTH secretion)

Idiopathic hypoparathyroidism is rare; it usually presents at puberty, where it is associated with increased calcium demand, and is often associated with candidiasis and other endocrine abnormalities.

The commonest cause of hypoparathyroidism is thyroid surgery which may result in transient hypocalcaemia occurring soon after the operation or fully developed hypoparathyroidism occurring later, in some cases up to 10 years after the operation.

Hypocalcaemia due to suppressed PTH secretion is common in severe magnesium depletion (serum magnesium <0.4 mmol/L). It is characteristically unresponsive to calcium therapy until the patient becomes magnesium-replete.

Table 6.3. Causes of the vitamin D deficiency syndromes.

Environmental
 Inadequate exposure to UV light
Nutritional
 Decreased intake (dietary deficiency)
 Malabsorption syndromes
Decreased 25-hydroxylation
 Liver disease
 Anticonvulsant therapy (phenytoin)
Decreased 1α-hydroxylation
 Renal disease
Endorgan resistance to 1,25-DHCC
 Renal disease
 Anticonvulsant therapy
Increased clearance of 1,25-DHCC
 Nephrotic syndrome, Alcohol,
 Aminoglutethimide, Phenytoin

A rare and unusual cause of hypocalcaemia is that due to pseudohypoparathyroidism. This is due to end organ resistance to PTH and is associated with high plasma levels of this hormone. Clinically these patients are short, stocky, mentally dull, and have short 4th metatarsal bones.

Renal failure

Mild hypocalcaemia (1.70-1.90 mmol/L) occurs in acute renal failure and in most cases of chronic renal failure. It is of multifactorial origin, some of the causes being:

- Decreased intestinal uptake due to:
  (a) decreased 1,25-DHCC production
  (b) precipitation of calcium in the gut as insoluble phosphates
- *In vivo* precipitation of calcium phosphate
- Decreased renal reabsorption of calcium
- Bone resistance to PTH (uraemic toxins)

The low plasma ionised calcium level stimulates PTH synthesis (secondary hyperparathyroidism) resulting in very high plasma levels of the hormone. Often prolonged stimulation of the parathyroid gland can result in an autonomous functioning gland (tertiary hyperparathyroidism) which may result in hypercalcaemia.

Increased bone uptake

When disorders that cause bone demineralisation such as primary hyperparathyroidism, thyrotoxicosis, and vitamin D deficiency are successfully treated the bone uptake of calcium may outstrip the rate of gut absorption and this can result in hypocalcaemia. This condition is termed the hungry bone syndrome.

Acute pancreatitis

One to two days after the onset of acute pancreatitis mild to moderate hypocalcaemia often occurs. The exact cause is unclear but may involve:

- deposition of calcium as calcium soaps around the damaged pancreas (lipases liberate fatty acids).
- release of glucagon which stimulates calcitonin release
- hypoalbuminaemia

- hypomagnesaemia

CONSEQUENCES OF HYPOCALCAEMIA

Acute hypocalcaemia results in excitation of neuromuscular activity which may present as muscle cramps, perioral paraesthesia, carpopedal spasm (tetany), and convulsions in infants. Tapping the facial nerve may elicit a facial twitch (Chvostek's sign) and the inflation of a sphygmomanometer cuff on the arm may cause carpopedal spasm (Trousseau's sign). These features are also seen in acute respiratory alkalosis which lowers the plasma ionised calcium by increasing calcium binding to protein.

Chronic hypocalcaemia in infants can result in mental retardation, poor teeth formation, cataracts, skeletal malformations (exostoses, premature closing of epiphyses), and basal ganglia calcification.

LABORATORY EVALUATION

A logical approach to the investigation of the patient with hypocalcaemia is:

1. Exclude the obvious and common causes such as hypoalbuminaemia, renal failure, and acute pancreatitis.

2. Estimate the serum PTH level: *High values* are consistent with secondary hyperparathyroidism (e.g., vitamin D deficiency), and pseudohyperparathyroidism; *Low or low 'normal' values* indicate hypoparathyroidism.

3. If there is secondary hyperparathyroidism (low calcium, high PTH) the patient's vitamin D status should be evaluated (serum 25-HCC and 1,25-DHCC).

4. In all cases of hypocalcaemia where the cause is unclear, particularly those unresponsive to calcium therapy, the serum magnesium level should be estimated.

Bone disease

The bone diseases which often present with characteristic biochemical patterns are Paget's disease, secondary malignancy, and osteomalacia. Osteoporosis, on the other hand, usually presents with normal serum biochemical parameters but the urinary excretion of various analytes may be increased.

PAGET'S DISEASE

Paget's disease is a disorder of uncertain aetiology caused by excessive osteoclastic bone resorption followed by formation of dense trabecular bone organised in a haphazard manner which results in deformed bones. The disorder may be localised (monostotic) or generalised (polyostotic). The localised disorder may be asymptomatic and only come to light when the patient is investigated for some other problem.

The prevalence is difficult to estimate because many subjects with the disorder are asymptomatic but autopsy surveys have indicated that 3-4% of subjects over 40 years and up to 10% over the age of 70 years have the disorder.

As stated above, the condition is often asymptomatic; the common presenting features are bone pain, bone deformities (bowed tibia, kyphosis, increasing skull size), and bone fractures.

The characteristic laboratory findings are:

1 Normal serum calcium and phosphate levels (immobilisation of patients with widespread disease can result in hypercalcaemia and hypercalciuria).

2 Moderate to markedly elevated serum alkaline phosphatase levels (values in excess of 1000 U/L are not unusual and values in excess of 2000 U/L have been recorded).

3 Normal serum PTH levels.

4 Increased urinary hydroxyproline excretion during active disease.

The diagnosis is made on the basis of the clinical and biochemical picture and confirmed by radiology. The differential diagnosis is secondary malignancy, particularly prostatic carcinoma, which can present with a similar biochemical and radiological picture.

BONE MALIGNANCY

Almost all tumours can metastasise to bone but the more common ones are carcinomas of the breast, prostate, thyroid, and kidney. They produce characteristic osteolytic or osteosclerotic lesions and present with either bone pain or pathological fracture. From the biochemical point of view they may be silent or associated with hypercalcaemia, or hyperphosphatasaemia, or both. The main differential diagnosis is Paget's disease.

Haematological malignancies such as multiple myeloma and leukaemia can also present with similar biochemical features but primary bone malignancies are generally biochemically silent.

OSTEOMALACIA

Osteomalacia (adults) and rickets (children) is due to defective mineralisation of newly formed cartilage or bone matrix or both which results in the accumulation of excess osteoid.

The clinical feature of rickets are bone pain, fracture, and skeletal deformities such as enlarged costochondrial joints (rachitic rosary), bow legs (genu varum), knock-knees (genu valgus), and cranial defects such as frontal bossing, and posterior skull flattening (craniotabes). The feature of osteomalacia in adults are non-specific and include bone pain, muscular weakness, and fractures associated with minimal trauma.

The basic cause is calcium or phosphate deficiency or both. Calcium deficiency is usually due to the vitamin D deficiency syndromes (Table 6.3). Phosphate deficiency is most commonly due to defective tubular phosphate reabsorption (e.g., familial X-linked hypophosphataemia, Fanconi syndrome) and phosphate malabsorption due to gut-binding by aluminium hydroxide antacids.

The characteristic biochemical features are: hypocalcaemia, hypophosphataemia, and elevated serum PTH levels (secondary hyperparathyroidism). In the vitamin D deficient syndromes there will be decreased serum vitamin D metabolites (normal in familial hypophosphataemia). The serum alkaline phosphatase is characteristically elevated but usually to values less than 300 U/L.

Renal osteodystrophy is a specific type of the disorder which occurs in chronic renal failure in which there is osteitis fibrosa, osteomalacia, secondary hyperparathyroidism and osteosclerosis (increased mineralisation). The most important causative factor is defective vitamin D metabolism but an increased PTH and the

100

consequent hyperphosphataemia due to phosphate retention may also play a role.

Table 6.4. Causes of osteoporosis.

Senile
Postmenopausal
Immobilisation
Hormone deficiency
    oestrogens (women), androgens (men)
Hormone excess
    glucocorticoids (iatrogenic, Cushing's syndrome)
    PTH (primary hyperparathyroidism)
    thyroid hormones (thyrotoxicosis)
Malignancy
    multiple myeloma
Miscellaneous
    protein-calorie malnutrition, alcoholism
    diabetes mellitus, liver disease
    prolonged heparin therapy
    rheumatoid arthritis

OSTEOPOROSIS

Osteoporosis describes a common bone condition where there is equal loss of osteoid and mineral resulting in decreased bone. The rate of formation is usually normal but the rate of resorption is increased and there is greater loss of trabecular bone than compact bone. It is the most common metabolic bone disease in Western society, being particularly common in women after the menopause. In the early stage it is asymptomatic but as the disease progresses bone pain (e.g., severe backache), spontaneous fractures and collapse of vertebrae, and fractures of the ribs and hips with minimal trauma occur. The commonest causes are postmenopausal osteoporosis in women, senile osteoporosis in men, and immobilisation (Table 6.4).

The serum biochemistry is usually unhelpful in diagnosis because the levels of calcium, phosphate, and PTH are generally normal. Markers of increased bone turnover such as serum alkaline phosphatase, serum osteocalcin, and urinary hydroxyproline excretion rate (see below) may be positive. The diagnosis depends on the clinical picture and radiological examination.

MARKERS OF BONE TURNOVER

Bone is constantly undergoing formation and resorption (remodelling) with the two processes occurring in equal amounts. A number of diseases can affect this balance and resorption can outstrip formation resulting in bone loss and demineralisation, e.g., osteoporosis, hyperpara-thyroidism. The routine tests available for the estimation of bone turnover are limited but if used in the context of the clinical picture can provide useful information.

Markers which indicate bone formation (osteoblastic activity) are the serum levels of alkaline phosphatase and osteocalcin. The available markers of bone destruction are urinary hydroxyproline and urinary pyridinoline.

Alkaline phosphatase (ALP). The bone contributes some 15-30% of the total serum alkaline phosphatase, the remainder coming from liver, gut, and other minor sources. In the bone it is localised in the osteoblast membrane and is released during osteoblast turnover; hence it is a marker of bone formation. The problem with this marker is that special techniques (e.g., electrophoresis, iso-electrofocusing) are required to separate the bone ALP from the other isoenzymes.

Osteocalcin. Osteocalcin, or bone Gla protein (BGP), is a non-collagenous protein synthesised by osteoblasts and released into the plasma during bone formation; hence it is a marker of bone formation. It can be measured by radioimmunoassay techniques and is available in some routine laboratories.

The model for its accumulation in bone and serum shown in Figure 6.5 indicates that the post-translational synthesis of γ-carboxyglutamic acid (Gla) residues is required for osteocalcin to bind to the hydroxyapatite of bone. The non-γ-carboxylated form of osteocalcin which is secreted by warfarin-treated animals cannot bind to bone mineral and is released directly into the circulation. These experimental evidences support the claim that serum osteocalcin or BGP concentrations reflect the amounts synthesised by osteoblasts and not those released from bone matrix during bone resorption.

Hydroxyproline. This amino acid is a component of collagen which is released and excreted in the urine during bone reabsorption (it is reutilised in collagen

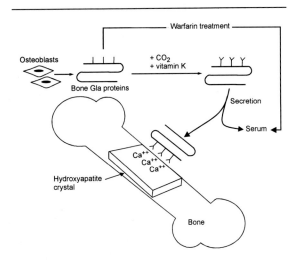

Figure 6.5. Probable relationship between bone Gla protein (osteocalcin) secretion by osteoblasts and its accumulation in bone and serum. Glutamic residues are represented by vertical lines, and γ-carboxyglutamic acid residues by Y. Redrawn from: Price PA. New bone markers. In: *New Frontiers in Bone Research. Triangle* 1988,27:22.

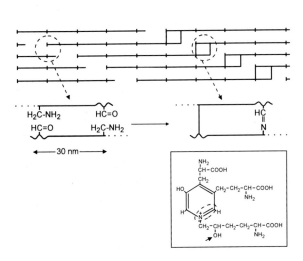

Figure 6.6. Location of intermolecular pyridinium crosslinks in collagen fibrils. The inset shows the structure of a pyridinium crosslink. The compound depicted is pyridinoline. In deoxypyridinoline, the OH-group marked with the arrow is replaced by H.

synthesis). Free hydroxyproline released from the bone is metabolised in the liver and does not appear in the urine. However, some 10% of the hydroxyproline

released during bone destruction is in the form of oligopeptide fragments and these are excreted in the urine and can be estimated after suitable hydrolysis.

Pyridinium crosslinks. Pyridinoline and deoxypyridinoline are collagen crosslinks found in bone and cartilage (Figure 6.6). They are released during bone resorption and the urinary levels can be used as markers of bone resorption. The urinary pyridinoline can be estimated by high performance liquid chromatography (HPLC) and radioimmuno-assay, the latter now becoming available on a commercial basis.

REFERENCES/FURTHER READING

DelmasPD. Biochemical markers of bone turnover for the clinical assessment of metabolic bone disease. Endocrinol Metab Clinics North Am 1990;19:1-18.

Heath DA. Parathyroid hormone related protein Clin Endocrinol 1993;38:135-136.

Hutchinson FN, Bell NH. Osteomalacia and rickets. Semin Nephrol 1992;12:127-141.

Nusshaum SR. Pathophysiology and management of severe hypercalcaemia. Metab Clinics North Am 1993;22:343-362.

Price CP, Thomson PW. The role of biochemical tests in the screening and monitoring of osteoporosis. Ann Clin Biochem 1995;32:112-22.

Reichel H, Koeffler HP. The role of the vitamin D endocrine system in health and disease. N Engl J Med 1989;320:980-991.

Seyedin SM, Kung VT, et al. Immunoassay for urinary pyridinoline: the new marker of bone reabsorption. J Bone Mineral Research 1993;8:635-641.

Walls J, Ratcliffe WA, Howell A, Bundred NJ. Parathyroid hormone and parathyroid hormone related protein in the investigation of hypercalcaemia in two populations. Clin Endocrinol 1994;41:407-13.

Wood PJ. The measurement of parathyroid hormone. Ann Clin Biochem 1992;29:11-21.

Chapter 7

Phosphate

Hitherto phosphate has not played a vital role in clinical medicine, but recent developments in total parenteral nutrition have indicated its importance and shown that chronic phosphate depletion can have deleterious effects on a number of body functions. Its metabolism is closely related to that of calcium and parathyroid hormone and a proper interpretation of disordered calcium metabolism often requires a knowledge of phosphate homeostasis.

The biological roles of phosphate include:

- Combination with calcium to form the mineral component (hydroxyapatite) of bones and teeth
- Participation as essential agents (high energy phosphate bonds) in energy transfer and in the metabolism of carbohydrate and fat
- Crucial urinary buffer ($HPO_4^{2-}/H_2PO_4^-$) constituting most of the titratable acidity
- Maintenance of cell wall integrity
- Enzyme regulation
- Regulation of oxygen transport through 2,3-diphosphoglycerate

Normal homeostasis

It is important to recognise that in the clinical laboratory only serum and urine inorganic phosphate is routinely estimated and that this represents only a tiny fraction of the total body phosphate content which is mainly in the form of bone mineral and other organic compounds.

Distribution

The total body content is ~25 moles with ~80% complexed with calcium in bones, 10% incorporated into organic compounds, and 10% combined with carbohydrates, proteins, and lipids. In its various forms, it comprises the principal intracellular anion; less than 1% is found in the extracellular fluid.

Intake

About 80% of the dietary phosphate intake of 20-40 mmol/day is absorbed in the small intestine. The rate of absorption is increased by parathyroid hormone and 1,25-dihydroxyvitamin D.

Cell uptake

Most of the extraskeletal phosphate resides in the cells as organic phosphate. Cell uptake is influenced by the rate of glycolysis and the acid-base status. Increased glycolysis, e.g., upon insulin and glucose administration, increases cell uptake to meet the demands of phosphorylation and formation of compounds with high energy phosphate bonds (ATP, etc). Alkalaemia has a similar effect, presumably due to stimulation of the pivotal glycolytic enzyme phosphofructokinase. In fact very low serum phosphate values (e.g., <0.4 mmol/L) may be associated with insulin therapy and with respiratory alkalosis (see below). Insulin deficiency and acidaemia induce the opposite effect (leakage of phosphate from cells).

Output

The major route of phosphate excretion is the kidney. About 100-200 mmol of phosphate is filtered daily by the glomerulus, 80-90% is reabsorbed in the proximal tubule and the remainder excreted in the urine. The two major factors influencing renal phosphate excretion are PTH and the intake; other factors include the extracellular volume (ECV), growth hormone, calcitonin, and sodium intake.

Increased renal excretion is associated with:

- Increased PTH secretion
- Increased phosphate intake
- Increased ECV
- Increased sodium intake
- Calcitonin

Decreased renal excretion occurs with:

- Decreased PTH secretion
- Decreased phosphate intake
- Decreased ECV
- Increased growth hormone secretion

Renal phosphate excretion. It is often useful to have a quantitative measure of the urinary excretion of phosphate. This may be obtained by measuring the *urinary phosphate concentration per day* (this requires a 24 h urine collection) or by calculating the *fractional excretion (FE) of phosphate, a la* that of sodium (see page 7). The FE_{PO4} computes the amount of phosphate excreted in the urine as a percentage of the amount filtered, and has the advantage of requiring only a spot (untimed) urine sample in addition to a blood sample.

Two other parameters which have been found useful in relation to the handling of phosphate by the nephrons are the *tubular reabsorption of phosphate (TRP)* and the *maximum renal tubular reabsorption capacity for phosphate (TmP/GFR)*.

The tubular reabsorption of phosphate is related to the fractional excretion, and can be calculated as shown below. The TRP is a fraction and has no units. The maximum renal tubular reabsorption capacity for phosphate (TmP/GFR) may be derived from the plasma phosphate concentration and the TRP value, using the following nomogram (Figure 7.1).

$$FE_{PO4} = (U_{PO4} \times P_{Cr}) / (P_{PO4} \times U_{Cr}) \times 100\%$$
$$= (C_{PO4} / C_{Cr}) \times 100\%$$

$$TRP = 1 - (C_{PO4} / C_{Cr})$$

U_{PO4} urine phosphate concentration; P_{Cr} plasma creatinine concentration; P_{PO4} plasma phosphate concentration; U_{Cr} urine creatinine concentration; C_{PO4}, phosphate clearance; C_{Cr}, creatinine clearance.

PLASMA PHOSPHATE

In the adult subject the plasma inorganic phosphate concentration is around 0.60 to 1.25 mmol/L with 12 to 15% bound to protein. The level varies with age, being higher during infancy and childhood, i.e.,

Neonates	1.20-2.80 mmol/L
<7 years	1.30-1.80 mmol/L
<15 years	0.80-1.30 mmol/L
Adults	0.60-1.25 mmol/L

Disordered homeostasis

In clinical practice the only readily available indicator of disordered phosphate homeostasis is the plasma level and this does not necessarily reflect the total body phosphate content or even the extraskeletal content. For example, in untreated diabetes mellitus the patient is usually phosphate depleted (as evidenced by a positive phosphate balance during treatment), but presents with hyperphosphataemia (a direct effect of insulinopaenia). Similarly, during acute respiratory alkalosis, although the patient may be phosphate replete, the plasma phosphate may be very low due to an intracellular shift.

Notwithstanding these problems, estimation of the plasma phosphate can be clinically useful because:

- low plasma phosphate values associated with conditions known to cause phosphate depletion indicates the presence of significant depletion (e.g., in parenteral nutrition), and

- a high or low plasma phosphate may, in association with other abnormal plasma analytes, help to confirm a diagnosis, e.g., low plasma calcium and phosphate in vitamin D deficiency, low plasma phosphate and high plasma calcium in primary hyperparathyroidism.

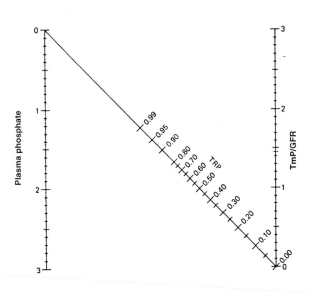

Figure 7.1. Nomogram for the derivation of the maximum renal tubular reabsoption capacity for phosphate (TmP/GFR). See text for details.

Hyperphosphataemia

Hyperphosphataemia is often encountered in clinical medicine but it is usually of a factitious nature and associated with hyperkalaemia and a high plasma lactate dehydrogenase level, e.g., haemolysis-related artifact.

CAUSES/PATHOPHYSIOLOGY

The commonest cause of a high plasma phosphate is *in vitro* seepage from red cells or haemolysis (factitious hyperphosphataemia); the commonest pathological aetiology is renal failure. Table 7.1 lists the causes most often encountered in clinical practice.

Table 7.1. Causes of hyperphosphataemia.

Factitious
  Haemolysis
  Delay in separation of plasma from red cells
Physiological
  Age-related (infancy, childhood)
Increased intake
  Oral/IV therapy, Vitamin D overdose
Cell release
  Tissue destruction (rhabdomyolysis, crush injury,
    malignancy, chemotherapy of malignancy)
  Bone release (malignancy)
  Starvation
  Acidaemia (lactic acidosis)
  Diabetes mellitus (insulin deficiency)
Decreased renal excretion
  Renal failure
  Hypoparathyroidism
  Growth hormone excess
  Volume contraction
  Tumour calcinosis
  Post-menopause

Increased intake. This is usually associated with hyperphosphataemia only if there is concomitant decreased renal excretion.

Renal failure. Early in renal insufficiency the plasma phosphate level remains normal because of increased excretion by the remaining functional nephrons. The plasma level begins to rise when the GFR falls to below 20 mL/min (or the plasma creatinine is >0.35 mmol/L).

Tumour calcinosis. This is a rare recessive inherited disorder characterised by hyperphosphataemia, normocalcaemia, and deposits of calcium phosphate about the large joints. The basic lesion is renal phosphate retention (? tubular insensitivity to PTH).

Postmenopausal and juvenile hypogonadism. These states are associated with mildly elevated plasma phosphate levels due to decreased renal excretion.

Acromegaly. Growth hormone increases renal phosphate reabsorption which may be the cause of hyperphosphataemia in acromegaly and in age-related instances (higher paediatric and childhood values).

Cell destruction. Very high plasma phosphate levels may occur during chemotherapy of malignancy, rhabdomyolysis, and crush injuries, particularly if there is also some degree of renal insufficiency where values in excess of 4.0 mmol/L are not uncommon.

Lactic acidosis. Diabetic ketoacidosis and lactic acidosis are commonly associated with hyperphosphataemia. For a given degree of acidaemia lactic acidosis produces a more severe hyperphosphataemia than the diabetic variety. This may be due to an associated tissue anoxia which causes the breakdown of ATP to AMP and inorganic phosphate.

CONSEQUENCES

Persistent hyperphosphataemia influences calcium metabolism and may result in:

- Metastatic calcification due to *in vivo* precipitation as calcium phosphate.

- Hypocalcaemia due to (a) *in vivo* precipitation, (b) decreased gut absorption of calcium (precipitation in the gut lumen as insoluble calcium phosphate).

LABORATORY EVALUATION

Most causes of hyperphosphataemia are obvious from the clinical picture and plasma electrolyte and calcium levels. If the aetiology is obscure the following scheme should be followed.

1 Exclude hyperphosphataemia of childhood and that caused by haemolysis or delayed separation of blood cells (repeat the estimation on a fresh blood sample).

2 If the plasma creatinine is <0.35 mmol/L, proceed to step 3; if >0.35mmol/L, consider renal failure.

3 If plasma calcium is normal or increased, consider vitamin D excess, bone malignancy, untreated diabetes mellitus, acidaemia (lactic acidosis). If plasma calcium is low, hypoparathyroidism is the most likely cause.

4 Estimation of the urinary phosphate excretion rate may be helpful in difficult cases. If <50 mmol/day, consider hypoparathyroidism; if >50 mmol/day, consider increased intake, *in vivo* cell destruction, and malignancy.

Hypophosphataemia

This disturbance, although not as common as hyperphosphataemia, has the potential to cause more damage to the patient because of the importance of phosphate sufficiency for optimisation of various metabolic processes.

CAUSES/PATHOPHYSIOLOGY

The causes are numerous (Table 7.2) but in most cases the condition is mild and of little clinical significance. Severe hypophosphataemia (<0.25 mmol/L) may occur in:

1. Phosphate binding in the gut (medication with aluminium hydroxide)
2. Hyperalimentation
3. Nutritional recovery syndrome
4. Respiratory alkalosis
5. Treatment of diabetic ketoacidosis
6. Treatment of acute alcoholism
7. Recovery from burns

Decreased intake. Phosphate is widely distributed in foods and deficiency due to inadequate intake is rare; there are, however, two situations where hypophosphataemia may occur as a consequence of decreased intake -- parenteral nutrition and medication with aluminium hydroxide.

Parenteral nutrition. In the early days of this therapy hypophosphataemia was common due to inadequate phosphate supplement in the IV fluids. Now that the problem is widely recognised it occurs with less frequency.

Aluminium hydroxide therapy. Aluminium hydroxide binds phosphate in the gut lumen and may result in severe hypophosphataemia.

Table 7.2. Causes of hypophosphataemia.

Decreased intake
Starvation, inadequate IV nutrition, malabsorption syndromes, vomiting, aluminium hydroxide therapy

Increased cell uptake
High carbohydrate meal, insulin therapy, nutritional recovery syndrome, respiratory alkalosis

Increased renal excretion
Diuretic therapy, magnesium depletion, renal phosphate leak (Fanconi syndrome, vitamin D-resistant rickets), hyperparathyroidism (primary and secondary)

Multiple causes
Alcoholism, diabetes mellitus, burns, hyperalimentation

Increased cellular uptake. Two common causes of severe hypophosphataemia are insulin therapy and respiratory alkalosis.

Insulin. Increased glycolysis, as occurs with insulin therapy or after a carbohydrate load, causes increased cellular phosphate uptake and hypophosphataemia (often severe). This is due to the increased production of phosphorylated carbohydrates and can occur in the treatment of diabetic ketoacidosis with insulin and during refeeding after a period of starvation (nutritional recovery syndrome, e.g., post-starvation or alcoholism).

Respiratory alkalosis. Intracellular alkalaemia stimulates glycolysis and cellular uptake of phosphate by stimulating phosphofructokinase. The cellular pH is less apt to fall in extracellular metabolic alkalosis because bicarbonate has difficulty crossing the cell membrane; on the other hand, carbon dioxide (which is low in respiratory alkalosis) crosses the cell wall easily and diffuses out readily when the extracellular concentration is low.

Increased renal excretion. In the Fanconi syndrome (page 80) and familial hypophosphataemic rickets (vitamin D resistant type), the tubular reabsorption mechanism for phosphate is defective. Diuretics, including osmotic diuretics, and hypomagnesaemia increase renal phosphate excretion. The metabolic and biochemical sequelae of primary and secondary hyperparathyroidism are discussed in Chapter 6.

CONSEQUENCES

Short-term hypophosphataemia, even though severe, does not appear to cause any dramatic clinical problems; the following have been described in long-term phosphate deficiency.

- Paresthesia, ataxia, coma
- Muscle weakness, rhabdomyolysis
- Increased susceptibility to infection (? defective phagocytosis)
- Haemolysis (? decreased 2,3-diphosphoglycerate)
- Decreased platelet aggregation
- Osteomalacia

LABORATORY EVALUATION

The first approach is to exclude the common causes of severe hypophosphataemia, such as respiratory alkalosis, alcoholism, hyperparathyroidism, based on clinical observation and routine biochemical tests. If the aetiology is not obvious then determination of the urinary phosphate excretion rate, or fractional excretion (FE_{PO4}, page 76) can be useful (Figure 7.2).

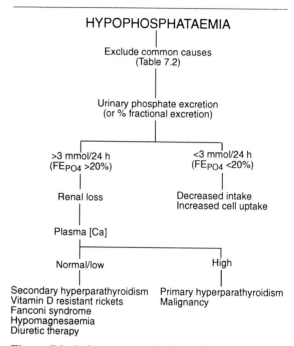

Figure 7.2. Laboratory evaluation of hypophosphataemia. FE_{PO4}, fractional excretion of phosphate.

REFERENCES/FURTHER READING

Knochel JP. The clinical status of hypophosphataemia: An update. N Engl J Med 1985;31:447-449.

Stoff JS. Phosphate homeostasis and hypophosphataemia. Am J Med 1982;72:489-495.

Yu GC, Lee DB. Clinical disorders of phosphorus metabolism. West J Med 1987;147:569-576.

Chapter 8

Magnesium

Magnesium is the fourth commonest cation in the body. The greater portion is found in bone but it is otherwise located in the cells, with less than 1% residing in the extracellular fluid (ECF). It is important in clinical medicine because:

- It is a co-factor for many enzymes, particularly those concerned with energy metabolism.
- It is required for normal DNA function, cell membrane permeability, and neuromuscular excitation.
- Its metabolism is closely associated with that of calcium and it is necessary for the synthesis and secretion of parathyroid hormone (PTH).

Hypomagnesaemia and hypermagnesaemia are common in the hospital population but it is important to note that because less than 1% of the total body magnesium is found in the ECF, plasma levels do not necessarily reflect the total body content.

Normal metabolism

Figure 8.1 presents an overview of basic magnesium metabolism in the body, which primarily is controlled by the renal handling of magnesium (Figure 8.2).

DISTRIBUTION

The total body magnesium content of 900-1200 mmol is distributed as follows. Approximately two-thirds is in the skeleton (half of which is exchangeable); of the remaining third ~20% is in muscle tissue and ~10% in the soft tissues. Less than 1% is in the ECF (including the plasma).

PLASMA MAGNESIUM

In normal adults the plasma magnesium concentration is around 0.7-1.0 mmol/L and is made up of the following fractions:

ionised   ~55%

protein-bound   ~32% (mainly to albumin)
complexed   ~13% (as phosphate, citrate)

INTAKE

The average dietary intake is about10-15 mmol/day, 30-40% of which is absorbed in the small gut. Phosphate inhibits absorption by precipitating magnesium as insoluble complexes.

CELLULAR UPTAKE

The cellular uptake of magnesium is an energy dependant process which may be related to calcium transport. There is some evidence that, like potassium ions (page 26), its uptake is stimulated by the catecholamines acting via the β-adrenergic receptors.

EXCRETION

Magnesium homeostasis is due mainly to control of the rate of renal excretion of the ion (see Figure 8.2);

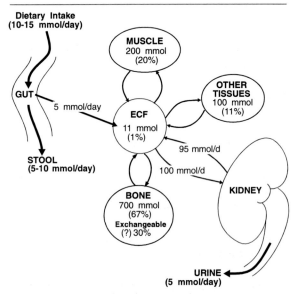

Figure 8.1. Magnesium homeostasis. See text for details

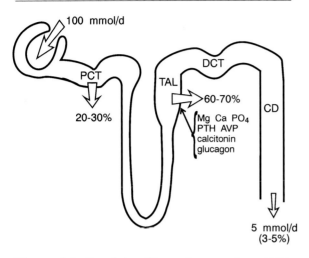

Figure 8.2. Renal handling of magnesium. PCT, proximal convoluted tubule; TAL, thick ascending loop of Henle; DCT, distal convoluted tubule; CD, collecting duct.

little else is lost from the body via other excretion routes. The glomerulus filters some 100-150 mmol of magnesium daily; only about 3-5% (2.5-5 mmol) appears in the urine. About 20-30% is reabsorbed in the proximal tubule and 60-70% in the thick ascending limb of the loop of Henle.

Unlike calcium, there are no well defined mechanism controlling magnesium balance but the rate of excretion is influenced by many factors including:

• *body magnesium:* a low intake or deficiency causes increased reabsorption

• *plasma calcium levels:* hypercalcaemia decreases reabsorption

• *phosphate:* depletion decreases reabsorption

• *parathyroid hormone (PTH), calcitonin, antidiuretic hormone (ADH), glucagon:* all of which increase reabsorption

• *Extracellular volume:* an increased ECV increases renal excretion

• *Drugs:* Alcohol and a number of drugs such as diuretics and various chemotherapeutic agents (see below) also increase the excretion rate.

Provided renal function is adequate, increased magnesium intake is associated with increased renal excretion and decreased magnesium intake (and magnesium depletion) is associated with decreased excretion, e.g., to less than 0.5 mmol/day. Hence:

• A low plasma magnesium level associated with a urinary output of less than 0.5 mmol/day suggests extrarenal loss (renal loss is associated with values in excess of 0.5 mmol/day).

• Oral and intravenous magnesium therapy will be associated with ongoing urinary loss, and this should be considered when planning therapy.

Hypomagnesaemia

Hypomagnesaemia (plasma [Mg] <0.70 mmol/L) has a prevalence in the hospital population of 5-11%). As the plasma magnesium represents less than 1% of the total body magnesium it is likely that hypomagnesaemia can occur in the absence of magnesium deficiency and that magnesium depletion may be associated with a normal plasma level. Estimations of the tissue levels (e.g., muscle, bone, red cells) would probably give a better indication of the patient's magnesium status than the plasma concentration but these investigations are impractical in the routine clinical situation and therefore the clinician has to manage the patient on the basis of the plasma concentration.

CAUSES/PATHOPHYSIOLOGY

Magnesium depletion and hypomagnesaemia have a wide range of causes (Table 8.1). The commonest clinical situations where magnesium depletion should be considered are:

• alcoholism
• drug therapy (especially diuretics, gentamicin, amphotericin B, and cis-platinum)
• gastrointestinal disorders (vomiting, diarrhoea, malabsorption)
• renal loss (osmotic diuresis, alcoholism, renal tubular acidosis, hypercalcaemia)

Decreased intake. Although magnesium is widely

distributed in foods an inadequate intake can occur in chronic alcoholism, the malabsorption syndromes, and with infusion of magnesium-poor fluids. In these cases there may be associated magnesium depletion, particularly if there is increased renal excretion (as occurs in alcoholism).

Table 8.1. Causes of magnesium deficiency and hypomagnesaemia

Decreased intake
Starvation (protein-calorie malnutrition)
Malabsorption syndrome
Prolonged gastric suction
Inadequate parenteral nutrition
Specific magnesium absorption defect (neonates)

Increased cell uptake
Stress conditions

Extrarenal losses
Diarrhoea (prolonged)
Laxative abuse
Loss from gut fistula
Excessive lactation (rare)

Renal losses
Alcoholism
Interstitial nephropathy
Diuresis: osmotic (diabetic ketoacidosis),
    post-obstructive nephropathy,
    post-acute tubular necrosis
Drugs: diuretics (loop, not thiazides), amphotericin B,
    gentamycin, cis-platinum, tobramycin, viomycin,
    carbenecillin
Hypercalcaemia
Renal tubular acidosis
Bartter's syndrome
Endocrine: primary hyperaldosteronism,
    hypoparathyroidism, hyperthyroidism, SIADH

Miscellaneous
Acute pancreatitis (sequestration)
Multiple transfusions (precipitation)
Insulin administration (redistribution)
Hungry bone syndrome: post-parathyroidectomy,
    post-thyroidectomy

Increased cell uptake. Many acutely ill patients present with moderate hypomagnesaemia (not less than 0.60 mmol/L) which corrects itself over the next few days without intervention. This may be due to cell uptake due to stress-induced catecholamine release. There is good evidence that β-adrenergic receptor stimulation induces cellular magnesium uptake as it does potassium (page 26).

Renal loss. This is a common cause of deficiency (Table 8.1) and includes alcoholism, diuretic therapy, cis-platinum and gentamicin administration, and hypercalcaemia.

Alcoholism. This is a common cause of severe hypomagnesaemia due to increased renal excretion (alcohol-induced), inadequate intake, vomiting and diarrhoea.

Diuretic therapy. Hypomagnesaemia is seen in thiazide and loop diuretic therapy but not with the potassium-sparing diuretics.

Cis-platinum. This cytotoxic agent induces renal magnesium wasting and is almost always associated with moderate to severe hypomagnesaemia.

Gentamicin. A nephrotoxic antibiotic which may be associated with both hypomagnesaemia and hypokalaemia due to increased renal excretion of both ions.

Hypercalcaemia. Many hypercalcaemic states are associated with hypomagnesaemia as a result of PTH suppression and competitive interaction between the two divalent cations in the renal tubule.

CONSEQUENCES

Clinically hypomagnesaemia may be silent or it may present manifestations similar to those of hypocalcaemia. Biochemically the important associations are hypokalaemia and hypocalcaemia, both of which are resistant to specific treatment until the patient is magnesium-replete.

Clinical: Severe hypomagnesaemia can cause muscle weakness, fasciculation,, and tremors, positive Chvostek's and Trousseau's signs, and tetany. However, some of these symptoms may also occur in patients with hypocalcaemia and hypokalaemia, both of which may be associated with hypomagnesaemia.

Biochemical: The associated hypokalaemia is due to increased renal potassium excretion, possibly reflecting diminished ATPase activity; hypocalcaemia, the other associated biochemical abnormality, is due to decreased PTH secretion, or to diminished PTH activity at the bone level, or both (see below).

MANAGEMENT

In the acute situation magnesium can be given intravenously (25 mmol of magnesium sulfate in one litre of normal saline over six to twelve hours, repeated if necessary). It is usually necessary to continue the treatment for three to four days (up to 50 mmol/day) because (a) much of the infused magnesium is lost in the urine, and (b) distribution through out the body takes up to three days. The plasma level should be monitored regularly particularly if the patient has renal insufficiency.

Note: Some studies have shown that hospitalised patients with mild hypomagnesaemia (plasma [Mg] <0.6 mmol/L) usually normalise their plasma levels within two to three days of admission without specific therapy. The reason is unclear but could reflect a transient abnormal distribution due to stress -- ? catecholamine related.

LABORATORY EVALUATION

In the majority of cases the cause of magnesium deficiency is obvious from the clinical picture. If the cause is obscure some or all of the following tests may be useful:

1. 24 h urinary magnesium excretion rate
2. plasma calcium
3. plasma electrolytes
4. tests of malabsorption

Urinary magnesium. The daily urinary excretion of magnesium depends on the intake but is about 0.5-12.0 mmol. In magnesium-depleted states not due to renal loss the level will fall to less than 0.5 mmol/day. Thus, if hypomagnesaemia is associated with a urinary excretion rate greater than 0.5 mmol/day then renal wastage is indicated.

Plasma calcium. *Hypercalcaemia:* Calcium loading and chronic hypercalcaemia, including that due to primary hyperparathyroidism, may increase renal magnesium excretion and result in low plasma magnesium levels. *Hypocalcaemia* may be associated with diseases that also cause hypomagnesaemia (e.g., hypoparathyroidism) and hypocalcaemia may also be the result of hypomagnesaemia.

Plasma electrolytes. Low plasma potassium values may indicate causes of the magnesium depletion such as primary hyperaldosteronism, diuretic therapy, diarrhoea (overt and covert), and laxative abuse. A low plasma sodium associated with hypomagnesaemia may indicate SIADH.

Tests of malabsorption. These are performed to confirm malabsorption as the cause of magnesium deficiency.

Hypermagnesaemia

The prevalence of hypermagnesaemia (plasma [Mg] >1.00 mmol/L) in the hospital population is around 4-5% . Severe hypermagnesaemia (>1.5 mmol/L) only occurs in patients with renal failure who have an increased intake. Acutely increased levels will occur after rapid intravenous infusion but the kidney is efficient at excreting excess loads (90% within 24-48 hours).

CAUSES/PATHOPHYSIOLOGY

The common causes of hypermagnesaemia are listed in Table 8.2. The commonest cause is renal failure which is usually associated with mild hypermagnesaemia (e.g.,<1.25 mmol/L) and this is usually symptomless and of little clinical importance. Severe hypermagnesaemia (>1.50 mmol/L) associated with

Table 8.2. Causes of hypermagnesaemia

Increased intake*
Oral: antacids, laxatives
IV magnesium therapy, e.g., treatment of eclampsia
Dialysis fluids containing high magnesium content

Cell release
Diabetic ketoacidosis
Severe hypoxia, e.g, birth asphyxia
Cell necrosis/catabolism

Decreased excretion
Renal failure: acute, chronic
Familial hypocalciuric hypercalcaemia
Mineralocorticoid deficiency
Hypothyroidism

* usually only when associated with decreased renal excretion

magnesium excess, which may require treatment, may be found in:

- IV magnesium therapy, such as treatment of eclampsia
- Increased magnesium intake in patients with renal insufficiency, e.g., chronic renal failure patients who take magnesium-containing laxatives or antacid preparations.

Increased intake. Acutely administered magnesium is rapidly eliminated by the normal kidney with 50% excreted in 24 hours and 90% excreted in 48 hours; only with the addition of renal impairment will chronic hypermagnesaemia occur.

Increased cell release. In diabetic ketoacidosis and tissue hypoxia magnesium will leak out of cells and increase the plasma level. Cell necrosis, e.g., crush injury, can result in the release of large amounts of extracellular magnesium, but if renal function is unimpaired this is easily excreted.

Decreased renal excretion. In progressive renal

failure normal magnesium excretion is maintained until the GFR drops to below 10-20 mL/min, due to an increased workload by the remaining nephrons. The mildly increased serum magnesium levels associated with mineralocorticoid deficiency probably reflects a decreased ECV.

CONSEQUENCES

Acute elevations depress the central nervous system and neuromuscular activity resulting in muscle weakness, and depression of the deep tendon reflexes. Flaccid quadriplegia, cardiac arrhythmias, and respiratory paralysis have also been described. It also causes flushing and hypotensive episodes may occur.

LABORATORY EVALUATION

The common causes of hypermagnesaemia are listed above and these are usually evident from the clinical picture. However, there are only two conditions associated with severe hypermagnesaemia (>1.5 mmol/L):

1 Magnesium therapy, e.g., treatment of eclampsia

2 Increased magnesium intake in the face of renal insufficiency, e.g., patients with chronic renal failure who take laxatives or antacid preparations containing magnesium.

REFERENCES/FURTHER READING

Buckley JE. Clark VL, Meyer TJ, Pearlman NW. Hypomagnesaemia after cisplatinum combination therapy. Arch Intern Med 1984;144:2347-2348.

Chase LR, Saltopolsky E. Secretion and metabolic efficiency of parathyroid hormone in patients with severe hypomagnesaemia. J Clin Endocrinol Metab 1974;38:363-371.

Croker JW, Walmsley RN. Routine plasma magnesium estimation: a useful test? Med J Aust 1986;145:71-75.

Reinhart RA. Magnesium metabolism: a review with special reference to the relationship between intracellular content and serum levels. Arch Intern Med 1988;148:2415-2420.

Shils ME. Experimental human magnesium depletion. Medicine 1969;49:61-85.

Wacker WEC, Parisi AF. Magnesium metabolism. N Engl J Med 1968; 278:658-775.

Whang R, Oei TD, Aikawa JK, et al. Predictors of clinical hypomagnesaemia: hypokalaemia, hypophosphataemia, hyponatraemia, and hypocalcaemia. Arch Intern Med 1984;144:1794-1796.

Zaloga GP. Interpretation of the serum magnesium level. Chest 1989;95:257-258.

Chapter 9

Urate and Gout

Urate, high plasma levels of which may result in gout and renal disease, is the end product of purine metabolism. The purine nucleotides of adenine and guanine are essential components of both DNA and RNA; additionally adenine has a wide distribution in the form of adenosine triphosphate (ATP). The sources of purines in the body are *de novo* synthesis, degradation of nucleic acids due to cell turnover, and the diet.

hypoxanthine, derived from adenine, can be re-converted to purine nucleotides by a salvage pathway involving the enzymes hypoxanthine-guanine phosphoribosyl transferase (HGPRT) and adenine phosphoribosyl transferase (APRT). The other substrate in both cases is PRPP. This salvage pathway does not require ATP.

Purine metabolism

The purine bases (adenine, guanine, etc) are assembled from a variety of precursors including glutamine, glycine, aspartate, tetrahydrofolate, and bicarbonate. In addition to *de novo* synthesis from these substrates, there is a salvage pathway whereby nucleotides are resynthesized from purine bases (Figure 9.1).

DE NOVO SYNTHESIS

Starting with ribose-5-phosphate and ATP, 5-phospho-ribosyl-pyrophosphate (PRPP) is synthesized by the enzyme phosphoribosylpryrophosphate synthetase (PRPPS). The conversion of PRPP and glutamine to 5-phosphoribosylamine by phosphoribosyl-pyro-phosphate amidotransferase (PRPP-AT) is the rate-limiting step in purine synthesis, being subjected to negative feedback by purine nucleotides. After a number of intermediate steps requiring energy in the form of ATP, inosine monophosphate (IMP), which can be converted to guanosine monophosphate (GMP) and adenosine monophosphate (AMP), is formed.

The purine nucleotides GMP, IMP, and AMP are broken down during cellular turnover to the respective purine bases guanine, hypoxanthine, and adenine. These are converted to xanthine, and further to uric acid, both steps catalysed by the enzyme xanthine oxidase (Figure 9.1).

SALVAGE PATHWAY

The free purine bases (guanine and adenine), formed by the hydrolytic degradation of nucleic acids, and

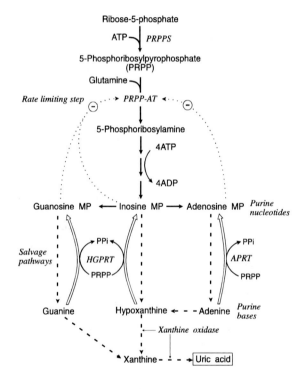

Figure 9.1. Purine metabolism. See text for details.

Urate Metabolism

Urate, the dead-end product of purine metabolism, is excreted from the body by both renal and alimentary routes.

Production

The overall production rate of urate, on a normal diet, is 5 to 6 mmol/day of which 3 to 4 mmol are derived from the *de novo* route. One to two mmol are derived from the diet, particularly meat, fish and yeast products.

Excretion

About one third of the urate produced is secreted into the gastrointestinal tract where it is destroyed by bacterial uricases. The remaining two thirds is excreted by the kidney.

Renal Handling of Urate. The renal clearance of urate is about 8-12 mL/min or around 5-10% of inulin clearance. Most of the filtered urate (~98%) is reabsorbed in the proximal tubule. The remaining portion passes through the tubule and is augmented by urate secreted by the tubules. The final amount excreted (~5 mmol/day) is 20% derived from the glomerular filtrate and 80% derived from tubular secretion.

Factors influencing urinary urate excretion

A number of factors can increase or decrease the renal clearance of urate, and some of these can be important determinants of the plasma urate level.

Decreased excretion.

* *Lactic acids and ketoacids.* These small acid anions compete with renal tubular secretion of urate.

* *Low-dose salicylates.* Low doses inhibit tubular urate secretion.

* *Hypovolaemia.* A decrease in the GFR results in increased proximal urate reabsorption.

* *Diuretics.* Thiazides and furosemide, but not the potassium-sparing diuretics, increase renal tubular urate reabsorption.

Increased excretion.

* *High-dose salicylates.* High doses inhibit tubular urate reabsorption.

* *Uricosuric agents,* e.g., probenecid, promote renal excretion.

* *? hypervolaemia,* e.g., in SIADH. An increased urine flow rate results in decreased reabsorption.

PLASMA URATE

The upper limit of the plasma urate reference range is 0.42 mmol/L for men and 0.36 mmol/L for women. As the plasma level reflects a balance between urate production and excretion it follows that hyperuricaemia can be due to increased production, or decreased excretion, or both (Figure 9.2).

Increased production. High production rates may reflect four basic situations.

* High *de novo* synthesis, e.g., inborn errors of metabolism.

* Increased endogenous nucleoprotein degradation, e.g., malignancy, myeloproliferative disorders, blood dyscrasias.

* Increased ATP turnover. Normally ATP is degraded to AMP most of which is re-utilised. However, if there is a high turnover rate, it can be further degraded to purine bases and finally to urate, e.g., with excessive alcohol consumption, during exercise, and in hypoxia.

* High dietary intake.

Decreased renal excretion. In addition to renal failure, a number of acid anions and drugs (see above) can decrease renal excretion. Up to 80% of subjects with primary gout have decreased renal urate clearance in an otherwise normal kidney, the exact cause of which is yet to be elucidated.

Inborn errors of purine metabolism

Congenital disorders of purine metabolism are rare. The three best known are xanthine oxidase deficiency which produces hypouricaemia, and disorders of PRPPS and HGPRT both of which result in hyperuricaemia. In addition, the better known von Gierke's disease (glucose 6-phosphatase deficiency) is associated with hyperuricaemia (see below).

Xanthine oxidase. Deficiency of this enzyme is an autosomal recessive disorder associated with increased urinary excretion of xanthine and hypoxanthine, xanthine stones, and hypouricaemia. The only clinical manifestation is xanthine stones.

Hypoxanthine-guanine phosphoribosyl transferase Deficiency of this enzyme eliminates the salvage pathway and accelerates *de novo* purine synthesis (? decreased feedback inhibition of PRPP-AT by nucleotides). Severe deficiency results in the Lesch-Nyhan syndrome whilst partial deficiency results in severe X-linked gout.

   Lesch-Nyhan Syndrome. This rare disease is a X-linked recessive disorder due to a severe deficiency of HGPRT. It is characterised by hyperuricaemia, mental deficiency, spasticity, choreoathetosis, and self-mutilation.

Phosphoribosyl pyrophosphate synthetase. An X-linked disorder due to *excessive* activity of PRPPS and resulting in purine overproduction and gout has been described. The increased enzyme activity seems to be due to resistance to feedback inhibition by purine nucleotides.

Glucose-6-phosphatase. Deficiency of glucose-6-phosphatase (von Gierke's disease) results in glycogen accumulation in the liver and kidneys, fasting hypoglycaemia, lactic acidosis, hypertriglyceridaemia, and hyperuricaemia. The hyperuricaemia is due to increased *de novo* synthesis and decreased renal urate secretion as a consequence of the lactic acidosis. The increased *de novo* synthesis may be due to excessive production of ribose-5-phosphate as a consequence of shunting of glucose-6-phosphate through the pentose phosphate pathway.

Hyperuricaemia

Hyperuricaemia is defined as a serum urate concentra-tion greater than 0.42 mmol/L in the male and 0.36 mmol/L in the female.

CAUSES/PATHOPHYSIOLOGY

The plasma urate concentration reflects the balance between urate production and excretion and high values may occur during periods of increased production, or decreased excretion, or both. Furthermore, these two basic defects can be either primary, or of a genetic nature, or secondary to a number of acquired disease processes (Figure 9.2).

Genetic factors

Overproduction. HGPRT deficiency and PRPPS overactivity can cause defective purine metabolism resulting in overproduction of urate. This may lead to hyperuricaemia, gout, and high renal excretion rates of urate.

Renal underexcretion. About 80% of gouty subjects have a primary defect in the renal excretion of urate, i.e., there is no, or little, evidence of overproduction but the 24-hour renal excretion rate is <6.0 mmol on a mixed diet (<3.6 mmol/24hour on a purine-free diet). This group has been termed non-secretors (the remaining 20% of gouty subjects who have evidence of overproduction only are called secretors).

Acquired causes

As for the primary group the secondary, or acquired, causes of hyperuricaemia can be classified into overproduction and underexcretion groups but it should be noted that the aetiology may be multifactorial in many cases.

Overproduction. The major causes in this group are those patients who have excessive cellular prolifera-tion and those who have a high rate of ATP degradation.

   Cellular proliferation. Increased cell turnover, and associated high nucleoprotein degradation leading to hyperuricaemia, occur in haematological diseases such as the myeloproliferative disorders including polycythaemia vera, leukaemia, and infectious mononucleosis. It also occurs when malignancies are treated with chemotherapy or irradiation and during severe psoriasis.

High purine diet. A diet rich in purines such as flesh (meats, fish, etc) and yeast products (including beer) may only result in a high urinary urate excretion rate. However, if there is an associated defect in renal urate excretion (see below) hyperuricaemia can occur.

Increased ATP turnover. The metabolism of alcohol to acetyl-CoA utilises considerable amounts of ATP which is degraded to AMP, which in turn may be converted to urate. Similarly, during severe exercise and tissue hypoxia, excessive ATP can be degraded to AMP with an increase in urate production.

Decreased renal excretion.

Renal disease. A fall in the GFR will result in decreased urate clearance which can lead to urate retention. In uncomplicated chronic renal failure the plasma urate begins to rise when the GFR falls below 20 mL/min which is equivalent to a serum creatinine of approximately 0.35 mmol/L. As the failure progresses the plasma urate rises further but plateaus off at a concentration of around 0.60 to 0.70 mmol/L, presumably due to increased secretion into the gut.

Drugs. Therapy with the thiazide diuretics and furosemide is often associated with hyperuricaemia. This may reflect volume contraction (see below) rather than a direct effect of the drugs. Salicylates, *in small doses*, decrease renal urate excretion by inhibiting renal tubular secretion (high doses are associated with hypouricaemia because of inhibition of tubular urate reabsorption).

Organic acidaemia. The organic acid anions -- lactate, acetoacetate, and β-hydroxybutyrate, are competitive inhibitors of tubular urate secretion and hence can result in renal urate retention. These factors operate to a certain extent in alcoholism and starvation.

Alcohol. Excessive alcohol ingestion is often associated with hyperuricaemia, not only because of increased urate production (see above) but also because of decreased renal urate excretion. This latter effect may be due to the lactic acidosis and ketoacidosis which can be associated with alcohol abuse.

Hypertension. Hyperuricaemia commonly accompanies uncontrolled hypertension. The cause is unclear but is thought to be due to altered intrarenal distribution of blood flow.

Dehydration. Volume contraction due to any cause, including diuretic therapy, results in renal urate retention presumably due to a drop in the GFR which stimulates increased proximal tubular reabsorption.

Factors Contributing to Hyperuricaemia

Persistent hyperuricaemia occurs not only in patients with primary gout but also in many subjects presenting at medical examinations for other reasons (asymptomatic hyperuricaemia). Many of these will have a number of factors which are potentially correctable.

Alcohol. As stated above regular alcohol consumption is a major contributor to hyperuricaemia.

Obesity. Many obese people are hyperuricaemic and appropriate loss of weight will result in reduction of the plasma urate level. The cause is unclear.

Hypertriglyceridaemia. Up to 30% of gouty subjects have hypertriglyceridaemia. There may be a genetic link between the two but hypertriglyceridaemia, like hyperuricemia, is common in obese patients and those who overindulge in alcohol.

Hypertension. Correction of poorly controlled hypertension, by drugs other than diuretics, will improve an associated hyperuricaemia.

Diuretics. Therapy with the non-potassium-sparing diuretics (thiazides, furosemide) is a common cause of hyperuricaemia, particularly in the elderly (e.g., those with cardiac failure and hypertension).

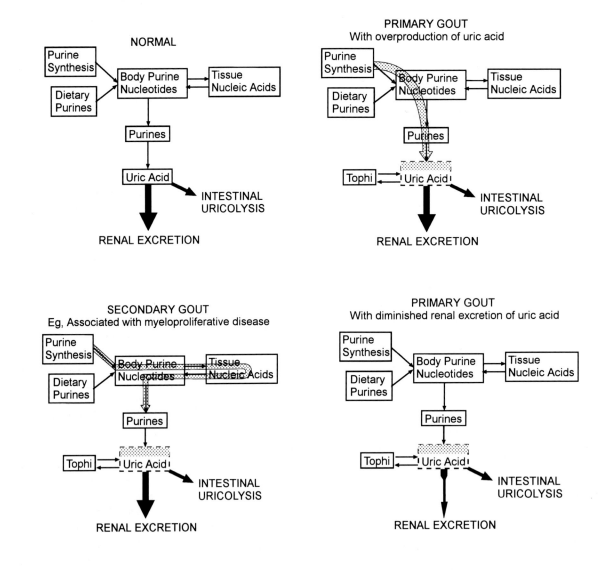

Figure 9.2. Normal and abnormal urate metabolism and pathophysiologic schemes of hyperuricaemia. See text for details.

Starvation. Prolonged starvation, e.g., religious fasting, anorexia nervosa, can result in quite severe hyperuricaemia. This is due to increased producton (increased cell turnover due to endogenous protein utilisation) and decreased renal excretion as a consequence of starvation ketosis.

Low urine volume. Extracellular volume contraction increaseas the renal reabsorption of urate

and an adequate urine flow is necessary for the optimal excretion of urate.

Gout

Gout is a metabolic disorder associated with hyperuricaemia and deposition of urate crystals in tissues. Over 90% of gouty subjects are men (prevalence of about 3 per1000) over the age of 30 years. In women gout is uncommon and it usually does not occur until after the menopause. The majority of gouty subjects have the primary (genetic) disorder reflecting either renal urate underexcretion, or urate overproduction, or both. Secondary gout, due to an acquired hyperuricaemia (e.g., myeloproliferative disorders, myeloma, renal failure) is less common.

There are four recognisable stages in the development of gout: asymptomatic hyperuricaemia, acute gouty arthritis, intercritical gout, and chronic tophaceous gout.

Asymptomatic hyperuricaemia. Hyperuricaemia is usually present for many years before the development of clinical gout. However, only one in twenty patients with hyperuricaemia will go on to develop gout.

Acute gouty arthritis. Around 70% of patients present with the classical acute inflammation of the metatarso-phalangeal joint of the big toe; other joints may be involved later. Urate crystals may be found in the synovial fluid, the periarticular tissues, and cartilage.

Intercritical gout. Most patients have recurrent attacks at shorter intervals. Between attacks the subject is usually normal except for the hyperuricaemia.

Chronic tophaceous gout. Following recurrent acute attacks tophi, swellings containing urate crystals, may develop in the periarticular tissue. Tophi can also occur at other sites such as the helix of the ear, bursae, and tendons.

CONSEQUENCE

If treatment is not adequate the subject may develop urolithiasis, or renal disease, or both.

Urolithiasis. Around 5% of all renal stones are of urate composition and about 10-20% of gouty subjects develop kidney stones.

Renal disease. Progressive chronic renal failure is an important cause of morbidity in untreated gout (deposition of urate crystals about the renal tubules) and acute renal failure due to obstructive uropathy can occur during the severe hyperuricaemia which develops during cytotoxic therapy for malignancy.

Note: There are several points about gout that are

useful to keep in mind:

- Hyperuricaemia is not synonymous with gout (only 1 in 20 people with hyperuricaemia develop the disorder).

- Acute gout can be associated with a normal plasma urate level, although repeated estimations will reveal hyperuricaemia at some stage.

- The demonstration of urate crystals in tissues (e.g., in white cells of synovial fluid, in tophi) is essential for the definitive diagnosis of gout. Asymptomatic hyperuricaemia can be incidental in a patient who has developed arthritis due to a non-gouty cause, e.g., infection, pseudogout.

- Chronic renal failure is a complication of gout and chronic renal failure is a cause of hyperuricaemia. In the latter case the serum urate level seldom rises beyond 0.65 mmol/L.

Asymptomatic hyperuricaemia

In general and hospital practice hyperuricaemia, in the absence of gout or any of its recognised complications, is a common finding. This is not surprising considering the high prevalence of factors such as obesity, alcohol overconsumption, hypertension, and diuretic use in the community. The majority of subjects with hyperuricaemia are asymptomatic but the risks of developing the manifestations of gout increases with rising urate levels. In men this risk rises from 0.5% per annum at urate levels of 0.42 mmol/L to 5.5% per annum at levels of 0.54 mmol/L. Hence no patient with asymptomatic hyperuricaemia should be ignored, particularly since most of the causes are treatable. The plasma urate level at which active urate-lowering drugs should be administered is a matter of controversy but it is generally acknowledged that plasma levels above 0.80 mmol/L should be treated as a matter of urgency.

EVALUATION OF HYPERURICAEMIA

In all subjects with hyperuricaemia, whether gouty or not, there should be a thorough clinical examination to determine the presence of any contributing factors and, in addition, relevant laboratory tests to evaluate renal function and the renal handling of urate excretion.

Figure 9.3 is a checklist for the evaluation of hyperuricaemia.

Hyperuricaemia

Exclude — Potentially correctable contributory factors:
- Obesity
- Alcohol
- Hypertriglyceridaemia
- Drugs (esp. thiazides)*
- Hypertension
- Low fluid intake

Consider —

High Purine Intake
Diet (meats, yeast pdts.)

Increased Urate Production
PRIMARY
- Idiopathic
- Enzyme defects
SECONDARY
- Blood dyscrasias
- Infectious mononucleosis
- Malignancy
- Cytotoxic therapy
- Psoriasis
- Alcoholism
- Exercise (prolonged)

Decreased Renal Excretion
PRIMARY
- Idiopathic
SECONDARY
- Renal failure†
- Dehydration
- Diuretics
- Ketonaemia
  - starvation
  - diabetes mellitus
- Hyperlactataemia
  - alcohol
  - toxaemia of pregnancy
- Drugs*
- Hyperparathyroidism

If cause obscure consider 24 h urinary excretion rate before and after a 5-day low purine diet

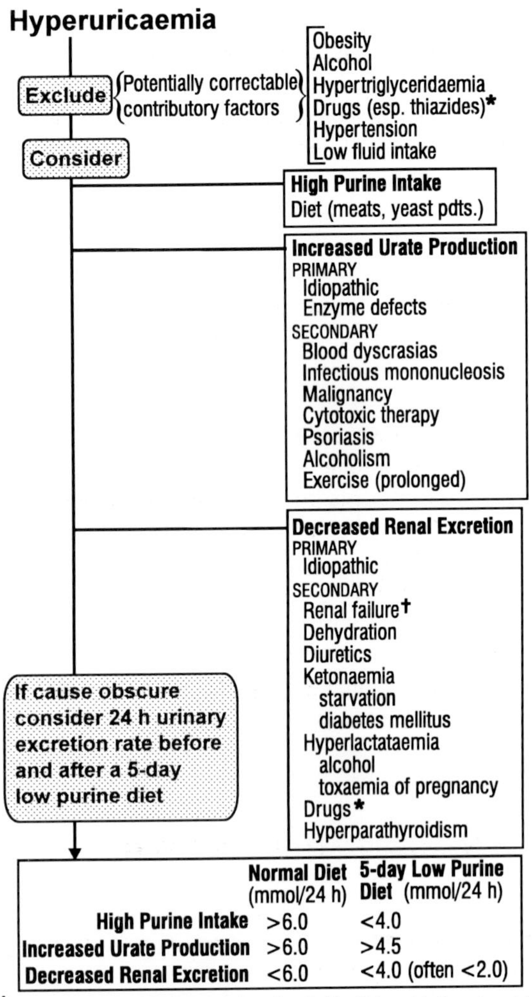

	Normal Diet (mmol/24 h)	5-day Low Purine Diet (mmol/24 h)
High Purine Intake	>6.0	<4.0
Increased Urate Production	>6.0	>4.5
Decreased Renal Excretion	<6.0	<4.0 (often <2.0)

*Drugs: Diuretics, Salicylates (low dose), Nicotinic acid, Pyrazinamide, Ethambutol, Cyclosporin.

†Renal failure: If cause, then serum [creatinine] will be >0.40 mmol/L, serum [urate] <0.65 mmol/L & urine urate:creatinine ratio <0.7. If hyperuricaemia causing the renal failure then serum urate >0.7 mmol/L & urine urate:creat ratio >0.7.

Figure 9.3. Checklist for the evaluation of hyperuricaemia.

Clinical aspects. During the clinical examination particular attention should be given to the factors contributing to hyperuricaemia as noted above -- diet, alcohol consumption, obesity, diuretic therapy, etc.

Laboratory aspects. The questions that need to be answered are:

- Is there renal disease?
- Is there urate overproduction?
- Is there a high dietary purine intake?
- Is there renal underexcretion of urate?

These questions can be answered by estimating the urinary creatinine clearance, the 24-hour urate excretion rate, and the urinary urate clearance on a 24-hour urine collected during the period of the patient's normal diet and one collected after the patient has been on a purine-free diet for at least five days. The normal values for these parameters are of the following order:

Creatinine clearance: 90-120 mL/min
24-hour urate excretion rate:
    (a) normal diet <6.0 mmol/day,
    (b) purine-free diet <3.6 mmol/day,
    (c) fall in urate excretion after a 5-day
        purine-free diet: ~1.2 mmol/day
Urate clearance: 8-12 mL/min

Interpretation

- *Primary renal disease.* This is manifested by a low creatinine clearance.

- *Urate overproduction.* On a purine-free diet the urate excretion rate will be >3.6 mmol/day.

- *Excessive purine ingestion.* The fall in urate excretion after a purine-free diet will be in excess of 1.5 mmol/day.

- *Primary urate underexcretion.* The creatinine clearance will be normal, the urate clearance will be below 8 mL/min, and on a purine-free diet the urate excretion will be <3.6 mmol/day.

Plasma Urate Lowering Drugs

Three groups of drugs are available for the management of gout and hyperuricaemia.

Allopurinol and derivatives. These are structural analogues of hypoxanthine and xanthine which inhibit the enzyme xanthine oxidase, thus producing low plasma and urine urate levels (Figure 9.4).

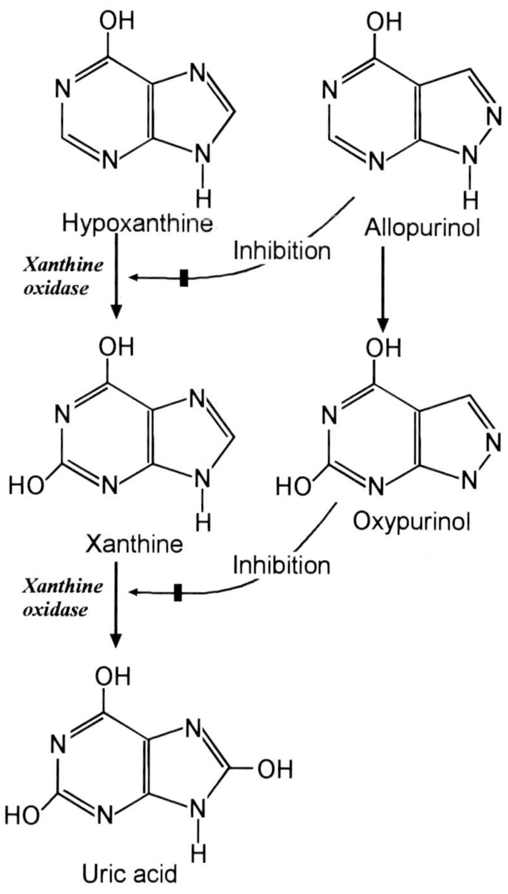

Figure 9.4. Structures and sites of action of allopurinol and oxypurinol, competitive inhibitors of xanthine oxidase activity used in treatment of hyperuricaemia.

Uricosuric agents. These drugs, e.g., Probenecid, lower the plasma urate by inhibiting renal tubular urate reabsorption.

Anti-inflammatory agents. These agents, e.g., colchicine, indomethacin, are used to relieve the pain of gouty arthritis and have no effect on the plasma urate level.

Hypouricaemia

Hypouricaemia, unlike hyperuricaemia, is of little clinical importance but such a finding may provide the clue to some unrecognised disorder. The commonest cause is allopurinol therapy.

Causes

Decreased urate production
    Xanthine oxidase deficiency
    Allopurinol therapy

Increased urate excretion
    Fanconi syndrome
    Uricosuric agents (inc. high doses of salicylates)
    SIADH (inappropriate anti-diuresis)
    Isolated tubular defects
    Early pregnancy

Factitious
    High plasma vitamin C levels, due to high dietary intake, can interfere with plasma urate estimation.

REFERENCES/FURTHER READING

Alvsaker JO. Metabolic aspects of gout. Scand J Rheumatol 1984;53:54-63.

Boss GR and Seegmiller JE. Hyperuricemia and gout. N Engl J Med 1979;300:1459-1468.

Emerson BT. Identification of the causes of persistent hyperuricaemia. Lancet 1991;337:1461-1463.

Roubenoff RR. Gout and hyperuricaemia. Rheumat Dis Clinics North Am 1990;16:539-551.

Chapter 10

Glucose, Lactate and Ketones

Glucose metabolism

The metabolic pathways of glucose metabolism and their regulation are more appropriately dealt with in textbooks of biochemistry. Only an outline, with emphasis on the more important aspects relating to pathophysiological processes met with in medical practice, will be covered in this section.

Glucose is the most important source of energy for most tissues. Many tissues can also utilise fatty acids as fuel but tissues lacking mitochondria (e.g., the red blood cells) or are deficient in mitochondria (e.g., renal medulla, testes) cannot utilise fat for energy (fatty acid oxidation takes place within the mitochondria). Such tissues are dependant solely on glucose as fuel; thus maintenance of the blood glucose level is essential for survival. The brain is unique in that it can utilise both glucose and ketone bodies, but not fatty acids, as metabolic fuels. Homeostatic mechanisms governing glucose metabolism serve to maintain fuel supply to the central nervous system.

In the postprandial state excess glucose is converted to both glycogen (glycogenesis) and triglycerides (lipogenesis), and stored as such. In the fasting, or starvation, state the lack of exogenous glucose is overcome by production of endogenous glucose by gluconeogenesis (formation of glucose from amino acids, lactate and glycerol) and glycogenolysis (glycogen breakdown). The major regulators of these metabolic processes are insulin (Figure 10.1) and the counter-regulatory hormones, glucagon, cortisol, and the catecholamines.

Glycolysis

This is the metabolic pathway by which glucose is oxidised to pyruvate with the production of 2 ATP molecules. The control of this process is complex but the main factors are insulin, which enhances, and glucagon, which suppresses. These two hormones act by influencing enzyme complexes along the glycolytic pathway. Further oxidation of pyruvate in the tricarboxylic acid (TCA) or citric acid cycle produces a further 36 molecules of ATP (Figure 10.2).

In the presence of sufficient energy (ATP) for metabolic requirements the pyruvate is converted to

acetyl-CoA but this is not channelled into the TCA cycle; rather, acetyl CoA which is the first building block for the formation of fatty acids and hence triglyceride production, is an important intermediate in the interrelationships between carbohydrate and lipid metabolism (Figure 10.1).

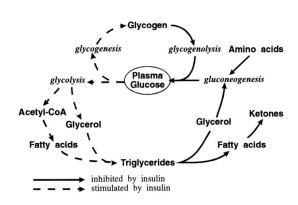

Figure 10.1. Metabolic factors controlling the blood glucose level.

Gluconeogenesis

This process, which occurs in the liver and renal cortex during glucose-starved states, produces glucose from pyruvate which is in turn derived from protein (alanine) and lactate. It is an energy-requiring process which is basically a reversal of glycolysis but for three steps -- those catalysed by the enzymes *hexokinase, phosphofructose kinase,* and *pyruvate kinase.* These irreversible steps are circumvented by alternate reactions catalysed by the gluconeogenic enzymes: glucose-6-phosphatase, 1,6-bisphosphatase, pyruvate carboxylase, and phosphoenolpyruvate carboxykinase. Conversion of pyruvate to phosphoenol-pyruvate is a two-step process involving the last two enzymes (Figures 10.2 and 10.3).

The process occurs during fasting so that predominant glucose-requiring tissues (brain, red cells, etc) have a ready supply of energy. The main controllers

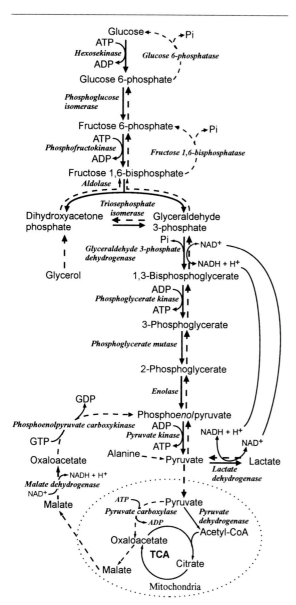

Figure 10.2. Metabolism of glucose. The pathways of glycolysis and the citrate (TCA) cycle are drawn with unbroken lines, the steps for gluconeogenesis are depicted by the broken, dashed lines. The citrate cycle reactions take place inside the mitochondria. Names of key enzymes are in italics.

are insulin (which inhibits), glucagon (which stimulates), and cortisol (which stimulates the process by mobilising muscle amino acids). Glycerol, an end-product of triglyceride breakdown, can also be converted to glucose.

Glycogenesis and glycogenolysis

Glycogen synthesis (glycogenesis) from glucose occurs during a plentiful glucose supply (fed state). It is stimulated by insulin (by its action on glycogen synthetase) and inhibited by glucagon. The breakdown of glycogen to glucose-6-phosphate (glycogenolysis) occurs during glucopenic states and is stimulated by glucagon and catecholamines and inhibited by insulin.

In the fed state the liver contains about 70-80 grams of glycogen; muscle tissues contain an additional 150 grams. The hepatic glycogen stores represents a readily convertible source of glucose for all tissues -- glycogen is broken down to glucose-6-phosphate which is then converted to glucose by glucose-6-phosphatase. Because muscle tissues lack the latter enzyme, glucose is not produced from

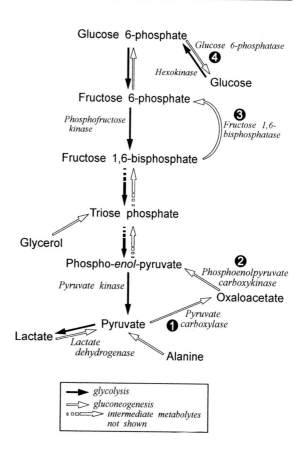

Figure 10.3. Key gluconeogenic reactions catalysed by specific gluconeogenic enzymes.

muscle glycogen. Rather, glycogen is converted to lactate which can then be transported to the liver to be converted to glucose via gluconeogenesis, a process known as the Cori cycle. These glycogen stores are limited and are depleted after 18-24 hours of fasting.

Fatty acid β-oxidation

The conversion of fatty acids to acetyl-CoA with the production of energy is referred to as β-oxidation and takes place in the mitochondria. It occurs during glucopenic states and plays an important role in energy supply for many tissues during fasting. The acetyl-CoA can either enter the citric acid (TCA) cycle and produce more energy (ATP) or may be diverted to the production of ketone bodies which are a major source of energy for the brain during prolonged fasting.

Ketogenesis

The formation of ketone bodies (acetoacetate, β-hydroxybutyrate and acetone) from acetyl-CoA during glucopenic states occurs almost exclusively in the liver although the renal cortex is also capable of ketogenesis. It will be discussed in later sections (see page 00).

Carbohydrate digestion and absorption

On average, around 40-45% of dietary calories are derived from carbohydrates. In a young adult male, for example, this represents about 300-350 g which is mainly in the form of starch (plant sources) and glycogen (animal sources); in addition there may be significant amounts of the disaccharides sucrose and lactose.

Salivary and pancreatic amylases convert starch and glycogen to a mixture of D-glucose and maltose; the latter is in turn cleaved into two D-glucose molecules by intestinal maltase located in the brush border of the small bowel epithelial cells. The D-glucose is actively transported across the epithelial cells to the portal venous system and carried to the liver. In the liver it is phosphorylated and enters one of several possible metabolic pathways responsible for its disposition.

Sucrose and lactose are also acted upon by brush border-located disaccharidases -- sucrase converts sucrose to D-glucose and D-fructose and lactase transforms lactose to D-glucose and D-galactose. As in the case of D-glucose, D-galactose and D-fructose are actively absorbed across the gut epithelial cells, transported to the liver, and then phosphorylated.

The liver and glucose metabolism

D-glucose is transported into the hepatocyte by an insulin-independant process and phosphorylated to glucose-6-phosphate by the enzymes hexokinase and glucokinase. Further metabolic processes depend on the prevailing nutritional status and the action of the counter-regulatory hormones (glucagon, growth hormone, cortisol, catecholamines). Although glucose does not require insulin to enter the hepatocyte the ensuing disposition is markedly insulin-sensitive.

In the fed state, and resultant high insulin activity, anabolic activities predominate with glucose entering several metabolic ventures:

↑ glycogen synthesis and ↓ glycogen breakdown →
    ↑ glycogen storage

↑ fatty acid and triglyceride synthesis → fat storage

inhibition of gluconeogenesis → protein conservation

The energy for these activities are, in part, provided by the oxidation of glucose via glycolysis and the citric cycle. The net effect is storage of glucose as glycogen and triglyceride, and protein conservation.

During starvation, as a result of relative insulinopenia and increased activity of the counter-regulatory hormones, the liver reverts into a glucose-producing organ. The immediate stimulus for this activity is a low insulin:glucagon ratio and increased cortisol and catecholamine activity, which result in:

↓ glycogen synthesis and ↑ glycogen breakdown →
    ↑ glucose

↑ glucose formation from protein (gluconeogenesis)

↓ fatty acid and triglyceride synthesis from glucose and ↑ breakdown of fat stores (lipolysis) → energy and ketone bodies via β-oxidation of the fatty acids

Hence in the absence of a sustained exogenous glucose supply, there is hepatic production of glucose from glycogen and protein and most of the required energy is derived from fat (β-oxidation of fatty acids and formation of ketone bodies).

Extrahepatic tissues and glucose metabolism

All body tissues utilise glucose for energy production, although most can also oxidise alternative fuels. Insulin is necessary for glucose uptake by the nonhepatic tissues (cf liver). This is effected through an insulin receptor which, when activated, mobilises a transmembrane glycoprotein-glucose transporter which cycles between the plasma membrane and intracellular compartments. Once inside the cell the glucose is phosphorylated by hexokinase to glucose-6-phosphate and then diverted to the same processes that operate in the liver.

Hormones regulating carbohydrate metabolism

Insulin. Insulin, secreted by the β-cells of the pancreas in response to a high blood glucose, is a peptide hormone (MW ~6000) consisting of two chains (a 21 amino acid A chain and a 30 amino acid B chain) joined by two disulphide bridges. It is produced as proinsulin which contains an additional 31 amino acid residue connecting peptide (C-peptide) joining the A and B chains. This is transported into the Golgi complex where it is proteolysed to form the biologically inactive C-peptide and active native insulin, both of which are secreted in equimolar amounts.

Control of insulin secretion. Glucose is the most important stimulus for insulin secretion but it can also be stimulated by physiological concentrations of amino acids, ketone bodies, fatty acids, acetylcholine, and adrenaline. Blood glucose concentrations above 5.5 mmol/L produce an immediate response with secretion occurring in two phases:

- an immediate burst with peak levels occurring at one minute, followed by a fall-off to low secretion levels of variable duration
- a second, more prolonged peak of secretion which lasts 15 to 30 minutes

Insulin action. Insulin diffuses from the capillaries and binds to specific cell surface receptors which are activated to produce its blood glucose-lowering and anabolic effects by stimulating glucose transport into cells and inducing, or inhibiting, a number of enzyme complexes. The major activities are:

1. Stimulation of anabolic processes

a. Promotes entry of glucose and amino acids into muscle cells and glucose into adipose tissue cells.
b. Stimulates glycolysis by induction of the enzymes hexokinase, phosphofructokinase, and pyruvate kinase thus increasing the building blocks (acetyl CoA, ATP, NADPH) for macromolecules.
c. Stimulates glycogen and fatty acid synthesis in the liver, triglyceride synthesis in adipose tissues, and glycogen and protein synthesis in muscle tissues.

2. Inhibition of catabolic processes

a. Inhibits gluconeogcnesis.
b. Inhibits fat breakdown and β-oxidation of fatty acids and ketogenesis.
c. Inhibits glycogenolysis.

3. Potassium homeostasis
Insulin increases the cellular uptake of potassium ions. This is independent of its action on glucose.

Counter-regulatory hormones. This group of hormones are so called because they oppose the action of insulin and excess production of any of them results in hyperglycaemia. They are 'starvation hormones' which are called into play when exogenous glucose intake is low and consequently stimulate the production of glucose from glycogen (glycogenolysis) and protein (gluconeogenesis), and generation of energy from fatty acids via β-oxidation.

Glucagon. This straight chain polypeptide of 29 amino acids (MW 3500) is secreted by the α-cells of the pancreas in response to hypoglycaemia (and inhibited by hyperglycaemia). Its main action is to increase glucose release by the liver but, in association with a low insulin, it also stimulates free fatty acid release and increases ketogenesis (page 136). In summary, glucagon *stimulates* glycogenolysis, gluconeogenesis, β-oxidation of fatty acids and ketogenesis; and *inhibits* glycogenesis, fatty acid synthesis (lipogenesis), and glycolysis.

Cortisol. Cortisol, secreted by the adrenal cortex, increases glucose production by:

a. Decreasing glucose and amino acid uptake by muscle

b. Mobilising muscle protein to increase delivery of amino acids to the liver for gluconeogenesis

c. Increasing gluconeogenesis

Catecholamines. Adrenaline (and to a lesser extent noradrenaline) is secreted by the adrenal medulla and the sympathetic nerve endings in response to hypoglycaemia. In the context of glucose metabolism, catecholamines:

a. Increase release of fatty acids from adipose tissue
b. Stimulate glycogen degradation to glucose
c. Inhibit cellular glucose uptake
d. Stimulate glucagon secretion and depresses insulin secretion.

The end result is increased glucose production by the liver.

Growth hormone. The relationship between growth hormone and glucose metabolism is unclear but excessive secretion, as in acromegaly, is often associated with hyperglycaemia. Growth hormone secretion responds to the blood glucose levels -- hyperglycaemia suppresses, and hypoglycaemia stimulates, secretion.

Hyperglycaemia

Hyperglycaemia is defined as either a fasting blood glucose level greater than 7.8 mmol/L or a random level in excess of 11.1 mmol/L. There are many causes but these can be conveniently divided into two groups, *diabetes mellitus* and *non-diabetic causes*.

Non-diabetic causes of hyperglycaemia

- postprandial
- factitious
- drug-related
- non-pancreatic endocrine disease
- pancreatic disease other than diabetes mellitus
- stress

Postprandial. After a carbohydrate meal blood glucose levels may exceed 12.0 mmol/L (in the first

hour) in patients with gastrectomy (page 00), and in non-diabetic subjects with liver disease, obesity, acromegaly, Cushing's disease, phaeochromocytoma, or on steroid therapy (all due to tissue insensitivity to insulin); and also in patients with pancreatitis and those on thiazide diuretics and phenytoin (all due to reduced insulin secretion).

Factitious. If the blood sample is mistakenly taken from a vein above a glucose infusion very high glucose levels (e.g., >100 mmol/L) can be obtained.

Drug-related. Some drugs (e.g., glucocorticoids, nicotinic acid, sympathetomimetic drugs) can cause hyperglycaemia by producing tissue insensitivity to insulin; others (e.g., thiazide diuretics and phenytoin), by inhibiting insulin secretion.

Non-pancreatic endocrine disease: Excessive production of the 'anti-insulin' hormones such as growth hormone (acromegaly), cortisol (Cushing's syndrome), and catecholamines (phaeochromocytoma) may result in hyperglycaemia and indeed produce a diabetic picture (secondary diabetes mellitus).

Pancreatic disorders: Decreased insulin secretion and secondary diabetes mellitus may be associated with partial pancreatectomy, chronic pancreatitis, and haemochromatosis. Total pancreatectomy, of course, will result in diabetes mellitus.

Stress: Stress (physical and psychogenic) increases the secretion of a number of hormones, including cortisol and the catecholamines, which may induce fasting hyperglycaemia. However, the blood glucose level reached is usually less than 10 mmol/L. Hence 'stress-related' hyperglycaemia, as may occur during an acute myocardial infarct, in excess of 10.0 mmol/L usually indicates underlying diabetes mellitus. Such patients should be appropriately re-evaluated after the period of stress has resolved.

Diabetes mellitus

Diabetes mellitus is defined as a state of chronic hyperglycaemia. It is a syndrome of disordered metabolism resulting in hyperglycaemia due to either absolute insulin deficiency or reduced tissue response to insulin, or both. To establish the diagnosis, any of the following three conditions need to be demonstrated.

- A random plasma glucose >11.1 mmol/L in the setting of classical symptoms and signs of diabetes (polyuria, polydipsia, weight loss, etc)
- Two fasting blood glucose exceeding 7.8 mmol/L.
- A blood glucose >11.1 mmol/L 2 hours after an oral 75 g glucose load.

Diabetes is usually classified into three major types, *type I or insulin dependant diabetes mellitus, type II or non-insulin dependant diabetes mellitus,* and *gestational diabetes mellitus.* A closely related disorder is *impaired glucose tolerance.*

Type I diabetes mellitus (insulin-dependant diabetes mellitus, IDDM)

This type represents 5-10% of all diabetics and usually presents in juveniles although adults are occasionally involved. It is caused by autoimmune destruction of the pancreatic β-cells causing decreased or absent insulin secretion which results in hyperglycaemia (and ketoacidosis if untreated). It is a catabolic disease which, in addition to hyperglycaemia and glycosuria, presents with weight loss, polyuria (nocturia), polydipsia, ketonuria, and ketonaemia.

Circulating islet cell antibodies have been detected in up to 85% of such patients and the majority also have detectable anti-insulin antibodies prior to receiving insulin therapy. Most of the islet cell antibodies are directed against *glutamic acid decarboxylase*, an enzyme located in the pancreatic β-cells.

The exact cause of the disease is unknown but it is thought to result from an infectious or toxic insult to the pancreatic islet cells. Some human leucocyte antigens (HLA) have a strong association with this disorder, e.g., 95% possess either HLA-DR3 or HLA-DR4. HLA-DQ gene associations are even more specific (HLA-DQw3.2 is found in the DR4 patients).

Type II diabetes (non-insulin dependant diabetes mellitus, NIDDM)

This is a heterogeneous group of diabetic patients who usually present in adulthood although juvenile cases (maturity-onset diabetes of the young, MODY) have been described. These constitute 90-95% of all diabetics and the disorder differs from IDDM in that significant amounts of insulin can be demonstrated in the blood (presumably this prevents the development of ketosis which is characteristic of IDDM). It is usually described as a non-ketotic form of diabetes not linked to HLA markers, that has no associated islet cell antibodies, and is not dependant on insulin for management. Most patients are over the age of 40 years and polydipsia and polyuria are unusual presentations. Hypertension, hyperlipidaemia and atherosclerosis are common accompaniments.

The cause is unknown but there is tissue insensitivity to insulin and a defect in pancreatic β-cell response to glucose, e.g., early in the disease there is delayed and excessive insulin secretion. Peripheral insulin resistance induces the pancreas to hypersecrete the hormone, resulting in hyperinsulinism which has been linked to complications such as accelerated atherosclerosis and hypertension. One such condition is the recently described syndrome X (insulin resistance syndrome) consisting of hyperglycaemia, hyperinsulinism, hyperlipidaemia, and hypertension which leads to coronary artery disease and stroke.

Two subgroups of type II diabetes mellitus are distinguished by the absence, or presence, of obesity:

- *Non-obese type II* in which, in addition to insulin resistance, there is an absent or blunted early phase of insulin release in response to glucose (see page 00). Some of these patients may be mild type I diabetics.

- *Obese type II* in which the major factor is insensitivity to insulin which is believed to be due to a post-receptor defect in insulin action related to over-distended storage deposits in the cells. When overfeeding is corrected, improvement occurs (storage deposits become less saturated).

Heredity has a stronger role in type II diabetics than in type I, e.g., monozygotic twin studies of NIDDM probands showed a concordance rate of diabetics in excess of 90%, in IDDM the rate is around 50%.

Gestational diabetes

A diabetic woman may become pregnant and a pregnant woman may develop diabetes during her pregnancy. The latter situation, glucose intolerance first detected during pregnancy, is termed gestational diabetes. Such subjects should not be labelled 'diabetic'

Impaired glucose tolerance (IGT)

An oral glucose tolerance test using a 75 g glucose load (see below) is considered normal if the 2-hour blood glucose is less than 7.8 mmol/L, and diabetic when this level exceeds 11.1 mmol/L. If the value falls between 7.8 and 11.1 mmol/L, then the term impaired glucose tolerance (IGT) is applied. Various surveys conducted over a ten-year period have revealed that 2-5% of patients with IGT revert to normal, 20-50% (average 25%) become diabetic, and the remainder maintain the IGT state.

PATHOPHYSIOLOGY AND METABOLIC CONSEQUENCES OF DIABETES MELLITUS

As stated above the basic defect in diabetes mellitus is insulin deficiency (absolute or relative) which affects glucose, lipid, protein, potassium, and phosphate metabolism and, in addition, indirectly influences water and sodium homeostasis. In severe cases of (untreated) type I diabetes there is hyperglycaemia, ketoacidosis, and high blood levels of triglycerides, fatty acids, potassium, and phosphate in addition to disturbances of acid-base balance, and of sodium and water metabolism.

Hyperglycaemia. This is due to increased hepatic glucose production and decreased cellular glucose uptake.

Increased hepatic production: Insulin lack and the unopposed actions of glucagon and adrenaline cause decreased glycogenesis and increased glycogenolysis. In addition, the unopposed action of cortisol (low insulin) increases gluconeogenesis (Figure 10.4).

Decreased peripheral uptake: Insulin deficiency inhibits cellular glucose uptake and glycolysis. Substrates other than glucose (fatty acids, ketones) are substituted for energy production.

The consequences of hyperglycaemia are:

• Increased urinary glucose which results in osmotic diuresis and consequent loss of water, sodium, potassium, and phosphate ions, hence body depletion of these four substances.

• Increased tonicity of the extracellular fluid which draws water out of the cells producing cellular dehydration and, if the subject is still able to take water orally, dilution of the extracellular analytes which may result in hyponatraemia (hypertonic hyponatraemia, page 19).

Disturbances of protein metabolism. Diabetes mellitus is a catabolic state associated with protein wasting due mainly to increased gluconeogenesis -- for each 100 g of glucose produced, around 175 g of proteins are destroyed (Figure 10.4).

Disturbances of fat metabolism. Insulin lack and the unopposed action of glucagon and adrenaline stimulate lipolysis and the release of fatty acids into the circulation (Figure 10.4). These are taken up by the cells and converted to energy (β-oxidation), ketones (page 136), and triglycerides which are released from the liver in the form of very low density lipoproteins (VLDL, page 193). In addition, insulin deficiency inhibits lipoprotein lipase activity which depresses the clearance of both VLDL and chylomicrons, further increasing the blood triglyceride level.

Hyperkalaemia. A direct action of insulin is the cellular uptake of potassium ions. In insulin deficiency potassium leaks out of the cells, resulting in hyperkalaemia. Some of this potassium is lost in the urine, as a consequence of osmotic diuresis, causing potassium depletion which may be of the order of 200-400 mmol. When insulin is administered, the extracellular potassium returns to the cells and this may result in severe hypokalaemia unless potassium supplements are administered.

Hyperphosphataemia. Insulin, by stimulating glycolysis which utilises inorganic phosphate (production of ATP, etc), increases cellular phosphate uptake. In insulin lack this ion leaks out of the cells, resulting in high plasma levels. Like potassium, some is lost in the urine causing a body deficit and, like potassium, when insulin is administered it moves back into the cells, resulting in severe hypophosphataemia.

Acid-base disturbances. The characteristic acid-base disturbance in type I diabetes is a high anion gap metabolic acidosis due to diabetic ketoacidosis (page

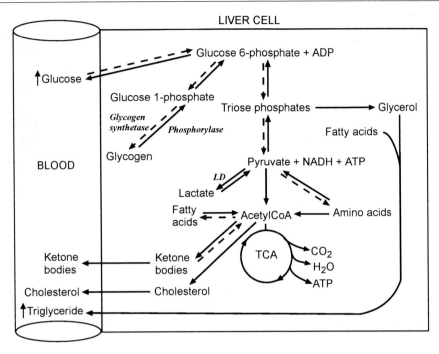

Figure 10.4. Characteristic changes in carbohydrate, fat, and protein metabolism associated with diabetes mellitus.

51). The plasma bicarbonate concentration can fall to below 5 mmol/L with pH values as low as 6.80. There may also be an associated moderate lactic acidosis.

Sodium and water disturbances. As stated above hyponatraemia may occur as a consequence of the extracellular hyperglycaemia. In addition, there may be an element of pseudohyponatraemia due to hyper-lipidaemia (page 19). Also, there is usually total body sodium depletion due to urinary sodium loss as a consequence of osmotic diuresis.

If the patient's consciousness is adequate and he can respond to thirst, any water lost as a result of osmotic diuresis will be replaced by oral intake. As the patient becomes very ill and confused he may not respond to thirst and become dehydrated and, depending on the degree of dehydration, the plasma sodium level may rise and hypernatraemia may occur.

COMPLICATIONS OF DIABETES MELLITUS

From a biochemical point of view the important complications are:

- diabetic ketoacidosis
- lactic acidosis
- hyperosmolar coma
- renal disease
- hyperlipidaemia

Diabetic ketoacidosis. In type I diabetes, ketoacid-osis may be the original presenting problem or may result from increased insulin requirements during the course of stress situations such as infections, trauma, and surgery. It is uncommon in type II diabetes but may occur if there is severe stress, such as infections. The subjects appear severely ill, often very dehydrated, and have rapid deep breathing with the odour of acetone on their breath (Kussmaul respiration). Hypotension, tachycardia, and abdominal pain are common. If untreated, they progress through mental stupor to coma.

The characteristic laboratory findings are:

- hyperglycaemia -- usually >20 mmol/L but values can be as low as 15 mmol/L
- high anion gap metabolic acidosis with blood pH <7.30 and plasma bicarbonate <10 mmol/L

- serum and urine positive for ketones -- the serum levels can be of the order of 5-20 mmol/L (total)
- hyperkalaemia
- hyperphosphataemia

The pathophysiology of ketosis is discussed on page 136 but, basically, it is related to insulin lack and a low insulin:glucagon ratio which increases lipolysis in adipose tissue with fatty acid release. These are taken up by the liver and converted to ketone bodies (acetoacetate, β-hydroxybutyrate, and acetone) by stimulated liver ketogenesis.

It is important to recognise that in diabetic ketoacidosis the major ketone body in the serum is β-hydroxybutyrate with lesser amounts of acetoacetate, and that only acetoacetate is detected by the nitroprusside reaction (Acetest, Ketostix). This can be misleading if serum is being tested by the nitroprusside method, e.g., during circulatory collapse the formation of lactic acid (page 140) can shift the redox state to increase β-hydroxybutyrate at the expense of the detectable acetoacetate. Hence it is possible to have severe ketoacidosis and only a slightly positive serum nitroprusside reaction.

Two other points of biochemical interest concern serum amylase and creatinine.

- An elevated serum amylase, often of both salivary and pancreatic origin, is common during diabetic ketoacidosis and, as these patients often have abdominal pain, the mistaken diagnosis of acute pancreatitis can be made.

- The serum creatinine levels are usually elevated because of dehydration, but also because acetoacetate will give a positive interference in its estimation by the Jaffe reaction. Hence serum creatinine concentrations (if measured by the above method) are not a reliable guide to renal function early in the disease process.

Lactic acidosis. Lactic acidosis (page 140) is not uncommon in any seriously ill patient and this holds for diabetes, particularly during ketoacidosis, where up to 50% of patients also have high blood lactate levels. The cause is of multiple origin but is probably due to poor tissue perfusion as a consequence of both dehydration and the vascular complications of diabetes.

Hyperosmolar non-ketotic hyperglycaemic coma. In the middle-aged and elderly patients with mild diabetes hyperglycaemic coma with no, or minimal, ketosis is commoner than ketoacidosis. It presents with slowly developing lethargy, confusion, and dehydration with the following characteristic biochemical features:

- hyperglycaemia with values in excess of 40 mmol/L
- very high serum osmolality: >320 mosmol/kg
- no or minimal acidaemia: blood pH >7.30 and plasma bicarbonate >15 mmol/L
- normal serum anion gap

The cause is not completely clear but it is suggested that there is sufficient circulating insulin to prevent excessive hepatic ketogenesis but insufficient to maintain normal glucose homeostasis. The resulting severe hyperglycaemia causes massive glycosuria and osmotic diuresis with excessive water loss. The hyperosmolality (due to hyperglycaemia) causes mental confusion and the subject is unable to respond to thirst to replace his water losses -- hence dehydration.

The high extracellular osmolality draws water out of the cells. This water dilutes the extracellular analytes and can result in hyponatraemia but, as the patient becomes severely water depleted (urinary loss plus decreased intake), the serum sodium will rise and hypernatraemia often occurs. Sodium levels in excess of 170 mmol/L are not uncommon.

Renal disease. Around 10-25% of patients being treated for end-stage renal disease have diabetic nephropathy. This is basically due to the diabetes-associated disease of the small blood vessels and is initially manifested by proteinuria and the nephrotic syndrome; subsequently, as renal function declines, there is a rise in the serum urea and creatinine, leading eventually to fully developed renal failure. Urinary microalbumin estimations are useful in the early detection of the disorder (see below).

Hyperlipidaemias. The lipid abnormalities associated with diabetes mellitus include:

Hypertriglyceridaemia due to high circulating VLDL: Insulin deficiency inhibits lipoprotein lipase which decreases the clearance of the VLDL and, in addition, there is increased hepatic synthesis of VLDL (stimulation of lipolysis releases fatty acids from the adipose tissue and some of these are converted to triglycerides and VLDLs in the liver).

130

Hypercholesterolaemia: Type II diabetes, glucose intolerance, and tissue insulin insensitivity are commonly associated with hypercholesterolaemia (Syndrome X, see above) and if the diabetic patient develops the nephrotic syndrome, hypercholesterolaemia will occur as it is a part of this complex (page 84).

CLINICAL AND LABORATORY EVALUATION

Clinical evaluation:

The characteristic features of type I diabetes are polyuria, polydipsia, and rapid weight loss in a young subject. Often the presenting picture is ketotic coma with nausea, vomiting, and mental stupor associated with dehydration and the characteristic deep breathing of metabolic acidosis. Type II diabetes characteristically occurs in obese subjects over the age of 40 years. Polyuria and polydipsia are often present but most patients have few or minimal symptoms and are initially recognised on the basis of an incidental finding of glycosuria or hyperglycaemia.

Laboratory evaluation:

(1) *Diagnosis.* The accepted criteria for the diagnosis of diabetes mellitus is the demonstration of a fasting plasma glucose value in excess of 7.8 mmol/L on at least two occasions. If the fasting level is less than 7.8 mmol/L in a subject suspected of the disorder (glycosuria, polyuria, polydipsia, etc) a standard oral glucose tolerance test is appropriate.

(2) *Monitoring therapy:* In addition to regular plasma glucose estimations, other useful tests include glycosylated haemoglobin, serum fructosamine, and urinary microalbumin excretion rate.

Oral glucose tolerance test (OGGT)

The usual protocol for carrying out an OGGT is:

- Ensure that the patient is on a normal mixed diet for at least 3-days prior to the test. Normal subjects deprived of carbohydrate may show glucose intolerance and mild diabetics on a high carbohydrate diet can produce a near normal response. This reflects enzyme induction (or suppression) affecting the glycolytic pathway. Acute illness and

drugs such as diuretics, contraceptive medications, glucocorticoids, nicotinic acid, and phenytoin may also impair glucose tolerance.

- The patient fasts overnight and presents for the test between 0800 and 0900 hours. During the test the patient should sit quietly and refrain from cigarette smoking.

- A blood sample is obtained for measurement of the fasting glucose value after which a drink containing 75 g of glucose in solution is administered. Blood samples are taken at 60 minutes and 120 minutes after the glucose administration. Urine samples for glucose are not necessary but may be useful to exclude renal glycosuria.

Interpretation: (plasma glucose values in mmol/L, from venous blood samples)

	normal response	impaired glucose tolerance	diabetes mellitus
Fasting	<6.8	6.8-7.8	>7.8
1-hour	<11.1	<11.1	>11.1
2-hour	<7.8	7.8-11.1	>11.1

The most important measurement is the 2-hour glucose level as the diagnosis depends on this value.

Note: A 75 g glucose meal is a fairly non-physiological challenge and the response varies with age which makes interpretation difficult at times. For these reasons many clinicians depend on the documentation of fasting hyperglycaemia rather than the glucose tolerance test for the diagnosis of diabetes mellitus.

Glycosylated haemoglobin (haemoglobin A_{1c})

Chronic hyperglycaemia is associated with non-enzymatic condensation of glucose with free amino groups of basic amino acids on the globin chains of haemoglobin. The major form of this complex is haemoglobin A_{1c} which comprises 4-6% of the total haemoglobin. The synthesis of haemoglobin A_{1c}

(Figure 10.5) is a two-step process with initial formation of an aldimine or Schiff base (labile pre-A_{1c} component) which then undergoes molecular rearrangement to form the stable ketoamine.

Haemoglobin A_{1c} levels in excess of 6% indicate chronic hyperglycaemia and the higher the prevailing glucose level, the higher this percentage will be. Hence it has been found to be a useful analyte in the evaluation of the efficacy of diabetic therapy, e.g.,

- To judge the degree of chronic glucose control in both Type I and II diabetic patients, especially those who are non-compliant or uncooperative

- To obtain information on chronic diabetic control during intercurrent illness

- To monitor the efficacy of changes in therapy

- To differentiate transient glucose intolerance associated with stress (e.g., post-surgical stress) from previously unrecognised diabetes

- To identify insulin-treated subjects at higher risk for hypoglycaemia (see below)

Since the life span of red cells is around 120 days the glycosylated haemoglobin level reflects the state of glycaemia over the previous 8-12 weeks; thus, measurements should be made at 2-3 month intervals to monitor the patient's progress.

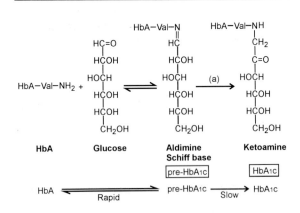

(a) Amadori rearrangement

Figure 10.5. Reaction pathway for the synthesis of haemoglobin A_{1c}.

Available methods differ in the measurement of *total* haemoglobin A_1 (including A_{1a}, A_{1b}, and A_{1c}) or of A_{1c} only, and whether the measurement includes the labile pre-A_{1c} component. The most commonly used methods are based on electrical charge differences, structural characteristics, and chemical reactivity. There are no established reference method or single haemoglobin A_{1c} standard that can be used for all assays, and reference values vary depending on the method employed.

Well-controlled diabetics usually have values which are slightly than the upper limit of the reference range; those with values falling within the reference interval may experience more frequent episodes of hypoglycaemia. Those conditions with shortened red cell survival times such as haemolytic anaemias, pregnancy, and repeated phlebotomy, may produce decreased values.

Serum fructosamine

Non-enzymatic glycosylation of serum proteins (mainly albumin) can be estimated as serum fructosamine which has a similar application in diabetes mellitus to that of the glycosylated haemoglobins. However, albumin has a shorter half-life (about 20 days) than red cells and fructosamine only reflects the glycaemic status over the past 2-3 weeks. Normal values are of the order of 1.5-2.5 mmol/L.

The test is sensitive to variations in specific proteins, e.g., in patients receiving only parenteral nutrition, the results fluctuate widely despite stable plasma glucose levels. There is a 1.3% increase in fructosamine for every 3 g/L increase in serum protein concentration. Severe hypoproteinaemic states (serum albumin <30 g/L) may falsely lower serum fructosamine values.

Urinary microalbumin

Microalbuminuria (small amounts of albumin, not small molecules) is defined as small elevations of urinary albumin excretion not detected by conventional means. In diabetes mellitus an elevated albumin excretion rate (AER) is associated with other complications such as elevated arterial pressure, proliferative retinopathy, lipoprotein abnormalities, and is predictive of insidious development of diabetic nephropathy, which will only be clinically apparent at a later stage.

The test can be performed on a random spot urine but an *overnight timed collection*, to determine the

AER, is the preferred method because there is a dramatic increase in the AER in diabetics on exertion or exercise. However, estimation of the albumin: creatinine ratio on the first morning urine sample is also a useful procedure.

Normal values in adult urines are:

Albumin concentration: <20 mg/mL
Albumin:creatinine (mg/mL:mmol/L) ratio: <3.5
Albumin excretion rate (AER): <15 mg/min

AERs greater than 20 mg/min are considered abnormal and values in excess of 30 mg/min are predictive of subsequent renal failure and correlate with increased blood pressure.

Hypoglycaemia

Hypoglycaemia is an acute medical condition characterised by the following three features first described by Whipple in 1938:

1. Symptoms/signs characteristic of hypoglycaemia
2. Biochemical hypoglycaemia
3. Relief of symptoms by glucose administration

Clinical features. The clinical manifestations are due to activation of the autonomic nervous system (adrenergic) and deprivation of the brain of glucose (CNS dysfunction, neuroglycopenic).

Adrenergic: sweating, tachycardia, weakness, anxiety, tremor, vomiting

Neuroglycopenic: headache, visual disturbances, altered mental state, aberrant behaviour, confusion, convulsions, coma.

Biochemical hypoglycaemia. The blood glucose level that constitutes hypoglycaemia has been variously defined but a value less than 2.8 mmol/L is a general consensus figure. However, it must be recognised that:

- When hypoglycaemia is induced in normal subjects by insulin infusion, symptoms may not begin to appear until the glucose level falls to between 2.0 and 3.0 mmol/L.

- After a prolonged fast (36-72 hours) the blood glucose levels in normal male subjects can drop to around 2.6 mmol/L, whilst in children and pre-menopausal females values as low as 2.2 mmol/L can be reached, with the subjects usually remaining asymptomatic.

- Hypoglycaemic symptoms, which are identified by the patient and are relieved by eating, can occur at blood glucose levels greater than 2.8 mmol/L.

Relief of symptoms by glucose administration (eating). This is the third component of Whipple's triad -- it identifies true hypoglycaemia with great specificity and results in few false positives.

CAUSES

Hypoglycaemia is the commonest metabolic emergency seen in clinical practice. Most cases (>95%) are due to inappropriate insulin or oral hypoglycaemic drug therapy in diabetics. A useful diagnostic classification recognises three groups: *Medication/toxins, fasting hypoglycaemia, and reactive hypoglycaemia.*

Medications/toxins:
    Insulin, Oral hypoglycaemics, Ethanol,
    Drugs: salicylates, β-adrenergic blockers

Fasting Hypoglycaemia:
    Insulinoma, Non-pancreatic neoplasms,
    Adrenocortical deficiency, Hypopituitarism,
    Liver failure, Renal failure, Sepsis,
    Autoimmune

Reactive:
    Idiopathic (functional), Early diabetes mellitus,
    Alimentary (gastric surgery)

Medications/toxins. Use of several drugs are known to cause hypoglycaemia -- only the main ones are discussed here.

Insulin overdose. In clinical practice, unintended or accidental insulin overdose in insulin-dependant diabetics is the commonest cause of hypoglycaemia and the cause is usually obvious from the clinical history. On the other hand, surreptitious insulin administration may be difficult to diagnose; simultaneous estimation of the serum insulin and C-peptide values during the hypoglycaemia generally provides the diagnosis (see below).

Oral hypoglycaemics. Most of the oral hypoglycaemics, e.g., sulphonylurias, act by stimulating the pancreatic secretion of insulin. C-peptide is also secreted in parallel and hence hypoglycaemia due to these agents will be associated with raised serum levels of both analytes. This biochemical picture is similar to that of insulinoma (see below). Thus the patient who surreptitiously ingests oral hypoglycaemics can be difficult to evaluate and it may be necessary to search for the offending drug in the urine.

Ethanol-induced hypoglycaemia. Ethanol excess in malnourished chronic alcoholics can result in severe hypoglycaemia because of depleted glycogen stores or suppression of gluconeogenesis by excess NADH derived from ethanol metabolism (see page 351).

Other drugs. Salicylates and propanolol have both been known to cause hypoglycaemia in children but rarely do so in adults. Both drugs decrease glucose flux from the liver. In addition, salicylates can enhance insulin secretion.

Reactive hypoglycaemia

Hypoglycaemia occurring within 5-hours of a carbohydrate meal (e.g., oral glucose load) has been described in three situations.

a. in otherwise normal subjects (functional hypoglycaemia)
b. in early adult-onset diabetes mellitus
c. in patients who have had gastric surgery (alimentary hypoglycaemia)

The usual investigative procedure in subjects complaining of 'hypoglycaemic' symptoms soon after a meal is the 5-hour glucose tolerance test (see below).

Functional hypoglycaemia.

This classically occurs two to four hours after meals when the otherwise normal subject complains of adrenergic symptoms, and a serum glucose less than 2.8 mmol/L is demonstrated. There is some doubt that this condition really exists because adrenergic type symptoms (e.g. anxiety) are not uncommon, the symptoms can occur in the absence of a significant lowering of the blood glucose, and 10-20% of normal subjects will develop 'biochemical hypoglycaemia' (blood glucose <2.8 mmol/L) after a glucose load and still be asymptomatic.

Alimentary hypoglycaemia. In subjects with a partial or complete gastrectomy there is rapid transfer of nutrients to, and absorption from, the small gut. This results in a rapid and high elevation of the blood glucose and a consequent outpouring of insulin. An 'over-shooting' of insulin occurs and the hyperinsulinism causes a rapid drop in the blood glucose level one to three hours after ingestion of carbohydrates. In glucose tolerance testing this response has been called the lag-storage curve.

Diabetes mellitus. Early in the course of adult-onset diabetes mellitus (Type II), often when the patient is in the impaired glucose tolerance stage, hypoglycaemia may occur three to five hours after meals. It reflects late, but excessive, secretion of insulin in response to postprandial hyperglycaemia.

Fasting hypoglycaemia

Insulinoma: Insulinomas (tumours of pancreatic β-cells) are the commonest hormone-secreting islet cell tumour of the pancreas. They secrete insulin which is unresponsive to a falling blood glucose so that hypoglycaemic symptoms usually develop after a 4-5 hour fast. During attacks the blood glucose is low and the plasma insulin and C-peptide levels are inappropriately high for the corresponding blood glucose level. Hence the appropriate test is to fast the patient (up to 72 hours) and demonstrate hypoglycaemia associated with hyperinsulinism and high serum C-peptide levels. These tumours are rare but should be considered when fasting hypoglycaemia occurs in an otherwise healthy well-nourished adult.

Non-pancreatic tumours. Fasting hypoglycaemia has been described in association with a number of tumours including those of mesothelial origin (fibroma, fibrosarcoma) originating in the abdomen and thorax, hepatomas, adrenal carcinomas, gastrointestinal neoplasm, and carcinoid tumours. The cause is unclear and the possibilities include excessive glycolytic activity by the tumour and the production of insulin-like substances by the neoplasm (e.g. insulin-like growth factor II). The serum insulin level in these patients during the hypoglycaemia is appropriately low.

Endocrine disorders. Disorders associated with deficiency of the 'anti-insulin' hormones may feature fasting hypoglycaemia, e.g., hypopituitarism (deficiency of growth hormone and cortisol), adrenocortical deficiency (deficiency of cortisol). Ketosis, which is absent in patients with insulinomas, often occurs in association with the hypoglycaemia found in these disturbances.

Liver failure. Massive hepatocellular destruction (>80%) may result in severe hypoglycaemia and, occasionally, acute hepatitis may be accompanied by hypoglycaemia (? impaired gluconeogenesis and glycogen depletion). Hypoglycaemia has also been described during the acute liver congestion caused by congestive heart failure. Although the liver has an important central role in glucose homeostasis, hypoglycaemia is not a common accompaniment of liver disease, presumably because of the large reserve capacity.

Sepsis. Severe hypoglycaemia has been described in patients with septic shock due to gram-negative septicaemia. The cause is unclear but is most likely multifactorial, e.g., starvation, hepatic dysfunction, increased glucose utilisation due to fever.

Renal failure. Uraemic patients are inclined to develop hypoglycaemia because of a number of factors: decreased renal inactivation of insulin, decreased renal gluconeogenesis, protein wasting resulting in decreased supplies of alanine (precursor of gluconeogenesis), and defective glucose reabsorption.

Autoimmune hypoglycaemia. This is a rare cause of hypoglycaemia which has been documented in the odd case report. Two types have been described: *(i) Insulin receptor antibodies* which mimic insulin by stimulating the receptor. *(ii) Antibodies to anti-insulin antibodies:* These have been described in a number of Japanese women treated for autoimmune thyroiditis with propylthiouracil. It has been suggested that an antibody to an anti-insulin antibody may biochemically resemble insulin and act as such.

LABORATORY EVALUATION

Assessment, in the first instance, depends on a thorough clinical evaluation with emphasis on the patient's drug history (overt and the possibility of covert drugs), and the relationship of the symptoms to meals.

In the *reactive* type a 5-hour glucose tolerance test may be useful but can also be misleading because 10-20% of normal subjects will show biochemical hypoglycaemia two to five hours after a glucose load.

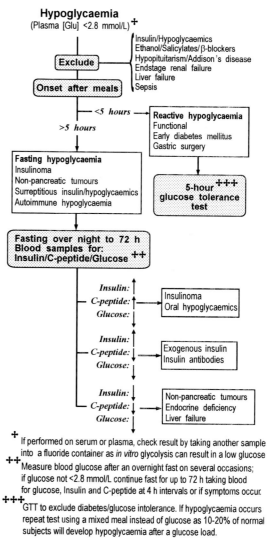

Figure 10.6. Checklist and suggested scheme for the evaluation of hypoglycaemia.

If this approach is used and 'reactive' hypoglycaemia occurs in a patient who has not had a gastrectomy or does not have impaired glucose tolerance, it is useful to repeat the test using a complex carbohydrate load.

If *fasting* hypoglycaemia is a possibility then determine the blood glucose and insulin levels on several occasions after an overnight fast. If this does not demonstrate hypoglycaemia then continue the fast for up to 72-hours, taking blood samples for glucose, insulin and C-peptide at 6-8 hour intervals (exercising the patient during this period can be useful).

- An insulinoma is characterised by a low blood glucose associated with 'normal' or high insulin and C-peptide levels (i.e. insulin values inappropriately high for the glucose level).

- In surreptitious insulin administration the serum insulin will be high but is accompanied by a low C-peptide.

- Hypoglycaemia due to self-administration of oral hypoglycaemics will be associated with high insulin and C-peptide levels (see above).

If endocrine disorders, liver failure, renal failure, or sepsis is the cause of the hypoglycaemia the diagnosis is usually not difficult because the features of the primary disorder will be predominant.

Ketosis (ketogenesis)

Ketogenesis is part of a normal metabolic response to starvation where the initiating factor is glucose deficiency which suppresses insulin secretion. The insulin lack acts at multiple enzyme loci resulting in:

- Elevated glucagon and growth hormone secretion
- Increased lipolysis and decreased fat synthesis
- Increased β-oxidation of fatty acids
- Increased hepatic ketogenesis
- Gluconeogenesis (from protein)

The aim is to switch energy production from carbohydrate (glucose) to fat whereby:

- the majority of energy is derived from β-oxidation of fatty acids
- the brain, normally dependant on glucose, switches to ketone utilisation

- just sufficient glucose to maintain the obligatory glucose-dependant tissues (e.g., red cells) is produced from tissue protein by gluconeogenesis with maximal protein conservation

Thus, in the absence of exogenous fuels, energy is derived mainly from fat and ketogenesis is brought into play to conserve tissue protein.

Ketogenesis is initiated and controlled by a low insulin:glucagon ratio which results from a falling blood glucose.

Fasting (starvation) → ↓ low glucose →
↓↓ insulin and ↑ glucagon →
↓ insulin:glucagon ratio →

- Stimulation of adipose tissue hormone-sensitive lipase release free fatty acids (FFA) which are transported to the liver attached to plasma albumin.

- In the hepatocyte the FFA is converted to acyl-CoA by acyl-CoA synthetase, an enzyme located in the outer mitochondrial membrane.

- The next step, the important rate-limiting step for β-oxidation, is the transfer of acyl-CoA (palmitoyl-CoA) across the inner mitochondrial membrane. This involves carnitine and two enzymes *carnitine palmitoyl transferase I (CPT-I)* located on the outer surface of the inner mitochondrial membrane and *carnitine palmitoyl transferase II (CPT-II)* located on the inner surface (Figure 10.7). The action of CPT-I is influenced by the cellular level of malonyl-CoA, an intermediate in the pathway for fatty acid synthesis (see below).

- Once in the mitochondria the fatty acid (acyl-CoA) enters the β-oxidation cycle producing ATP and acetyl-CoA.

Acetyl-CoA normally enters the TCA cycle to produce ATP by reacting with oxaloacetate to form citrate (catalysed by citrate synthetase). If the TCA cycle is inhibited due to generation of ATP (inhibitor of cycle) from the reducing equivalents (NADH) produced by β-oxidation, then acetyl-CoA will be diverted towards ketogenesis (Figure 10.7).

The first reaction in ketogenesis is the formation of acetoacetyl-CoA from two molecules of acetyl-CoA by a thiolase. Hydroxymethylglutaryl-CoA (HMG-CoA) is then formed by the condensation of acetyl-CoA and acetoacetyl-CoA (HMG-CoA synthetase).

During this reaction a hydrogen ion is released -- thus the acidaemic part of ketoacidosis. HMG-CoA is then split to acetoacetate (ketone body) and acetyl-CoA by HMG-CoA lyase.

The second ketone body, β-hydroxybutyrate, is formed from acetoacetate by β-hydroxybutyrate dehydrogenase. This reaction converts NADH to NAD+ thus allowing β-oxidation to proceed (Figure 10.7). Some acetoacetate is non-enzymatically converted to acetone by the irreversible loss of carbon dioxide. Ketogenesis occurs almost exclusively in the liver although the renal cortex is also capable of ketogenesis.

Note: The major factor controlling β-oxidation and

ketogenesis is the cellular concentration of malonyl-CoA. Low values, which are the result of inhibition of *acetyl-CoA carboxylase* by a low insulin:glucagon ratio, stimulate CPT-I activity and consequently increase ketogenesis and β-oxidation.

Fatty acids and ketones as fuel

Fatty acids constitute the major fuel reserves of the body and one molecule of palmitate, if completely oxidised, will generate 129 molecules of ATP. As noted above fatty acid oxidation occurs in the mitochondria and therefore those organs lacking mitochondria (e.g., red blood cells) and deficient in

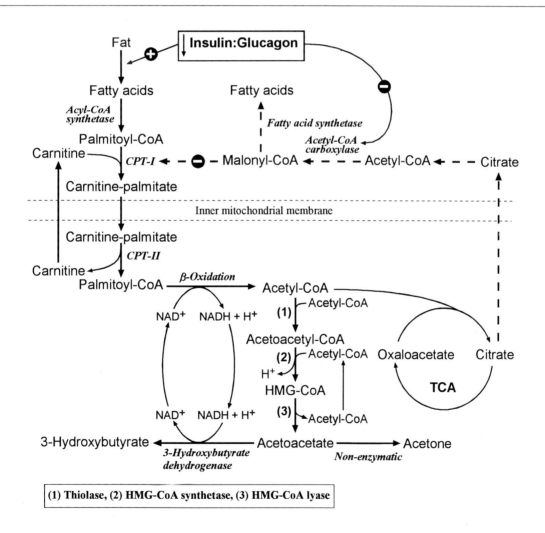

(1) Thiolase, (2) HMG-CoA synthetase, (3) HMG-CoA lyase

Figure 10.7. Ketogenesis. CPT-I and CPT-II, carnitine palmitoyl transferase I and II

mitochondria (e.g., renal medulla, testes) cannot utilise fat for energy -- they are dependant on glucose and gluconeogenesis. The brain is another tissue which is unable to use fatty acids as fuel. The fatty acid-albumin complex cannot penetrate the blood brain barrier but ketones can, as they are not bound to proteins, and are used by the brain cells during glucose-starved states.

Skeletal and cardiac muscle can also use ketones for fuel. In fact, early in starvation these tissues use ketones in preference to glucose to conserve the latter for the brain cells -- later in starvation they use fatty acids to conserve the ketones, again for the brain cells.

Acetoacetate is taken up by the appropriate cell and converted to acetyl-CoA by two enzymes: (i) *acetoacetyl:succinyl-CoA CoA transferase* converts acetoacetate to acetoacetyl-CoA, (ii) *ketothiolase* breaks acetoacetyl-CoA to two molecules of acetyl-CoA. The liver is interesting in that it does not contain acetoacetate:succinyl-CoA CoA transferase but contains large amounts of *hydroxymethylglutaryl-CoA synthetase* (low in other tissues); thus liver produces but does not use ketones.

Diabetic ketoacidosis

Diabetic ketoacidosis (DKA) occurs in patients with IDDM prior to diagnosis and treatment and if insulin is withdrawn in diagnosed cases, i.e., a fall in the insulin:glucagon ratio stimulates ketogenesis, as stated earlier. The absolute lack of insulin will also result in uncontrolled gluconeogenesis and consequently hyperglycaemia. The characteristic features are:

- *Hyperglycaemia:* plasma glucose values are usually around 12-25 mmol/L.

- *Metabolic acidosis:* low plasma bicarbonate level due to overproduction of H^+ during ketogenesis, levels as low as 5 mmol/L are not uncommon.

- *High anion gap:* Usually greater than 30 mEq/L and may be as high as 40 mEq/L. The major contributor is usually β-hydroxybutyrate but acetoacetate, lactate, and other non-specific anions also play a part.

- *Ketone anions:* levels are usually of the order of 5-15 mmol/L for β-hydroxybutyrate, and 2-5 mmol/L for acetoacetate, the ratio of β-hydroxybutyrate: acetoacetate is usually around 3:1 to 5:1.

- 10-30% of the acetoacetate is non-enzymatically converted to acetone which is excreted via the lungs and kidneys.

The ketone production rate in a number of insulin-dependant diabetics has been estimated during insulin therapy and after insulin withdrawal (Miles JM et al, 1980) with the following results:

	Pre-insulin withdrawal	Post-insulin withdrawal
Ketone production rate (mmol/day)	~540	~1830
Ketone utilisation rate (mmol/day)	~550	~1470
Plasma ketones (mmol/L)	0.9-1.9	5.7-8.7
Net gain of ketones (mmol/L)	---	~360

Starvation ketosis

In the well-fed post-absorptive state the approximate fuel stores in a 70 kg man are:

Glucose:	20 g (extracellular fluid)
Glycogen:	75 g in liver, 150 g in muscle
Fat:	15 kg
Protein:	3-6 kg (converted to glucose by gluconeogenesis)

In the absence of exogenous glucose energy is derived at first from the liver glycogen stores and, when these are depleted (in 12-18 hours), from β-oxidation of fatty acids. Tissues that preferentially utilise glucose (brain, red cells, etc) receive their nutrients from tissue protein (and glycerol derived from fat) by way of gluconeogenesis.

In the basal state some 100-180 grams of glucose is required for the glucose-dependant tissues daily. Around 1.75 grams of protein is required to manufacture 1 gram of glucose by gluconeogenesis and thus the daily protein requirement to synthesise 100 grams of glucose is 175 grams. Hence if there is a tissue protein reserve of 3 kg, this protein reserve will decrease by 50% in about 8 days. However, as fasting proceeds the brain switches its energy precursor from glucose to ketones to the extent that, in late fasting (after 7-10 days), about two thirds of the energy requirements are met by ketones. This allows a reduction in gluconeogenesis to the point where only 16-20 grams of protein are utilised daily (Note: In the context of energy ketones can be considered as the soluble and easily transportable form of fat.)

As stated above the instigator of this starvation process is a low plasma glucose which results in a low insulin:glucagon ratio. The stimulus which initiates the switch whereby the brain utilises ketones in preference to glucose is unclear.

Although the ketone production and utilisation rate during starvation is high (up to 100 g/day or 800-1000 mmol/day) the plasma levels do not generally rise beyond 5.0 mmol/L and then only after two to three weeks. On the other hand, subjects who have low glycogen reserves such as infants, pregnant women, and chronic alcoholics, will often develop significant ketosis during a short (12-24 hour) fast.

Alcoholic ketosis

Alcoholic ketoacidosis (AKA) has a characteristic clinical onset:

(a) An alcoholic binge with cessation of alcohol intake some 2-3 days prior to admission
(b) Moderate/severe vomiting since the binge
(c) No food (starvation) for several days

Hence the setting is of acute starvation resulting in:

> low plasma glucose
> ↓ insulin:glucagon ratio
> β-oxidation and hepatic ketogenesis

Ingestion of ethanol tends to prevent gluconeogenesis from lactate in the liver because the oxidation of ethanol competes for the NAD⁺ necessary for the oxidation of lactate, as shown below.

The ***differential diagnosis*** includes diabetic ketoacidosis (DKA). The characteristic differences are:

(1) Plasma [glucose]
DKA: >15.0 mmol/L
AKA: variable: it could be hypoglycaemia, normoglycaemia, or hyperglycaemia but usually <15.0 mmol/L

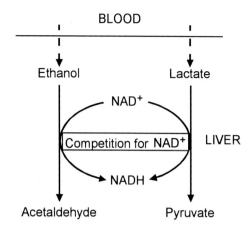

(2) Plasma [K]
DKA: hyperkalaemia
AKA: normal or hypokalaemia

(3) β-OHB:AcAc*   (β-OHB: β-hydroxybutyric acid; AcAc: acetoacetate)
DKA: 3:1-5:1
AKA: >6:1

(4) Acid-base status **
DKA: simple metabolic acidosis
AKA: variable: simple metabolic acidosis, mixed metabolic acidosis and alkalosis, mixed metabolic acidosis and respiratory alkalosis

*The β-OHB:AcAc depends on the NADH:NAD⁺ ratio which is high in the alcoholic because of the activity of alcohol and aldehyde dehydrogenases, i.e.,

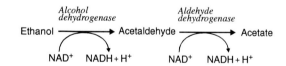

**The basic acid-base state in AKA is simple metabolic acidosis but to this may be added respiratory alkalosis due to hyperventilation of alcohol withdrawal, metabolic alkalosis due to vomiting, or both, resulting in a triple acid-base disturbance.

CLINICAL AND LABORATORY EVALUATION

Ketoacidosis presents as a high anion gap metabolic acidosis (page 00), the differential diagnosis being:

(1) Ketoacidosis
(2) Lactic acidosis
(3) Renal failure
(4) Intoxications: salicylate, methanol, ethylene glycol

Toxic conditions can usually be excluded on the basis of the clinical story and renal failure will be evident from the serum creatinine level (values usually greater than 0.40 mmol/L). The differentiation between lactic acidosis and ketoacidosis may require estimation of the serum lactate, or serum ketones, or both.

Determination of the cause of ketoacidosis is usually evident on the basis of the clinical presentation and the serum glucose level (see above). It may be difficult to differentiate between diabetic and alcoholic ketosis if the serum glucose is only moderately raised (e.g., to less than 15 mmol/L). In such cases the response to therapy may be the only indicator although a β-hydroxybutyrate:acetoacetate in excess of 6:1 argues for the alcoholic variety.

Lactic Acid

Lactate is a by-product of glycolysis which is produced when the metabolism of pyruvate through the TCA cycle is impeded.

Normal lactate metabolism

The conversion of one glucose molecule through the glycolytic path to two pyruvate molecules produces two molecules of ATP (actually 4 produced, but 2 are reutilised). If the glucose is derived from glycogen three ATP molecules are produced (only one is reutilised). Further metabolism of pyruvate via the TCA cycle produces a further 36 molecules of ATP.

The TCA cycle requires molecular oxygen to proceed; thus in the presence of oxygen a molecule of glycogen-derived glucose produces 39 molecules of ATP, whilst in the absence of oxygen (anaerobic metabolism) only 3 ATP molecules are produced. However, glycolysis can proceed at about 25-times the speed of the TCA cycle and thus can produce ~75 ATP molecules whilst the TCA cycle is producing ~36 molecules. Such occurs in rapidly contracting muscle.

Therefore, in hypoxic tissues, rapidly contracting muscles, and in tissues containing few or no mitochondria (the intracellular location of TCA cycle reactions) such as red cells, white cells, testes, renal medulla, and

skin, energy (ATP) is produced mainly by glycolysis. However, for glycolysis to proceed an adequate supply of NAD^+ is necessary for the conversion of glyceraldehyde-3-phosphate to glycerate 1,3-bisphosphate by glyceraldehyde-3-phosphate dehydrogenase. This problem is resolved by the conversion of NADH to NAD^+ during the transformation of pyruvate to lactate under the influence of lactate dehydrogenase (LD). This results in the accumulation of lactate (Figure 10.8).

A hydrogen ion is produced concomitantly with the lactate ion (lactic acid is not produced as such -- it has a pK of 3.8 and thus at tissue pH of 7.2-7.4 it exists as lactate, not lactic acid). The hydrogen ion originates from ATP hydrolysis.

During anaerobic glycolysis ADP is converted to ATP which is immediately hydrolysed:

$$2ATP^{4-} + 2H_2O \rightarrow 2ADP^{3-} + 2HPO_4^{2-} + 2H^+$$
$$\text{Thus: Glucose} \rightarrow 2Lactate^- + 2H^+$$

When lactate is metabolised by either gluconeogenesis (Cori cycle) or oxidation after conversion to pyruvate, hydrogen ions are consumed in a reverse manner.

Under resting conditions about 1400 mmols of lactate are produced daily (~20 mmol/kg/day) by tissues such as skin, red cells, white cells, renal medulla, and intestinal mucosae. This lactate diffuses out of the tissues to the blood and is transported to the liver, and to a certain extent the renal cortex, where it is converted back to glucose by gluconeogenesis. This process is known as the Cori cycle.

The plasma lactate concentration results from the balance between production and removal; hence the level will rise if there is increased production or decreased utilisation or both. If the blood lactate concentration exceeds 5 mmol/L (normal range <2.0 mmol/L) and the arterial pH falls below 7.35 then lactic acidosis is said to occur.

Lactic acidosis

Lactic acidosis results from a disturbance of pyruvate metabolism and an imbalance between ATP production and ATP hydrolysis, i.e. for some reason, e.g. hypoxia, pyruvate builds up and is converted to lactate in order to generate NAD^+ which enables glycolysis to proceed and produce ATP. The disorder is generally classified into two groups (Table 10.1):

Type A: hypoxic group in which the tissue oxygen is insufficient to meet metabolic needs

Type B: 'non-hypoxic' group in which factors other than hypoxia are the major cause

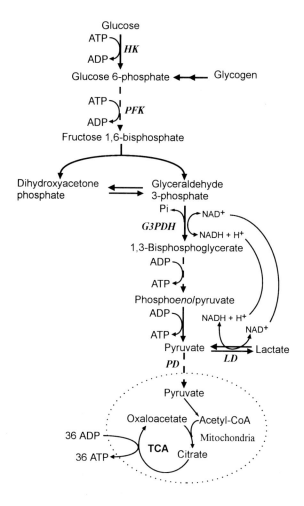

Figure 10.8. Anaerobic glycolysis and lactate metabolism. HK, hexokinase; PFK, phosphofructokinase; G3PDH, glyceraldehyde-3-phosphate dehydrogenase; PD, pyruvate dehydrogenase; LD, lactate dehydrogenase.

Type A: Hypoxic lactic acidosis is the commonest variety resulting mainly from poor tissue perfusion (shock etc) which increases the peripheral production of lactate. In addition, there is decreased hepatic removal of lactate due to an associated decrease in liver perfusion and the severe acidosis which impairs the ability of the liver to extract lactate from the blood. Shock is perhaps the most widely recognised cause of lactic acidosis. The lactic acidosis associated with severe exercise (or generalised convulsions) can also be quite severe, with blood lactate levels of 30-40 mmol/L being achieved (characteristically, within two to three hours after cessation of exercise the blood lactate, and bicarbonate, levels are back to normal or near normal levels).

Table 10.1. Causes of lactic acidosis.

Type A: With overt evidence of hypoxia
Severe exercise, Convulsions
Poor tissue perfusion: hypotension, cardiac failure, cardiac arrest
Reduced arterial oxygen content: asphyxia, hypoxaemia, carbon monoxide toxicity, severe anaemia

Type B: No overt evidence of hypoxia
Drugs/toxins/infusions: ethanol, methanol, nitroprusside, phenformin, catecholamines, fructose, sorbitol (infusions)
Predisposing disease: respiratory alkalosis, diabetes mellitus, liver failure, renal failure, sepsis, neoplasms
Congenital lactic acidosis: Defects in:
 - gluconeogenesis, e.g., glucose-6-phosphatase or pyruvate carboxylase deficiency;
 - pyruvate metabolism, e.g., pyruvate dehydrogenase deficiency;
 - mitochondrial oxidative phosphorylation
D-Lactic acidosis
Short bowel syndrome

Type B: Lactic acidosis occurring without overt evidence of tissue hypoxia may occur in association with a wide variety of diseases and toxins/chemicals (Table 10.1). In most cases the cause is unclear but it is postulated that tissue oxygen utilisation is impaired.

D-Lactic acidosis: The lactic acid produced by mammalian tissues is of the laevo variety (L-lactate).

Dextro (D-)lactate, a metabolic product of some bacteria, may be produced in excess if there is an overgrowth of such organisms in the gut. This can occur when a large section of the small gut is lost and the remaining gut is colonised by D-lactate-producing bacteria. This lactate is absorbed from the small gut and causes a high anion gap metabolic acidosis. It is not metabolised by the native L-lactate dehydrogenase and is excreted unchanged in the urine.

CLINICAL ASPECTS AND LABORATORY EVALUATION

Clinical: The clinical features are determined by the underlying cause but a common feature is the hyperventilation (Kussmaul respiration) due to the metabolic acidaemia.

Laboratory: The characteristic laboratory features are:

1. *Acidaemia:* pH <7.35
2. *Metabolic acidosis:* plasma [HCO_3] <20 mmol/L (and can be as low as 5 mmol/L)
3. *High anion gap:* >25 mEq/L (and can be as high as 40 mEq/L)
4. *Plasma lactate*: >5.0 mmol/L (values greater than 40 mmol/L are not uncommon)
5. *Plasma potassium*: usually normal
6. *Plasma phosphate:* characteristically increased

Note: Special care should be taken when handling specimens for lactate analyses to prevent *in vitro* accumulation of lactate. Heparinised blood may be used if it is kept on ice and the plasma is quickly separated. Iodoacetate, which inhibits glycolysis without affecting coagulation is a satisfactory additive.

REFERENCES AND FURTHER READING

Field JB (ed) Hypoglycaemia. Endocrinol Metab Clinics North Am 1989;18:1-257.

Flekman AM. Diabetic ketoacidosis. Endocrinol Metab Clinics North Am 1993;22:181-209.

Foster DW, McGarry JD. The metabolic derangements and treatment of diabetic ketoacidosis. N Engl J Med 1983;309:159-169.

Harris MI, Hadden WC, Knowler WC, Bennett PH. International criteria for the diagnosis of diabetes and impaired glucose tolerance. Diabetes Care 1985;8: 562-566.

Karam JH (ed) Diabetes mellitus. Endocrinol Metab Clinics North Am 1992;21(2).

Kitabchi AE, Wall BM. Diabetic ketoacidosis. Med Clinics North Am 1995;79:9-37.

Lorber D. Nonketotic hypertonicity in diabetes mellitus. Med Clinics North Am 1995;79:39-52.

Mizock BA, Falk JL. Lactic acidosis in critical illness. Crit Care Med 1992;20:80-91.

Service FJ. Hypoglycemia. Med Clinics North Am 1995;79:1-8.

Stern HJ. Lactic acidosis in paediatrics: clinical and laboratory evaluation. Ann Clin Biochem 1994;31: 410-419.

Wiener K. The diagnosis of diabetes mellitus, including gestational diabetes. Ann Clin Biochem 1992;29:481-493.

Chapter 11

The Hepatobiliary System

The liver plays a major and central role in protein, carbohydrate, and lipid metabolism, subjects which are dealt with elsewhere in this book and more appropriately in texts on basic biochemistry. The liver is also an important site for detoxification (of drugs, poisons, etc) and excretion of many end products of metabolism (e.g., bilirubin, bile acids) as well as the site of synthesis of many compounds (e.g., lipoproteins, clotting factors, and most other serum proteins except immunoglobulins).

Despite its essential role in overall metabolism, liver disease generally does not result in dramatic metabolic disturbances until the disease is well advanced; this reflects the immense reserve of its metabolic capacity. In fact most of the so-called 'liver function tests', a notable example being the liver enzymes, focus on structural integrity rather than metabolic status. An exception is the serum bilirubin estimation which, to a certain extent, reflects the role of the liver in bilirubin metabolism and is a true liver function test.

Bilirubin metabolism will be considered in some detail; other liver functions, such as albumin synthesis and bile acid metabolism, will only be discussed in relation to their influence on various laboratory tests.

Bilirubin metabolism

Haem, derived from aged or injured red cells, maturing cells during erythropoiesis, and degraded hepatic haemoproteins, is converted to biliverdin in the reticuloendothelial system. Biliverdin is reduced to bilirubin which is secreted into the plasma where it is reversibly bound to albumin and transported to the liver. The bilirubin is taken up by the hepatocytes, conjugated with glucuronic acid and excreted in the bile. Further metabolism takes place in the gut and a small proportion of the metabolites are recirculated via the enterohepatic circulation. These sequential stages in bilirubin metabolism (Figure 11.1) are discussed in greater detail below.

Production. One gram of haemoglobin produces about 620 μmol of bilirubin. Of the 250-350 mg (4-6

mmol) of bilirubin produced daily, 15 to 20% is derived from immature red cells and nonerythroid haemoproteins; the remainder comes from senescent red cells. Using radioactive haem precursors to study the rate of production and turnover, three excretion periods are recognised -- two so-called early labelled fractions and a late labelled fraction.

- *1-3 hours:* bilirubin produced in the liver from haemoproteins, e.g., cytochromes, enzymes.
- *1-3 days:* bilirubin produced from prematurely destroyed erythrocytes in the bone marrow.
- *90-150 days:* bilirubin produced from senescent red cells by the reticuloendothelial system, particularly the spleen.

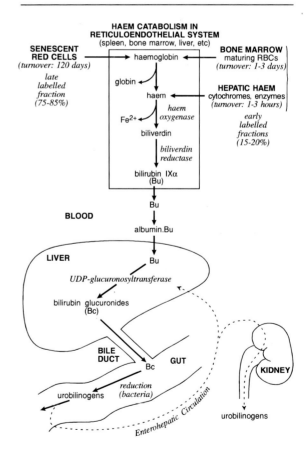

Figure 11.1. Bilirubin metabolism. See text for details. Bu, unconjugated bilirubin; Bc, conjugated bilirubin

Haem is converted to bilirubin in the reticulo-endothelial system by two enzymes, *haem oxygenase* and *biliverdin reductase*. Haem oxygenase breaks the α-CH= bridge of protoporphyrin IX to produce biliverdin IXα, which is then reduced to bilirubin IXα by biliverdin reductase (Figure 11.2). Although bilirubin IXα has two polar propionic acid side chains it is poorly soluble in water because of intramolecular hydrogen bonding between the propionic acid residues and other parts of the molecule (Figure 11.3). This

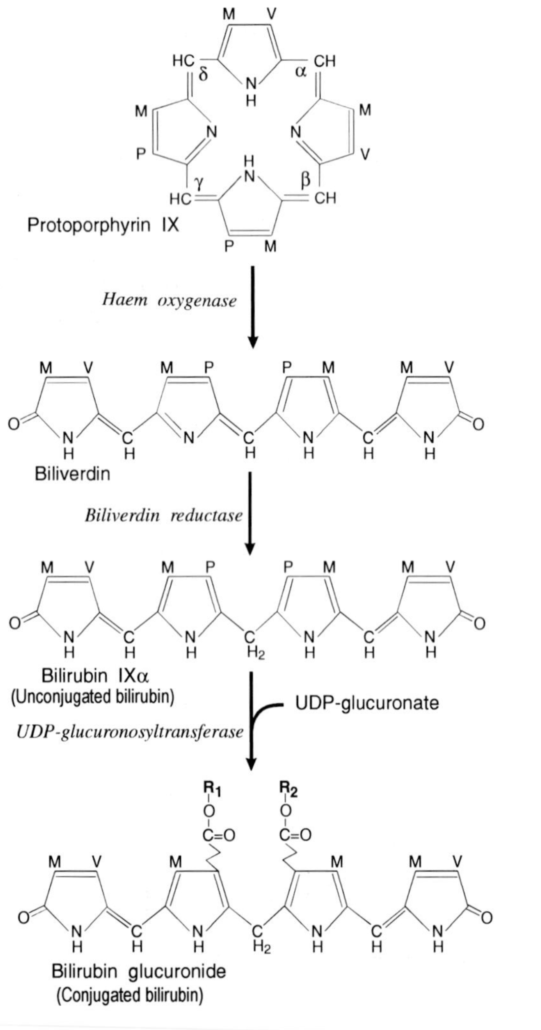

open structure   V = -CH=CH$_2$ (vinyl)
M = -CH$_3$ (methyl)

intramolecularly hydrogen bonded

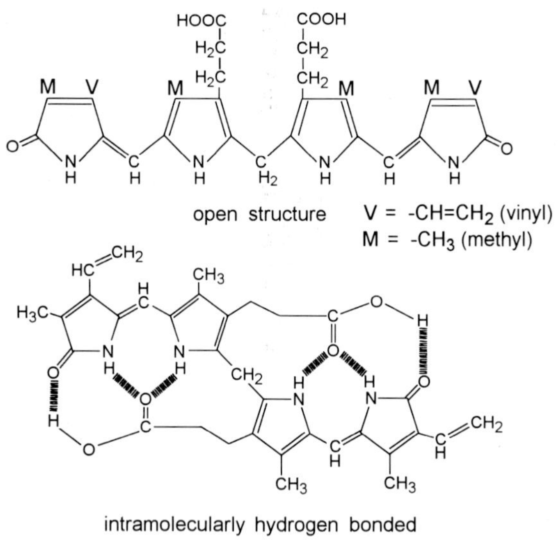

Figure 11.3. Structure of unconjugated bilirubin (Bu). *Top:* Open linear structure (Bilirubin IXα). *Bottom:* Intramolecularly hydrogen-bonded (ZZ) configuration. The extensive hydrogen bonding is responsible for the low solubility of Bu in water at pH 7.4. Bu is far more soluble at alkaline pH and in serum because it is bound to albumin. Bu is not excreted in urine.

Protoporphyrin IX

Haem oxygenase

Biliverdin

Biliverdin reductase

Bilirubin IXα
(Unconjugated bilirubin)

UDP-glucuronosyltransferase   UDP-glucuronate

Bilirubin glucuronide
(Conjugated bilirubin)

P -CH$_2$-CH$_2$-COOH (propionic) V -C=CH$_2$ (vinyl) M -CH$_3$ (methyl)
Monoglucuronide: R$_1$ = Sugar   or   R$_1$ = H
                R$_2$ = H   R$_2$ = Sugar
Diglucuronide: R$_1$ = R$_2$ = Sugar (Glucuronic acid)

Figure 11.2. Conversion of protoporphyrin to conjugated bilirubin. See text for details.

bonding may also account for the necessity for conjugation with glucuronic acid prior to biliary excretion, the conjugates being more water-soluble.

Transport to the liver. The newly formed bilirubin is referred to as unconjugated bilrubin (Bu) or indirectly reacting bilirubin. Most of it is transported in the blood reversibly bound to albumin; only a very tiny fraction remains unbound (~4 nmol/L in a total plasma bilirubin concentration of 20 µmol/L). The bilirubin-albumin complex, by virtue of its large molecular size, is not filtered at the renal glomerular membrane -- hence bilirubinuria does not occur in patients with unconjugated hyperbilirubinaemia. Compounds such as free fatty acids, sulphonamides, salicylate, and ampicillin compete with and displace bilirubin from its binding sites on the albumin molecule.

Hepatocyte uptake. At the hepatic sinusoidal membrane, the bilirubin-albumin complex dissociates, with selective uptake of bilirubin into the cell where it is reversibly bound to cytosolic proteins, one such protein being *ligandin*. The function of these proteins appears to be prevention of efflux of bilirubin from the cell.

Conjugation. Bilirubin is conjugated in the smooth endoplasmic reticulum with glucuronic acid and, to a lesser extent, with glucose and xylose. The enzyme responsible is *UDP-glucuronosyltransferase* which esterifies one or both the propionic acid side chains to produce mono- and diglucuronides, the former predominating.

Biliary secretion. The bilirubin conjugates are actively secreted into the bile canaliculi. This transport mechanism differs from that responsible for the biliary excretion of bile acids.

Gut degradation and excretion: Bacterial flora in the gut reduce the bilirubin conjugates to urobilinogens which are mainly excreted in the faeces. A portion of the urobilinogens are reabsorbed back into the blood stream and later re-excreted by the liver (enterohepatic circulation). Urobilinogens are water-soluble and can be excreted by the kidney but this is normally an unimportant excretory route (about 4 mg or 70 µmol per day). Conjugated bilirubin is more prone to the reductive processes in the gut lumen than unconjugated bilirubin; unconjugated bilirubin is readily reabsorbed from the gut. Thus, if bacterial flora are absent (e.g, in the neonate or due to antibiotic therapy) deconjugation of bilirubin glucuronides by intestinal mucosal β-glucuronidase may occur and reabsorption of the unconjugated compounds may result in an increase in the plasma unconjugated bilirubin (Bu) level.

BILIRUBIN FRACTIONS IN PLASMA

The total plasma bilirubin concentration in adults is usually less than 20 µmol/L; clinical signs of jaundice appear when the plasma total bilirubin rises beyond 40 µmol/L. Analysis of normal plasma using high-performance liquid chromatography has demonstrated the presence of four bilirubin fractions -- α, β, γ, and δ (Figure 11.4).

- *α-fraction:* This fraction is unconjugated bilirubin which is water-insoluble (see above) and bound to albumin. It is also called indirect (reacting) bilirubin because the diazo reaction used in the bilirubin measurement occurs only after the

addition of accelerators. It is the major bilirubin fraction in normal plasma (>90%). It does not appear in the urine because of its attachment to albumin and can only be cleared by the liver.

- *β- and γ-fractions:* The β-fraction is composed of bilirubin monoglucuronides; the diglucuronides constitute the γ-fraction. These conjugated bilirubins (<10% in normal plasma) are water-soluble and will appear in the urine if present in the blood in excess amounts. They are called direct (reacting) bilirubins as they react with the diazo reagent without the addition of accelerators.

- *δ-fraction:* The δ-fraction, usually referred to as 'delta' bilirubin, has the following characteristics: (a) it is direct reacting, (b) it is covalently bonded to albumin, and (c) its plasma level is increased in diseases associated with high plasma levels of conjugated bilirubin. It appears to be derived from conjugated bilirubin as it can be produced by incubating bilirubin glucuronides with plasma albumin. As it is tightly bound to albumin it has a half-life comparable to that protein (~20 days).

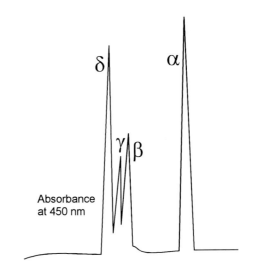

α = unconjugated = Bu
β = monoconjugated = mBc
γ = diconjugated = dBc
δ = albumin-bound (covalent-bonded) = Bδ

Figure 11.4. High performance liquid chromatographic separation of the four plasma bilirubin fractions.

URINARY BILE PIGMENTS

The bile pigments that may be found in the urine are urobilinogen and conjugated bilirubin. Unconjugated bilirubin is not filtered across the glomerular membrane.

- *Urobilinogen:* The normal subject excretes 1-4 mg (2-7 µmol) of urobilinogen daily in the urine (derived from the enterohepatic circulation). Increased amounts occur in liver disease (inability to re-excrete the small amounts reabsorbed from the gut into the bile) and in haemolytic anaemia (increased bilirubin production). Bile duct obstruction or cholestasis is associated with decreased or undetectable levels.

- *Bilirubin:* Bilirubin appears in the urine when the plasma level of conjugated bilirubin rises as in hepatocellular disease and cholestasis.

Inborn errors of bilirubin metabolism

There are four clinically significant congenital disorders of bilirubin metabolism: Gilbert's disease, Crigler-Najjar syndrome, Dubin-Johnson syndrome, and Rotor syndrome. All are associated with decreased hepatic clearance of bilirubin. Patients with the Gilbert's and Crigler-Najjar syndromes present with unconjugated hyperbilirubinaemia whilst the Dubin-Johnson and Rotor syndromes are characterised by conjugated hyperbilirubinaemia.

Gilbert's disease. This disorder, associated with mild fluctuating unconjugated hyperbilirubinaemia and an absence of bilirubin in the urine, is innocuous and occurs in up to 7% of the population. The most probable cause is decreased activity of UDP-glucuronosyl-transferase but other factors such as increased red cell turnover and decreased hepatic uptake of bilirubin have been observed. These subjects present with mild jaundice without bilirubinuria. The plasma bilirubin level is usually less than 100 µmol/L (often <50 µmol/L) and characteristically fluctuates, being increased during reduced calorie intake (fasting) and during illness associated with nausea and vomiting.

Crigler-Najjar syndrome. In the Crigler-Najjar syndrome (an autosomal recessive disorder) there is defective UDP-glucuronosyltransferase activity but of greater severity than in Gilbert's syndrome. Two types of the disorder have been described. Both types are associated with unconjugated hyperbilirubinaemia and no bilirubinuria.

- *Type 1:* Absolute deficiency of the transferase which results in kernicterus and death soon after birth.

- *Type 2:* Partial deficiency of the transferase which is not fatal but results in life-long unconjugated hyperbilirubinaemia. The residual enzyme activity can be increased marginally by phenobarbital (enzyme induction by drug action) which will lessen the degree of jaundice.

Dubin-Johnson syndrome: This syndrome, characterised by chronic fluctuating conjugated hyper-bilirubinaemia, is due to a defect in the biliary excretion of conjugated bilirubin. There is also an associated abnormality in porphyrin metabolism (of unknown aetiology). The liver has a characteristic black appearance due to the deposition of a melanin-like pigment. Most patients are asymptomatic with plasma bilirubin levels ranging from 30 to 90 µmol/L and bilirubinuria. The urinary excretion of copro-porphyrins (page 278) is normal in quantity but with increased levels of isomer III and decreased levels of isomer I; the significance of this is unclear.

Rotor syndrome: This disorder, first described in the Philippines, is similar to the Dubin-Johnson syndrome but differs in that (a) there is no pigmentation of the liver, and (b) the urinary copro-porphyrin excretion is increased but with normal proportions of the I and III isomers.

HEPATOBILIARY DISEASE

The following is not a complete list of the diseases processes affecting the hepatobiliary system but it covers most of those seen in clinical practice. There is considerable overlap between the disease processes and two or more can be found in the same patient.

- Jaundice
- Hepatocellular disease

- Cholestasis
- Infiltrations
- Cirrhosis
- Alcoholic liver disease
- Drug-induced liver disease
- Fatty liver
- Cholecystitis/cholelithiasis

Disorders of the hepatobiliary system usually present with one or more of the following:

- jaundice
- abnormal liver function tests (expected or unexpected)
- symptoms and signs related to the hepatobiliary system (hepatomegaly, right upper quadrant pain, etc).

Jaundice. Jaundice is detected in the sclera of the eye long before development of the classical picture and it becomes clinically conspicuous only when the serum bilirubin rises beyond 40 μmol/L. The differential diagnosis includes carotenaemia, (e.g., myxoedema, dietary excess) which may require a serum bilirubin estimation for exclusion.

Liver Function Tests. (These are discussed fully on page 156). As a minimum these will include the serum or plasma levels of bilirubin, total protein, albumin, a transaminase (e.g., aspartate aminotransferase, AST), and alkaline phosphatase (ALP). The levels of bilirubin, AST, and ALP will usually be sufficient to discriminate between the three main hepatobiliary disease processes -- hepatocellular disease, cholestasis, and infiltrations.

Table 11.1.

	Hepatocellular	Cholestasis	Infiltrations
Bili	0 - +++	0 - +++	0 - + (<100 μmol/L)
AST	++ - +++ (>400 U/L)	0 - + (<400 U/L)	0 - + (<400 U/L)
ALP	0 - + (<300 U/L)	++ - +++ (>300 U/L)	++ - +++ (>300 U/L)

Bili, total bilirubin; AST, aspartate aminotransferase; ALP, alkaline phosphatase; 0, normal; +, degree of increase.
The figures are rule-of-thumb levels assuming upper reference limits for AST of 40 U/L and ALP of 120 U/L.

Jaundice

As stated above, clinical jaundice indicates a hyperbilirubinaemia in excess of 40 μmol/L. It is often divided into two types, depending on the serum bilirubin component elevated: conjugated (direct) hyperbilirubinaemia and unconjugated (indirect) hyperbilirubinaemia. They differ clinically in various respects.

Patients with unconjugated hyperbilirubinaemia rarely have serum bilirubin values in excess of 100 μmol/L (neonatal jaundice is a notable exception) and do not have a dark urine due to bilirubinuria (page 00). On the other hand, conjugated bilirubin is water-soluble and appears in the urine. (Patients are often alarmed by the dark urine and clay-coloured faeces).

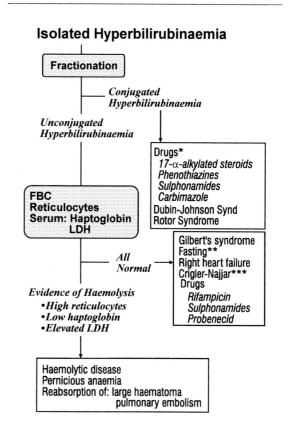

*Usually associated with increased ALT and ALP
**Bilirubin usually <40 μmol/L and fasting >24 hours
***Uncommon disorder usually diagnosed at birth

Figure 11.5. Suggested scheme for the evaluation of isolated hyperbilirubinaemia.

Severe jaundice with serum bilirubin values in excess of 200 μmol/L is usually due to hepatocellular disease or cholestasis and is of the conjugated variety. In certain situations, isolated hyperbilirubinaemia may be observed, the other "LFTs" being either normal (within reference ranges) or only slightly abnormal. A suggested scheme for the evaluation of patients with isolated hyperbilirubinaemia is presented in Figure 11.5.

CLASSIFICATION

Unconjugated hyperbilirubinaemia
    Starvation
    Haemolytic disease
    Resorption of haematoma/extravascular blood
    Inborn errors: Gilbert's syndrome
                            Crigler-Najjar syndromes
    Congestive cardiac failure
Conjugated hyperbilirubinaemia
    Inborn errors: Dubin-Johnson syndrome
                            Rotor syndrome
    Hepatocellular disease (see below)
    Cholestatic disease (see below)

Starvation. Calorie deprivation for 24 to 48 hours will result in a doubling of a normal subject's serum bilirubin level but the increase is rarely sufficient to produce jaundice (rarely above 35 μmol/L). The cause is unclear.

Haemolytic disease. Increased haemoglobin turnover, as occurs in *in vivo* haemolysis, may increase the bilirubin load sufficiently to overload the liver's excretory capacity. The serum level reached, in adults, is usually less than 100 μmol/L and the bilirubin is of the unconjugated variety. As there is no liver disease the liver function tests are usually normal. Serum analyte abnormalities that suggest haemolysis are a raised lactate dehydrogenase (LD is found in red cells) and a low haptoglobin concentration (haptoglobins attach to free serum haemoglobin and transport it to the reticulo-endothelial cells for metabolism).

Resorption of haematoma or extravascular blood. The resorption of large haematomas and blood lodged in extravascular spaces may, like haemolytic disease, produce sufficient bilirubin to overwhelm the excretory capacity of the liver.

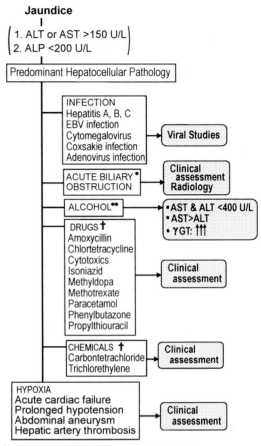

Figure 11.6. Check list for the evaluation of predominant hepatocellular disease.

Hepatocellular Disease

Liver cell damage can be caused by a wide variety of virus infections, drugs, chemicals, and toxins. Regardless of the cause, the basic lesion and biochemical characteristics are similar. A check list for the evaluation of patients with predominant hepatocellular pathology is given in Figure 11.6.

BIOCHEMICAL CHARACTERISTICS

The serum biochemical abnormalities associated with

148

hepatocellular damage are similar, regardless of the aetiology, although some subtle differences do exist.

Bilirubin. Jaundice, reflecting the hyperbilirubinaemia, is a characteristic feature. The serum bilirubin level is variable, e.g., in fulminating hepatitis, it may range from normal values to levels in excess of 1000 µmol/L. It is mostly of the conjugated variety, reflecting cholestasis due to local oedema of hepatocytes.

ALP. Serum ALP levels are usually normal but may be slightly increased to values less than 300 U/L.

AST (or ALT). A high serum transaminase level is characteristic of liver cell death with values above 400 U/L and often in excess of 1000 U/L. The highest levels occur early in the disease process, often before the onset of jaundice, and decline in parallel with the serum bilirubin level during later stages.

Albumin. The serum albumin concentration is variable depending on the severity of the process. Very low values indicate severe liver cell damage which results in depressed albumin synthesis.

CAUSES/PATHOPHYSIOLOGY

- **Viral agents:** Hepatitis A, B, C (non A, non B), Epstein-Barr virus, Cytomegalovirus, Coxsackie virus
- **Drugs** (see page 155)
- **Alcohol** (see page 154)
- **Toxins:** Mycotoxins (alfatoxins, toadstool poisoning)
- **Chemicals:** Carbon tetrachloride, trichlorethylene

The commonest cause of hepatocellular destruction is probably drug-related (including alcohol) but the most dramatic presentations are those due to viral hepatitis caused by the A and B viruses. In general practice, however, hepatitis due to the Epstein-Barr virus (EBV), e.g., infectious mononucleosis, is more common than that due to the hepatitis A and B viruses.

Acute viral hepatitis

The characteristic features of acute viral hepatitis are fever, anorexia, nausea, jaundice and hepatomegaly associated with markedly raised transaminases. Three clinical phases are recognised.

- *Prodromal phase.* This is a period of general malaise usually associated with fever, vomiting, and abdominal pain. Often the urine is dark, due to bilirubinuria, even though jaundice is not as yet clinically evident and the hyperbilirubinaemia is relatively mild. At this stage the serum transaminase activities are very high.

- *Icteric phase.* Clinical jaundice and marked hyperbilirubinaemia occur after 5 to 10 days and may last up to 2 to 3 weeks. As the jaundice begins to abate, the serum transaminases also drop.

- *Convalescent phase.* As the jaundice disappears so do the abdominal pain and tenderness.

The disease course lasts around 2-3 weeks in hepatitis A infection with complete clinical and biochemical recovery in 9 to 10 weeks (cf: 15-20 weeks in hepatitis B and C infections). Around 1-2% of patients may experience a severe acute fulminating course.

Hepatitis A. The Hepatitis A virus (HAV) is usually spread by the faecal-oral route causing sporadic or epidemic disease. Blood and stools are infectious during the incubation period (2-6 weeks). The mortality rate is low, chronic infection does not occur, but acute fulminating disease is a recognised complication.

Hepatitis B. The Hepatitis B virus (HBV) is usually spread by inoculation of infected blood or blood products. The incubation period varies from 6 weeks to 6 months. Acute infection can proceed to chronic hepatitis and 5-10% of infected individuals become carriers (Figure 11.7).

Hepatitis C. The hepatitis C virus (HCV) is a recently described agent about which information is still elementary. It is thought to be responsible for some 80% of post-transfusion cases of hepatitis and an unknown number of sporadic cases. It is detectable only by demonstration of antibody to HCV.

Non-A, Non-B Hepatitis. This term was used to describe those hepatitis patients who had neither HAV nor HBV infection. It is now generally recognised that most of these cases had infection with HCV.

149

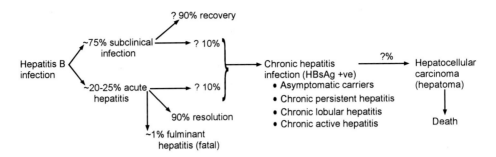

Figure 11.7. Clinical outcomes of hepatitis B infection.

Epstein-Barr virus. This virus causes infectious mononucleosis, a disease of young adults which is associated with fever, sore throat, lymphadenopathy, and a blood picture showing characteristic atypical lymphocytes. Liver involvement producing a hepatocellular picture is common. The liver disease is usually mild (e.g., AST <400 U/L, bilirubin <100 µmol/L) and self-limiting but can, in occasional cases, be severe and prolonged.

Chronic hepatitis

Chronic hepatitis is defined as hepatic inflammation continuing without improvement for longer than 6 months as demonstrated by persistently abnormal liver function tests. It may follow acute hepatitis B and C infection; it has been associated with drug reactions (e.g., methyldopa, isoniazid); it may occur in the absence of these causes, e.g., autoimmune hepatitis. Two distinct types are recognised: *chronic persistent hepatitis* and *chronic active hepatitis*.

Chronic persistent hepatitis. This is a benign, non-progressive condition with a good prognosis. The clinical and biochemical features are similar to chronic active hepatitis but the histology does not reveal the necrosis that is characteristic of active hepatitis. Definitive diagnosis requires a liver biopsy.

Chronic active hepatitis (CAH). This form usually progresses to cirrhosis and is characterised by liver cell necrosis and hepatic fibrosis. The serum bilirubin may be normal or only slightly increased but the

transaminases and serum globulin levels are usually significantly elevated, a five- to ten-fold increase in transaminases and a two-fold increase in gamma globulins being typical.

Hepatitis B CAH. In this disease the patients, usually males, are HBsAg positive and usually have a history of acute hepatitis B infection (see Figure 11.7).

Autoimmune CAH. This disorder, also called lupoid hepatitis, occurs predominantly in young women who may not have experienced an attack of acute hepatitis. They are negative for the usual hepatitis markers (HBV, HAV, etc) but some 80% will be positive for ANA (antinuclear antibody) and 60% positive for SMA (antismooth muscle antibody). There is an apparent increased incidence in patients with histocompatibility antigens HLA-A1 and HLA-B8. The patients often have hepatomegaly, spleno-megaly, jaundice and ascites.

Cholestatic Disease

Cholestasis is usually defined as impaired bile formation and flow due to a block in the excretion route anywhere in the area extending from the sinusoidal (excretory) surface of the hepatocyte to the ampulla of Vater. Biochemically it is characterised by disproportionate elevation of either serum alkaline phosphatase, or bilirubin, or both, relative to elevation of the serum transaminases. Two broad varieties are recognised -- *intrahepatic and extrahepatic cholestasis*. Additionally cholestasis may be associated with a normal serum bilirubin level (i.e., moderate to severe increase in ALP and a normal or slightly increased transaminase, associated with a normal bilirubin). This process has been termed *localised cholestasis* and usually indicates a localised infiltration (see below). The classical picture of cholestasis is a dark urine, pale stools, and pruritis.

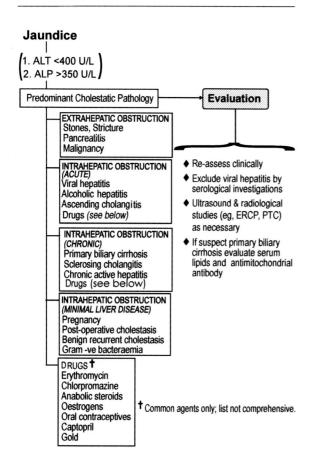

Figure 11.8. Check list for evaluation of predominant cholestatic disease.

BIOCHEMICAL CHARACTERISTICS

The characteristic serum biochemistry picture of cholestasis is:

Bilirubin. The bilirubin level depends on the degree of obstruction and varies from mildly elevated (<100 µmol/L) to grossly elevated values approaching 1000µmol/L; generally levels are of the order of 150-300 µmol/L. The major portion of the bilirubin will be

of the conjugated (direct reacting) variety.

ALP. Usually in excess of 300 U/L and can reach up to over 1000 U/L.

AST. This is generally normal or only slightly elevated (<400 U/L). If obstruction is severe and prolonged there may be significant hepatocellular destruction and values may then exceed 400 U/L.

Albumin. In the context of liver disease this analyte reflects the number of functional liver cells. In uncomplicated cholestatic disease the serum albumin level will be normal.

Note: The differentiation between intrahepatic and extrahepatic cholestasis can not be determined on the basis of the above tests which will be similar in both disorders. Discrimination between the two has to be based on the clinical picture and other procedures such as diagnostic imaging (e.g., ultrasound scans, refer to Figure 11.8); a definite diagnosis may require a liver biopsy in difficult cases.

CAUSES/PATHOPHYSIOLOGY

The common causes are:

Extrahepatic

- Biliary obstruction caused by stones, strictures, malignancy (e.g., carcinoma of the head of the pancreas), pancreatitis, biliary atresia, cholangitis

Intrahepatic

- Associated with structural liver damage: Acute hepatocellular disease, primary biliary cirrhosis, sclerosing cholangitis

- No associated structural liver damage: Postoperative cholestasis, benign recurrent cholestasis, total parenteral nutrition, pregnancy, steroid cholestasis, systemic infections

Extrahepatic cholestasis

Obstruction of the common bile duct can be due to a variety of causes (see above) but in all cases the serum biochemistry picture is similar and is not useful for differentiation. In some instances the clinical picture can be helpful, for example, stones are usually associated with biliary colic and painless progressive jaundice often indicates a malignant obstruction. Prolonged severe obstruction will result in hepatocellular destruction and a gross increase in the serum transaminase levels, producing a mixed hepatocellular and cholestatic picture (Table 11.2).

Table 11.2.

Mixed Hepatocellular & Cholestatic Pathology
Biochemical characteristics   ALT/AST: >150 U/L   ALP: >200 U/L   Bilirubin: variable
Causes   **Hepatitis:** Acute (cholestatic variety)   Chronic active   Alcoholic   **Biliary obstruction** (prolonged)   **Cirrhosis** (decompensated)\   **Ascending cholangitis**   **Malignancy** (secondary)   **Drugs:** *p*-Amino salicylic acid   Chlorambucil   Halothane   Ibuprofen   α-Methyldopa   Nitrofurantoin   Penicillamine   Phenylbutazone   Sulfonamides   Valproate
NB **The other possibility is bone disease (high ALP) associated with hepatocellular disease (high AST/ALT). An ALP fractionation should resolve the issue.**

Intrahepatic cholestasis with liver damage

Acute hepatocellular disease. Although hepatocellular disease typically produces a high serum transaminase relative to alkaline phosphatase (ALP), a prominent cholestatic picture with very high ALP values may occasionally be encountered in type A viral hepatitis and alcoholic hepatitis. In addition a similar situation, i.e., a mixed hepatocellular and cholestatic picture, may be associated with a number of drug reactions, particularly chlorpromazine (see below).

Primary biliary cirrhosis. Primary biliary cirrhosis (PBC) is a chronic progressive disease, which usually occurs in women age 40-60 years, that may be associated with complications such as steatorrhoea, osteoporosis, osteomalacia, xanthomata, and portal hypertension. The characteristic laboratory findings are cholestasis with a high ALP often being a chance early finding, hypercholesterolaemia, and, in up to 95% of cases, high titres of antimitochondrial antibodies. The serum IgM concentration is elevated in 80-90% of cases. Patients present with pruritis, dark urine (bilirubinuria) and hepatomegaly.

Sclerosing cholangitis. This fairly rare disorder is characterised by inflammation of the biliary tracts (intra- and extrahepatic) which leads to fibrosis and stricture. It presents with progressive obstructive jaundice and the characteristic cholestatic biochemical picture. Two-thirds of the patients have an associated ulcerative colitis (although only 1-5% of patients with ulcerative colitis will develop the disorder). The differential diagnosis includes cholangiocarcinoma and primary biliary cirrhosis and the definitive diagnosis depends on demonstration of diffuse thickening and obliteration of major bile ducts by endoscopic retrograde cholangiography (ERCP), transhepatic cholangiography and, in difficult cases, liver biopsy.

Intrahepatic cholestasis without liver damage

Postoperative cholestasis. On the second or third postoperative day, jaundice is a frequent complication and can be due to a variety of causes:

- increased bilirubin production due to transfusion of stored blood, resorption of blood from haematomas and extravascular spaces, haemolysis
- hepatic dysfunction due to halothane and hepatotoxic drugs used pre-operatively
- post-operative infections

When all such causative factors have been excluded the term *benign postoperative intrahepatic cholestasis* is usually applied.

Benign recurrent cholestasis. This is an uncommon (~100 cases reported) familial syndrome of recurrent intrahepatic cholestasis characterised by recurrent episodes of jaundice, pruritis, anorexia, and weight loss, lasting three to four months. In between episodes the serum biochemistry of hyperbilirubin-aemia and elevated ALP activity returns to normal.

Total parenteral nutrition. A mild cholestatic reaction with slightly elevated (e.g, two-fold) bilirubin, ALP, and AST levels is occasionally encountered in patients on total parenteral nutrition (commoner in neonates than in adults). The cause is unclear but it appears to occur predominantly in patients receiving large amounts of carbohydrates as the only source of energy.

Intrahepatic cholestasis of pregnancy. This benign disorder characteristically occurs in the third trimester and presents with pruritis and the features of mild cholestasis. The differential diagnosis includes all other causes of jaundice but viral hepatitis and cholelithiasis should be particularly excluded. The disorder tends to recur in subsequent pregnancies and when these women are given oral contraceptives. The occurrence in the third trimester suggests a role for oestrogens in its pathogenesis.

Steroid induced cholestasis. Pruritis which may progress to jaundice occurs in some subjects on the contraceptive pill and these patients will often develop cholestasis in pregnancy. Occasionally contraceptive administration will unmask disorders such as primary biliary cirrhosis and sclerosing cholangitis.

Systemic infections. Cholestatic jaundice is a well recognised complication of Gram-negative infections (presumably related to bacterial exotoxins). It is characterised by a high fever (due to the infection), moderate increase in serum conjugated bilirubin (up to 150 µmol/L), two to three-fold elevations of the ALP and, usually, a normal AST.

Infiltrations/space-occupying lesions

Space-occupying lesions of the liver and infiltrations present with characteristic biochemical features:

Bilirubin. Normal

ALP. Moderately to grossly elevated, e.g., 300-1500 U/L

AST. Normal or slightly increased, e.g., <200 U/L

Albumin. Normal

Often there may only be an isolated elevated serum ALP in which cases further tests are required to determine its origin (pages 157, 179). A useful test is the serum γ-glutamyltransferase (pages 158, 183) but one should be aware that this analyte can be elevated in the absence of liver disease, e.g., due to alcohol or drug enzyme induction; and severe liver disease can be associated with normal serum levels.

CAUSES/PATHOPHYSIOLOGY

- Carcinoma: primary, secondary (particularly metastatic GI tumours)
- Cysts
- Abscess
- Granuloma
- Infiltrations: leukaemia, myeloma, lymphoma

The biochemical features are due to obstruction of the small bile ducts (localised cholestasis) and damage to hepatocytes as the lesion enlarges. As the lesions generally do not occupy or involve the whole liver there is usually sufficient healthy parenchyma left to maintain bilirubin excretion and albumin synthesis. However, as lesions such as secondary tumours enlarge they replace more and more liver tissue (with decreased albumin synthesis) and often obstruct major bile ducts producing moderate to severe elevations of bilirubin (cholestatic jaundice). In these situations the patient's serum biochemistry can become indistinguishable from late stage cirrhosis (see below).

Cirrhosis

Cirrhosis is a chronic progressive disorder characterised by progressive hepatic fibrosis and localised nodules of regenerating liver tissue. Both the clinical manifestations and the serum biochemistry are variable but the characteristic presenting features are localised cholestasis (jaundice, portal hypertension), and hypoalbuminaemia and a bleeding tendency, reflecting the loss of hepatic cells.

Bilirubin. Usually normal but can be increased during the active phase.

ALP. Increased and usually >300 U/L

AST. Depends on the disease activity. Varies from normal to values >300 U/L.

Albumin. Normal in early stages but decreases as the disease progresses. May reach as low as 15 g/L, with development of ascites and oedema.

CAUSES/PATHOPHYSIOLOGY

The major aetiological factors are alcoholism, chronic active hepatitis (page 150), post hepatitis B and non-A, non-B infections, prolonged biliary obstruction, primary biliary cirrhosis (page 152), hepatotoxins, drug reactions, long-term hepatic congestion, haemochromatosis (page 276), hepatolenticular degeneration (Wilson's disease, page 159), and α_1-antitrypsin deficiency. The reader is referred to other sections elsewhere in the book and more specialised texts for more details of these causes and for discussions of methods used to establish the aetiology and to assess the nature and extent of complications.

However, regardless of the aetiology, the basic lesion in developing cirrhosis is localised areas of cell destruction (caused by viral infections, toxins, etc) which are replaced by fibrous tissue (scarring). As the disease progresses the fibrosis becomes extensive and adjacent areas merge producing isolated pockets of normal hepatocytes. These patches of normal liver cells attempt to regenerate and this produces the characteristic nodularity. Three phases of the disease can be recognised:

• *Quiescent (compensation) phase.* The disease is temporarily halted and the only biochemical features may be a high plasma ALP level (cholestasis due to fibrosis) and a moderately decreased serum albumin (loss of healthy liver parenchyma).

• *Active phase.* In this stage there is progessive liver cell necrosis (high serum transaminases) and fibrosis (cholestasis).

• *Decompensation phase.* This is the stage of liver failure and in addition to high levels of AST and ALP there is hyperbilirubinaemia and severe hypo-albuminaemia.

Alcoholic liver disease

The consequence of alcohol consumption on the liver may vary from an isolated induced elevation in the serum γ-glutamyltransferase (γGT, page 183) to severe alcoholic cirrhosis with liver failure. There are four well recognised liver responses any of which may be active at presentation.

• Enzyme changes without overt liver disease
• Fatty liver
• Alcoholic hepatitis
• Alcoholic cirrhosis

Enzyme changes without liver disease. Acute alcohol consumption in otherwise normal subjects is not usually associated with any significant serum abnormality although increases in the γGT have been reported. Thirty to 90% of chronic drinkers, who do not have overt liver disease, will exhibit an increased serum γGT which falls during abstinence (plasma half-life of 26 days). Some will also have mildly increased levels of ALT or ALP or both, but this should be considered as evidence of hepatic damage.

Fatty liver. This is the most frequent hepatic abnormality linked to alcohol usage. The disorder, due to triglyceride accumulation, results in an enlarged liver and variable serum enzyme changes but is believed to be reversible with abstinence from alcohol, if it occurs without concomitant alcoholic hepatitis (see below). The pathogenesis is likely to be a combination of increased influx of fatty acids from body fat stores, enhanced hepatic synthesis of triglyceride-rich very low density lipoproteins, and decreased fatty acid oxidation in the liver. A liver biopsy is required to diagnose the condition.

Alcoholic hepatitis. Alcoholic insults to the liver can result in hepatocellular necrosis presenting as acute hepatitis or even fulminating liver disease with severe hepatic decompensation. The serum biochemistry changes are similar to those described above for acute hepatocellular disease but usually with high transaminase and high ALP levels (i.e., usually a mixed hepatocellular and cholestatic disorder, Table 11.2). The transaminase values are usually less than 400 U/L with the AST being greater than the ALT. The serum γGT value, which is characteristically disproportionally increased relative to the ALP, often gives a clue to the diagnosis. A decrease in serum albumin level and an increase in serum IgA level are frequently seen. Liver biopsy reveals fatty infiltration, cell necrosis and the presence of Mallory bodies (perinuclear eosinophilic inclusions).

Alcoholic cirrhosis. After 5-15 years of heavy alcohol use, some 5-10% of practising chronic alcoholics will develop cirrhosis, usually after several bouts of acute alcoholic hepatitis, although it may be an insidious development. The clinical and biochemical features are again variable and depend on the activity of the disease. A liver biopsy is important in establishing the diagnosis and in staging the disease.

Drug-induced liver disease

Liver pathology due to drug toxicity is a common clinical problem and perhaps the commonest cause of abnormal liver function tests seen in general practice. Drug-related liver problems can vary from the innocuous isolated raised γGT due to enzyme induction through to severe hepatocellular disease. There are four types of responses and some of the more common drugs related to these responses are listed below.

Isolated elevation of serum γGT. This is due to liver enzyme induction and the drugs commonly responsible are *phenytoin, barbiturates, warfarin, amitriptyline, oral contraceptives (high oestrogen variety)*. Other causes and associations of an isolated raised serum γGT level are alcohol ingestion, obesity, diabetes mellitus, and hypertriglyceridaemia.

Predominant hepatocellular disease. This is biochemically characterised by a raised serum AST and normal or near normal serum ALP, and may present with or without jaundice.
Drugs responsible: *aspirin, chlortetracycline, cytotoxics, danthrolene, isoniazid, methotrexate, paracetamol, phenytoin sodium, propylthiouracil.*

Predominant cholestasis. Patients present with a cholestatic biochemical picture: Normal or near normal AST, elevated serum ALP, with or without jaundice.
Drugs causing cholestasis: *carbamazepine,*

chlorpromazine, erythromycin, indomethacin, oral contraceptive steroids, tolbutamide.

Mixed hepatocellular and cholestatic disease. This will result in significantly elevated levels of both serum AST and ALP; clinical jaundice may or may not be evident.
Drugs involved: *chlorambucol, halothane, α-methyldopa, nitrofurantoin, phenylbutazone, valproate.*

Fatty liver

A patient with a fatty liver presents with hepatomegaly which is due to accumulation of fat in the hepatocytes. The serum biochemistry results are variable but usually there are mild abnormalities.

Bilirubin. Usually normal but 25% of patients with alcoholic fatty liver have been reported to have elevated levels, but less than 100 μmol/L.

AST. Normal to mildly elevated (<200 U/L)

ALP. Normal to mildly elevated (<200 U/L). The exception is alcohol-induced fatty liver which may have an additional cholestatic element.

Albumin. Normal, providing there are no extrahepatic causes for hypoalbuminaemia, e.g., malnutrition.

γGT. In many cases the only abnormality may be an isolated raised serum γ-glutamyltransferase.

CAUSES

The commonest associated disorder is alcohol-related liver disease. Other associated causes include prolonged starvation, diabetes mellitus, obesity, corticosteroid therapy, total parenteral nutrition, and hyperlipidaemia.

Cholecystitis/cholelithiasis

Other diseases of the biliary tract which may present with abnormal serum biochemistry results are cholelithiasis, cholecystitis, and cholangitis.

Cholelithiasis. It has been estimated that in the USA some 10% of men and 20% of women over the age of 65 years have gall stones. Whilst inhabiting the gall bladder they are usually asymptomatic but they may be instrumental in causing cholecystitis and if they enter the common bile duct obstructive jaundice can occur (see above).

Cholecystitis. 90% of cases of cholecystitis (inflammation of the gall blader) are associated with gall stones. It presents with pain, fever, and often mildly abnormal serum biochemistry with elevated AST or ALP levels or both. The values of both enzymes is usually less than 300 U/L. Mild hyperbilirubinaemia (<80 µmol/L) may also be found.

Cholangitis. Bacterial infection of the bile ducts (ascending cholangitis) is usually associated with either cholecystitis or, more commonly, stone(s) in the common bile duct. The characteristic features are fever, chills, upper quadrant pain, and jaundice with a cholestatic biochemistry picture.

Laboratory evaluation of hepato-biliary disease

There are two broad groups of laboratory tests available for the evaluation of liver disease: the routine tests of liver function (LFTs) and the more specific tests which help in determining the cause of the disease.

- The *routine tests* include: serum bilirubin, transaminases (AST, ALT), alkaline phosphatase, γ-glutamyltransferase, total protein, albumin, urinary bilirubin and urobilinogen, coagulation factors.

- *Specific aetiological tests* that may be useful are serum α_1-antitrypsin, α-fetoprotein, hepatitis serological markers, specific autoantibodies, immunoglobulins, caeruloplasmin and copper, and serum iron studies.

ROUTINE TESTS OF LIVER FUNCTION

Besides the routinely available 'liver function tests' mentioned above, other liver function tests that have been used in the past or may be used in special situations are coagulation studies, plasma bile salts, bromosulphthalein (BSP) excretion test, and plasma ammonia. The basic front-line 'liver function tests' (LFTs) should include serum total bilirubin, a serum transaminase, serum alkaline phosphatase, and serum albumin. The use of this group of tests for the evaluation of suspected liver disease was discussed earlier in relevant sections. In the next section the clinical significance of the more frequently requested tests is summarised.

Serum bilirubins

As stated earlier, bilirubin circulates in the serum in two forms, unconjugated (85% of total in the normal subject) and conjugated bilirubin (most laboratories only measure the total level routinely). Unconjugated hyperbilirubinaemia occurs in haemolytic disease, Gilbert's syndrome, and the Crigler-Najjar group of disorders. Conjugated hyperbilirubinaemia occurs in the Dubin-Johnson and Rotor syndromes, and in hepatocellular and cholestatic liver disease.

Urinary bilirubin

Unconjugated bilirubin circulates attached to albumin and is neither filtered by the glomerulus nor found in urine. On the other hand conjugated bilirubins are water-soluble and appear in the urine if the plasma level is raised, i.e., bilirubinuria is an indicator of the blood conjugated bilirubin level. Bilirubinuria produces a dark urine and this may be the earliest manifestation of acute hepatitis.

Urinary urobilinogen

Urinary levels of this pigment are increased if there is (a) increased bilirubin production (e.g., haemolysis), or (b) there is impaired re-excretion due to liver damage. It disappears from the urine if there is complete cholestasis (no bile reaching the gut).

Serum albumin/total protein

The liver is the sole site of albumin synthesis (~12 g/day); thus low levels in the context of liver disease indicates severe dysfunction. However, the serum albumin level in liver disease can be misleading because (a) serum albumin has a half-life of ~21 days, hence normal levels prevail in the early phase of severe acute disease, (b) there are other common causes of a low serum albumin such as malnutrition and the nephrotic syndrome, (c) dehydration (haemoconcentration) increases the serum albumin concentration and may give a false impression. The serum total protein value minus the albumin value gives the serum total globulin level. The serum globulin levels can increase dramatically in chronic hepatitis and cirrhosis and this, in the presence of hypoalbuminaemia, can produce a normal total protein level, emphasing the importance of measuring both albumin and total protein under these conditions.

Serum transaminases

Traditionally the LFT enzyme profile has included one transaminase, either aspartate aminotransferase (AST) or alanine aminotransferase (ALT). The transaminases are located in the hepatocyte and high plasma levels indicate release from the cells during damage (hepatocellular disease). Values in excess of 400 U/L occur in hepatocellular disease whilst in cholestasis the level is normal or only slightly raised (<400 U/L.).

AST has a wide distribution and a raised serum value is a non-specific event with the possibilities including destruction of hepatocytes, myocardium, skeletal muscle, or erythrocytes. ALT also has a wide distribution in the body but a raised serum level is most likely to reflect liver cell damage, i.e., for clinical purposes a high serum ALT indicates liver pathology.

In the hepatocyte ALT is located only in the cytosol whereas AST is found in the cytosol and in the mitochondria and thus it has been suggested, particularly in the German literature, that in the context of liver disease a serum AST value in excess of the serum ALT value indicates a severe disease process. The reasoning behind this is as follows: Most of the raised transaminases in liver disease reflects 'seepage' of enzymes through damaged cell membranes, i.e., the cytosol components escape leaving the mitochondria behind. Hence the serum ALT level will exceed the AST level. If damage is severe and many hepatocytes are destroyed then, in addition to the cytosol component, the mitochondrial enzymes are released as well, giving an AST value higher than the ALT value.

There is good evidence in the literature, and personal experience confirms this, that alcoholic liver disease is associated with a high AST:ALT ratio; and it is further suggested that when the serum transaminase concentrations are raised, but less than ten-fold the upper reference limit (i.e., <400 U/L), an AST:ALT ratio greater than 2 is strong evidence for alcoholic liver disease. A paper by Cohen and Kaplan in 1969 showed that of 104 patients with alcoholic liver disease, 70% had ratios above 2, whereas of 167 patients with non-alcoholic liver disease only 9.6% has ratios above 2 (using a cut-off of 1.5 the proportions were 85% and 25% respectively).

The cause of the high ratio is unclear; it is unlikely to be due to the mitochondrial AST component because liver biopsies show the same pattern as serum. A suggested reason is reduced hepatic pyridoxal-5-phosphate which is a co-factor for both enzymes but its deficiency has a greater impact on ALT activity.

Serum alkaline phosphatase (ALP)

ALP is located on the sinusoidal surface of the hepatocyte and in the microvilli of the bile canaliculi. It is not a specific liver enzyme as it is also found in bone, the placenta, and some malignancies (page 178). During cholestasis (obstruction) the serum ALP level rises making it the indicator enzyme for this condition. The rise mainly results from increased synthesis (? enzyme induction) rather than from obstructed outflow. The increase in cholestasis is usually to values greater than 300 U/L whereas in hepatocellular disease the levels remain normal or are only slightly increased (to less than 300 U/L).

Subjects presenting with an isolated increased serum ALP may be difficult to evaluate if the clinical picture is unhelpful. The ideal approach is to determine the tissue of origin by separating and measuring the ALP isoenzymes using electrophoretic techniques (page 179). If this test is not available estimation of the serum γ-glutamyltransferase can be helpful -- a normal serum level makes liver disease unlikely; on the other hand a high value does not necessarily indicate liver disease because of enzyme induction (see below). A useful test, if available, is the serum 5'-nucleotidase which originates predominantly from the liver and is usually only increased in subjects with liver disease.

Serum γ-glutamyltransferase (γGT)

This enzyme is discussed on page 183. The plasma level is increased in both hepatocellular and cholestatic liver disease and is a sensitive marker of hepatic disease. However, two other characteristics can cause difficulties in interpretation. Firstly, on odd occasions, severe liver disease can be associated with normal serum γGTP levels and secondly, increased serum levels, due to enzyme induction, can present in the absence of liver disease (as occurs in chronic alcoholism, with the drugs phenytoin sodium, barbiturates, warfarin, and amitriptyline, and in disorders such as obesity, diabetes mellitus, and hypertriglyceridaemia). Despite these problems, it is a useful test which often provides the first indication of a patient's increased alcohol consumption, even though its specificity for this disorder is low.

Serum bile salts

Bile acids, which play an important role in fat absorption (page 215), are synthesised in the liver from cholesterol and conjugated with glycine or taurine prior to being excreted in the bile (cholic acid and chenodeoxycholic acid are primary acids whilst the secondary acids, deoxycholic and lithocholic acids, are formed in the intestine by bacteria). Over 95% of the 15 to 30 g excreted in the bile daily is reabsorbed in the distal ileum (enterohepatic circulation, see Figure 11.9). In hepatobiliary disease excretion is compromised and the plasma levels rise (the 2-hour postprandial plasma levels have been used as an

indicator of hepatobiliary disease). However, as a test of liver function, this estimation has not gained wide acceptance, mainly due to technical difficulties.

Coagulation factors

The coagulation factors II, VII, IX, and X are vitamin K dependant and are synthesised in the liver. Decreased plasma levels of these factors and blood clotting problems (raised *prothrombin time*) may occur during (a) severe liver disease, and (b) vitamin K deficiency (vitamin K is fat-soluble and requires bile acids in the gut for absorption; its level would be low in cholestasis).

Bromosulphthalein excretion test (BSP)

The ability of the liver to clear the blood of BSP after an intravenous injection of the dye is a sensitive test of hepatic function. It is most useful in those patients who have normal LFTs but who may have liver dysfunction because they have disorders known to cause liver disease, e.g, ulcerative colitis. One of the problems with the test is that a number of anaphylaxic reactions to the dye have occurred.

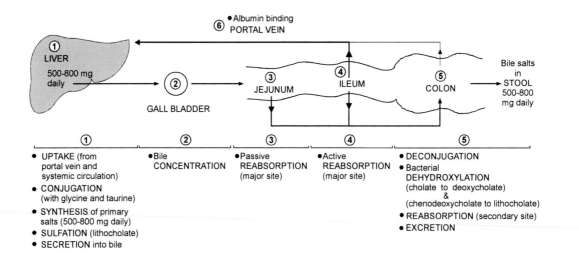

Figure 11.9. The enterohepatic circulation of bile salts.

Blood ammonia

The liver detoxifies gut-produced ammonia (action of enterobacteria on dietary protein) which is presented to it via the portal venous flow. If there is severe liver disease or a portal-systemic shunt (as in cirrhosis) the ammonia escapes the liver and the blood level rises (Figure 11.10). There is a loose association between the blood ammonia level and the degree of hepatic encephalopathy in severe liver disease, but it is not sufficiently close to be of clinical importance.

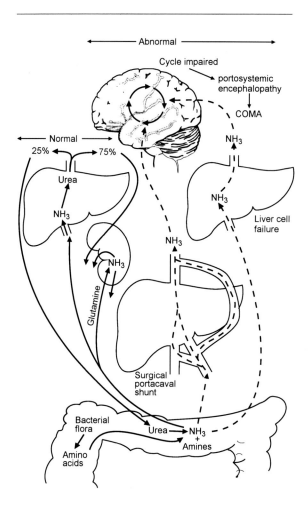

Figure 11.10. Normal and abnormal ammonia metabolism. Redrawn, with kind permission of McGraw-Hill, from Price SA and Wilson LM: *Pathophysiology: Clinical Concepts of Disease Processes, 3rd edn,* McGraw-Hill, New York, 1986. (Reappears also as Figure 27.2 on page 341).

SPECIFIC AETIOLOGICAL TESTS

α_1-Antitrypsin

This is an acute phase protein with anti-protease activity that constitutes 90% of the a_1-band on protein electrophoresis. Deficiency, which is evident by a decreased intensity of the α_1-band, is associated with lung (emphysema) and liver disease. The liver disease, hepatitis leading on to cirrhosis, usually develops in the neonatal period (see page 166). Most patients with liver disease have the PiZZ genotype, with only 15-20% of the normal α_1-antitrypsin activity in their sera.

α-Fetoprotein

This is the major serum protein in early foetal life but very low levels may be found in adults (<50 µg/L). Raised serum values are found in 75% of patients with primary hepatocellular carcinoma, in chronic hepatitis and in alcoholic liver disease.

Caeruloplasmin and copper studies

Hepatolenticular degeneration or Wilson's disease, due to a defect in copper metabolism, results in liver cirrhosis (page 153). A characteristic feature is a low serum level of the copper-binding protein, caeruloplasmin, an increase in hepatic copper (>250 µg/g tissue dry weight) and an increase in urinary copper excretion. The total serum copper level is usually reduced (due to the decreased circulating caeruloplasmin level) but the free (unbound) copper level is markedly increased.

Iron studies

The iron overload disorders, including haemochromatosis (page 276), can be associated with liver pathology, particularly cirrhosis. Serum iron studies indicating iron overload are characterised by (a) a high serum ferritin level, (b) an elevated serum iron level, (c) high saturation (e.g., >80%) of plasma transferrin by iron (page 276), and (d) demonstration of increased tissue iron stores on liver biopsy (>10 mg/g tissue dry weight). High plasma ferritin values may also occur in malignancy, chronic infections, haemolytic disorders, and acute hepatocellular disease.

Note: The other liver function tests are not particularly useful for the diagnosis of this condition, often showing near normal results when considerable tissue damage is already present.

Hepatitis serology

Hepatitis due to infective agents should be excluded in all patients with hepatocellular disease. The following markers identify infection with the known viruses and Table 11.3 lists the serological markers seen in symptomatic patients.

Table 11.3. Serological markers seen in symptomatic patients.

	Symptomatic Panel			
HBsAg	Anti-HBc IgM	Anti-HAV IgM	Anti-HCV	Interpretation
−	−	+	−	Acute hepatitis A infection
+	+	−	−	Acute hepatitis B infection
+	−	−	−	Acute or chronic hepatitis B infection (requires further serological investigation to determine chronicity)
−	−	−	+	Hepatitis C infection
+	+/−	−	+	Hepatitis B & hepatitis C coinfection or superinfection
−	−	−	−	Possible hepatitis C infection (requires follow-up testing for confirmation)

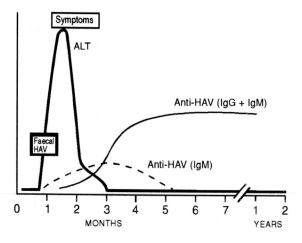

Figure 11.11. Serological events in acute (self-limiting) hepatitis A infection relative to alanine transaminase (ALT) peak. See text for details.

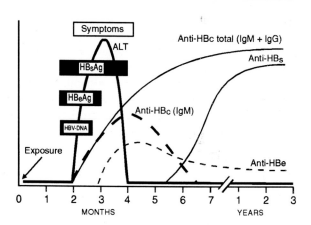

Figure 11.12. Serological events in acute (self-limiting) hepatitis B infection relative to ALT peak. See text for details.

Hepatitis A. The hepatitis A virus (HAV) can be identified in the stool up to two weeks prior to the illness but is rarely found after the first week of illness. The diagnosis is confirmed by finding IgM or IgG antibodies in the serum. They appear early in the disease with IgM occurring during the first week and disappearing within 8 weeks. The IgG antibody peaks at one month and may persist for years (Figure 11.11).

Hepatitis B. The hepatitis B virus (HBV) consists of an outer shell and an inner core. The first marker to appear is the surface antigen (**HBsAg**), occurring before evidence of liver disease. It persists though out the illness and disappears as the disease resolves. Persistence means either a carrier state or chronic hepatitis (its presence infers infectivity). The specific antibody to HBsAg, **Anti-HBs**, appears after the clearance of HBsAg and indicates recovery from HBV and noninfectivity. It also indicates successful immunisation for hepatitis B. An IgM antibody to the core antigen (**Anti-HBc**) appears shortly after HBsAg is detected and can persist up to two years; as it can often be demonstrated after HBsAg has disappeared and before anti-HBs appears, it is a useful marker for recent infection (Figure 11.12).

Delta agent (Hepatitis D). This viral agent has only been identified in association with HBsAg and is

160

cleared at the same time. It may increase the severity of the HBV infection.

Hepatitis C (HCV). This agent is responsible for 80 to 90% of cases of transfusion hepatitis and is also found in sporadic disease. A routine test to identify the antibody to the C virus is now available; a positive test indicates previous or ongoing infection, however it may not appear until 10 to 12 weeks after exposure.

Epstein-Barr virus (EBV). This is the agent of infectious mononucleosis and used to be demonstrated by the Paul Bunnell test. Some 10-15% of patients with infectious mononucleosis become jaundiced and up to 30% will have abnormal liver function tests.

Immunoglobulins

Non-specific polyclonal increases in serum gamma-globulins are associated with chronic hepatitis and cirrhosis, including alcoholic cirrhosis. Mild increases also occur in acute hepatitis but decline to normal values within 3 to 4 months. Increased IgA values may occur in alcoholic liver disease and IgM values increase in primary biliary cirrhosis.

Autoantibodies

Antibodies to mitochondria, smooth muscle and nuclei are often found in the sera of patients with primary biliary cirrhosis and autoimmune chronic active hepatitis and in some cases are diagnostic.

Anti-mitochondrial antibodies. Positive in 90 to 95% of patients with primary biliary cirrhosis (high titres are highly specific for this disease). They may also be positive in autoimmune chronic active hepatitis (~70%).

Anti-smooth muscle antibodies. A high titre is characteristic of autoimmune chronic active hepatitis.

Anti-nuclear antibodies. 80% of patients with autoimmune chronic active hepatitis have high titres.

REFERENCES/FURTHER READING

Chopra S and Griffin PH. Laboratory tests and diagnostic procedures in evaluation of liver disease. Am J Med 1985;79:221-230.

Cohen JA and Kaplan MM. The SGOT/SGPT ratio-- an indicator of alcoholic liver disease. Dig Dis Sci 1979;24:835-838.

Fevey J, Vanstaple F, Blanckert N. Bile pigment metabolism. Bailiere's Clin Gastroenterol 1989;3:283-306.

Johnson PJ. Role of the standard liver function tests in current practice. Ann Clin Biochem 1989;26:463-471.

Lauff JJ, Kasper ME, Wu TW, *et al*. Isolation and preliminary characterization of a fraction of bilirubin in serum that is firmly bound to protein. Clin Chem 1982;28:629-637.

Chapter 12

Plasma and CSF Proteins

There are more than a hundred different proteins in the plasma, the majority of which are enzymes and polypeptide hormones. While some plasma proteins have a specific role in blood, e.g., the clotting factors, many others represent cellular proteins shed into the circulation as a result of degradative processes, and a number of proteins found in circulation do not as yet have ascribed or proven functions. All the transcellular fluids such as urine, cerebrospinal fluid (CSF), synovial fluid, pleural fluid, and saliva also contain a considerable number of proteins, many or most of them derived from the plasma by transudation; some are secreted specifically into the fluid, e.g., the Tamm Horsfall protein found in urine and some immunoglobulins in CSF which are produced intrathecally.

Most of the changes involving proteins in blood and other body fluids are secondary to disease processes affecting either protein synthesis, distribution, catabolism or clearance but some changes are genetically determined. The secondary changes vary markedly in clinical usefulness, some are important to diagnosis (e.g., the finding of a paraprotein in myeloma), others are less informative. Clinical manifestations of the genetic disorders are due to abnormality or deficiency in specific proteins, which are primarily catalytic enzymes involved in metabolic pathways.

The measurement of proteins in body fluids is an integral part of any chemical pathology service in an acute patient care hospital. This chapter deals with plasma and CSF proteins; proteinuria is discussed in the chapter on renal function.

Plasma proteins

The plasma contains some 60-80 g/L of proteins. They are mostly synthesised in the liver, with the notable exception of immunoglobulins which are synthesised by cells of the lymphoreticular system, and cell-surface proteins such as β_2-microglobulin which are made by many different cell types. The structural heterogeneity of plasma proteins is parallelled by their functional diversity. Plasma proteins are involved in:

(a) the intravascular transport of various substances, such as hormones (thyroxine, cortisol), metals (calcium, iron, copper), bilirubin and certain drugs

(b) the inflammatory response and immunological defence against infection
(c) the control of extracellular fluid distribution
(d) blood clotting and fibrinolytic mechanisms
(e) intermediary metabolism (as hormones, enzymes, repressors, inhibitors)
(f) nutrition
(g) tissue and cell structure (as contractile, fibrous and keratinous proteins)
(g) repair mechanisms

PROTEIN MEASUREMENTS

A variety of techniques, both qualitative and quantitative, have been used to measure proteins in body fluids. They include chemical and immunochemical methods and physical separation methods such as electrophoresis and chromatography.

The most established methods for the measurement of albumin in serum use chemical reactions based on the bromcresol green or purple dyes. However, in the detection and quantitation of microalbuminuria, more sensitive methods based on antigen-antibody interaction, are needed. Such immunochemical methods using polyvalent or monovalent antibodies and sensitive detection systems (immunoturbidimetric assays, immunonephelometric assays, radioimmunoassays, etc) are also increasingly used in the clinical laboratory to quantitate other individual proteins in serum and other body fluids.

The above trend notwithstanding, the measurement of serum total proteins as a group by the Biuret reaction, remains a frequently performed test, either on its own or together with electrophoresis of serum, urinary or CSF proteins. Separations of proteins by electrophoretic techniques are regularly carried out as they provide useful information of changes in the relative proportions of individual proteins or groups of proteins.

Serum protein electrophoresis

Electrophoresis makes use of the fact that the constituent amino acids of proteins carry both positive and negative charges. If a mixture of serum proteins, buffered at pH 8.6, is subjected to an electric current

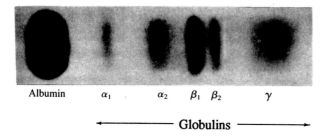

Figure 12.1. Serum electrophoretic patterns of normal human serum. **Top.** Cellulose acetate electrophoresis (only 5 or 6 bands are discernable). **Bottom.** High resolution agarose gel electrophoresis (A typical electrophoretogram of normal human serum would show fourteen major proteins; in case of plasma, an additional fibrinogen band).

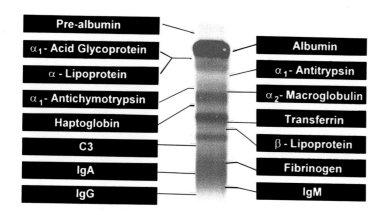

the individual proteins will migrate at varying speeds towards the positive electrode (anode) according to their net negative charges, e.g., albumin moves rapidly whilst γ-globulins hardly move at all. In practice, this separation is carried out on an inert support medium such as an agarose gel film or a cellulose acetate strip, and the protein fractions are visualised by staining with a suitable protein stain.

In serum or plasma, five main groups are seen on electrophoretic separation (Figure 12.1.Top). These are, from the anodic end, albumin, α₁-, α₂-, β-, and γ-globulins. The albumin fraction is essentially homogeneous, with prealbumin running ahead of it as a very faint minor band. Each of the globulin fractions contains a number of different proteins of which only the main ones are listed below:

- α₁-*globulins:* α₁-antitrypsin, α-lipoproteins, α₁-acid glycoprotein (orosomucoid)
- α₂-*globulins:* caeruloplasmin, haptoglobins, α₂-macroglobulin

- β-*globulins:* β-lipoprotein, transferrin, C₃ complement, fibrinogen (plasma only)
- γ-*globulins:* immunoglobulins, C reactive protein (CRP)

Using high resolution agarose gel electrophoresis, as many as 12-15 distinct bands may be observed in the stained gel (Figure 12.1.Bottom). **Note**: If plasma is used instead of serum, fibrinogen appears as an extra band between the β- and γ-globulin zones and may be misinterpreted as a paraprotein band by the unwary.

Plasma proteins in health and disease

We will discuss the following clinically important plasma proteins: albumin, α₁-antitrypsin, α₂-macroglobulin, caeruloplasmin, haptoglobin, β₂-microglobulin, CRP and the immunoglobulins, and the associated disorders. In addition, we will consider a

Figure 12.2. Top. A single gel run depicting single and multiple protein changes that may be discernable from electrophoretograms.

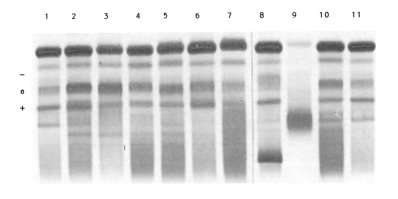

Lane

1: Normal serum.

2: Increased α-β interzone staining in a haemolysed sample due to haptoglobin haemoglobin complex formation.

3: Nephrotic syndrome (decreased albumin and transferrin, increased α2-macroglobulin)

4: Acute phase reaction - increased α_1 and α_2 globulins, decreased albumin, transferrin.

5: Inflammatory response -- acute on chronic, (acute phase reaction changes and polyclonal hypergammaglobinaemia).

6: Degraded sample (due to prolonged storage) with no C3 complement band.

7: Polyclonal hypergammaglobulinaemia with β-γ fusion in patient with cirrhosis.

8: Monoclonal hypergammaglobulinaemia (IgG, kappa paraproteinaemia), serum from patient with multiple myeloma.

9: Urine from same patient as lane 8, showing free kappa light chain paraproteinuria.

10: Polyclonal hypergammaglobulinaemia.

11: Normal serum.

Figure 12.2. Bottom. A composition of various protein electrophoretic patterns to illustrate multiple protein changes. *Unlike Figure 12.2. Top, this is not a single gel run.* Lanes are numbered consecutively from left to right.

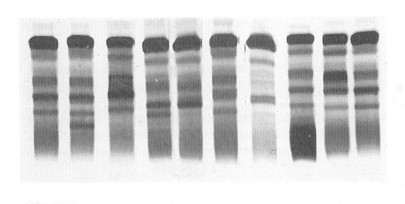

Lane

1': Normal serum.

2': Normal plasma (note additional fibrinogen band in fast gamma zone).

3': Haemolysed sample (see comments for Figure 12.2 Top, Lane 2).

4': Effect of sample storage on C3 -- degradation by extended refrigeration for >72 h. Note decreased C3; appearance of faint band in fast γ-zone.

5': Prolonged sample storage at room temperature, with disappearance of C3 band and appearance of faint band at anodic end of transferrin band (β_1 zone).

6': Genetic variation: Bistransferrinaemia (note altered electrophoretic mobilities).

7': Bistransferrinuria (urine sample).

8': Serum protein changes in a patient with an acute on chronic inflammation (see comments for Lane 4 above).

9': Acute phase response (see Lane 5 above)

10': Normal serum.

characteristic plasma protein response to inflammation known as the acute phase response, and the role of the cytokines. The lipoproteins (page 193) and transferrin (page 272) are discussed elsewhere and readers are referred to textbooks of haematology for discussions of complements and clotting factors.

Serum total protein

A quantitativemeasure of the serum total proteins is most often carried out as part of the serum protein electrophoresis profile or a liver panel; single measurements of the plasma total protein levels are of limited clinical application. This stems largely from the fact that acute changes are more likely to be due to the changes in the intravascular protein-free fluid rather than of the proteins. In addition, a change (e.g., a decrease) in the concentration of one protein may be masked by a compensatory change (e.g., an increase) in another constituent protein or proteins. Nonetheless, as a screening procedure, measurement of total protein may alert to some specific protein abnormality, if concentration changes are marked. This will be manifested as hyperproteinaemia or hypoproteinaemia.

Hyperproteinaemia. This is found in two situations:

1   Haemoconcentration (e.g., in dehydration or after prologed application of a tourniquet when collecting blood) causes an increase in all protein fractions by the same percentage.
2   Hypergammaglobinaemia.

Hypoproteinaemia. This can reflect one of three problems:

1   Haemodilution (gain in intravascular protein-free fluid) e.g., water overload, blood sample taken from a vein proximal to an IV infusion
2   Hypoalbuminaemia
3   Hypogammaglobulinaemia

Albumin

This protein (MW 40000-60000) is the most abundant single species in the plasma (30-55 g/L). It is an important controller of the water distribution between the intra- and extravascular fluids (predomi-nant contributor to the plasma oncotic pressure) and an important carrier of various plasma constituents, e.g., calcium, magnesium, thyroid hormones, unconjugated bilirubin, fatty acids and some drugs. The total body content is around 3-5 g/kg (250-350 g in a 70 kg adult); 35-40% is found in the intravascular space (30-55 g/L) and the remainder in the extravascular portion of the extracellular fluid.

Table 12.1. Causes of hypoalbuminaemia.

Haemodilution
　　Water overload, sample from IV infusion arm, pregnancy
Decreased synthesis
　　Deficient precursors: malnutrition, malabsorption
　　Severe liver disease: chronic hepatitis, cirrhosis
　　Analbuminaemia
Loss from the body
　　Skin:　burns, exudative lesions
　　Gut:　protein-losing enteropathy
　　Renal:　nephrotic syndrome
Miscellaneous
　　Acute phase response
　　Chronic illness:　infection, malignancy
　　Pregnancy

NORMAL METABOLISM

Albumin is synthesised by the liver at the rate of ~200 mg/kg/day (10-18 g/day in a 70 kg adult); the rate of synthesis being influenced by the oncotic pressure of the hepatic extracellular fluid, the amino acid supply, and plasma levels of cortisol, anabolic steroids, and thyroxine (these hormones increase both the synthesis and catabolism of albumin). Under normal circumstances only about 20% of the total synthetic capacity of the liver is utilised. The plasma half-life of albumin is about 21 days, degradation occuring in most cells of the body including the capillary endothelial cells.

CHANGES IN PLASMA ALBUMIN LEVELS

The only known cause of hyperalbuminaemia is haemoconcentration. Hypoalbuminaemia, on the other hand, has a wide variety of causes (Table 12.1).

Factors influencing plasma albumin concentration are, in order of importance:

- changes in body fluids, their distribution and amount
- changes in capillary permeability
- changes in lymphatic return
- losses (in nephrosis, protein-losing enteropathy, blood loss, extravasation as in burns, etc)
- changes in synthesis
- changes in metabolism (catabolic rate)

Analbuminaemia. This is a rare inborn error of metabolism in which there is deficient synthesis of albumin. Surprisingly, the clinical consequences are slight: there may be very mild dependant oedema.

Protein-losing enteropathy. In this condition there is pathological loss of proteins including albumin and globulins into the lumen of the gastrointestinal tract. It occurs in a variety of ulcerative conditions (such as peptic ulcer, ulcerative colitis, bowel malignancy), in lymphatic obstruction, and in intestinal lymphangiectasia. The clinical features are due to hypoalbuminaemia.

CONSEQUENCES OF HYPOALBUMINAEMIA

Hypoalbuminaemia affects the fluid distribution of the body and the plasma concentrations of substances normally transported in the plasma bound to albumin.

Fluid distribution: Albumin is the most important contributor to the plasma oncotic pressure and decreased plasma levels result in oedema (page 11).

Carrier function: In hypoalbuminaemia the concentration of substances normally carried by albumin will be decreased. Thus, there will be, for example, hypocalcaemia (page 97) and decreased protein-bound bilirubin and drugs. Substances bound to albumin are physiologically inactive; binding of bilirubin prevents it from crossing the blood-brain barrier. Thus, decreased plasma protein binding of bilirubin increases the "free" bilirubin levels in the plasma and their deposition in brain tissues (kernicterus in neonatal jaundice).

EVALUATION OF HYPOALBUMINAEMIA

In the absence of haemodilution, a low plasma level may be due to decreased protein synthesis (malabsorption, liver disease) or increased protein loss (renal, protein-losing enteropathy). A urinary protein excretion rate will exclude (or confirm) renal loss and liver function tests (page 156) will indicate the probability of a liver disorder, causing the hypoproteinaemia (Figure 12.3).

If these two tests are negative, the possibilities include protein-losing enteropathy or malabsorption.

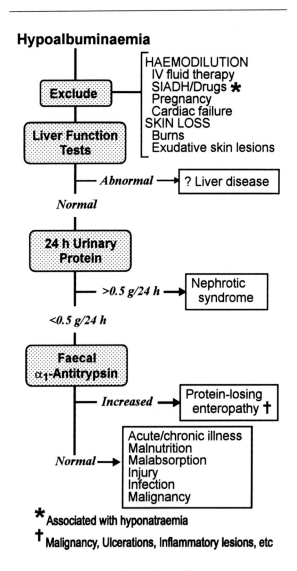

Figure 12.3. Evaluation of hypoalbuminaemia.

These possibilities should be further evaluated by (a) tests for malabsorption (page 220) and (b) tests to determine gut protein loss, e.g., radioactive chromium-labelled albumin studies and faecal α_1-antitrypsin excretion.

α_1-antitrypsin

This is a protease inhibitor with a molecular weight of ~50,000 which is distributed throughout the extracellular fluid. It is increased during the acute phase response (page 173, see also Figure 12.2), probably to restrict proteolytic activity to localised sites. Decreased levels, seen as a greatly reduced or missing α_1-globulin band on the protein electrophoretogram, occur as a result of an inborn error of metabolism and are also seen in protein-losing states (nephrotic syndrome, protein-losing enteropathy).

The congenital defect is caused by inheritance of abnormal alleles of the α_1-antitrypsin gene which exhibits polymorphism; about 30 such genetic variants have been identified. The normal allele is PiM (Pi for protease inhibitor). The most serious defects are caused by the abnormal alleles called null (there is no synthesis of the protein) and Z (the synthesised protein cannot be secreted and accumulates in the liver).

Individuals who are homozygous for both these alleles, especially the former, often develop pulmonary emphysema in childhood and young adulthood; the PiZZ phenotype may predispose to hepatic damage, which may present as hepatitis in the neonate and as cirrhosis in children or young adults.

Faecal α_1-antitrypsin: α_1-antitrypsin, being a relatively low molecular weight protein, will be excreted into the gut if there is any protein-losing abnormality. As a trypsin inhibitor, it will not be destroyed by the digestive proteases and will appear intact in the faeces. A measure of the enzyme activity in the stool will give some indication of the proteins leaking into the gut, as in protein-losing enteropathy.

α_2-macroglobulin

This is a large molecular weight protein (~900,000) which functions as a protease inhibitor. It is often increased in plasma in protein-losing states, presumably due to increased synthesis, or to relative retention by the glomerulus (compared to proteins of lower molecular size), as occurs in the nephrotic syndrome (Figure 12.2, lane 3).

Haptoglobins

These proteins bind haemoglobin which is released into the intravascular space during intravascular haemolysis and transport it to the cells of the reticuloendothelial system where it is catabolised (with salvage of iron and amino acids). High plasma levels are seen during the acute phase response (Figure 12.2, lanes 4, 5, 8', and 9'). However, if there is extensive intravascular haemolysis or haemorrhage into tissues,

the haptoglobin levels drop as a consequence of excessive utilisation, at times to undetectable levels (page 175).

Caeruloplasmin

In the plasma most of the circulating copper is complexed to the protein caeruloplasmin. The physiological significance of caeruloplasmin is uncertain; it contains oxidase activity and may be associated with the oxidation of Fe^{2+} prior to the incorporation of iron into haemoglobin. Its concentration is raised in plasma as part of the acute phase response. Low plasma levels may be associated with Wilson's disease and malnutrition. Pregnant women and those on oestrogen-containing oral contraceptives often have increased plasma caeruloplasmin levels.

Wilson's disease: This is an inborn error of copper metabolism associated with deposition of this metal in:

- the liver producing cirrhosis
- the brain causing basal ganglia degeneration
- the cornea producing the characteristic Kayser-Fleischer rings
- the proximal renal tubules causing the Fanconi syndrome

The plasma copper and caeruloplasmin levels are often low, while that of the urinary free copper is probably high as the urinary excretion rate is known to be increased.

β_2-microglobulin

This small protein (molecular weight ~120,000) is a component of the HLA complex found on the surfaces of all nucleated cells. Most of the β_2-microglobulin in the plasma is derived from myeloid and lymphoid cells and removed from it by glomerular filtration. The filtered protein is reabsorbed at the proximal tubule and degraded by lysosomal enzymes. Increased levels are thus seen in patients with proliferation of the above cell types, e.g., myeloma patients, as well as those with renal failure (reduced GFR).

The immunoglobulins

The immunoglobulins (IgG, IgA, IgM, IgD, IgE), which are found mainly in the plasma γ-globulin fraction, but are occasionally found in the α_2- and β-globulin fractions, comprise the body's antibodies and are also involved in hypersensitivity reactions. They have two primary functions: recognition of antigens and initiation of effector mechanisms to destroy them. Immunoglobulins as a group are characterised by their remarkable structural heterogeneity, and the fact that their synthesis is an adaptive response to antigenic stimulation.

Whereas most plasma proteins are produced in the liver, immunoglobulins are produced by B lymphocytes or mature plasma cells, either in the bone marrow or in lymphatic tissue. As the progenitor stem cells undergo progressive differentiation into early and late B lymphocyte stages (Table 12.2), they develop numerous receptor immunoglobulins on the surfaces of their cell membranes, and circulate into the lymphatic system and the blood. Upon encountering antigen, B lymphocytes proliferate and develop into plasma cells.

Each plasma cell line synthesises and secretes into the blood a highly specific antibody, i.e., each plasma cell line produces antibodies with a single specificity. A complex antigen is capable of eliciting a multiplicity of antibodies with different specificities which are derived from different cell lines. The immunogens (or antigens that elicit immune responses) are normally

foreign bodies, but may occasionally be host antigens that result in autoimmune diseases.

The basic immunoglobulin structure is shown schematically in Figure 12.4. All immunoglobulins consist of one or more basic units, each comprised of two identical heavy (H) chains and two identical light (L) chains joined together by a variable number of disulphide bonds. Each chain is organised into a series of globular regions or domains -- each L chain with two, each H chain with five. The N-terminal domains of both H and L chains encompass the hypervariable regions and contain the variable amino acid sequences which determine antigenic specificity; there are thus two antigen-combining sites per unit. The characteristic features of the remaining domains, which constitute the constant (C) region, allow the classification of immunoglobulins into 5 classes and a number of subclasses. They also contain the effector sites which enable them to interact with cells and complement.

IgG. *Molecular weight:* 160,000
Function: Protects extravascular tissue spaces
Synthesis: Synthesised in response to soluble antigens. At birth the baby has a full-strength complement due to transfer from the mother's blood across the placenta. Over the next 3-6 months IgG levels fall and then increase as the endogenous synthesis occurs. Adult levels (5-13.5 g/L) are reached by 3-5 years.

IgA. *Molecular weight:* Circulating IgA: 160,000; "secretory" IgA: 400 000. Secretory IgA is a dimer of two subunits joined by a peptide chain and with a "secretory" piece attached (circulating IgA does not have the "secretory" piece).
Function: "Secretory" IgA serves to protect body surfaces
Synthesis: Synthesised in the lamina propria of intestinal and respiratory tracts. IgA levels are low at birth and gradually increase to reach adult levels (0.5-3.5 g/L) by the age of 15.

IgM. *Molecular weight:* 900,000 (pentamer)
Function: IgM protects the blood stream (where they are mostly confined due to their large size) against particulate antigens such as foreign organisms.
Synthesis: The foetus can synthesise IgM but levels are usually low at birth: high levels indicate intrauterine infection. Adult levels (0.5-2.5 g/L) are reached by nine months.

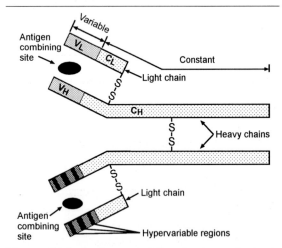

Figure 12.4. A diagram of the structure of a basic immunoglobulin unit. The terms variable, hypervariable, and constant regions denote regions of amino acid sequence variability in the antibody molecule: V_L and C_L, variable and constant regions on the light chain; V_H and C_H, corresponding regions on the heavy chain. For each specific immunoglobulin unit, each pair of heavy chains are identical, as are each pair of light chains.

Table 12.2. Types of immunoglobulins and malignant neoplasms associated with the B lymphocyte series.

Stages in Maturation and Proliferation	Principal Site	Immunoglobulin		Associated Malignant Neoplasms
		Surface Receptor	Secreted into Blood	
Stem cell	Bone marrow	None	None	Acute lymphocytic leukaemia
Early B lymphocyte	Lymph nodes	IgM, IgD	None	Lymphoma, chronic lymphocytic leukaemia (85%)
Late B lymphocyte	Lymph nodes	IgM	IgM	Lymphoma, chronic lymphocytic leukaemia (15%), and Waldenstrom's macroglobulinaemia
Plasma cell	Lymphatic tissue bone marrow	IgG, IgA	IgG, IgA	Multiple myeloma

Antigen → Primary immune response (Early B lymphocyte)

Antigen → Secondary immune response (Late B lymphocyte); H-chain changes

Adapted, with permission of W.B. Saunders, from: Silverman LM, Christenson RH and Grant GH. Amino acids and proteins. In: Burtis CA and Ashwood ER (eds), *Tietz Textbook of Clinical Chemistry, 2nd edn.* W.B. Saunders, Philadelphia, 1994.

IgE: *Molecular weight:* 200,000
Function: Involved in hypersensitivity reactions
Synthesis: Produced by plasma cells situated in the respiratory tract, the gastrointestinal tract, and the nasopharynx. It is bound to the surfaces of cells such as mast cells and basophils. Adult levels (<0.005 g/L) are reached by the age of 15.

IgD: *Molecular weight:* 190 000,
Little is known about its function or synthesis. <0.1 g/L are found in plasma in normal adults.

Circulating levels of the immunoglobulins, which make up the bulk of the γ-globulins, may be increased (hypergammaglobulinaemia) or decreased (hypogammaglobulinaemia). In hypergammaglobulinaemia, there will be an associated hyperproteinaemia (an exception occurs if there is a concurrently low albumin concentration when the total protein level may be normal). Hypogammaglobulinaemia is usually associated with hypoproteinaemia.

Hypogammaglobulinaemia

Low levels of immunoglobulins sufficient to produce hypoproteinaemia may be transient (infants), primary, or secondary to a number of disorders (Table 12.3).

Transient hypogammaglobulinaemia: This is due to low levels of IgG and is seen in premature babies (full quota of IgG has not crossed the placenta), and in normal infants between three to six months of age (normal drop prior to synthesis of IgG, see above).

Table 12.3. Causes of hypogammaglobulinaemia.

Decreased synthesis
Transient
 Prematurity, First 3-6 months of life
Primary
 IgA deficiency
 Genetically defective immune system
Secondary
 Haematological disorders: myeloma, chronic lymphatic leukaemia, lymphosarcoma
 Toxins: uraemia, diabetes mellitus, immunosuppressive drugs
Protein loss (secondary)
 Skin: burns, exudative lesions
 Gut: protein-losing enteropathy
 Renal: nephrotic syndrome

Primary hypogammaglobulinaemia: This is a rare condition. There are two types: (1) an isolated deficiency in IgA (1 in 500 people), and (2) that associated with some hereditary immunoglobulin deficiency syndromes, e.g., Bruton's sex-linked agammaglobulinaemia, Swiss agammaglobulinaemia.

Secondary hypogammaglobulinaemias: These are fairly common, occurring in about 4-5% of the hospital population. The commonest causes are the protein-losing conditions and immunosuppression due to haematological malignancies.

Hypergammaglobulinaemia

The hypergammaglobulinaemias can be classified as either monoclonal or polyclonal in type (Figure 12.5). The causes of the hypergammaglobulinaemias are listed in Table 12.4.

Table 12.4. Causes of hypergammaglobulinaemia.

Polyclonal
Chronic liver disease: cirrhosis, chronic active
    hepatitis
Chronic infections: bronchiectasis, leprosy, brucellosis
    tuberculosis, parasites (malaria, kala-azar)
Inflammatory disease of bowel: Crohn's disease,
    ulcerative colitis
Autoimmune disorders: rheumatoid arthritis,
    systemic lupus erythematosis
Granulomas: sarcoidosis

Monoclonal
Benign: idiopathic, secondary (diabetes mellitus,
    chronic infections, cirrhosis, connective tissue
    disorders)
Malignant: multiple myeloma, macroglobulinaemia,
    soft tissue plasmacytoma, heavy chain disease,
    lymphoreticular malignancy

Polyclonal hypergammaglobulinaemia

This condition is characterised by a diffuse increased intensity of staining in the gammaglobulin portion of the electrophoretic pattern (Figure 12.5, Top). This is due to the immune stimulation of many plasma cell clones, producing a variety of immunoglobulins, although usually a particular immunoglobulin class predominates. It represents the normal B cell response to antigenic stimulation and indicates the presence of a chronic infection or autoimmune process. In some instances, the immunoglobulin classes may give some indication of the aetiology, as illustrated by the following examples:

- *Predominantly IgG:* chronic active hepatitis, systemic lupus erythrematosus
- *Predominantly IgA:* cryptogenic cirrhosis, Crohn's disease, tuberculosis, sarcoidosis
- *Predominantly IgM:* primary biliary cirrhosis, parasitic disease
- *Equivalent increase in IgA, IgG, IgM:* longstanding chronic infections

Monoclonal hypergammaglobulinaemia

In this situation there is only one clone of B lymphocytes which proliferates, producing the single offending immunoglobulin (also called a paraprotein) in excess. This results in a discrete, well-demarcated band of protein in the globulin area of the electrophoretogram. The paraproteins vary in electrophoretic mobility and band appearance from case to case (Figure 12.5, Bottom). The condition may be benign or malignant.

Benign monoclonal hypergammaglobulinaemia. The benign condition may be secondary to a number of diseases (Table 12.4) or idiopathic. The characteristic features of this condition are:

- Serum paraprotein concentration of less than 20 g/L (<10 g/L if the paraprotien is an IgA)
- Normal serum concentrations of albumin and other immunoglobulins
- Present for five years or more without increase in paraprotein concentration
- More common in the elderly, e.g., the prevalence rate is 2% between 60-80 years, 10% between 80-90 years, and 20% for those >90 years old.

Malignant monoclonal hypergammaglobulinaemia. The causes are listed in Table 12.4. The features that suggest malignancy are:

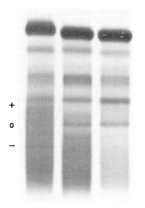

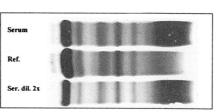

Hypergammaglobulinemia

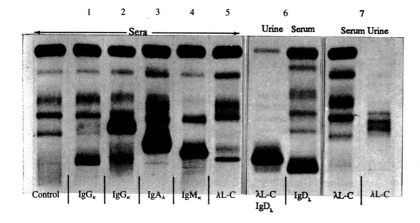

Figure 12.5. Serum protein electrophoretic patterns in polyclonal hypergammaglobinaemia (**Top Left and Right**) and monoclonal hypergammaglobinaemia (**Bottom**).

Top Left (from left to right): Polyclonal hypergammaglobinaemia with β-γ fusion, polyclonal hypergammaglobulinaemia, and normal serum.

Top Right: Ref = normal serum

Bottom:
Lanes 1-5 are paraproteins found in 5 different patients. The immunotype of the paraprotein is shown below the gel.

Gel #6 shows the urine protein (left) and serum protein (right) patterns for a patient with IgDλ paraproteinaemia and Bence-Jones proteinuria.

The 2 lanes in Gel #7 depict serum and urine protein patterns from a patient with light chain disease and Bence-Jones proteinuria.

Note variations in size and positions of paraprotein bands for the different cases (L-C=light chains).

- Paraprotein concentration in excess of 20 g/L and increasing with time.
- Immune paresis (suppression of activity of other plasma cells, hence low serum concentrations of other immunoglobulins).
- Bence-Jones protein (BJP) present in urine (BJP are free monoclonal light chains, or fragments thereof, which freely pass through the glomerulus and cause tubular cell damage).
- Characteristic bone marrow and X-ray findings (see below).

Multiple myeloma. This condition which is due to malignant proliferation of abnormal plasma ("myeloma") cells is characterised by an onset between 40 to 60 years, bone pain, normochromic, normocytic anaemia, and raised ESR. There is a characteristic bone X-ray pattern showing punched-out areas of radiotranslucency. There may also be pathological fractures, impaired renal function, amyloidosis, and infections such as pneumonia. Diagnosis depends on haematological, biochemical and radiological findings. The definitive diagnosis depends on demonstration of an increased proportion of plasma cells and the presence of atypical "myeloma" cells in the bone marrow. Relevant biochemical investigations and findings include:

- ***Serum protein electrophoresis:*** 80% have a high serum total protein level and a monoclonal paraprotein band in the protein pattern. The secreted paraprotein has been typed as an IgG in 55%, IgA in 25%, IgD in 1%, IgM in 0.5% of myeloma patients; 20% do not have a demonstrable paraprotein band in the serum pattern. Of this group, the majority are those who produce only light chains. In light-chain myeloma, a paraprotein band may not be seen in the serum protein electrophoresis gel pattern (being of small molecular weight, they readily filter across the glomerular membrane and thus do not have the critical mass to show up as a discernable band) but the filtered light chains are excreted in the urine as Bence-Jones protein. Thus a concomitant urine protein electrophoresis will reveal their presence and minimize missed diagnoses. In the remaining cases, the paraprotein bands may be masked by proteins normally present in serum which have the same or overlapping electrophoretic mobility.

- *Urine protein electrophoresis.* Urine positive for BJP; 20% have BJP only. Provided the urine is optimally concentrated, a paraprotein band should be demonstrable on electrophoresis.

- *Other serum protein levels.* Hypoalbuminaemia is usually present; serum levels of immunoglobulins (other than that produced by the proliferating malignant clone) are usually low due to suppressed production (immune paresis).

- *Serum calcium levels.* Hypercalcaemia is common (bone resorption).

- *Serum uric acid levels.* Hyperuricaemia occurs in most cases (increased cellular turnover in malignancy).

- *Serum alkaline phosphatase.* As there is little osteoblastic activity around the bone lesions, the alkaline phosphatase activity is usually normal.

Multiple myeloma accounts for most of the cases of malignant paraproteinaemias. Rare cases involve only the soft tissues, without marrow changes. Progress of such soft tissue plasmacytoma, which are usually localised, is slow and surgical removal of the solitary tumour often terminates the spread.

Waldenstrom's macroglobulinaemia. This is associated with IgM paraproteinaemia and, in the majority of cases, with the hyperviscosity syndrome (production of large molecular weight paraproteins). Anaemia and lymphadenopathy are common but bone changes are rare. It usually occurs in older people (60-80 years), being more common in men than in women.

LABORATORY EVALUATION OF MONOCLONAL HYPERGLOBULINAEMIAS

Multiple myeloma has been used as a paradigm to discuss the laboratory tests of diagnostic relevance in the evaluation of monoclonal hypergammaglobin-aemias in general. Biochemically, these disorders present with hyperproteinaemia. Investigation of suspected cases of paraproteinaemia usually includes biochemical, haematological and radiological investigations, as well as lymph node/bone marrow biopsies.

They should be confirmed by protein electrophoresis (on serum *and* urine). Once a paraprotein has been detected, it can be further investigated by specific immunotyping techniques, e.g., immunofixation or immunoelectrophoresis, to type its H and L chains (the clinical significance of immunoglobulin typing is discussed below). Quantitative estimations of individual immunoglobulin classes can be performed by radioimmunoassays (IgE), non-isotopic immunoassays (IgE), immunonephelometric methods (IgG, IgA, IgM), and radial immunodiffusion (IgD), and are useful in monitoring progress of the disease or the response to therapy.

The biochemical tests which have proven useful for detection, characterisation and quantitation of the paraprotein and for subsequent monitoring of the progress of the disease are:

First-line tests

- *Serum and urine protein electrophoresis.* Fresh specimens are essential to avoid erroneous results due to specimen deterioration on storage. A random urine specimen is adequate for characterisation of the monoclonal paraprotein and demonstration of Bence-Jones proteinuria. In addition, the urine protein pattern will indicate the presence of glomerular or tubular proteinuria.

- *Quantitative determinations of the paraprotein and other serum immunoglobulins* help in the differentiation of benign and malignant hypergammaglobulinaemia.

Further investigations

- *Immunoelectrophoresis or immunofixation of the serum and urine proteins*, to determine the type of paraprotein. Some examples of immunofixation gels are shown in Figures 12.6 and 12.7.

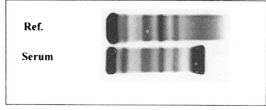

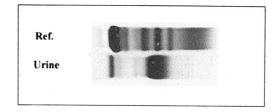

Monoclonal Gammopathy

Light Chain Disease

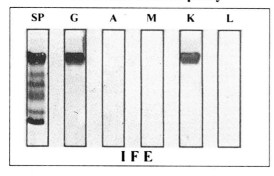

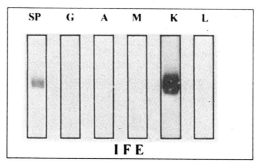

Figure 12.6. Immunotyping of paraproteinaemia (**Left**) and paraproteinuria (**Right**) by immunofixation. **Insets** show the corresponding high resolution protein electrophoretic patterns (reference lanes are normal sera).

Lane 1 was fixed with acid and stained with Coomassie blue; lanes 2-6 were incubated with specific antibodies to various heavy and light chains (Lane 2: anti-IgG antibody; Lane 3: anti-IgA antibody; Lane 4: anti-IgM antibody; Lane 5: anti-kappa light chains antibody; Lane 6: anti-lambda light chains antibody).

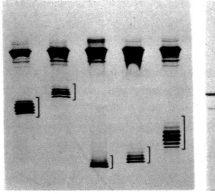

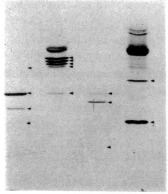

Figure 12.7. Immunotyping of paraproteinaemia by immunofixation following iso-electrofocusing. **Left.** Six patients with monoclonal IgG (indicated by brackets). **Right.** Four patients with monoclonal kappa or lambda light chains (indicated by arrows).

- *Serum β₂-microglobulin* quantitation to monitor the progress of the disease; high levels of this protein indicate a poor prognosis.
- *Serum urea and creatinine* estimations to assess renal function.
- *Serum calcium, alkaline phosphatase and uric acid* measurements as indices of the extent of bone

involvement and cell turnover, respectively.

The acute phase response

This is a non-specific change in the synthesis and plasma levels of various liver-derived proteins following tissue damage (trauma, infarction, malignancy) and infections. It is a physiological response to inflammation, providing increased blood and tissue concentrations of proteins integral to the inflammatory process, many of which are actively consumed in the performance of their functions.

The acute phase response is now believed to be mediated by the release of cytokines from activated macrophages. In bacterial infections this is induced by bacterial endotoxins, eliciting massive responses. It is accompanied by a variety of systemic effects of inflammation such as fever, leucocytosis, endocrine changes, alterations in fluid and electrolyte balance, and muscle proteolysis.

The acute phase proteins

The term "acute phase proteins" is used to denote all the plasma proteins which change in concentration by 25% or more in the week following tissue damage -- amongst them are C-reactive protein (CRP), α_1-antitrypsin, α_1-antichymotrypsin, haptoglobin, complement factors, and fibrinogen. These proteins subserve a variety of roles in inflammation, acting variously as mediators, modulators, inhibitors, scavengers, and repair agents.

Most of these acute-phase reactants register increases in concentration whilst others, such as albumin and transferrin, show a decrease. Clinically, interest lies in the measurement of these changes to indicate the presence of inflammation and organic disease and its extent or severity. The changes can be detected by quantitative measurement of the individual proteins or qualitatively by observation of the characterististic pattern in serum protein electrophoresis (Figure 12.2, lanes 4, 5, 8', 9'). Table 12.5 shows the acute phase proteins which are often measured.

The major finding is an increase in several proteins of the α_1- and α_2-globulin fractions, such as α_1-antitrypsin, caeruloplasmin, and haptoglobin, as well as β-globulins such as fibrinogen and complement factors. The C-reactive protein is also increased.

Proteins which may show decreased concentrations include albumin, prealbumin, and transferrin, due predominantly to an associated alteration in capillary membrane permeability. Secondary decreases of haptoglobin and complement factors may occur, reflecting excessive utilisation (see below).

The rate of increase in plasma concentration following an inflammatory stimulus varies between the different proteins. A typical pattern of changes seen in the 24 hours following a surgical trauma will be:

CRP > α_1-chymotrypsin > α_1-antitrypsin > α_1-acid glycoprotein > haptoglobin > albumin

These variations result from a combination of the different sensitivities to induction of hepatic synthesis by cytokines and the different distribution and catabolic characteristics of each protein. In some types of inflammatory disease, certain acute phase proteins protein(s), relative to the others. This applies to the low levels of fibrinogen in intravascular coagulation, may be more actively catabolised, resulting in a disproportionately low concentration of the particular

Table 12.5. Major human acute phase proteins.

Protein	Normal plasma concentration (g/L)	Typical plasma concentration in inflammation (g/L)	Response time (h)
Group III up to 1000 × increase			
C-reactive protein	0·00007–0·008	0·4	6–10
Serum amyloid A	0·001–0·030	2·5	6–10
Group II, 2–4 × increase			
α_1-antichymotrypsin	0·3–0·6	3·0	10
α_1-antitrypsin	1·0–2·0	7·0	
α_1-acid glycoprotein	0·5–1·4	3·0	24
Haptoglobin	1·0–3·0	6·0	
Fibrinogen	2·0–4·5	10	
Group 1 about 50% increase			
Ceruloplasmin	0·15–0·6	2·0	
C3	0·55–1·2	3·0	48–72
C4	0·2–0·5	1·0	

Data from Kushner I and Mackiewicz A. Acute phase proteins as disease markers. *Disease Markers* 1987;5:1-11.

Table reproduced, with kind permission from the main author, fromThompson D, Milford-Ward A, Whicher JT. The value of acute phase proteins in clinical practice. *Ann Clin Biochem* 1992; 29:123-131.

and haptoglobin in intravascular haemolysis. Such "dysharmonic responses" detract from the value of these proteins as markers of inflammation.

Nonetheless, despite various limitations, acute phase protein measurements can be very useful for diagnosing the presence of inflammation and in monitoring its activity. They are particularly useful in monitoring the responses of chronic inflammatory diseases, such as connective tissue diseases, to therapy. Many of these diseases (e.g., rheumatoid arthritis) are difficult to monitor clinically.

Mention must be made of two other related measurements -- the erythrocyte sedimentation rate (ESR) and cytokine measurements, although a detailed discussion is outwith our scope.

Erythrocyte sedimentation rate. Despite the wide availability of measurements of individual acute phase proteins, and although its use in recent years has gradually declined, the ESR still remains the most used measurement of the acute phase response. Changes in the ESR encompasses changes in several proteins (fibrinogen, α_2-macroglobulin, immunoglobulins and albumin) as well as in erythro-cyte membrane characteristics and numbers. It is especially useful in monitoring chronic inflammation.

Cytokine measurements. The recently established role of cytokines, interleukin 1, interleukin 6 and tumour necrosis factor, in stimulating the acute phase response argues strongly for their measurement in inflammatory conditions. Both bioassays and immunoassays for these effector molecules are currently available. However, their adoption in clinical practice is hampered by various technical problems related to interferences (by cytokine inhibitors and binding proteins) in the case of bioassays, and to sensitivity and cost in the case of immunoassays (unable to detect normal plasma concentrations, and very costly).

Cerebrospinal fluid (CSF) protein

The CSF is secreted by the choroid plexus located in the lateral and fourth ventricles of the brain. It flows outwards across the cerebellum, where it is absorbed by the arachnoid villi, and downwards through the spinal canal. The mechanism of secretion is not clear, the fluid probably represents a modified filtrate of plasma. A sample drawn from the lumbar region of a young adult will have a protein concentration within the range 0.15-0.45 g/L (which is 100-300 times less than that of plasma), containing mostly albumin and other small MW proteins.

This great difference in the protein concentration of CSF versus plasma contrasts starkly to the glucose and chloride concentrations in the two body fluids:

- glucose concentration (1.7-3.9 mmol/L), about 1-2 mmol/L less than that of plasma
- chloride concentration (120-130 mmol/L), higher than that of plasma probably due to a Donnan equilibrium defect.

The total amount of protein in CSF varies with age and the site of fluid withdrawal, being higher in infants and older individuals (>40 years of age), and lower in fluids drawn from the ventricular and cisternal regions as compared to those given above, which are for lumbar samples from adults less than 40 years of age.

The CSF protein levels may be increased due to increased capillary permeability, mechanical obstruction of CSF circulation, increased secretion of immunoglobulins within the CNS by inflammatory or other invaliding cells, and if there is blood contamination of the CSF specimen (Table 12.6).

Changes in the CSF protein composition are best assessed by separating the individual proteins by high resolution electrophoresis on samples which have been concentrated 80- to 100-fold. In Figure 12.8, the contrast between the protein electrophoresis patterns of a normal CSF sample and those from patients with multiple sclerosis is clearly demarcated.

Quantitation of CSF immunoglobulins, particularly IgG, are often requested for patients with suspected multiple sclerosis. IgG is usually increased in this

---

Table 12.6. Causes of high CSF protein concentration.

Increased capillary permeability
Infections: bacterial and viral meningitis
Intracranial tumours: meningiomas, gliomas
Obstruction
Usually obstruction of the spinal area, leading to
Froin's syndrome (very high CSF protein content)
Increased immunoglobulin production
Chronic infections: tuberculosis, meningitis,
    neurosyphilis
Degenerative disorders: multiple sclerosis,
    chronic alcoholism

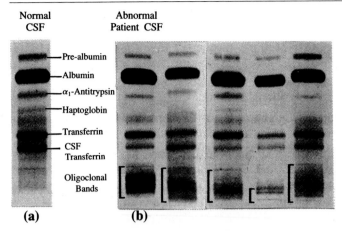

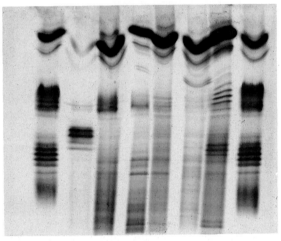

Figure 12.8 (Top). High resolution agarose gel electrophoresis of CSF proteins from (a) a normal subject and (b) from patients with multiple sclerosis.

The brackets indicate the oligoclonal bands.

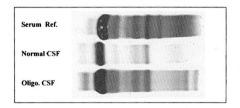

(Bottom). Iso-electrofocusing of serum and CSF proteins and control specimens.

Lane 1: Positive CSF control.
Lane 2: Haemoglobin standard extract.
Lane 3: Normal serum.
Lane 4: CSF from patient (?multiple sclerosis), showing oligoclonal bands.
Lane 5: Serum from same patient (Lane 4).
Lane 6: CSF from patient (negative sample, no oligoclonal bands).
Lane 7: Positive CSF control from patient with diagnosed multiple sclerosis.
Lane 8: Abnormal (positive) CSF sample.

disorder but it is not a specific finding. However, the phenomenon known as "oligoclonal banding" in which multiple bands, largely of IgG, appearing in the gamma zone, are observed in at least 90% of patients with multiple sclerosis at some time during the course of their disease. These bands can occur in various forms, ranging from a few faint bands to many intense bands (Figure 12.8). Banding can only be shown by the use of high resolution electrophoretic or iso-electrofocusing techniques.

Despite its importance as a diagnostic tool, the oligoclonal banding pattern is not pathognomonic of multiple sclerosis, being associated in varying extents with subacute sclerosing parencephalitis, neuro-syphilis, viral or meningo-encephalitis, and bacterial meningitis. Its use as a prognostic indicator for multiple sclerosis is not recommended, as the intensity of the bands does not appear to correlate well with the subsequent course of the disease.

REFERENCES AND FURTHER READING

Beetham R, Cattell WR. Proteinuria: pathophysiology, significance and recommendations for measurement in clinical practice. Ann Clin Biochem 1993;30:425-434.

Oken MM. Multiple myeloma. Med Clin North Am 1984;68:757-787.

Thompson D, Milford-Ward A, Whicher JT. The value of acute phase proteins in clinical practice. Ann Clin Biochem 1992;29:123-131.

Thompson EJ, Keir G. Laboratory investigation of cerebrospinal fluid proteins. Ann Clin Biochem 1990; 27:425-435.

Whicher JT. The laboratory investigation of para-proteinaemia. Ann Clin Biochem 1987;24:119-139.

Chapter 13

Enzymes in Diagnosis

Enzymes are proteins that act as catalysts in metabolic reactions. With the exception of the coagulation factors, the enzymes of the renin-angiotensin system, and the digestive enzymes secreted into the gut, most enzymes are located primarily in the cells. They are released from the cells as a result of cell membrane leakage or cell death caused by natural decay. Thus the plasma activities of enzymes are normally low (but measurable) and reflect the balance between the rate of egress from cells and the rate of degradation or clearance from the circulation.

The biological half-lives of tissue enzymes following their release into plasma vary considerably -- in the case of the enzymes often measured for diagnostic purposes, this may vary from a few hours to about a week. In health plasma enzyme activities remain fairly constant, reflecting the balance between these processes. Changes in plasma enzyme levels occur in situations in which this balance is altered.

Increases are most commonly caused by:

1 Increased release into the plasma consequent to:

- Extensive cell damage, e.g., the raised CK-MB isoenzyme activity after a myocardial infarction. Cell damage is usually caused by ischemia or cell toxins.

- Cell proliferation and an increased cell turnover rate, e.g., elevated alkaline phosphatase from increased osteoblastic activity during active growth spurts or tissue repair after multiple bone fractures.

- Enzyme induction (increased enzyme synthesis), e.g., markedly raised γ-glutamyl-transferase activity after alcohol ingestion.

- Duct obstruction: this affects enzymes normally found in exocrine secretions e.g., amylase and lipase in pancreatic juice. These enzymes may be regurgitated into the bloodstream if the pancreatobiliary duct is blocked.

2 Decreased removal from plasma due to renal impairment affecting enzymes excreted in urine, e.g., amylase may be high in renal failure.

Decreased plasma enzyme levels, which are much less common, can occur when there is:

1 Reduced enzyme synthesis, e.g., low plasma cholinesterase in severe liver failure (decreased hepatocyte numbers).

2 Congenital deficiency of the enzyme, e.g., low plasma alkaline phosphatase activity in congenital hypophosphatasaemia.

3 Inherited enzyme variants with low biological activity, e.g., abnormal cholinesterase variants (page 187).

CLINICAL APPLICATION OF ENZYME ASSAYS

The diagnostic usefulness of measuring plasma enzyme activities lies in the fact that changes in their activities provide very sensitive indicators of tissue damage or cell proliferation. These changes not only help to detect and, in some cases, localise the tissue damage but also to monitor treatment and progress of disease. However, their usefulnes is diminished by the lack of specificity, i.e., the difficulty of identifying an increased enzyme activity with the tissue which has been damaged. This is because most, if not all, enzymes are not confined to specific tissues or organs, rather most of them are widely distributed and their plasma activities may be raised in disorders involving different tissues.

In practice, this problem of lack of specificity is partially overcome by measuring several parameters which may include several enzymes, as the relative concentrations of enzymes in different tissues vary considerably. For instance, although both alanine and aspartate transaminase (ALT and AST) are equally abundant in liver tissue, AST is present in much greater concentration than ALT (20:1) in heart muscle. Simultaneous measurement of both enzymes can thus provide a clearer indication of the probable site of tissue damage.

The diagnostic specificity can also be enhanced by performing isoenzyme analyses. Isoenzymes are different molecular forms of an enzyme which have the ability to catalyse the reaction characteristic of that enzyme. They are often organ-specific in origin, e.g., of the lactate dehydrogenase (LD) isoenzymes, LD_5 is found mainly in the liver whilst LD_1 occurs mainly in cardiac muscle.

Awareness of the time course of the elevation of various enzymes after certain pathological events may be applied judiciously to provide additional useful information, e.g., in the interpretation of the cardiac enzyme profiles in post-myocardial infarction. The basis of this is that each individual enzyme has a fairly constant half-life which is characteristic of that enzyme; a knowledge of the half-lives of the different enzymes affected by the acute illness will be of help in assessing the time of its onset.

In this chapter we will discuss some individual enzymes which are of diagnostic importance and some of the enzyme patterns found in specific disease processes.

Non-pathological factors affecting results of plasma enzyme assays

There are a number of factors, other than disease processes, that will affect results of plasma enzyme assays. These factors may be considered under three categories:

- Pertubations in results due to some physiological state which may mislead if the physiological state goes unrecorded or unnoticed, e.g., exercise increases serum CK activity and pregnancy causes elevation of ALP activity (contribution from placental ALP isoenzyme). The presence of macro forms due to polymerisation of enzyme molecules (e.g., macroamylase) or due to the formation of complexes with other proteins such as immuno-globulins (e.g., LD and CK complexed with IgG) will delay the rates of their clearance from the circulation and raise their plasma activities in the absence of liver or renal disease.

- Most enzyme assays in current usage measure the enzyme activities rather than their concentrations. Analytical variations will affect the results of such assays, introducing both bias and imprecision. The lack of standardisation of assay conditions such as the choice of substrate, cofactor and product concentrations, the type and strength of buffer, the assay pH and reaction temperature as well as the spurious presence of inhibitors, activators or interferents in the samples or reagents are the main causes of analytical variability. Enzyme units used to report activity

are seldom well defined in terms of these factors, and results generated by different laboratories are often not comparable. Reference ranges are not universally applicable for the same reasons.

- The pharmacological effects of drugs taken by the patient may also affect the results, e.g., many drugs including the anticonvulsants phenytoin and phenobarbital cause elevated plasma GGT activities via microsomal induction.

Plasma enzyme results must be interpreted bearing in mind these and other relevant points, before attributing a change in the plasma enzyme activity to a specific disease process. Reference ranges of the issuing laboratory which are matched for the correct age, sex, and assay method, and preferably based on the local population, should be used for interpretation of the results.

Enzymes of clinical importance

Alkaline phosphatase (ALP)

ALP is not a single enzyme, rather it is the generic name for a group of enzymes that catalyse hydrolysis of phosphoric acid mono-esters at alkaline pH (9.0-10.5). It is found in most tissues, with different tissues having one or more isoenzymes or isoforms. The clinically important isoenzymes are those of the bone (osteoblasts), the liver (cells lining the biliary canaliculi), the intestine (epithelial cells), the kidney (renal tubular cells) and the placenta. Electrophoretic separation of the isoenzymes will enable one to determine the tissue of origin of an increased plasma total ALP activity (see Figure 13.1)

The physiological role of ALP is not known, although a role in membrane transport has been suggested as it is attached to the cell membrane in most tissues. It may also be associated with calcification of bone. Like many other plasma enzymes, ALP is removed from the plasma by the cells of the reticuloendothelial system.

CAUSES OF RAISED PLASMA ALP ACTIVITY

Physiological
 Age: neonate/children/young adults
 Pregnancy: third trimester

Liver disease

  Hepatocellular disease, cholestasis,
  space-occupying lesions

Bone disease

  Paget's disease (↑↑ to ↑↑↑ ALP)
  Malignancy: primary, secondary
  Hyperparathyroidism: primary, secondary (with bone disease)
  Chronic renal failure
  Rickets/osteomalacia
  Healing fractures

Malignancy

  Bone: primary, secondary
  Liver: primary, secondary
  Ectopic production : Regan isoenzyme

Miscellaneous

  Transient hyperphosphatasaemia of infancy
  Familial benign hyperphosphatasaemia

Physiological changes: Very often, what appears to be an abnormal ALP elevation could be due to a physiological state. Plasma ALP in adults is mainly derived from bone and liver (about equal contribution). In children and in young adults at puberty, the plasma levels are about 2-3 times the adult levels but levels up to 1000 U/L have been described in preterm infants, for instance. The increase is in the osteoblastic ALP fraction associated with the bone growth in these age groups. In the third trimester of normal pregnancy, release of the placental ALP isoenzyme causes a transient increase in the total plasma ALP activity. In the elderly, especially in postmenopausal women, there is also a slight increase in plasma ALP activity, originating from increased bone turnover.

Postprandial blood specimens taken after a meal containing fat are not recommended for plasma ALP estimations, due to the transient release of intestinal ALP. Blood should preferably be drawn from fasting subjects and it is important to take into account the above factors before ascribing a pathological reason to a raised plasma ALP result.

Liver disease: Very high levels (>500 U/L) may be seen in obstructive jaundice, primary biliary cirrhosis, and the space-occupying lesions, as a result of cholestasis. This causes increased synthesis of ALP by the cells bordering the biliary canaliculi and regurgitation of the hepatic enzyme into plasma following solubilization of the membrane-associated enzyme.

Bone disease: The highest plasma ALP levels have been recorded in Paget's disease (may be >2000 U/L). In the other bone diseases with increased osteoblastic activity listed above, the levels are usually in the range of 200-400 U/L.

Malignancy: High plasma ALP levels in malignancy may be due to:

- secondaries in the liver
- primary or secondary neoplasms in bone
- production of ALP by the tumour (ectopic enzyme production, Regan isoenzyme)

LOW PLASMA LEVELS OF ALP

This occurs in a rare autosomal recessive condition, familial hypophosphatasaemia, which is characterised by bone abnormalities, vitamin D-resistant rickets and the excessive excretion of phosphoethanolamine in the urine. Low levels of ALP may also occur in conditions of arrested bone growth such as cretinism.

ALP isoenzymes

Occasionally, the cause of an isolated raised plasma ALP activity is not apparent, prompting the need for further tests. Separation of the ALP isoenzymes (e.g., by high resolution gel electrophoresis) is currently the best method for determining the tissue of origin of increased ALP activities detected in the plasma. Measurement of certain other analytes may also indicate the cause, e.g., in liver disease the plasma activities of alanine aminotransferase (ALT), 5'-nucleotidase (5'-NT) and gamma-glutamyltransferase (GGT) are also increased. A concomitant increase of any of these enzymes suggests that liver is the likely origin of the raised ALP.

Alternative means of differentiating the ALP isoenzymes make use of physical or chemical properties such as differences in the sensitivity to inhibition by L-phenylalanine or urea and in heat stability. The main disadvantage of these simpler tests is the inability to make a clear distinction between liver and bone ALP isoenzymes, which is the most important clinical distinction needed.

To achieve this, one has to rely on separation of the isoenzymes by electrophoresis (Figure 13.1) or isoelectrofocusing. There are currently several commercial kits, some with pre-cast gels, which are available for ALP isoenzyme analysis. They differ in the degree of resolution that can be achieved. Those which utilise the isoelectrofocusing technique generally give better resolution but are yet to be adopted for routine diagnostic purposes.

In essence, it involves the following:

1. Exclude physiological causes (age, pregnancy)
2. Consider the possibility of liver diseases (measure bilirubin, GGT and other liver function tests).
3. Do an ALP isoenzyme analysis.

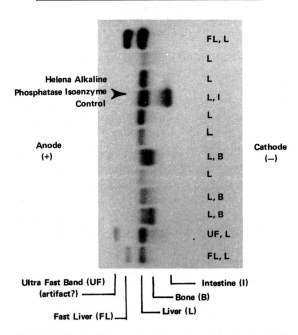

Figure 13.1. Electrophoretic separation of ALP isoenzymes using cellulose acetate membranes. (Top) A schematic representation of the electrophoretic mobilities of the various isoenzymes separated; (Bottom) Typical patterns of serum samples.

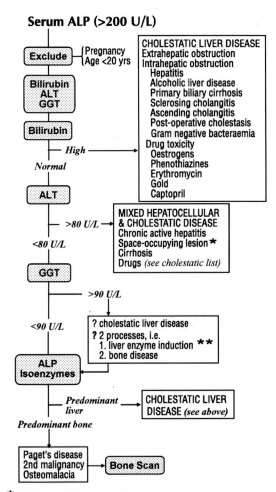

Figure 13.2. A suggested scheme for the evaluation of a high plasma ALP activity.

EVALUATION OF HYPERPHOSPHATASAEMIA

A suggested scheme for the evaluation of a high plasma of serum ALP activity is given in Figure 13.2.

5'-Nucleotidase (5'-NT)

5'-NT catalyses the hydrolysis of nucleotides in which a phosphate group is attached to the 5'-position of the pentose ring. Although of wide distribution, increased plasma levels are usually due to liver disease. Unlike GGT, it is not affected by enzyme-inducing agents. Thus it is useful in determining if a raised plasma ALP is of liver or of bone origin (see above).

Acid phosphatase (ACP)

ACP catalyses the hydrolysis of the mono-esters of phosphoric acid at an acidic pH. It is concentrated in the prostate gland (at 100-300 times the concentration found in other tissues), leucocytes, red blood cells, and platelets. Up to 14 isoenzymes have been described, but in clinical medicine only the prostatic isoenzyme is of importance and most laboratories measure this exclusively, e.g., by L-tartrate inhibition (which affects only the prostatic isoenzyme) or by the more recently available immunoassays.

CAUSES OF AN INCREASED TOTAL PLASMA ACP ACTIVITY

- Prostatic malignancy
- *In vitro* haemolysis (artefactual)
- Thrombocytopenia purpura
- Gaucher's disease
- Paget's disease
- Metastatic bone disease
- Following a rectal examination (artefactual)

Prostatic acid phosphatase. The main clinical uses of this enzyme are:

- diagnosis of prostatic malignancy
- monitoring therapeutic efficacy e.g., during treatment of carcinoma of the prostate

Diagnosis: The plasma ACP level depends on the extent of the malignancy and the degree of differentiation of the tumour. Eighty to 90% of patients with tumours limited to the gland will not show increased plasma levels; 70 to 80% of patients with metastatic disease will have a high plasma ACP. Poorly differentiated tumours may not produce ACP and hence plasma levels are not increased.

Treatment of malignancy: If the patient's plasma ACP was high on presentation then successful therapy will be accompanied by a rapid fall in the plasma level. However, the enzyme rises again if a relapse occurs.

Note: Blood specimens for prostatic ACP estimations need to be properly preserved and collected before a rectal examination. The latter procedure causes a temporary but significant increase in plasma ACP activity. Heparin is unsuitable as an anticoagulant as it inhibits ACP activity; *in vitro* haemolysis will invalidate the results as ACP is released from the red blood cells.

In the evaluation and treatment of prostatic cancer, prostatic specific antigen (PSA) will soon replace ACP as the analyte of choice. PSA is a more specific marker than ACP; total plasma ACP is relatively non-specific in disease association. In addition, although PSA is also an enzyme, it is much more stabile than ACP.

Prostatic specific antigen (PSA)

This is a glycoprotein enzyme (a serine protease) which is found in prostatic tissue (normal and malignant), seminal fluid, and plasma (small amounts, <4.0 mg/L). It is elevated in ~85% of patients with carcinoma of the prostate but also in up to 15% of subjects with benign prostatic hypertrophy (levels usually less than 10 mg/L). It is considered to be a useful screening test for prostatic cancer in patients 50 years and above and is very useful for following therapy of prostatic malignancy (Figure 13.3).

α-Amylase

Amylases are hydrolases that split complex carbohydrates constituted of interlinked α-D-glucose units, e.g., starch and glycogen. They are able to hydrolyse both linear and branched polyglycans:

Amylose → maltose
(linear)

Amylopectin/Glycogen → limit dextran + maltose
(branched)

The main amylase isoenzymes are those of the pancreas and the salivary glands, secreted into the pancreatic juice and saliva, respectively. These isoenzymes can be readily differentiated in the

181

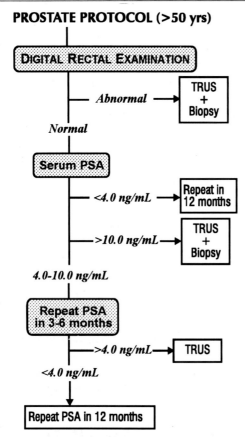

Figure 13.3. Suggested scheme for prostate evaluation after 50 years of age.

increase in the enzyme activity at its peak is, unfortunately, usually not clear cut (see page 00).

CAUSES OF HYPERAMYLASAEMIA

Pancreatic disorders
  Acute pancreatitis
  Trauma
  Pancreatic pseudocyst
  Carcinoma

Non-pancreatic abdominal disease
  Leakage of enzymes into the peritoneum:
    perforated ulcers, intestinal obstruction,
    ischaemia of small bowel
  Ruptured ectopic pregnancy
  Salpingitis

Miscellaneous
  Salivary glands: mumps, duct obstruction
  Ectopic enzyme production: carcinoma of the
    bronchus, ovary, colon
  Renal failure: decreased renal excretion
  Diabetic ketoacidosis: pancreatic in origin,
    cause unknown
  Macroamylasaemia: amylase bound to a plasma
    protein and unable to be excreted by the kidney
  Opiate drugs: morphine causes spasm of sphincter
    of Oddi

Urinary amylase

Urinary amylase measurements, though often requested simultaneously with plasma amylase, provide little additional diagnostic specificity in the diagnosis of acute pancreatitis. They are useful, however, in the recognition of macroamylasaemia and pancreatic pseudocysts.

Macroamylasaemia. This is a symptomless condition in which there is a persistent increase in the plasma amylase activity accompanied by a normal urinary amylase activity, despite normal glomerular function. This is due largely to reduced renal clearance of the larger enzyme macromolecules in circulation. These could be the result of polymerisation or formation of immune complexes (complex formation between amylase and an immunoglobulin). Because this harmless, rare condition may be confused with other causes of hyperamylasaemia, recognition of it

laboratory but the estimation is of limited clinical use and is not routinely available.

Plasma amylase has a half-life of 12-24 hours. Because of their relatively small size (MW of 40 000-50 000), both these amylase isoenzymes are partially filtered by the glomeruli and 25% of plasma amylase is excreted in the urine. Renal glomerular impairment alone may be associated with hyperamylasaemia. Other causes of hyperamylasaemia are listed below.

Plasma amylase is most frequently requested to assist in the differential diagnosis of acute pancreatitis in which surgery is not indicated, from other acute abdominal disorders with severe abdominal pain which may require immediate surgical treatment. In all these conditions, plasma amylase activity may be very much raised and the distinction using the extent of

will avert misdiagnosis and unnecessary further investigations.

Pancreatic pseudocyst. When urinary amylase levels are high and plasma amylase activities remain persistently high after an attack of acute pancreatitis, it may be due to leakage of pancreatic juice into a pancreatic pseudocyst. The high urinary amylase differentiates this condition from macroamylasaemia -- the two conditions being among the few indications for estimating urinary amylase excretion.

Aspartate aminotransferase (AST)

AST catalyses the following reaction which requires pyridoxal 5'-phosphate (vitamin B6) as a coenzyme:

$$AST$$
$$\text{L-aspartate} + \text{2-oxoglutarate} \longrightarrow \text{L-glutamate} + \text{oxaloacetate}$$

The reaction, a reversible one, has a pivotal role in amino acid metabolism. As it is difficult to measure either the reaction substrates or the products, the above reaction is usually coupled to a second reaction which utilises reduced nicotinamide adenine dinucleotide (NADH) as coenzyme. The oxidation of NADH is followed by measuring the decrease in absorbance at 340 nm.

```
2-Oxoglutarate          L-Glutamate
              \        /
         AST   )      (
              /        \                    MDH
L-Aspartate         Oxaloacetate  ------->  Malate
                              H+ + NADH   NAD+
```

AST is present in most tissues, and two organelle-specific (mitochondrial and cytosolic) isoenzymes have been found in heart and liver tissues. In terms of tissue distribution the heart has the highest concentration of AST, followed by the liver, skeletal muscle, pancreas, erythrocytes, and spleen. AST isoenzyme estimation has not found a place in diagnostic clinical chemistry; usually only total AST activity is measured.

CAUSES OF A HIGH PLASMA AST ACTIVITY

- Myocardial disease: infarction ($\uparrow\uparrow$)*
                       myocarditis ($\uparrow\uparrow$)

- Circulatory failure with shock and hypoxia ($\uparrow\uparrow$)
- Liver disease: hepatocellular damage caused by viral hepatitis and hepatic toxins ($\uparrow\uparrow$)
- Skeletal muscle disease: dystrophy, trauma, dermatomyositis, myoglobinuria
- Miscellaneous: pernicious anaemia ($\uparrow\uparrow$), renal infarction, acute pancreatitis, malignancy (cell death), infectious mononucleosis (due to liver involvement)
- Artefactual: *in vitro* haemolysis
- Physiological: neonates (about 1.5 to 2 times adult values)

* ($\uparrow\uparrow$) represents markedly elevated AST activities (10-100 times upper limit of adult reference range)

This enzyme has been used as a marker of liver, heart, and skeletal muscle disease. Increased AST activities in plasma (5-50 times the upper reference value at its peak) are valuable in the recognition of myocardial infarction and other conditions associated with myocardial damage (myocarditis). However, the more specific alanine aminotransferase (ALT) is generally a better marker for liver disease and likewise, creatine kinase (CK), for skeletal muscle disorders.

Alanine aminotransferase (ALT)

ALT catalyses the following reversible reaction:

$$\text{L-alanine} + \text{2-oxoglutarate} \leftrightarrow \text{L-glutamate} + \text{pyruvate}$$

The principle of the assay is similar to that of the AST assay except for the difference in substrates.

The predominant source of ALT is the liver, but it is also found, to a lesser extent, in the kidney, heart, skeletal muscle, and pancreas. Plasma ALT levels are elevated in a number of liver disorders, with very high levels found in viral or toxic hepatitis (see pages 149, 150), and moderately raised levels in cholestatic jaundice, infectious mononucleosis (due to liver involvement), liver congestion secondary to congestive cardiac failure and cirrhosis (ALT activities could also be normal in this last condition).

Gamma-glutamyltransferase (GGT)

GGT, which catalyses the transfer of γ-glutamyl groups from one peptide to another, is involved in the transport of amino acids across cell membranes. An amino acid about to enter a cell reacts with the tripeptide, glutathione (γ-glutamylcysteinylglycine) as follows:

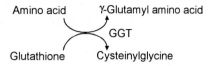

This is the initial reaction in the internalisation of amino acids at the cell membrane. Regeneration of glutathione (via the Meister cycle) is essential to sustain the process.

The liver, kidney, pancreas, and prostate are the main sources of GGT. Several isoenzymes have been described but have not yet been shown to be of clinical value. GGT is associated with the cell membrane fraction, which includes the microsomes, stimulation of which induces the synthesis of a host of enzymes. GGT can be induced by drugs such as phenytoin and phenobarbital and other xenobiotics such as alcohol.

CAUSES OF A RAISED PLASMA GGT

- Liver disease: all types
- Induction of microsomal enzymes by alcohol or drugs (e.g., phenytoin, barbiturates)

Although there is a wide distribution of GGT through out the body tissues, raised plasma levels are found mainly in liver disorders, both acute and chronic, with the largest increases occurring in cholestasis. However, although most types of liver disease are associated with high plasma levels of GGT, a high plasma GGT does not always indicate liver disease. As mentioned above plasma levels of this enzyme may increase due to drug induction of the liver enzyme and raised levels should be interpreted with care because of possible implications of alcohol or drug abuse. A suggested scheme for evaluating the finding of a high serum (plasma) GGT activity is shown in Figure 13.4.

Creatine kinase (CK)

CK catalyses the transfer of a high energy phosphate from adenosine triphosphate (ATP) to creatine:

$$\text{Creatine} + \text{ATP} \xrightarrow{\text{CK}} \text{Creatine phosphate} + \text{ADP}$$

Elevated serum GGT (>100 U/L)

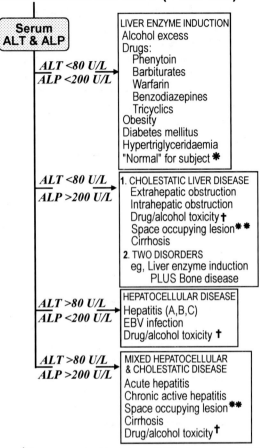

* Some normal subjects have GGT values up to 120 U/L
** Space occupying lesions: malignancy, abscess, cyst etc
† In alcoholic liver disease the AST is often > ALT

Figure 13.4. Suggested scheme for evaluating a high serum GGT activity.

The tissue with the highest concentration of CK is skeletal muscle, followed by brain and the myocardium. CK activity resides in dimeric protein molecules the subunits of which are of two types only, namely, the "M" and "B". It follows that there will be three CK isomers -- MM (CK-3), MB (CK-2) and BB (CK-1); the isoenzyme patterns from the various tissues are distinctive. The MM form is the predominant form in heart and skeletal muscle, BB is the predominant form in brain, and MB is a characteristic component in cardiac muscle, accounting for about 30-35% of total CK activity in that tissue. CK-MB is also found in skeletal muscle but in much lesser amounts (<5% of total CK activity).

In addition, there are at least three other forms of CK: CK-Mt is derived from the mitochondria of a variety of tissues and there are two "macro" forms -- one associated with immunoglobulins and the other, a polymer of CK-Mt. These forms are not as clinically important as the MM, BB and MB forms. CK isoenzyme analysis can be carried out using electro-phoretic or immunological assays.

In the plasma of normal people 95% or more of total CK activity is due to CK-MM and the remainder is CK-MB; CK-BB is not present. CK values are very age-dependant and, to a lesser extent, sex-dependant, related as they are to muscle mass. It is liable to be elevated in any sort of muscle trauma; thus, a specimen from a patient who has been subjected to numerous IM injections or strenuous physical activity may well give an artefactual result.

Isomeric forms of the CK enzyme may also be formed as a result of post-translational modifications. Of special clinical interest is the family of CK-MM isoforms referred to as CK-MM$_3$, CK-MM$_2$ and CK-MM$_1$. CK-MM$_3$ is the nascent tissue form and is first converted in the peripheral circulation to CK-MM$_2$ by serum carboxypeptidase-N (which cleaves off the carboxy-terminal amino acid, lysine, from the M subunit), and then to CK-MM$_1$. Clinical interest in these isoforms relates to their potential use in the early diagnosis of AMI and in monitoring the response to antithrombolytic therapy. Measurement of the serum levels of the CK-MM isoforms may provide an earlier indication of the success of the antithrombolytic agents.

CAUSES OF AN INCREASED PLASMA CK

- Heart: infarction, myocarditis
- Skeletal muscle: dystrophy, trauma, IM injections, strenuous physical activity, grand mal convulsions, dermatomyositis, myopathy
- Miscellaneous: hypothyroidism, cerebrovascular accidents, hyper- or hypothermia, septicaemia, diabetic ketoacidosis

Both total CK and CK-MB activity measurements and CK isoenzyme analysis are used most often for the diagnosis of acute myocardial infarction. The largest increases in total CK activity are seen, however, in patients with muscular dystrophy, especially the

Duchenne variety and in patients with rhabdomyolysis. In general raised CK activity is found whenever there is skeletal muscle damage, which could be caused by trauma (accidents, surgery), inflammation, ischemia, or metabolic disorders. CK-MB activity may be increased in skeletal muscle disorders but it will account for <5% of the total CK activity.

In the muscular dystrophies, plasma CK (and to a lesser extent, AST) activities are markedly increased. CK results are the more specific for these conditions (plasma aldolase activity is also raised and may sometimes be requested). The enzyme elevations are most pronounced in the early stages of the disease, presumably because of the extreme muscle wasting in the later stages, their levels fall, in some cases back to normal values. Similar, but less marked, changes are observed in patients with dermatomyositis.

Additional tests which may be useful in the evaluation of an elevated CK activity include serum LD, AST, CK isoenzymes, troponin T or I , myosin light chains, urinary myoglobulin and autoimmune immunology.

Lactate dehydrogenase (LD)

LD catalyses the reversible reaction:

$$NAD^+ \quad NADH + H^+$$
$$Lactate \xrightarrow[LD]{} Pyruvate$$

The substrate, lactate, has an absolute affinity for LD and the above reaction is an example of the "blind alleys" of metabolism. It is an important "shunt" during anaerobic metabolism when there is a relative lack of oxygen, e.g., in conditions of rapid glucose catabolism.

The LD enzyme is ubiquitous but the highest concentrations are found in the heart, skeletal muscle, liver, kidney, and erythrocytes. There are at least five isoenzymes in the serum (LD$_1$-LD$_5$).

CAUSES OF HIGH PLASMA LD ACTIVITIES

Plasma LD is elevated in a wide variety of diseases:

- Heart : infarction, myocarditis (↑↑)
- Circulatory failure with shock and hypoxia (↑↑)
- Liver : hepatocellular destruction

- Skeletal muscle : trauma, dystrophy, myositis, myoglobinuria
- Haematological: megaloblastic anaemia (↑↑), leukaemia (↑↑), pernicious anaemia, myeloproliferative disorders
- Miscellaneous:
    Malignancy - all types
    Renal infarct (↑↑)
    renal transplant rejection (↑↑)
    Pulmonary embolism
    Hypothyroidism
    Acute pancreatitis
- Artefactual: in vitro haemolysis, delayed separation of plasma from the red blood cells
- Physiological: Very young children**, drugs++

(↑↑): LD activities >5 times upper reference value
** Very young children have higher plasma LD activities. At birth levels of some 3-9 times adult values are common, gradually falling to adult values by the age of ten.
++ Any drug that is hepatotoxic or which causes muscle damage or haemolysis is liable to increase LD activity.

As can be seen from the above list a high plasma LD level is a very non-specific marker of cell damage. A proposed scheme for the evaluation of a high plasma LD activity is presented in Figure 13.5.

LD isoenzymes

The five isoenzymes (LD_1-LD_5) have the following origins: LD_1 and LD_2 are primarily from cardiac muscle, red blood cells (including premature cells), and kidney; LD_5 is mainly derived from the liver, but is also found in malignant tissues and skeletal muscle.

Certain changes in the LD isoenzyme distribution are of diagnostic use:

- ***Diagnosis of a myocardial infarct.*** Normally the concentration of LD_2 is greater than that of LD_1; in myocardial infarction the LD_1 level may exceed that of LD_2. This is called the 'flipped' pattern (Figure 13.6B). It is, however, not specific for myocardial infarction as it may also occur in pernicious anaemia, haemolysis, and acute renal infarction.

- ***Damage to the liver.*** The pattern would show a distinct LD_5 elevation (Figure 13.6F, G, H)

- ***Evaluation of a high plasma total LD of obscure***

origin. Patients with malignancies (e.g., acute leukaemia) often have an isolated increase in LD_3 alone or LD_2 and LD_3.

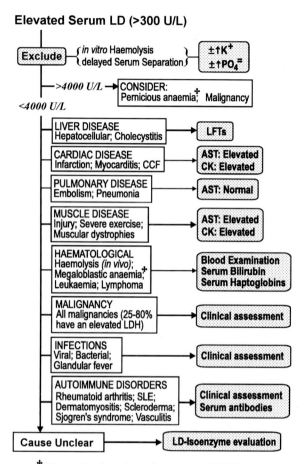

Elevated Serum LD (>300 U/L)

+ Values in Pernicious Anaemia may exceed 9000 U/L.

Figure 13.5. Evaluation of a high serum LD activity.

Cholinesterase

There are two cholinesterases, the 'true' acetyl-cholinesterase enzyme found in nervous tissue and the 'pseudo' cholinesterase enzyme found in the liver, heart, muscle, and plasma which catalyses the hydrolysis of choline esters. Here we are concerned only with the pseudocholinesterase measurable in plasma.

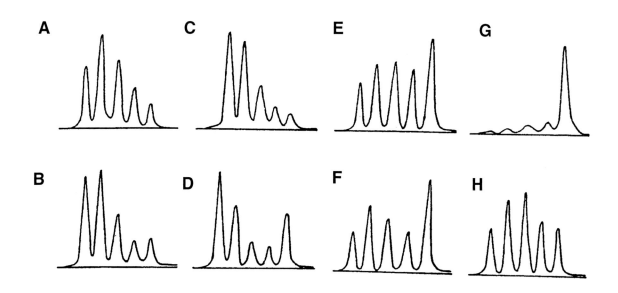

Figure 13.6. Serum LD isoenzyme patterns (densitometric scans). (A) Normal pattern. (B) Acute myocardial infarction (AMI) with the $LD_1:LD_2$ reversal (LD 'flip'). (C) AMI not showing the LD flip. (D) AMI with left heart failure, liver congestion, and a fatal outcome. (E) Sepsis. (F) Intrahepatic cholestatic jaundice. (G)Acute circulatory shock showing very severe hepatic anoxia. (H) Infectious mononucleosis with involvement of platelets or lymphatic tissue. The anode and LD_1 are on the left in all cases.

CAUSES OF DECREASED PLASMA (PSEUDO)CHOLINESTERASE

- Inherited abnormal variants (suxamethonium sensitivity)
- Secondary causes:
  - (a) liver disease: decreased synthesis
  - (b) organophosphate toxicity
  - (c) severe anaemia
  - (d) myocardial infarction

Suxamethonium sensitivity. The muscle relaxant suxamethonium is destroyed by pseudocholinesterase. In subjects with congenital decreased levels and abnormal variants of this enzyme prolonged apnoea follows suxamethonium administration (used as an anaesthetic for patients undergoing surgery).

The subjects with inherited suxamethonium sensitivity have low plasma levels of the enzyme and a dibucaine number of 15-30 (the dibucaine number is the percentage inhibition of the enzyme by dibucaine). They are homozygous for the atypical gene. Genetically normal individuals with low plasma enzyme levels due to disease have a normal dibucaine number.

Normal homozygote: dibucaine number 75 - 80
Atypical homozygote: dibucaine number 15 - 30
Heterozygote: dibucaine number 40 - 70

As the condition is an inherited disorder it is important to evaluate other members of the family if an index case presents.

Angiotensin converting enzyme (ACE)

ACE converts angiotensin I to angiotensin II (page 64). It is widely distributed throughout the body but the highest concentrations are found in the capillary endothelial cells of the lung. It is also found in plasma in measurable amounts.

In granulomatous conditions of the lung such as sarcoidosis, asbestosis, silicosis, Gaucher's disease, and leprosy, the plasma ACE level is raised, presumably due to increased synthesis. This factor has been utilised in the diagnosis and management of sarcoidosis. Ninety-two per cent of patients with sarcoidosis have an increased plasma ACE level which will become normal upon successful treatment.

Conditions associated with abnormal enzyme profiles

Acute pancreatitis

Acute pancreatitis classically presents with abdominal pain radiating to the back and a high plasma amylase level (e.g. >5 times the upper limit of normal). The plasma amylase begins to rise within hours of the attack, reaches a maximum in 12-24 hours and, if there are no complications, falls back to normal in 3-5 days Its plasma half-life is of the order of 12-24 hours.

In certain situations the plasma amylase level may be misleading and may give rise to a wrong diagnosis, for example:

1 Normal or near normal plasma amylase levels may be found in patients with acute pancreatitis if:

    (a)   it is acute haemorrhagic pancreatitis
    (b)   the blood sample is taken after the enzyme level has returned to normal.

2 High plasma amylase levels can occur in pain-associated, non-pancreatic, intra-abdominal diseases as in:

    (a)   perforating ulcers of the gut
    (b)   an obstructed gut
    (c)   a ruptured ectopic pregnancy
    (d)   diabetic ketoacidosis

3 Abdominal pain, non-pancreatic in origin (e.g. appendicitis), can be associated with non-pancreatic disorders that have persistently high plasma amylase levels, for example:

    (a)   salivary gland : mumps, duct obstruction
    (b)   renal insufficiency
    (c)   macroamylasaemia

    (d)   carcinoma: bronchus, colon, ovary

Whilst the interpretation of a high plasma amylase level may appear fairly straightforward, there are a number of pitfalls that may confuse the unwary. The diagnosis of acute pancreatitis remains essentially a clinical one.

Myocardial infarction

Following a myocardial infarct many enzymes, including AST, CK, and LD, are released into the blood stream. These three enzymes, which have been called the cardiac enzymes, differ in their time of appearance, time of peaking, and time of normalisation in the plasma during and after an infarct (Figure 13.7). They also differ in their specificity. The appropriate test to use depends on the time (known or estimated) which has elapsed since the onset infarction.

CK: appears 3-6 hours post-infarct, peaks at 12-24 hours, normalises in 3-4 days; specificity: found in heart, skeletal muscle, brain.

AST: appears after 6-8 hours, peaks at 24-48 hours, normalises in 5-7 days; specificity: found in heart, skeletal muscle, liver, pancreas.

LD: appears after 6-12 hours, peaks at 24-48 hours, normalises in 8-12 days; specificity: very wide distribution.

Note: It is obvious (but the fact is often overlooked) that the plasma activities of all the 'cardiac' enzymes may remain normal for up to about four hours after an infarct has occurred. There is little advantage (and a potential risk of misdiagnosis) in performing enzyme estimations during this 'quiescent' period.

The plasma activities of these enzymes have been shown to be raised at the appropriate times in more than 90% of cases of AMI and very high levels may be reached. The extent of the rise, however, does not correlate closely with the size of the infarct. This is not a serious setback as the prognosis is often more dependant on the site rather than the size of the infarct. In patients who subsequently develop congestive cardiac failure or who suffer a second infarct shortly thereafter, a late resurgence of AST and LD activities

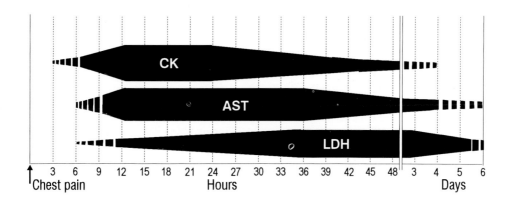

Figure 13.7. Changes in cardiac enzyme activities in the plasma after an acute myocardial infarct.

after returning to normal levels may be seen. In contrast, no increases in enzyme activities are evident in patients with angina pectoris.

Despite their proven worth in the diagnosis of AMI, none of these enzymes are specific for heart disease. Generally this is not a major problem as the patient will show other evidences of myocardial infarction, e.g., typical clinical history, typical ECG changes. (**Note**: Plasma enzymes should only be used for confirming the diagnosis of myocardial infarction and they should be measured over three to four days to observe the characteristic rises and falls.)

If the diagnosis is equivocal, for example, if there are other possible causes for the raised enzyme values or if the ECG changes are masked by some conduction defect, then the LD and CK can be made more specific by estimating their isoenzymes.

LD-isoenzymes: increased levels of LD_1 and LD_2 with $LD_1 > LD_2$ (see above)

CK-MB: cardiac muscles contains 10-15% CK-MB and skeletal muscle contains ≈ 5%, therefore in cardiac infarct there is an increased absolute level of CK-MB which will be equivalent to 10-15% of the total CK, in skeletal muscle damage there will also be an increase in the CK-MB but it will be <10% of the total CK.

Hydroxybutyrate dehydrogenase (HBD) assay:
The principle of this assay is based on the fact that LD_1 (and to a lesser extent LD_2) can use an alternate

substrate, 2-hydroxybutyrate, while the more cathodic LD isoenzymes cannot. Thus the HBD assay gives a measure of the LD_1 activity. It is a simpler and faster test to run than the LD isoenzyme separation and is amenable to automation.

Skeletal muscle disease

The skeletal muscles contain large amounts of the following enzymes: CK, AST, LD and aldolase. The plasma CK shows the biggest elevation in muscle disorders and is the enzyme of choice when investigating suspected muscle disease.

Plasma CK levels in excess of 100 times normal (e.g. >30 000 U/L) can occur in Duchenne muscular dystrophy. In the other dystrophies such as the limb-girdle variety, and fascioscapulohumeral dystrophy, the plasma CK levels do not rise quite as high (but reach levels of about 10-20 times the upper limits of normal). In polymyositis and dermatomyositis plasma CK levels may rise by 10-100 times normal.

Liver disease

The use of enzymes as diagnostic tools in differential diagnosis of liver disease is discussed in Chapter 11.

Haemolysis and red cell enzymes

A number of erythrocyte enzyme deficiencies may result in haemolytic anaemia. They are rare, the two commonest being glucose-6-phosphate dehydrogenase deficiency, and pyruvate kinase deficiency. Other enzyme deficiencies which may result in haemolysis involve hexose kinase, triosephosphate isomerase, diphosphoglycerate mutase, and ATPase.

Glucose-6-phosphate dehydrogenase (G-6-PD) deficiency. The red cell is constantly being oxidised and if its reducing mechanism is inefficient, haemoglobin is converted to methaemoglobin which can be further denatured to form Heinz bodies. These bodies, and the cells containing them, are removed by the spleen; hence the scene is set for haemolytic anaemia.

Normally the reduced glutathione of the cell prevents this oxidation. The reduction of glutathione is dependant on an adequate supply of NADPH which is produced by the pentose phosphate pathway. The central enzyme in this pathway is glucose-6-phosphate dehydrogenase and a deficiency of this enzyme exposes the red cell to damage.

G-6-PD deficiency occurs as an inborn error of metabolism in many races and can result in:

- Chronic haemolytic anaemia
- drug-induced haemolytic anaemia, (oxidant drugs - primaquine, sulphonamides)
- favism (following ingestion of the fava bean)

Pyruvate kinase deficiency. This defect is rare and causes neonatal and recurrent jaundice. The direct cause of the haemolysis is unclear but may be related to the accumulation of phosphoenol-pyruvate and 2,3-diphosphoglycerate in the red cell.

REFERENCES AND FURTHER READING

Alkaline phosphatase

Posen S, Doherty E. Serum alkaline phosphatase in clinical medicine. Adv Clin Chem 1981; 22:163-245.

Price CP. Multiple forms of human serum alkaline phosphatase: detection and quantitation. Ann Clin Biochem 1993;30:355-372.

Amylase

Geoaks MC. Acute pancreatitis: Davis conference. Ann Intern Med 1985;103:86-100.

Koop H. Serum levels of pancreatic enzymes and their clinical significance. Clin Gastroentr 1984;13:739-61.

Lott JA. Inflammatory disease of the pancreas. CRC Reviews Clin Lab Sciences 1982;17:201-228.

Creatine kinase

Goto I. Serum creatine phosphokinase isoenzymes in hypothyroidism, convulsions, myocardial infarction and other disease. Clin Chim Acta 1974;52:27-30.

Griffiths PD. CK-MB: A valuable test? Ann Clin Biochem 1986;23:238-242.

Lott JA, Strang JM. Serum enzymes in the diagnosis and differential diagnosis of myocardial ischaemia and necrosis. Clin Chem 1980;26:1241-1250.

γ-glutamyltransferase

Penn R, Worthington DJ. Is serum γ-glutamyl-transferase a misleading test? Br J Med 1983;286: 531-535.

Chapter 14

Plasma Lipids and Lipoproteins

Lipids, like proteins, carbohydrates, and nucleic acids are ubiquitous constituents of all living cells. They function as a primary source of energy, as precursors for the steroid hormones, prostaglandins, leukotrienes, and lipoxins, and as important structural components of cell membranes. Dietary sources as well as endogenous synthesis contribute to the lipid pool in the body and steady-state levels are normally maintained within certain limits.

From a metabolic viewpoint, the major classes of lipids are the fatty acids, neutral glyceridcs (acylglycerols), sterols (cholesterol), sterol esters, phospholipids, and bile acids. These different lipids vary considerably in their chemical and physical properties. One common characteristic is their relative insolubilty in water. Most lipids, with phospholipids as the exception, are hydrophobic molecules and have to be packaged with proteins to ensure their carriage and transport in the plasma. Free fatty acids are carried tightly bound to albumin; other lipids circulate in the form of lipoproteins, complexed with specific proteins known as apolipoproteins.

Advances in our understanding of lipid metabolism have had a considerable impact on current views of the pathophysiology of cardiovascular diseases. While many issues regarding lipids and cardiovascular disease remain unresolved, an unassailable body of evidence indicates that abnormalities in plasma lipoprotein concentrations are a major risk factor for the development of atherosclerosis, coronary heart disease (CHD) and stroke. Raised low density lipoproteins (LDL) and reduced high density lipoproteins (HDL) are separately and jointly responsible.

Raised levels of cholesterol in blood, which exist mainly in the form of LDL cholesterol, leads to atheroma formation; in general, the higher the level, the greater the extent of atheromatous involvement. Evidence of the benefit of reducing hypercholesterolaemia, culled from five major primary prevention trials, is impressively congruous. The data show that it is possible to reduce the incidence of CHD in individuals with initially high plasma concentrations of cholesterol and LDL through appropriate remedial measures.

Both intrinsic characteristics such as age, gender and inheritance, and modifiable factors such as diet, body weight, and lifestyle habits are involved in causing hyperlipidaemia. A high dietary intake of saturated fat has emerged as a leading cause of high blood cholesterol and of CHD. Inheritance is a potent determinant of blood cholesterol and lipoprotein concentrations and of lipoprotein receptor acitivity: indeed, genetic influences probably determine more than half of the variability in plasma lipoprotein concentrations.

In this chapter, we will briefly discuss the properties and clinical significance of plasma lipids, lipoproteins, and apolipoproteins, and present current views on lipoprotein metabolism, various lipoprotein disorders, and the role of lipids in the pathogenesis of cardiovascular diseases, emphasising the diagnostic aspects. Tests used in the investigation of dyslipidaemia and lipoprotein disorders will be discussed.

Plasma lipids

Fatty acids

Fatty acids are linear, single-chain, monocarboxylic acids, containing between 12 to 24 carbon atoms per molecule. The most abundant fatty acids found in man are the C16 (palmitic) and C18 (stearic, oleic and linoleic) acids. Fatty acids are amphipathic molecules containing a hydrophobic hydrocarbon side chain and a polar carboxyl group. The hydrocarbon chain may be saturated, as in palmitic acid, or unsaturated, with one, two, or three double bonds, as in oleic, linoleic, and linolenic acid, respectively. The polyunsaturated fatty acids are subdivided into ω-3, ω-6 and ω-9 subtypes, depending on the position of the double bond closest to the methyl terminal (ω) end of the fatty acid chain.

Polyunsaturated fatty acids are precursors of prostaglandins, leukotrienes and lipoxins. Prostaglandins play an important role in platelet aggregation and CHD. Except for the so-called essential fatty acids, e.g., linoleic and linolenic acids, the rest can be synthesised in the body from carbohydrate precursors.

Fatty acids exist largely as esters, mainly in the form of neutral triglycerides (triacylglycerols) or phospholipids. Only traces occur as free or nonesterified fatty acids (FFA or NEFA) in cells. In plasma, FFA are transported covalently bound to albumin to sites of utilisation or storage (after re-esterification) in the liver and muscle.

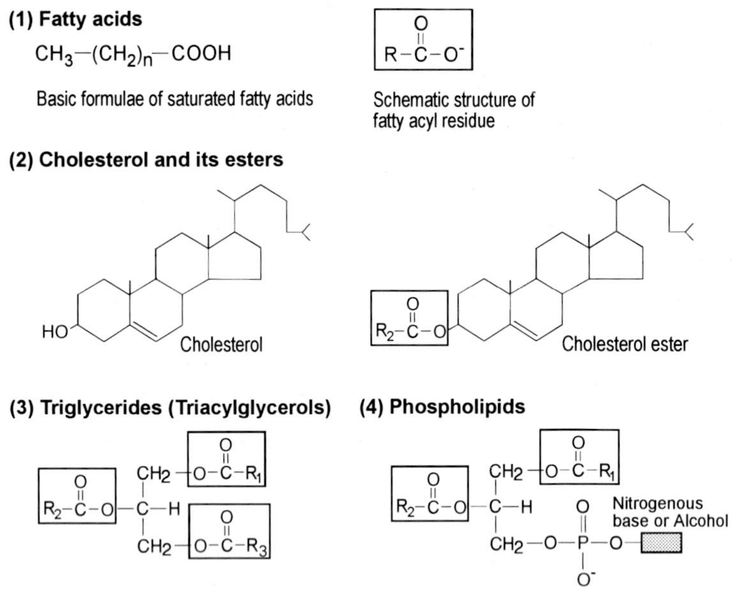

(1) Fatty acids

$$CH_3-(CH_2)_n-COOH$$

Basic formulae of saturated fatty acids

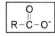

Schematic structure of
fatty acyl residue

(2) Cholesterol and its esters

Cholesterol

Cholesterol ester

(3) Triglycerides (Triacylglycerols)

(4) Phospholipids

Nitrogenous
base or Alcohol

Figure 14.1. Structures of the major lipids of the human cells.

Cholesterol

Free cholesterol is a component of all cell membranes and the precursor steroid from which other steroid hormones including vitamin D_3 may be derived. It has a hydroxylated four-ringed steroid nucleus with an iso-octane side-chain (Figure 14.1).

The cholesterol content in the body is dependant on the balance between its intake in the diet, its synthesis within tissue cells, and its excretion by the liver. The proportion absorbed from the diet depends partly on the amount ingested, with less being absorbed when there is a higher intake. As the body cannot break down its sterol nucleus, cholesterol is either excreted unchanged or as bile acids in bile. Its transport in the plasma and its metabolism are intimately related to lipoprotein metabolism. More than two-thirds of plasma cholesterol is in the esterified form.

Triglycerides

Triglycerides are formed by the esterification of all three hydroxyl groups of the glycerol nucleus with identical or different fatty acid molecules. They are the major components of depot or storage lipids. Triglycerides are derived partly from dietary sources and partly from endogenous synthesis in the liver and adipose tissue. Normally about 70-150 g (80-170 mmol) is absorbed from the diet per day (>90% of a typical diet). In the plasma they are packaged and transported as part of the macromolecular lipoprotein particles.

Phospholipids

These are complex lipids, resembling the triglycerides in structure, but having a phosphate group attached to a polar organic molecule (nitrogenous base or an alcohol) in place of the third fatty acid residue (Figure 14.1). The polar group can be choline, ethanolamine, serine, inositol, inisitol phosphates, and glycerol; the two fatty acids are asymmetrically positioned. Because of the polar group, phospholipids are amphipathic, a property that allows them to form bilayers in aqueous media and makes them uniquely suited to form membranes.

The most abundant phospholipids in the body are phosphatidylcholine (lecithin) and phosphatidyl-ethanolamine. Phosphatidylserine is localised mainly in brain cells, and diphosphatidylglycerol (cardiolipin) occurs primarily in the inner mitochondrial membrane.

Another major type of phospholipid (sometimes called a sphingolipid) is sphingomyelin, which has

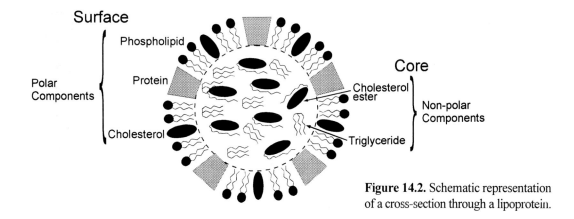

Figure 14.2. Schematic representation of a cross-section through a lipoprotein.

sphingosine as the 'backbone' molecule in lieu of glycerol. It is a major component of myelin, which forms a protective coating on certain brain and nerve cells.

In the plasma, phospholipids (mainly lecithin and sphingomyelin) occur as constituents of lipoproteins, where they play a key role, by virtue of their amphipathic property, in mediating the transport of non-polar lipids such as triglycerides and cholesterol esters in the aqueous plasma medium. Plasma levels range from 2 to 3 mmol/L in healthy subjects.

Plasma lipoproteins

Lipoproteins are synthesised by the liver and the intestines. Their main physiological function is that of transporting dietary and endogenously synthesised lipids in the blood. Before we discuss the metabolism of the various lipoprotein classes, it is necessary to review briefly their physical properties and those of their constituent apolipoproteins.

Lipoproteins are macromolecular complexes. Their constituents are arranged to form an outer shell or envelope, comprised of the amphipathic apolipoproteins, phospholipids and free cholesterol (polar groups facing outwards), surrounding an inner core containing the non-polar cholesterol esters and triglycerides (Figure 14.2). In normal plasma, there are five main lipoprotein classes, defined according to their behaviour upon ultracentrifugation (flotation rates), which depends on their hydrated densities.

They also differ in their lipid and apolipoprotein content as well as in electrophoretic mobility, as summarised in Table 14.1.

Chylomicrons

These are large triglyceride-rich complexes, formed from dietary lipids and apolipoproteins in the microvilli of the small intestines. They are released into the lacteals of the lymphatics, reaching the systemic system via the thoracic duct. For a few hours after each meal, they serve to transport exogenous lipids from the intestines to all cells but are virtually absent from normal plasma after a 12-hour fast. Chylomicrons are the largest of the lipoproteins, and therefore have the lowest density and electrophoretic mobility. They contain very little protein (1-2%) but their apolipoprotein components, especially apo B-48, are essential for their synthesis and secretion. This is illustrated by the complete absence of chylomicrons from the plasma of patients with abetalipoproteinaemia, in whom there is an inherited defect of apo B secretion.

Very low density lipoproteins (VLDL)

These are moderately large particles, with triglycerides as the main lipid component, and apo B-100, the main apolipoprotein. They are formed mainly in the liver, and to a lesser extent in the intestinal mucosa. Their main function is to transport endogenously synthesised lipids from the liver to extrahepatic cells for utilisation

Table 14.1. Properties, composition and functions of plasma lipoproteins.

Class	Diameter (A)	Density (g/mL)	Electrophoretic Mobility	Chemical Composition (% of dry mass)					Apoproteins
				TG	CE	Chol	PLs	Proteins	
Chylomicrons	800-5000	0.93-0.95	Origin (cathode)	80-95	2-4	1-3	3-6	1-2	A-I, A-IV, B-48,C-I
CLDL	300-800	0.96-1.006	Pre-beta	45-65	12-16	4-8	15-2	6-10	B-100, E, C-I, C-II
IDL	250-350	1.006-1.0	Slow pre-beta	15-32	25-35	6-10	16-2	17-20	B-100, E
LDL	180-300	1.019-1.0	Beta	4-8	40-50	6-8	18-2	18-22	B-100
HDL	50-120	1.063-1.210	Alpha	2-7	15-20	3-5	26-3	45-55	A-I, A-II, E, C-II

or storage. With a half-life of 2-4 hours, the rate of turnover of VLDL in humans is less rapid than that of chylomicrons. Two other classes of lipoproteins, the intermediate density and the low density lipoproteins, are derived from VLDL metabolism.

Intermediate density lipoproteins

The intermediate density lipoproteins (IDL), sometimes termed VLDL remnants, are transient intermediates formed during the conversion of VLDL to LDL. By virtue of their transient existence, IDL are not detected in normal plasma. However, in certain forms of hyperlipidaemia, IDL excess in the plasma may produce a characteristic 'broad β' band during lipoprotein electrophoresis (Figure 14.13, page 206), and thus can become a major determinant of both serum total cholesterol and triglyceride concentrations.

Low density lipoproteins (LDL)

These are relatively smaller, cholesterol-rich particles, derived mainly from the metabolism of VLDL; however, direct hepatic synthesis and secretion of LDL has been demonstrated in patients with familial hypercholesterolaemia and Type III hyperlipidaemia. LDL serve as the main cholesterol carrier in the plasma. They differ from their precursors, the VLDL, in their much lower triglyceride content and in retaining only *one* of the various apolipoproteins found in VLDL, namely, apo B-100.

High density lipoproteins (HDL)

These are the smallest of the lipoproteins and the most dense. Their lipid to protein ratio is 1:1. Cholesterol (25%) and phospholipids (20%) make up the bulk of the lipid fraction, there being very little triglycerides (5%) in these particles. They are involved in mediating the reverse transport of cholesterol from cells in peripheral tissues to the liver, for excretion from the body. Several subgroups have been recognised, designated HDL-1, HDL-2, HDL-3, and HDL-4, which differ in their protein and lipid content, shape, structure, and density. There is progressive loss of phospholipids, cholesterol, and cholesterol esters when HDLs are transformed from HDL-1 to HDL-4.

Lipoprotein (a) [Lp(a)]

This lipoprotein, a variant of LDL, was first discovered in 1963. Lp(a) is now known to be present in essentially all plasma, in concentrations varying from <1 mg/dL to >200 mg/dL. Studies have shown that high plasma levels of Lp(a) are strongly associated with atherosclerosis. Lp(a) closely resembles LDL in lipid composition but has a higher protein content. In addition to apo B-100, it has the unique apolipoprotein (a), which is bound to apo B-100 by a disulphide linkage (Figure 14.3). Despite its apo B-100 content, it remains unresolved whether Lp(a) is catabolised via the LDL receptor. If present in raised amounts, Lp(a) would give rise to a band in the region between LDL and VLDL in a lipoprotein electrophoretic run (page 206).

Note: It must be emphasised that each lipoprotein class represents a heterogeneous continuum of particles that are in continuous metabolic flux. There is rapid uptake, loss and interchange of components between different lipoprotein particles as well as between the lipoproteins and cells. Thus particles within each lipoprotein class vary in size, density and composition. However, certain properties and broad generalities still apply to lipoprotein classes as a whole.

- The triglyceride-rich lipoprotein complexes (chylomicrons and VLDL) are larger and less dense and have lower protein content. Because of their large size, chylomicrons and VLDL particles scatter light. This accounts for the turbid or milky appearance of plasma specimens containing high levels of these lipoproteins. On prolonged standing (hours or overnight) at 4°C (the refrigerator test), the larger and less dense chylomicrons rise to form a creamy layer on the surface (see Figure 14.13). VLDL particles, being relatively denser, do not float and samples with high VLDL concentrations remain diffusely turbid. Fasting samples from normal individuals do not contain chylomicrons.

- The smaller lipoproteins (LDL and HDL) have relatively lower triglyceride and higher protein and cholesterol in their composition, compared to chylomicrons and VLDL. This compositional difference is reflected in their increased density. These smaller particles do not scatter light and samples containing even very high levels of these lipoproteins are not turbid (Figure 14.13).

Plasma apolipoproteins

The apolipoprotein composition of the major lipoproteins is shown in Table 14.1. Their specific characteristics and functions are summarised in Table 14.2. Clinical interest in apolipoproteins stems from the greater appreciation of the structure-function relations of these proteins to an understanding of the mechanisms of lipoprotein metabolism and their possible relationship to disease states.

- In addition to being essential structural components of lipoprotein particles, apolipoproteins are also necessary for their synthesis and catabolism. The importance of apo B for VLDL and chylomicron secretion is underscored by the complete absence of these lipoproteins from the plasma of patients with abetalipoproteinaemia, who are believed to have a defect in apo B synthesis (page 210). It appears that apo B is essential for the incorporation of triglycerides into chylomicrons and VLDL.

- Apolipoproteins (e.g., apo A-I, apo C-I and apo C-II) also act as cofactors or activators of certain enzymes associated with lipid and lipoprotein metabolism (Table 14.2).

- They are also involved as transfer proteins, e.g., apo D is believed to be part of the cholesterol ester transfer protein complex of HDL, facilitating the exchange of cholesterol esters between different lipoprotein particles.

- Apolipoproteins (e.g., apo B and apo E) also play a part in receptor recognition of lipoproteins, thus controlling the rate of tissue uptake of cholesterol or triglycerides.

Salient points regarding the structure of apo B and apo(a) of relevance to their metabolic functions are briefly discussed below.

The apo B structure

Both chylomicrons and VLDL contain apo B which is essential for the assembly of these particles. Intestinal and hepatic apo B differ in size. The hepatic form, apo B-100, found in VLDL, has 4563 amino acids; the intestinal form, apo B-48, found in chylomicrons, is only 48% as large and contains only the amino terminal amino acids of apo B-100. This is due to a single nucleotide substitution in the messenger RNA, a cytosine-to-uracil change at codon 2153, giving rise to a premature stop codon. In individuals with the rare disease, abetalipoproteinaemia, both the apo B proteins are absent, a finding congruous with their common gene origin.

As it is the carboxy terminal domain of apo B-100 which enables LDL, derived from VLDL, to bind to the LDL receptors and become internalised, apo B-48 which lacks this domain will not bind to LDL receptors. For the chylomicron remnants, which contain apo B-48, receptor binding is mediated by recognition of apo E; the presence of apo B-48 is needed to allow for effective receptor-ligand binding.

Table 14.2. The human plasma apolipoproteins and their properties and functions.

Apolipoprotein	Major Sources	Lipoprotein Distribution	Function
A-I	Intestine, liver	HDL, chylomicrons	LCAT cofactor
A-II	Intestine, liver	HDL, chylomicrons	Unknown hepatic lipase cofactor?
A-IV	Intestine, liver	HDL, chylomicrons	LCAT cofactor?
B-48	Intestine	Chylomicrons	Chylomicron synthesis and secretion
B-100	Liver	VLDL, LDL	VLDL synthesis, secretion; LDL receptor recognition
C-I	Liver	Chylomicrons, VLDL, HDL	LCAT cofactor?
C-II	Liver	Chylomicrons, VLDL, HDL	Lipoprotein lipase cofactor
C-III	Liver	Chylomicrons, VLDL, HDL	Inhibition of (a) interaction with hepatic receptors (b) lipoprotein lipase
D	Liver	HDL	Unknown
E	Liver	Chylomicrons, VLDL, HDL	B,E receptor recognition

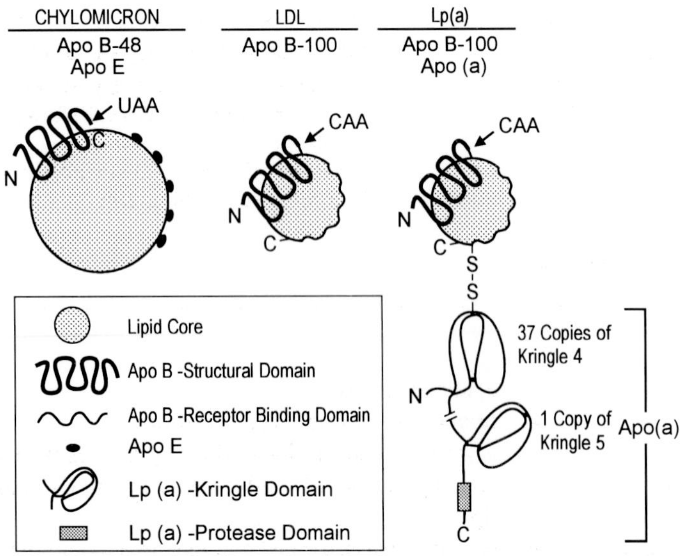

Figure 14.3. Three lipoproteins that contain apolipoprotein B in their structures.
Copyright © Macmillan Magazines Ltd. Printed by permission from Nature 1987;330:113.

The arrow denotes the site at which codon 2153 in the apo B gene is changed at the mRNA level from CAA to UAA in intestinal cells, creating a premature stop codon.

The apo(a) homology to plasminogen

Apo(a), one of the two apolipoproteins of Lp(a), is a high molecular weight glycoprotein which exhibits amazing heterogeneity. Phenotypes ranging in size from ~300,000 to ~700,000 Daltons have been reported. DNA sequencing has revealed a striking sequence homology of the apo(a) gene with that of human plasminogen, the precursor of the fibrinolytic enzyme plasmin. The serine protease domains and the 'kringle' domains of plasminogen are highly conserved in the apo(a) gene structure (Figure 14.4), with 37 copies of Kringle 4. From evidence from linkage studies in pedigrees, it is postulated that the apo(a) gene originated via gene duplication of the plasminogen gene with some deletions of exons at the NH$_2$-terminal end. Both the two genes have been located by in situ hybridisation to loci in close proximity on chromosome 6, at 6q 26-27. The size heterogeneity observed between different apo(a) phenotypes may represent alternative allelic variants of the apo(a) gene, and homologous recombination events resulting in varying numbers of tandemly repeated Kringle 4 sequences are the likeliest cause of the intra-individual size variation.

A large volume of epidemiological data shows that the 20% of the population with levels of Lp(a) greater than 300 mg/L have a two-fold increase in relative risk of developing coronary atherosclerosis. The risk associated with raised levels of Lp(a) are markedly influenced by the prevailing level of LDL cholesterol. Patients with Lp(a) >300 mg/L and LDL cholesterol >4.4 mmol/L have a two to four-fold higher odds ratio for CHD than those whose LDL cholesterol are not so elevated. Information emanating from studies on the apo(a) gene has resulted in possible structure-function relationships which may explain this close association between elevated levels of Lp(a) and atheromatous vascular disease (page 202).

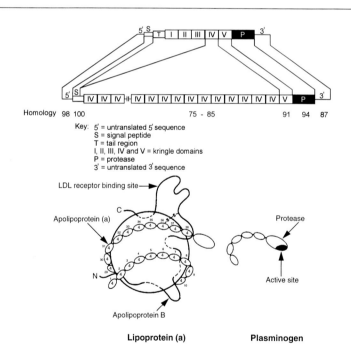

Figure 14.4. Top. Schematic representation comparing the sequences of the plasminogen and apolipoprotein (a) genes. Modified after McLean *et al*, *Nature* 1987;330:132-137.

Each gene is divided into structural domains; the percentage sequence homologies of the various domains are shown below the respective domains.

Bottom. Schematic representation of the structural homology of apolipoprotein (a) and plasminogen. Redrawn from: Durrington PN. *Hyperlipidaemia: Diagnosis and Management 2nd edn*, Butterworth Heinmann, Oxford, 1995, with kind permission of the author.

Lipoprotein metabolism

Lipoprotein metabolism involves the following:

- the synthesis and post-synthetic modification of apolipoproteins
- lipoprotein assembly and secretion
- enzymatic modification of their lipid components e.g., hydrolysis of triglycerides by lipoprotein lipase
- enzyme-catalysed transfer of their apolipoproteins

- receptor-mediated internalization and intracellular catabolism of the modified or remnant particles
- the reverse transport of cholesterol from the peripheral tissues to the liver.

Most of the apolipoproteins are synthesised by the liver and the intestine. Some of these proteins undergo post-translational alterations after they have been secreted into the plasma. For example, apo A-I is secreted with a six amino acid N-terminal extension, the cleavage of which may be important for the stability of the HDL molecule. Apo E is secreted as sialylated apo E and the sialic acid residues are subsequently removed.

Lipoproteins are assembled in the liver and the intestine. The chylomicrons, containing primarily dietary lipids, are secreted by the intestines and are metabolised via the exogenous lipid pathway (Figure 14.5). Most of the VLDL particles are formed in the liver from lipids derived from endogenous synthesis. The conversion of VLDL to IDL and LDL and their subsequent receptor-mediated catabolism constitute the endogenous lipid pathway (Figure 14.6). Both pathways involve HDL, lipolytic enzymes and transfer proteins.

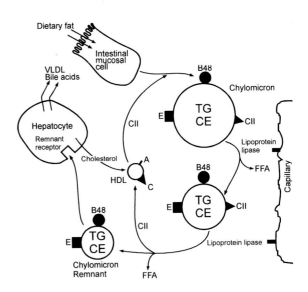

TG, triacylglycerol; CE, cholesterol esters; FFA, free fatty acids

Figure 14.5. The exogenous lipid pathway -- the synthesis and metabolism of chylomicrons.

Exogenous lipid pathway

Following a meal, the products of digestion of dietary fat (mainly free fatty acids, 2-monoglycerides and lysolecithin) are absorbed and re-esterified to form triglycerides and phospholipids in the microvilli of the small intestines. Dietary cholesterol is similarly absorbed and a portion is esterified. These lipids are assembled with apolipoproteins (mainly apo B-48, apo A-I and apo A-IV) into chylomicrons which are secreted into the mesenteric lymph, ultimately entering the systemic circulation; secretion depends on the presence of apo B. Nascent intestinal HDL containing apo A-I, apo C and apo E is also secreted via the lymphatics into the blood. In the blood, chylomicrons exchange apolipoproteins with other lipoproteins and with HDL in particular, transferring apo A-I to the latter and receiving apo C and apo E in return.

Chylomicrons are mainly metabolised in adipose and muscle tissue which contains high concentrations of the enzyme lipoprotein lipase. The enzyme is located on the luminal surface of the vascular endothelium and is activated by apo C-II. It catalyses the hydrolysis of triglycerides in the chylomicrons, releasing fatty acids and glycerol. These re-enter cells -- the bulk of the fatty acids are taken up by adipocytes

and stored as fat; glycerol is utilised in the liver for the synthesis of phospholipids and triglycerides.

The chylomicron remnants are rapidly removed by the liver and catabolised intracellularly within the hepatic lysosomes. They are taken up by receptor-mediated endocytosis, after binding to specific receptors on the surface of the hepatocytes, which recognise both the apo E and apo B-100 ligands. Apo B-48, although unable to bind to the receptor itself, allows for the effective binding of apo E. In newly formed chylomicron remnants, the apo E recognition site is 'obstructed' by the large complement of apo C proteins. Transfer of the apo C to HDL removes the steric hindrance and permits receptor binding.

In summary, exogenous lipid pathways deliver dietary triglycerides to peripheral tissues, mainly adipose and muscle tissues. The remaining constituents in the chylomicron remnants are re-circulated to the liver and may be used for the synthesis of VLDL and HDL by the liver cells. In addition, chylomicron remnants interact with HDL in the 'reverse transfer' of cholesterol, and participate in the removal of the cholesterol esters resulting from the LCAT reaction back to the liver for excretion as bile acids.

Endogenous lipid pathway

The liver is the primary site of endogenous VLDL synthesis (some VLDL originates from the intestine). The triglycerides of hepatic VLDL are synthesised in the post-absorptive period, either from glucose or from the fatty acids and glycerol mobilised from chylomicron metabolism (see above). The cholesterol is either synthesised de novo or derived from intracellular degradation of chylomicron remnants. These lipids are assembled with phospholipids and apolipoproteins, mainly apo B-100 and apo E, before secretion into the circulation via the lymphatic ducts.

The first step of VLDL metabolism is similar to that of chylomicroms. Nascent VLDL particles acquire more apo C from ciculating HDL or other lipoproteins. In peripheral tissues they are converted to IDL as triglycerides are progressively removed by the hydro-lytic action of lipoprotein lipase, activated by apo C-II.

Thereafter, the metabolism of IDL takes a different path. Whilst a small portion of IDL (VLDL remnants) are taken up by the liver cells through interaction with receptors that recognise their apo E components, in large part these particles are converted to LDL, with loss of more triglycerides and apolipoproteins (other than apo B-100) in the process. The cholesterol-rich LDL particles are much smaller, more dense and have a longer half-life than their precursors. LDL are the main carriers of cholesterol in plasma. Further uptake and metabolism of LDL by cells are dependant on the presence of the LDL receptor. This receptor recognises apo B-100. Most of the LDL in plasma is removed via this receptor-mediated path and defects in the LDL receptor results in diminished clearance of circulating LDL. However, some may enter cells by an unregulated receptor-independant mechanism, especially when plasma LDL levels are high. Figure 14.6 summarises the metabolism of VLDL via the endogenous lipid pathway.

Although the liver contains the highest concentration of LDL receptors, LDL are catabolised to a substantial extent in extrahepatic tissues that have a high demand for cholesterol. These include the adrenal cortex and the gonads, for steroid hormone synthesis, and loci of rapidly dividing cells, for cell membrane formation.

Many cells derive their cholesterol requirements from LDL uptake and degradation, as described above. However, most of them can also synthesise cholesterol from its precursors, when needed. The intracellular cholesterol pool is kept at a relatively constant level, with several mechanisms preventing its intracellular accumulation (Figure 14.7). Regulation of cellular

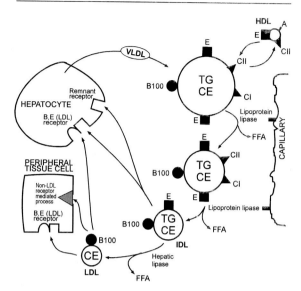

Figure 14.6. Endogenous lipid transport and metabolism. See text for details.

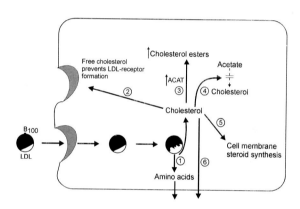

Figure 14.7. LDL metabolism and regulation of intracellular cholesterol flux in extrahepatic tissues. ACAT, acyl cholesterol acyltransferase. See text for details of the steps denoted by the numbers in the figure.

cholesterol metabolism is effected by:

- degradation by lysosomal enzymes (step 1, Figure 14.7)
- down-regulating and reducing further synthesis of LDL receptors (step 2)
- increasing the activity of acyl cholesterol acyltransferase, thus storing the excess cholesterol as its esters (step 3)

- inhibiting the activity of β-hydroxy-methyl-glutaryl coenzyme A reductase (HMG-CoA reductase), which catalyses the rate-limiting step of cholesterol synthesis, via product inhibition (step 4)
- increasing cholesterol utilisation, e.g., in forming new membranes, steroid synthesis (step 5)
- stepping up cholesterol egress from cells (step 6).

HDL and 'reverse cholesterol transport'

The only known route of cholesterol excretion is in the bile. Cholesterol from extrahepatic tissues has to be removed and transported to the liver, to prevent its accumulation in these cells. HDL mediates this transfer (Figure 14.8). Nascent HDL, synthesised by the liver, contain very little triglycerides and cholesterol esters. The downloading of cholesterol to these disclike particles is mediated by the enzyme, lecithin cholesterol acyltransferase (LCAT), located within the HDL particles. LCAT transfers an unsaturated fatty acid from lecithin (phosphatidlycholine) to the 3β-hydroxyl group of cholesterol, producing lysolecithin and a cholesterol ester.

LCAT is activated by apoA-I, apo A-II, apo A-IV, and possibly apo C-I. The LCAT enzyme is packaged inside the HDL particle as part of the cholesterol ester transfer protein (CETP) complex, which also contains apo A-I, the major cofactor for LCAT, and apo D.

The cholesterol for esterification by LCAT in the above reaction can come from the other plasma lipoproteins as well as from the extrahepatic cells. Most of the esterified cholesterol is transferred back to LDL, IDL and chylomicron remnants by the CETP and reaches the liver thus (Figure 14.8). A small amount is packed into the inner core of the HDL particle, gradually changing its shape from discoid to spherical. The conversion of polar cholesterol to nonpolar cholesteryl esters creates a gradient down which cholesterol moves to the CETP complex.

This pathway is termed the 'reverse cholesterol transport' and delivers cholesterol to the liver via receptor-mediated uptake of the IDL, LDL, and chylomicron remnants.

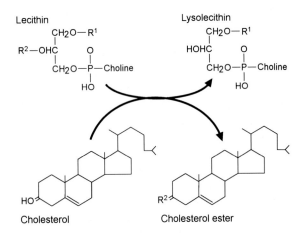

The LCAT reaction. In human plasma the fatty acid in the 2-position of lecithin (R_2) is mono- or polyunsaturated.

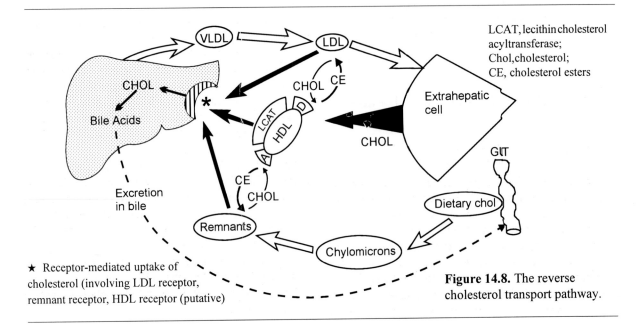

LCAT, lecithin cholesterol acyltransferase; Chol, cholesterol; CE, cholesterol esters

★ Receptor-mediated uptake of cholesterol (involving LDL receptor, remnant receptor, HDL receptor (putative)

Figure 14.8. The reverse cholesterol transport pathway.

Lp (a) metabolism

Relatively little is known about the synthesis and catabolism of Lp(a). The liver appears to be the most likely source of Lp(a) synthesis as the apo(a) cDNA used in many molecular studies was constructed from a library of hepatic mRNAs. Low plasma Lp(a) levels are found in people with chronic liver disease such as cirrhosis.

Data from *in vivo* turnover studies show that Lp(a) is not derived from VLDL, LDL or chylomicrons. Its metabolism appears to be independant from that of LDL, despite its close structural similarity with the latter. Data from *in vitro* studies indicate that Lp(a) is catabolised at a much slower rate than LDL and that uptake and degradation of Lp(a) may not be mediated by the LDL receptor pathway. Results from clinical trials with different pharmaceutical agents are in keeping with the *in vitro* experimental data. Both HMG CoA-reductase inhibitors and cholestyramine, which are used to lower plasma LDL levels, have no effect on plasma Lp(a) levels, suggesting alternative pathways of synthesis and clearance of the Lp(a) particle.

Plasma Lp(a) levels are largely genetically controlled and appears to be minimally influenced by metabolic, endocrine, or anthropometric variables. Available evidence points to polygenic control of the Lp(a) trait. Only about 40% of the variability observed appears to be determined by the apo(a) gene locus itself -- the strongest effect of a single polymorphic locus on plasma lipid and lipoprotein levels hitherto reported -- and a number of other gene loci and/or environmental factors may influence Lp(a) metabolism. Mutations in the LDL receptor gene has been clearly shown to influence plasma Lp(a) levels.

Lipids and cardiovascular disease

Atherosclerosis: the process

The basic pathology underlying the development of CHD, and other vascular disease, in patients with hyperlipidaemia is nearly always atherosclerosis. Atherosclerosis tends to affect large- and medium-sized arteries, auch as the aorta and the femoral, coronary and cerebral arteries, and is common at sites of turbulent blood flow such as arterial bifurcations. It involves a variable combination of changes in the intima (inner lining) of arteries consisting of the focal accumulation of lipids, other blood constituents and fibrous tissue, accompanied by changes in the media (middle layer) of the vessel wall. These changes are the result of interaction between the structural and metabolic properties of the arterial wall, components of the blood and haemodynamic forces.

The atherosclerotic process is often considered to be proliferative, rather than primarily degenerative, and is believed to begin early in life. The earliest recognizable lesion is the juvenile fatty streak, which occurs in the coronary arteries before the age of ten, in children of all societies, and increases during adolescence. It comprises an accumulation of monocytes and lipid-filled macrophages within the intima of the vessel. The issue of whether this lesion progresses to a fibrous plaque is still controversial.

The characteristic lesion of atherosclerosis is the fibrous plaque. Fibrous plaques are white lesions which often protrude into the vessel lumen, causing obstruction to blood flow. Each lesion consists of a core containing lipid, along with necrotic cells, and a cap of smooth muscle cells and fibrous tissue covered by a layer of endothelium. Up to 45% of the lesion consists of lipids, mainly cholesterol. This cholesterol is derived almost entirely from the plasma lipoproteins and not from local synthesis. The possible sequence of events leading to the development of fibrous plaques and thrombi is shown diagrammaically in Figure 14.9.

Based on studies of diet-induced hypercholesterolaemia in primates, the endothelial cell is identified as the site where the lesion is initiated (Figure 14.9a). An important event in the process is an alteration in the functional or structural barrier presented by the endothelial cell lining of the vessel (cf endothelial damage as the cornerstone of the 'response to injury' hypothesis).

Experimental damage of arterial endothelium, exposing connective tissue to the blood, causes platelet activation and aggregation on the surface. The release of thromboxanes by the platelets further enhances aggregation and leads to the contraction of the smooth muscle cells within the arterial wall. Lipid-filled monocytes (foam cells) can then enter the intima between endothelial cells. Growth factors released by the endothelial cells, monocytes, and especially the platelets (platelet-derived growth factor or PDGF) stimulate smooth muscle cell proliferation and subsequent migration to the intima, forming the fibrous plaque (Figure 14.9b).

Platelet aggregation and adherence to the damaged surface of the atherosclerotic plaque is intimately involved in mural thrombus formation (Figure 14.9c).

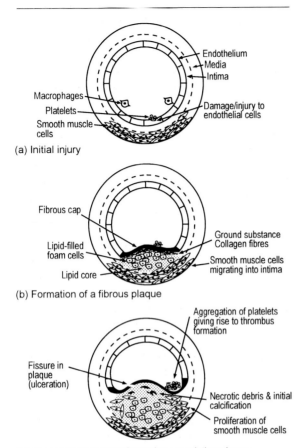

Macrophages
Platelets
Smooth muscle cells

Endothelium
Media
Intima

Damage/injury to endothelial cells

(a) Initial injury

Fibrous cap
Lipid-filled foam cells
Lipid core

Ground substance
Collagen fibres

Smooth muscle cells migrating into intima

(b) Formation of a fibrous plaque

Fissure in plaque (ulceration)

Aggregation of platelets giving rise to thrombus formation

Necrotic debris & initial calcification

Proliferation of smooth muscle cells

(c) Secondary thrombus formation on existing plaque

Figure 14.9. Sequential changes in the vessel wall giving rise to atheromatous lesions and potential vessel occlusion. Redrawn, with permission of Oxford University Press, from: Ball M and Mann J. *Lipids and Heart Disease: A Practical Approach.* Oxford University Press, Oxford, 1988.

Atherosclerosis: role of oxidised LDL

The causal role of hypercholesterolaemia (due primarily to an increase in LDL) in the aetiology of atherosclerosis implies that monocyte and macrophages become foam cells by LDL uptake, presumably via the LDL receptor-mediated pathway. However, *in vitro* experiments have shown that this is not the case. Monocytes do possess LDL receptors, but these become down-regulated as soon as the intracellular cholesterol content increases. It is now known that in addition to LDL receptors, monocytes also have receptors for various forms of modified LDL

(e.g., acetyl LDL, oxidised LDL) which are not down-regulated in the same manner as the LDL receptors. This receptor, called the scavenger receptor, has been cloned and its presence demonstrated in foam cell-packed areas of atheromatous lesions.

Various lines of direct experimental evidence have established the role of oxidised LDL in atherogenesis beyond reasonable doubt and support the concept that native LDL *in vivo* is avidly taken up by macrophages via this scavenger receptor-mediated pathway, *after oxidative modification*. The reader is referred to the work of Parthasarathy, Steinberg and Witztum (referenced on page 211) for a full review.

Atherosclerosis: the role of Lp(a)

The precise mechanism whereby elevated levels of Lp(a) increase risk of CHD remains uncertain. The recent finding of the high fidelity homology between the sequences of the plasminogen and apo(a) genes has stimulated much interest and focus into unraveling the functional consequence, if any, of this remarkable molecular mimicry. The tantalising question to be answered is whether these dramatic findings may provide the long-sought link between atherosclerosis, lipoproteins, and the clotting system. *In vitro* evidence suggests that Lp(a) has both thrombogenic and anti-fibrinolytic potential. However, *in vivo* evidence has thus far remained tenuous.

There is evidence, though still controversial to some extent, that microthrombi on the vessel wall become incorporated into atherosclerotic plaques. Fibrinogen and fibrin are found in these loci in roughly the same proportion as cholesterol; Lp(a) has also been shown to be present. Apo(a) is shown to have a higher tissue:plasma ratio than apo B, suggesting that Lp(a) has an even higher affinity for the vessel wall than has LDL, and thus confirms its atherogenecity.

The kringle 4 domain is known to bind to fibrinogen, although somewhat weakly. It is not unlikely that the apo(a) protein, with 37 copies of this kringle might bind to fibrinogen or fibrin under certain conditions *in vivo*. Thus when Lp(a) finds its way into the fissured arterial wall following endothelial damage, it might adhere to fibrin, forming a complex that precipitates out and remains within the vessel wall. Lp(a) might also block proteolysis of fibrin by inhibiting the activation of plasminogen by tissue plasminogen activator, thereby inhibiting cleavage of fibrin clots. The possible impact of Lp(a) on fibrinolysis is represented diagrammatically in Figure

14.10. These potential roles of Lp(a) are still under intensive study.

A conceptual overview of the role of the atherogenic lipoproteins in the development of the foam cell and more advanced atherosclerotic lesions is shown in Figure 14.11.

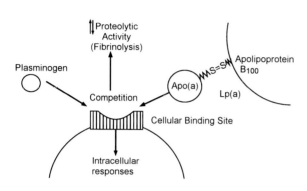

Figure 14.10. Proposed mechanism of competitive inhibition of fibrinolysis by Lp(a).

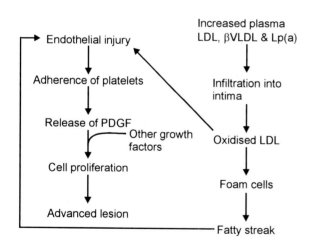

Figure 14.11. The roles of various plasma lipoproteins and growth factors (GF) in the development of an atherosclerotic lesion. PDGF, platelet-derived GF.

Atherosclerosis and CHD: major risk factors

The epidemiological delineation of risk factors has not

only provided a valuable means of identifying those at increasing risk of developing CHD, but has also contributed to an understanding of the pathogenesis of atherosclerosis. Two factors which have a major bearing on the occurrence of atherosclerosis are raised plasma lipid concentrations and high blood pressure. Thus the condition seldom affects individuals with serum cholesterol levels less than 4 mmol/L, nor does it affect veins unless these are exposed to arterial levels of blood pressure (e.g., saphenous veins used for coronary artery bypass grafts). Other important determinants of atherosclerosis include age and sex, which also influence, respectively, the concentration of cholesterol in plasma and its distribution between LDL and HDL.

The classic study by Smith and Slater in 1972 (see page 211) showed the close correlation between the concentration of LDL cholesterol in aortic intima at post mortem examination and the ante-mortem serum cholesterol level (in blood taken a week before death). This seminal finding has been confirmed by data from other studies in which the extent and severity of coronary atherosclerosis were shown to correlate with serum cholesterol concentrations measured as far back as nine years before death. The severity of atherosclerotic lesions found in individuals with familial hypercholesterolaemia (plasma LDL levels persistently 2-4 times higher than normal) underscores the role of hypercholesterolaemia in atheromatous involvement.

The association between hypercholesterolaemia and atherosclerosis is thus firmly established. Because it is the major carrier of cholesterol in plasma and

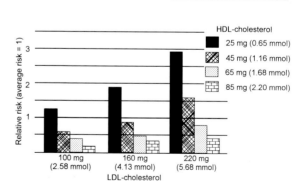

Figure 14.12. Correlation of serum LDL-cholesterol and HDL-cholesterol with risk of developing coronary heart disease in four years in men, aged 50-70 years. Source: Framingham Heart Study (reference on page 211).

because the mechanistic evidence relating it to atherosclerosis is strongest, LDL is regarded as the main culprit. However, other atherogenic lipoproteins such as Lp(a) and the triglyceride-rich VLDL and chylomicrons increase and compound the risk, when abnormally high levels are present in circulation. In contrast, individuals with elevated plasma HDL levels are not at increased risk of CHD. On the contrary, an inverse correlation exists between HDL cholesterol levels and risk of CHD (Figure 14.12).

INVESTIGATION OF THE HYPERLIPIDAEMIC PATIENT

The investigation of an individual with possible hyperlipidaemia or one shown to be hyperlipidaemic on a fasting sample on at least one previous occasion requires both clinical assessment and laboratory testing.

Clinical assessment

This involves taking a good history and conducting a full physical examination during the patient's first clinic visit.

History. The patient should be questioned about the following aspects of his own personal history:

- Symptoms of vascular insufficiency such as angina
- Results of any previous plasma lipid results
- Any previous complications, e.g., myocardial infarction
- Any previous surgical procedures, e.g., coronary artery bypass graft, angioplasty, cholecystectomy
- Dietary habits, especially alcohol consumption
- Lifestyle habits, such as smoking, exercise, drugs taken currently
- Any intercurrent disease such as diabetes, thyroid dysfunction, renal disease, gout

In addition, a family history should also be carefully recorded. This includes eliciting details of:

- premature CHD in immediate relatives, age of onset and death due to CHD
- history of hyperlipidaemia in family members
- presence of other risk factors for CHD, such as hypertension, diabetes, gout.

Clinical examination. Blood pressure measurements to exclude (or document) hypertension, and a search for external signs of hyperlipidaemia (corneal arcus, eruptive/tendonous xanthomata, xanthelesma) are particularly relevant in such patients.

Laboratory investigation

The first and most important concern is to confirm the presence of hyperlipidaemia in a sample taken after an overnight fast of at least 10 hours duration. The initial testing should include minimally measurements of total cholesterol, triglyceride and HDL cholesterol, which enables calculation of LDL cholesterol, as described below. Other tests, if indicated, can be performed after the results of the initial tests are available for interpretation.

In addition to assessing the nature and severity of the patient's hyperlipidaemia, a search should be made for underlying causes of secondary hyperlipidaemia before attributing it as a primary hyperlipidaemia. The appropriate biochemical tests depends on the history and presentation.

Tests for lipid analysis

Measurement of plasma or serum *total cholesterol* and *triglycerides* were traditionally used for the assessment of hyperlipidaemia and its attendant risks of CAD. For both analytes, chemical and enzymatic methods are available, the former being fast replaced by the latter.

In the last twenty years, methods for *plasma lipoproteins* have been automated and the measurement of plasma *HDL and LDL*, usually as their cholesterol equivalents, have been added to tests that can be performed routinely to assess the lipid profile of an individual at risk. In most laboratories the use of ultracentrifugation to isolate the various lipoprotein fractions is considered too impractical; instead precipitation protocols are used in the HDL cholesterol assays, and LDL and VLDL concentrations are derived by applying the Friedewald formula (see below).

Quantitation of HDL cholesterol (HDLc) depends on initial precipitation of the apo B-containing lipoproteins -- VLDL, LDL and Lp(a), usually with use of a polyanion-divalent cation mixture, followed by analysis of cholesterol in the supernatant (theoretically only the HDL fraction).

Users of the **calculated LDLc** values must be cognizant of the two assumptions on which the formula is based: (1) that most of the plasma triglyceride content resides in the VLDL fraction, and (2) that the molar ratio of triglyceride to cholesterol in VLDL is 2.2 to 1(mass ratio 5 to 1). When the ratio is exceeded, i.e., when the plasma triglyceride concentration is >4.5 mmol/L, the formula is invalid. If a non-fasting specimen is used, the VLDL triglyceride value may be inaccurate (contribution by chylomicron triglyceride) and LDL cholesterol is underestimated. If these caveats are borne in mind, the formula provides a reasonable estimate of the LDLc concentration.

LDLc = total cholesterol - HDLc - (triglyceride/2.2)
(Note: all three measured parameters in mmol/L)

Additional biochemical markers have been carefully evaluated for their clinical utility as diagnostic indicators of abnormal lipid metabolism and many of these are now available in most diagnostic laboratories as adjunct tests. They include the *serum apolipoproteins (apo A-I, apo B), Lp (a), subfractions of HDL, and apo E phenotypes or genotypes.*

Of these, the **apolipoproteins** have been the most intensively investigated with regards to their clinical use as independant biochemical markers for increased risk of developing CHD. An impressive amount of epidemiological data has been accumulated in recent years, citing low levels of **apo A-I**, especially in conjunction with high levels of **apo B**, as indicative of relatively greater risks in the individuals concerned. There are currently numerous methods for measuring these apolipoproteins; mostly immunochemical assays.

Suitable methods for routine measurements of **Lp(a)** are now available and the test is assuming increasing clinical importance in lipid profiling. This follows in the wake of growing evidence of the atherogenicity of this lipoprotein and its confirmation as an independent risk factor for development of CHD.

The **subfractionation of HDL** involves dual precipitation. The first precipitation step enables

quantitation of the total HDL cholesterol, as described earlier; this is followed by a second precipitation of the HDL_2 subfraction, which enables HDL_3 cholesterol to be measured. HDL_2 is then calculated as the difference.

Phenotyping or genotyping of apolipoprotein E polymorphism are labour-intensive techniques, and are currently only performed in specialised laboratories. Phenotyping can be carried out on delipidated VLDL using iso-electrofocusing gel electrophoresis; the genotyping assay uses molecular genetics techniques. The tests have specific application and provide useful information in selective cases, e.g., the association of the E2/2 phenotype with some cases of Type III hyperlipoproteinaemia (see page 206), and the association of the ε4 allele with higher cholesterol levels and thus higher CHD risk and with an increased predisposition to development of late-onset Alzheimer's disease. They are increasingly being used as a diagnostic tool in clinical practice.

Lipoprotein electrophoresis, although no longer advocated as a routine diagnostic procedure for hyperlipidaemia, remains a useful confirmatory test for Type III hyperlipoproteinaemia, in particular, to help differentiate it from other types of marked hypertriglyceridaemia. Electrophoretic separation and quantitation of β-VLDL (cholesterol-rich VLDL) has yet to find general application and is of only limited use at present.

Lipoprotein phenotyping (WHO classification)

The WHO classification is a modification of Fredrickson's scheme for the classification of hyperlipidaemia using lipoprtein phenotypes, introduced in 1967 and primarily based on the lipoprotein patterns obtained after serum lipoprotein electrophoresis using agarose gels (Table 14.3). Lipoprotein phenotyping is now considered to be of restricted use, primarily due to the lack of specific correlations between the phenotypic expression and the underlying lipid disorders. The same pattern (e.g., Type IIb) may be seen in patients with hyperlipidaemias of different causes. The corollary is also true -- the same patient may develop different phenotypes at different times, e.g., changing from a Type IIb pattern to a Type IV with disease progression, changes in diet or treatment. Other shortcomings of the classification are that it does not specify whether the cause is genetically determined or is secondary to underlying disease or environmental factors, nor does it take into account variations in HDL cholesterol which we now know is an equally important (negative) risk factor for CHD.

There are, however, situations in which knowledge of the lipoprotein phenotype is of diagnostic use, e.g., the Type III hyperlipidaemia pattern with its pathognomonic broad β band (see Figure 14.13). In current practice, lipoprotein electrophoresis is carried out only in such selected instances. A useful remnant feature of Fredrickson's

scheme is its neat correlation with information obtained from the appearance of the serum samples (Figure 14.13). Examination of the lipaemic serum or plasma left standing overnight at 4°C is a useful adjunct to the performance of other tests in the investigation of hyperlipidaemia.

Appearance of serum

Observation of the appearance of the plasma or serum samples may provide a clue to the extent of hypertriglyceridaemia, when present, and whether chylomicrons are present. This stems from the light-

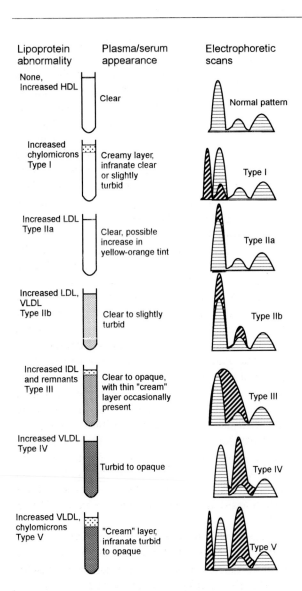

Table 14.3. WHO classification of lipoprotein phenotypes.

Type		[TC]	[TG]
I	Hyperchylomicronaemia	N	I++
IIa	Hyper-betalipoproteinaemia	I++	N
IIb	Hyper-betalipoproteinaemia, hyper-pre-betalipoproteinaemia	I++	I+
III	Broad-betalipoproteinaemia (Dysbetalipoproteinaemia)	I+	I+
IV	Hyper-pre-betalipoproteinaemia	N - I++	sl I
V	Chylomicronaemia and hyper-pre-betalipoproteinaemia	N - I++	sl I

N, normal
I, increased
I^+, moderately increased
I^{++}, greatly increased

Figure 14.13. Plasma appearance after 16 hours at 4°C in relation to WHO classification of lipoprotein phenotypes.

scattering properties of chylomicrons and VLDL (page 195), which in turn imparts turbidity to the plasma or serum. An opaque or lactescent sample is likely to contain >6 mmol/L of triglycerides in VLDL particles or chylomicrons (lipaemia ++). A simple test will determine whether chylomicrons are present -- the 'refrigerator' test. Chylomicrons float atop the serum or plasma, forming a creamy film or layer, when the sample is incubated at 4°C for several hours. This could mean, more often than not, a non-fasting sample or hyperchylomicronaemia (see Figure 14.13). Hypercholesterolaemic samples are translucent, with some bearing a slight orange tinge.

Sample collection: requirements and pitfalls

Both plasma and serum may be used for most of the lipid analysis. Some laboratories run lipid assays on plasma separated out from EDTA-anticoagulated blood samples; others run them on serum. Using EDTA-anticoagulated samples gives the added advantages of increased stability of the lipoproteins during storage (effect of EDTA) and the availability of the buffy coat for leucocyte DNA extraction, if needed. Lipid concentrations in serum are approximately 3% higher than those in plasma. Both serum and plasma samples (separated from the red cells) are stable at 4°C for up to 4 days or can be stored frozen at -20°C prior to analysis.

Investigation of hyperlipidaemia requires taking special precautions in the patient preparation and specimen collection. To obtain reliable results, it is important to ensure that the patient:

- takes a normal balanced diet for at least a week prior to the test
- fasts for 10-14 hours prior to blood sampling
- not be severely stressed before or during the blood sampling
- reports any current use of medication.

A *fasting* specimen is essential for triglyceride analysis because plasma triglyceride concentrations increase as soon as two hours postprandially (after ingestion of a meal containing fats) and reach a maximum at 4-6 hours post-meal. For the same reason, non-fasting samples are also not suitable for the determination of LDL estimations using the Friedewald calculation (see above). The chylomicron particles found in nonfasting specimens will cause volume displacement problems and produce a false lowering of most results.

Hyperchylomicronaemia also causes incomplete precipitation of the apo B-containing lipoproteins, leading to falsely elevated HDL values. Unlike triglycerides, plasma cholesterol levels do not rise acutely after a fatty meal.

Severe metabolic traumas such as a myocardial infarct adversely affect serum lipid levels. Plasma cholesterol results after an MI can be very misleading, often falling markedly due to the trauma. It normally takes 3-6 weeks for the cholesterol levels to return to pre-infarct levels. Stress also causes mobilisation of free fatty acids and results in artefactually elevated plasma triglyceride levels.

Reference ranges: special considerations

Another problem in plasma lipid analyses relates to reference ranges for plasma total cholesterol and LDL cholesterol. Relevant reference values are difficult to define as plasma lipids are affected by multiple factors, such as sex, age, life-style, and other physiological states. The use of a unimodal frequency distribution of values from a 'reference population' to derive either the mid 90th, or more commonly the mid 95th, percentile values, was previously employed to obtain the reference ranges for plasma lipids. This method is now replaced by the use of desirable reference values (see Table 14.4).

Epidemiological studies have shown that the upper cut-off limit for serum cholesterol (using the standard parametric methods to calculate reference ranges) may rise as high as 8.0 mmol/L in the fifth and sixth decades in many societies; this does not occur in other communities in which the incidence of CHD is much lower. Such findings have underscored the limitation of the above practice of defining the reference ranges for analytes such as plasma lipids.

Results from nationwide surveys carried out as part of the U.S. National Cholesterol Education Programme, by the Expert Panel on Detection, Evaluation, and Treatment of High Blood Cholesterol in Adults (National Blood Institute, U.S.A.), showed that the risk of developing CHD is pegged to serum cholesterol levels. Hence, they recommend that the interpretation of serum cholesterol values should use desirable cut-off limits as reference points (Table 14.4).

The above 1988 report also recommends that the presence of other CHD risk factors (hypertension, smoking, diabetes mellitus, obesity, and family history of CHD) should be documented and that in the clinical

Table 14.4. Recommendations* for patient classification according to statistical risk of developing coronary heart disease

Risk classification	Serum Concentrations[#]			
	Total cholesterol		LDL cholesterol	
	mg/dL	mmol/L	mg/dL	mmol/L
Desirable	<200	<5.17	<130	<3.36
Borderline high	200-239	5.17-6.18	130-159	3.36-4.11
High	≥240	≥6.21	≥160	≥4.13

*Source: *Report of the Expert Panel on Detection, Evaluation, and Treatment of High Blood Cholesterol in Adults, National Cholesterol Education Program, National Heart, Lung, and Blood Institute, 1990.*

[#] *To convert mg/dL cholesterol to mmol/L, divide cholesterol by 38.7 or multiply by 0.02586.*

management of patients of the relatively high risk groups, these other risk factors should also be addressed to complement the measures taken to modify plasma lipid levels.

Primary or secondary hyperlipidaemia

If a patient is found to be hyperlipidaemic, it is useful to determine whether it is a primary disorder, secondary to some other abnormality, or caused by a combination of genetic and environmental factors.

Hypercholesterolaemia

Hypercholesterolaemia, with little or no elevation of plasma triglycerides, is almost always due to raised plama LDL levels. Familial hypercholesterolaemia is due to deficiency of LDL receptors or to internalisation defects and may be a single gene or multigene defect.

In the monogenic type, homozygotes for the abnormal gene have very high plasma cholesterol; the plasma cholesterol levels or family members of afflicted individuals show the characteristic trimodal distribution, with three distinct peaks of expression for the homozygotes with either the normal or the

abnormal gene and the heterozygotes. In polygenic familial hypercholesterolaemia, the cholesterol values would show a continuous distribution, reflecting the variable expression of several gene abnormalities. The hypercholesterolaemia in the latter group is usually moderate.

The main causes of secondary hypercholesterolaemia which has a higher prevalence than primary or familial hypercholesterolaemia are hypothyroidism, diabetes mellitus, nephrotic syndrome, cholestatic liver diseases, and Cushing's syndrome. Treatment of the underlying disorder normally corrects the cholesterol abnormality.

Hypertriglyceridaemia

Elevated plasma triglyceride levels may be due to increased VLDL or chylomicrons or both. Primary hypertriglyceridaemia, e.g., hyperchylomicronaemia, is relatively less common; more often hypertriglyceridaemia is secondary to another condition or disorder. The most common of these causes are alcoholism, obesity (and excessive carbohydrate intake), diabetes mellitus, pregnancy or use of oral contraceptives, nephrotic syndrome, and acute pancreatitis.

Combined hyperlipidaemia

Secondary causes: Elevated plasma levels of both cholesterol and triglycerides are most common in patients with poorly controlled diabetes mellitus and nephrotic syndrome or those with florid hypothyroidism.

Primary causes: Familial combined hyperlipidaemia is the most common; dysbetalipoproteinaemia with excess IDL (page 194) is less common.

Primary hyperlipidaemias

Familial hypercholesterolaemia. This is a distinct clinical entity characterised by elevated levels of total cholesterol and LDL, tendonous xanthomata, xanthelesma, corneal arcus, and premature arteriosclerosis. The mode of inheritance is monogenic, autosomal dominant. The biochemical hallmark is a defect of the LDL receptor. There is a high frequency of heterozygotes (1 in about 500 Caucasians), the homozygous form is much rarer, being present in only about 1 in a million individuals. Almost all homozygotes die of a fatal myocardial infarction before the age of 30. In heterozygotes, the disease often presents in middle life, with a mean onset at 43 years in males and 53 years in females. Their risk of developing CHD is as much as 25 times greater than that in normal individuals above the age of 30 years.

The average plasma cholesterol level in heterozygotes is about 9.0 mmol/L; homozygotes have levels which are >15.0 mmol/L. Values for plassma LDL are also uniformly high and proportionate to the elevation in total cholesterol concentration.

Familial combined hyperlipoproteinaemia. This familial condition, the most common of the primary hyperlipidaemias, presents as a variety of hyperlipidaemic types in affected individuals within one family and is difficult to classify. The pathophysiologic mechanisms responsible for the disease are unknown, and the exact genetic inheritance is not clear but it is believed to be a monogenic, dominant trait. Patients identified with the disorder are at an increased risk (about 3-4 times) for premature atherosclerosis. Many of these patients have hypercholesterolaemia but only rarely do their plasma total cholesterol levels exceed 10 mmol/L. Tendonous xanthomas are rarely present

and hyperlipidaemia does not manifest itself until adulthood, unlike homozygotes with familial hypercholesterolaemia.

Polygenic hypercholesterolaemia. This classification refers to a disorder in a group of individuals with plasma levels of total cholesterol and LDL in the high risk range (see Table 14.4), but without an identifiable monogenic mode of inheritance. It is likely that a combination of environmental factors and poorly understood polygenic expression is involved. Manipulation of diet alone has produced significant reduction of plasma cholesterol levels in some of these patients. Metabolic defects identified in patients include increased LDL formation, defective LDL catabolism, or both. A large proportion of Type II hyperlipidaemic individuals (Fredrickson classification, page 206) may belong to this group.

Familial hyperchylomicronaemia. This is a rare autosomal recessive disorder characterised by eruptive xanthomatosis of the skin, lipaemia retinalis, recurrent bouts of abdominal pain with or without pancreatitis, and hepatosplenomegaly. Two separate biochemical defects have been identified, one due to a deficiency in lipoprotein lipase, the other due to a deficiency of its activator, apoC-II. There is no increased incidence of ischaemic heart disease. The plasma of fasting affected individuals are grossly lipaemic with floating creamy layers on storage at 4°C. Plasma triglyceride levels are always greater than 10 mmol/L. There are no effective drugs for the treatment of this disorder; the usual management option consists of putting the patients on a very low fat diet.

Familial endogenous hypertriglyceridaemia. This relatively common condition or, more likely, group of conditions, is associated with either defective production or catabolism of VLDL or both defects. It is inherited as an autosomal dominant trait. Characteristically plasma triglyceride and VLDL levels are much elevated, with TG levels usually in the range of 3.5-12.0 mmol/L (1.5-6 times the upper reference limit) and detectable early in life. There may be accompanying hyperchylomicronaemia. Whether this condition predisposes to premature atherosclerosis is debatable but patients have at most a slightly increased risk of early ischaemic disease. It can be exacerbated by diabetes mellitus, obesity, excessive alcohol consumption, hypothyroidism, and oestrogen therapy. Proper diagnosis of the condition and identification of drugs that can alter VLDL and triglyceride metabolism are integral components of the management of this condition.

Familial dysbetalipoproteinaemia. Patients with this uncommon disorder have elevated levels of total cholesterol (usually >7.5 mmol/L) and triglycerides (of similar magnitude). This is secondary to accumulation of cholesterol-rich lipoprotein remnants, due to defective catabolism of VLDL to LDL. On electrophoresis, the lipoproteins show a characteristic broad band (encompassing the zone of pre-beta and beta lipoprotein electrophoretic mobilities); this is due to increased IDL. Both HDL and LDL are reduced, the latter quite markedly. Many of the patients show a apo ε2/2 genotype, which results in diminished binding of the remnant particles to hepatic apo E receptors. The disorder is associated with a high risk of premature CHD and characterised by cutaneous xanthomas.

The condition can be aggravated by the concurrent development of several disorders, the chief of which are hypothyroidism, marked weight gain, uncontrolled diabetes mellitus, and excessive alcohol consumption. Prompt treatment of these exacerbating conditions will significantly control the lipid disorder in these patients and may avert the need for drug therapy for the lipid abnormalities.

Other inherited lipid disorders

Hyperalphalipoproteinaemia. As the name implies, individuals with this inherited disorder have increased plasma HDL (α-lipoproteins). The plasma total cholesterol levels are usually only slightly increased as the plasma LDL levels are normal. It is important to recognise that the hypercholesterolaemia is HDL- and not LDL-driven, and that no treatment is needed. Quite the contrary, as these individuals actually have a reduced risk for CHD.

The hypolipoproteinaemias

These rare familial conditions are of interest in that they provide models that have helped in the understanding of normal lipoprotein metabolism.

Tangier disease. (Familial alpha-lipoprotein deficiency). This is a rare autosomal recessive disorder of lipoprotein metabolism characterised by extremely low levels of plasma HDL and apo A-I and extensive cholesteryl ester storage. The disorder is caused by a post-translational modification of apo A-I, resulting in enhanced apo A-I catabolism, and not by defective apo A-I synthesis, as was originally ascribed. The circulating HDL levels are barely detectable; plasma LDL levels are also reduced but detectable. Excessive phagocytosis of the abnormal chylomicron and VLDL (deficient in their apo A-I content) has been proposed as an explanation for the large build-up of cholesteryl ester stores.

Abetalipoproteinaemia. This is a rare autosomal recessive disorder characterised by a complete absence of apolipoprotein B. Consequently lipoproteins that contain apo B as a structural component (VLDL, LDL, chylomicrons) are affected. Patients present clinically with fat malabsorption, failure to thrive, and ataxic neuropathy; only about 50 cases have so far been reported. The lesion can be caused by mutations of the apo B gene, either leading to defective apo B synthesis or producing an unstable aberrant variety.

Hypobetalipoproteinaemia. Patients homozygous for this condition are differentiated from those with abetalipoproteinaemia in having a dominant mode of inheritance, and subnormal (but detectable) plasma levels of apo B, LDL and VLDL. The parents of afflicted index cases have subnormal LDL levels whereas those of patients with abetalipoproteinaemia would have normal LDL levels.

REFERENCES AND FURTHER READING

Assmann G, von Eckardstein A, Funke H. High density lipoproteins, reverse transport of cholesterol, and coronary heart disease. Insights from mutations. Circulation 1993,87 (suppl III):28-34.

Castelli WP, Garrison RJ, Wilson PWF, Abbott RD, Kalousdian S, Kannel WB. Incidence of coronary heart disease and lipoprotein cholesterol levels. JAMA 1986,256:2835-2838.

Cowan LD, Wilcosky T, Criqui MH, Barrett-Connor E, Suchindram CM, Wallace R, Laskarzewski P, Walden C. Demographic, behavioural, biochemical and dietary correlates of plasma triglycerides. Lipid Research Clinics Program Prevalence Study. Arteriosclerosis 1985,5:466-480.

Davies MJ. Pathogenesis of atherosclerosis. Curr Opin Cardiol 1992,7:541-545.

Expert Panel: Summary of the Second Report of the National Cholesterol Education Program (NCEP) Expert Panel on Detection, Evaluation, and Treatment of High Blood Cholesterol in Adults (Adult Treatment Panel II). JAMA 1993,269:3015-3023.

Goldstein JL, Brown MS. Regulation of low density lipoprotein receptors: implications for pathogenesis and therapy of hypercholesterolaemia and athero-sclerosis. Circulation, 1987, 76:504-507.

Gotto AM, Pownall HJ, Havel RJ. Introduction to the plasma lipoproteins. In: *Methods in Enzymology*, Segrest JP, Albers JJ (eds). London: Academic Press, 1986, pp 3-41.

Green MS, Heiss G, Rifkind BM, Cooper GR, Williams OD, Tyroler HA. The ratio of plasma high density lipoprotein cholesterol to total and low density lipoprotein cholesterol: age-related changes and race and sex differences in selected North American populations: the Lipid Research Clinics Program Prevalence Study. Circulation 1985,72:93-104.

Gurr MI, James AT. *Lipid Biochemistry: An Introduction*. London: Chapman and Hall, 1971.

Heiss G, Tamir I, Davies CE, Tyroler HA, Rifkind BM, Schonfeld G, Jacobs D, Franz ID. Lipoprotein cholesterol distributions in selected North American populations: the Lipid Research Clinics Program Prevalence Study. Circulation 1980,61:302-315.

International Task Force for Prevention of Coronary Heart Disease, European Atherosclerosis Society. Prevention of coronary heart disease: Scientific background and new clinical guidelines. Nutr Metab Cardiovasc Dis 1992,2:113-156.

Leake DS. Oxidised low density lipoproteins and atherogenesis. Br Heart J 1993,69:476-478.

Libby P, Clinton SK. The role of macrophages in atherogenesis. Curr Opin Lipidol 1993,4:355-363.

Mahley RW, Innerarity TL, Rall SC Jr, Weisgraber KH, Taylor JM. Apolipoprotein E: genetic variants provide insights into its structure and function. Curr Opin Lipidol 1990,1:87-95.

McLean J, Tomlinson J, Kuang W-J, Eaton D, Chen E, Fless G, Scanu A, Lawn R. cDNA sequence of human apolipoprotein (a) is homologous to plasminogen. Nature 1987;330:132-137.

Morrisett JD, Guyton TR, Gaubatz JW, Gotto AM. Lipoprotein (a): structure, metabolism and epidemiology. In: *Plasma Lipoproteins*, Gotto AM (ed). Amsterdam: Elsevier Science Publishers, 1987, pp 129-152.

NIH Consensus Development Panel on Triglycerides, High-Density Lipoproteins, and Coronary Heart Disease. Triglyceride, high-density lipoprotein, and coronary heart disease. JAMA 1993,269:505-510.

Shipley MJ, Pocock SJ, Marmot MG. Does plasma cholesterol concentration predict mortality from coronary heart disease in elderly people? 18 year follow up in a Whitehall study. BMJ 1991,303:89-92.

Smith E, Slater RS. Relationship between low density lipoprotein in aortic intima and serum lipid levels. Lancet 1972,i:463.

Pathasarathy S, Steinberg D, Witztum JL. The role of oxidised low-density lipoproteins in the pathogenesis of atherosclerosis. Ann Rev Med 1992,43:219-225.

Chapter 15

The Gastrointestinal Tract

This chapter deals with the normal processes of digestion and absorption, the disorders of vomiting, diarrhoea, malabsorption, pancreatic and ileal disease and the gastrointestinal hormone-secreting tumours. Tests of exocrine pancreatic function and other biochemical tests used in the diagnosis of the malabsorption syndromes will be discussed.

Normal physiology

The main function of the gastrointestinal tract is the digestion and absorption of nutrients. Digestion depends on secretions from the stomach, pancreas, liver, and small intestine. For absorption to proceed normally there must be adequate digestion of nutrients by the gut secretions and normally functioning small and large intestines.

GASTRIC FUNCTION

Each day, in response to oral food intake, the stomach secretes about two litres of fluid (Table 15.1) containing hydrochloric acid (HCl) and pepsin which initiates the digestion of protein. The stomach also secretes intrinsic factor which facilitates the absorption of vitamin B_{12} by the ileum.

The 200 to 300 millimoles of HCl, which lowers the pH of the gastric juice to 1.0-2.0, is secreted by the parietal cells and derives from the intracellular action of carbonic anhydrase on carbon dioxide and water, producing hydrogen (H^+) and bicarbonate (HCO_3^-) ions.

$$CO_2 + H_2O \rightarrow H_2CO_3 \rightarrow H^+ + HCO_3^-$$

The H^+ is secreted into the lumen whilst the HCO_3^- is secreted into the blood. Thus, during meals, the fluid entering the small intestine is acidic and the blood leaving the stomach is alkaline (often referred to as the 'alkaline tide' as it may raise the peripheral blood bicarbonate level). If the gastric contents are removed as in vomiting, there would be a large positive HCO_3^- balance (see Figure 15.4, page 218).

Control of gastric secretion

The secretion of gastric juice is under the control of the vagus nerve and the hormone gastrin.

- **Vagus nerve.** Gastric secretion is in response to neural stimulation from the cerebral cortex via the vagus nerve, normally initiated by sight, smell, and taste of food (also by hypoglycaemia).

- **Gastrin.** Gastrin, released from the gastric antrum in response to gastric distension and an increase in the luminal pH (a low luminal pH suppresses secretion), also stimulates gastric fluid secretion.

The acidic gastric fluid is neutralised in the small intestine by the bicarbonate-rich secretions of the pancreas, liver, and small gut. The alkaline blood flowing from the stomach is eventually neutralised by the H^+ generated by the pancreas (and other gut organs) when they secrete bicarbonate (the reverse of the process discussed earlier).

PANCREATIC FUNCTION

The pancreas responds to the entry of food and acid into the duodenum by secreting bicarbonate (Table 15.1) and the important digestive enzymes amylase, lipase, and proteolytic enzymes (Figure 15.1). The basic unit of the exocrine pancreas is the acinus (Figure 15.1, inset) which terminates with a collection of acinar cells containing zymogen granules loaded with the proteolytic enzymes. Along the wall of the acinus duct are located special cells that contribute fluid and bicarbonate to the pancreatic juice.

Bicarbonate

Amount: 100-200 mmol/day.
Function: Neutralisation of gastric acid to provide the optimum pH for duodenal digestive enzyme activity.
Control: By secretin , produced and released by the S cells of the duodenal mucosa in response to the entry of acid and food into the duodenum.

Table 15.1. Approximate concentrations of gastrointestinal secretions

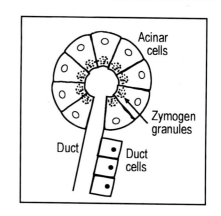

	Volume/day (L)	pH	Na⁺	K⁺	Cl⁻	HCO₃⁻
Saliva	1	7-8	60	15	30	40
Gastric juice	2	1-2	80	10	150	---
Bile	1	7-8	150	10	50	30
Pancreatic juice	2	7-8	110	10	40	100
Succus entericus	2	7-8	140	5	110	25
Ileostomy fluid	0.5-2	7-8	125	10	60	70

Concentration (mmol/L)

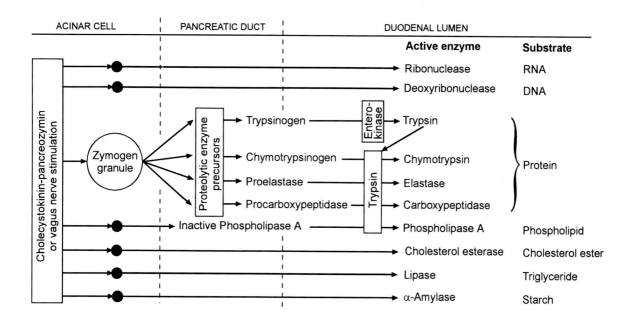

Figure 15.1. Pancreatic exocrine enzymes. **Inset:** The pancreatic exocrine unit, the acinus.

Amylase

Function: Hydrolysis of polysaccharides (starch, glycogen) to disaccharides (maltose, lactose, sucrose)

Control: By cholecystokinin (-pancreozymin) which is secreted by the I cells of the duodenal mucosa and proximal ileum in response to entry of acid and food into duodenum.

Proteolytic enzymes

These enzymes are produced in an inactive form and are activated in the gut lumen: trypsinogen to trypsin, chymotrypsinogen to chymotrypsin, proelastase to elastase, procarboxypeptidase to carboxypeptidase.

Function: Hydrolysis of peptides and proteins to small peptides and amino acids.

Control: By cholecystokinin, as for amylase.

213

The end result of the pancreatic enzymes is a fluid containing di- and monosaccharides, fatty acids and monoglycerides, amino acids and tri- and dipeptides. Further digestion and absorption requires the presence of bile salts and a normally functioning small gut mucosa.

Lipase, colipase

Function: Lipase hydrolyses triglycerides to fatty acids and monoglycerides.
Colipase prevents inhibition of pancreatic lipases by bile salts.

Control: By cholecystokinin, as for amylase.

BILIARY SECRETION

The most important digestive component of the bile is the bile salts, the metabolism of which is shown in Figure 15.2.

Function: Emulsification of fat to facilitate digestion by lipases and absorption by the small intestine.

Control: Bile is released by contraction of the gall bladder upon stimulation by cholecystokinin.

INTESTINAL ABSORPTION

The various nutrients are absorbed in specific parts of the small gut (Table 15.2).

* *Proximal portion (duodenum):* Iron, calcium, monoglycerides, fatty acids, amino acids, monosaccharides, water-soluble vitamins.
* *Mid portion (jejunum):* Amino acids, monosaccharides.
* *Distal portion (ileum):* Bile salts, vitamin B_{12}, amino acids.

Carbohydrates. The disaccharides (maltose, lactose, sucrose) produced by the action of amylase on dietary polysaccharides are hydrolysed to their constituent monosaccharides by disaccharidases located in the brush border of the intestinal cell, i.e., by maltase, lactase, and sucrase, respectively.

Lactose → glucose and galactose

Sucrose → glucose and fructose

Maltose → two glucose molecules

The monosaccharides are then actively absorbed by the mucosal cell. Glucose and galactose share a

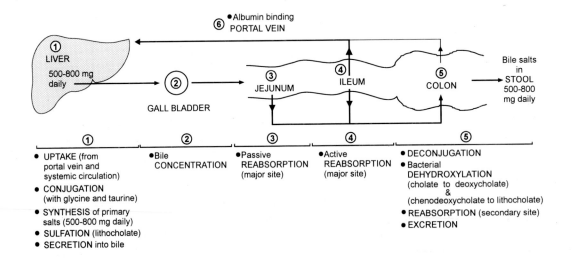

Figure 15.2. The enterohepatic circulation of bile salts.

Table 15.2. Sites of absorption and requirements for absorption of the principal dietary constituents.

Dietary constituent	Site of absorption	Requirements	Manifestations of insufficiency
Water and electrolytes	Mainly small bowel	Osmotic gradient	Diarrhoea, dehydration, cramps
Fat	Upper jejunum	Pancreatic lipase Bile salts Functioning lymphatic channels	Weight loss Steatorrhoea Fat-soluble vitamins deficiency
Carbohydrates			
Starch	Small intestine*	Amylase, maltase, isomaltase	Diarrhoea Flatulence
Sucrose	Small intestine*	Sucrase	Abdominal discomfort
Lactose	Small intestine*	Lactase	
Maltose	Small intestine*	Maltase	
Fructose, glucose	Small intestine*	--	
Proteins	Small intestine+	Pancreatic proteolytic enzymes	Loss in muscle mass Weakness, oedema
Vitamins			
A	Upper jejunum	Bile salts	Night blindness, dry eyes
B_{12}	Ileum	Intrinsic factor	Megaloblastic anaemia, glossitis, neuropathy
Folate	Duodenum and jejunum	-- (absorption may be impaired by anticonvulsants)	Megaloblastic anaemia, cheilosis, glossitis
D	Upper jejunum	Bile salts	Bone pain, fractures, tetany
E	Upper jejunum	Bile salts	?
K	Upper jejunum	Bile salts	Easy bruising and bleeding
Calcium	Duodenum	Vitamin D, Parathyroid hormone	Bone pain, fractures, tetany
Iron	Duodenum and jejunum	Normal pH (normal HCl secretion)	Iron-deficiency anaemia, glossitis

* mainly the proximal and mid portions; + entire length of small intestine.

common transport process whilst fructose is absorbed by a different mechanism.

Proteins. Protein digestion results in the formation of amino acids and small peptides; both are absorbed by an active process with the peptides undergoing further hydrolysis within the intestinal cell. Groups of amino acids have their own transport mechanisms in the proximal renal tubule, e.g., there is one mechanism for cystine and the other dibasic amino acids (ornithine, arginine, lysine), one for the Hartnup group of neutral amino acids, and so on (see page 300).

Fats. The end products of fat digestion are fatty acids, 2-monoglycerides, free cholesterol, and phospholipids. In the presence of bile salts, these compounds together with the fat-soluble vitamins (A, D, E, K) aggregate and form into water-miscible micelles. These micelles are small enough to pass into the microvillous spaces of the gut epithelium and be absorbed.

In the intestinal cells triglycerides are reformed from monoglycerides and fatty acids, and cholesterol is re-esterified. The triglycerides, cholesterol esters, phospholipids, and fat-soluble vitamins are then packaged into chylomicrons by a coating of apolipo-proteins (page 193). These particles then pass into the

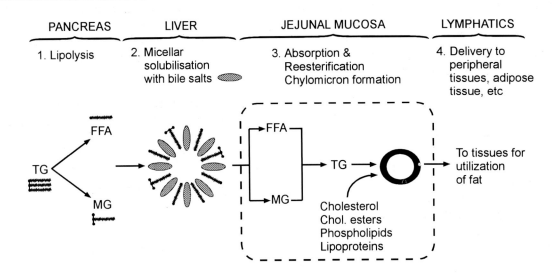

Figure 15.3. Mechanisms of intestinal fat absorption. Modified from Wilson FA, Dietschy JM. Gastroenterology 1971;61:911. Copyright 1971, The Williams and Wilkins Company,Baltimore, USA.

lymphatic circulation, finally entering the bloodstream by way of the thoracic duct. Some fatty acids, particularly the short and medium chain variety, pass across the intestinal cells to enter the portal blood stream directly. Figure 15.3 is a schematic representation of intestinal fat absorption, showing the roles of the pancreas, liver and intestinal mucosa in the process.

Vitamin B$_{12}$. After forming a complex with the intrinsic factor secreted by the stomach this vitamin is absorbed in the terminal ileum.

Calcium. Calcium is absorbed in the upper part of the small intestine in the ionic form. It requires the active metabolite of vitamin D for this process (page 88) and is inhibited by substances that form insoluble calcium salts (phosphate, oxalate, etc).

Iron. Dietary iron is converted to the ferrous form in the stomach (page 271), absorbed by active transport in the upper small gut and stored in the erythrocyte as ferritin.

Sodium chloride. The mechanism for electrolyte

absorption is poorly defined but a suggested process is:

1. In the intestinal cell H$^+$ and HCO$_3^-$ are formed from carbon dioxide and water (catalysed by cell-located carbonic anhydrase).

2. H$^+$ is secreted into the gut lumen in exchange for Na$^+$; and HCO$_3^-$ is secreted in exchange for Cl$^-$. The absorbed Na$^+$ and Cl$^-$ then pass into the blood.

3. In the gut lumen, under the influence of brush border-located carbonic anhydrase, the H$^+$ and HCO$_3^-$ combine to form carbonic acid and then CO$_2$ and H$_2$O. The generated CO$_2$ diffuses back into the mucosal cell and re-enters the cycle described in (1).

ROLE OF THE LARGE BOWEL

Each day about 0.5 to 2.0 litres of fluid containing the waste products of digestion and absorption and electrolytes passes from the small into the large intestine. Most of this (less the waste products) is absorbed and only about 100-200 mL containing very small quantities of electrolytes is finally passed in the faeces.

Sodium and chloride ions are absorbed in a manner similar to that described above and the sodium level falls to around 40 mmol/L. The potassium level increases to around 80 to 90 mmol/L due to intestinal secretion, possibly in exchange for luminal sodium ions. Chloride ions are reabsorbed in exchange for HCO_3^- via the Cl^--HCO_3^- pump.

Endocrine aspects of the gut

The gastrointestinal (GI) tract produces a large variety of hormonally active peptides, most of which are involved in the digestive process. Several of these are also found outside the GI tract, notably in the central and peripheral nervous system, where they may have neurotransmitter and neuroendocrine action. Only very brief mention of the known functions of the better characterised of the GI hormones is made here.

The endocrine cells of the gut are scattered throughout the entire GI tract in clusters forming a diffuse endocrine system. They were initially characterised by their affinity for silver (argentaffin) and amine precursor uptake and decarboxylation (APUD) ability; and thought to be of neural crest origin. It is well accepted that their products can act as both hormones and neurotransmitters. Over 25 peptides have been extracted from the GI tract and characterised. The more important and best known are the gastrins, secretin, cholecystokinin, gastrin inhibitory polypeptide, vasoactive intestinal polypeptide, and motilin. A number of others such as glucagon and somatostatin which occur in larger quantities elsewhere have also been located in the gut. No deficiency states are known for any of the GI hormones but several GI hormone-secreting tumours have been described.

Gastrin. This is produced by the G-cells of the gastric antrum and to a lesser extent, the duodenum. Two major (and several minor) forms are found in the gastrin-producing tissues and in the circulation, 'big' gastrin (G34, half-life ~40 min) and 'little' gastrin (G17, half-life ~8 min). Both forms stimulate the secretion of gastric acid and increase gastric antral motility. Excessive amounts are secreted by gastrinomas and are responsible for the Zollinger-Ellison syndrome (page 222).

Cholecystokinin. This hormone, also known as pancreozymin, is a 33 amino acid peptide produced by the small intestinal mucosal cells (mainly duodenum and proximal ileum). Significant amounts have been localised in brain tissue, suggesting a role as a neurotransmitter. It stimulates pancreatic enzyme secretion and gall bladder contraction.

Secretin. This hormone (a polypeptide of 27 amino acid residues), which stimulates pancreatic fluid and bicarbonate secretion, is produced by the S-cells located between crypts and villi of the upper intestinal mucosa. Elevated serum levels are found in chronic renal failure, cystic fibrosis, and the Zollinger-Ellison syndrome.

Vasoactive intestinal polypeptide. VIP was originally thought to be secreted by the endocrine gut as well as by the brain and peripheral nervous tissue; recent studies suggest that it may be localised exclusively in nerve fibres and nerve cells. It stimulates intestinal secretion; excess is found in patients with the WDHA syndrome (VIPoma, page 223).

Gastric inhibitory polypeptide. GIP (a polypeptide with 47 amino acid residues) is secreted by the duodenum and upper jejunum. When given together with intravenous glucose it potentiates insulin release and improves glucose tolerance.

Motilin. This is a 22 amino acid peptide released from the upper small intestine and concerned with interdigestive motor activity.

Disorders of GIT function

Vomiting, diarrhoea, and the malabsorption syndromes produce characteristic biochemical pictures; other gut disorders such as peptic ulcer and ulcerative colitis do not produce dramatic biochemical effects in the uncomplicated state and will not be discussed.

VOMITING

From a metabolic aspect there are two types of

vomiting, pre-pyloric and post-pyloric. Both result in loss of water, sodium, and potassium but differ in their effects on acid-base homeostasis.

Pre-pyloric vomiting

In this condition there is loss of excessive amounts of HCl from the stomach which results in a metabolic alkalosis (high plasma [HCO_3^-]). When H^+ is secreted into the gastric lumen an equimolar amount of bicarbonate is secreted back into the blood. During vomiting H^+ is continually secreted and lost in the vomitus and thus large quantities of bicarbonate are generated and produces metabolic alkalosis (Figure 15.4).

The hypovolaemia due to dehydration (water loss in vomitus) stimulates the renin-angiotensin complex resulting in secondary hyperaldosteronism and renal potassium loss (alkalosis *per se* also encourages renal potassium excretion); thus the hypokalaemia associated with vomiting is due mainly to renal potassium loss.

The characteristic biochemical picture of pre-pyloric vomiting is hypovolaemia, hypokalaemia, metabolic alkalosis (high plasma bicarbonate) and a low plasma chloride (see Figure 2.4, page 32).

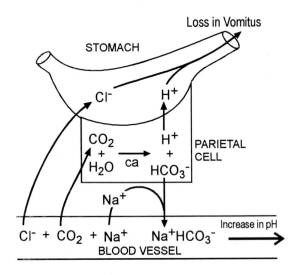

Figure 15.4. The pathogenesis of excess HCO_3^- with vomiting. See text for details. ca, carbonic anhydrase.

Post-pyloric vomiting

If the vomitus comes from the gut below the pyloric antrum (e.g., in a patient with intestinal obstruction) considerable bicarbonate is lost because of the high bicarbonate content of the small intestinal fluids (Table 15.1). Hence in this situation the bicarbonate generated by the stomach (following H^+ secretion) can be considered to be lost via the small gut fluid component of the vomitus and this will result in a normal plasma bicarbonate concentration. There is accompanying hypovolaemia and hypokalaemia, as in pre-pyloric vomiting.

If dehydration is severe, as can occur with prolonged obstruction, the resulting compromised circulation may produce sufficient tissue anoxia to cause a lactic acidosis; hence a low plasma [HCO_3^-] and metabolic acidosis may ensue.

DIARRHOEA

Diarrhoea is characterised by increased frequency and quantity of stools containing excessive amounts of water. The increased water (the basic lesion) is due to an increased total solute content in the gut lumen which may be a consequence of increased gut secretion or decreased gut absorption of these substances. The offending solute is often sodium but can be fatty acids (fat malabsorption), organic acids (carbohydrate malabsorption), chloride ions (chloride diarrhoea), or therapeutic substances, e.g., lactulose, magnesium sulphate. There are three recognised types of diarrhoea -- *osmotic, secretory,* and *that due to defective ion absorption.*

Osmotic diarrhoea

This is due to accumulation of non-ionic osmotically active substances in the gut caused by poorly absorbed solutes (e.g., $MgSO_4$), defective digestion (e.g., fatty acids in lipase deficiency), or malabsorption of non-electrolytes (e.g., disaccharides in disaccharidase deficiency). The osmotically active particles prevent the absorption of water from the gut and increase withdrawal of water through the gut wall.

Secretory diarrhoea

This is due to excessive secretion of solute, mainly sodium and its associated anions, into the gut lumen.

218

This may be due to toxic insult to the gut by bacteria (e.g., *E. coli, V. cholerae*), damage to the mucosa (e.g., ulcerative colitis), and hormonal causes (carcinoid syndrome, VIPoma, Zollinger-Ellison syndrome, etc).

Defective ion absorption

This rare cause is exemplified by chloride diarrhoea which is due to defective absorption of luminal chloride (page 333).

CONSEQUENCES OF DIARRHOEA

Diarrhoeal fluid has a similar electrolyte composition to that of ileostomy fluid (Table 15.1), i.e., high bicarbonate and potassium content. Hence a prolonged loss of this fluid will, in addition to causing dehydration, result in potassium depletion (hypokalaemia) and bicarbonate depletion (metabolic acidosis) with a characteristic hypokalaemic hyperchloraemic metabolic acidosis (page 51). The exception is chloride diarrhoea which is associated with a metabolic alkalosis.

LABORATORY EVALUATION

The routine investigation of the patient with diarrhoea should include plasma electrolytes, urea and creatinine, and evaluation of the acid-base status. To distinguish secretory diarrhoea from osmotic diarrhoea, it is useful to measure the diarrhoeal fluid osmolality and to calculate its osmolality from the measured [Na] and [K]. In secretory diarrhoea the major osmotic particles are sodium, potassium, bicarbonate, and chloride; thus the measured osmolality will be similar to the calculated osmolality $(2 \times \{[Na] + [K]\})$, or within 10-20 mmol/kg. In osmotic diarrhoea the major particles are non-electrolytes and thus the difference between the calculated and measured osmolalities (osmolal gap) will be greater than 20 mmol/kg.

MALABSORPTION SYNDROMES

The malabsorption syndromes can be classified according to the nature of the defect into those with general disease, usually associated with steatorrhoea, and those with specific defects which are not usually associated with steatorrhoea.

CAUSES/PATHOPHYSIOLOGY

The common causes of the malabsorption syndromes are listed in Table 15.3.

Table 15.3. Common causes of the malabsorption syndromes.

General defect (associated with steatorrhoea)
Pancreatic insufficiency
   Cystic fibrosis, chronic pancreatitis,
   haemochromatosis, pancreatic carcinoma,
   pancreatic resection.
Bile salt deficiency
   Deficient secretion: biliary obstruction, depletion
   due to loss in faeces (terminal ileal disease or
   resection)
   Loss of conjugation: bacterial overgrowth.
Small bowel disease
   Coeliac disease (gluten enteropathy), tropical
   sprue,
   infiltrations (lymphoma, amyloid, malignancy),
   resection, mesenteric vascular insufficiency.

Specific defects
Enzymes: disaccharidase deficiency
Transport defects: glucose/galactose, cystinuria,
   Hartnup disease.
Intrinsic factor deficiency: pernicious anaemia.

Clinical manifestations

General defects. Depending on the degree of malabsorption and the nutrients involved some or all of the following may occur:

- *Fat:* steatorrhoea, weight loss
- *Protein/carbohydrate:* weight loss, protein malnutrition (hypoalbuminaemia, osteoporosis etc).
- *Fat-soluble vitamins:*
  Vitamin D -- rickets, osteomalacia, hypocalcaemia;
  Vitamin K -- clotting abnormalities.
- *Folic acid/vitamin B_{12}:* megaloblastic anaemia, nervous system dysfunction.
- *Iron:* iron-deficiency anaemia.

Specific defects. The manifested defect will vary with the abnormality:

- *Intrinsic factor:* megaloblastic anaemia.
- *Disaccharidase deficiency:* explosive diarrhoea, borborygmi when offending sugar taken orally.
- *Cystinuria and Hartnup disease:* see page 300.

General defects

Pancreatic deficiency. The commonest causes of pancreatic insufficiency are chronic pancreatitis in the adult and cystic fibrosis in the infant.

Cystic fibrosis. This common inborn error of metabolism is a disease of uncertain aetiology (? membrane chloride transport defect) which is transmitted as an autosomal recessive trait with an incidence of 1 in 2500 (1 in 25 is a carrier) in Caucasians -- a mutation of the long arm of chromosome 7 (band q31) accounts for the majority of cases. It is characterised by exocrine and eccrine glands that secrete a very viscous mucus and sweat that has a high sodium content (>60 mmol/L). It may present as meconium ileus at birth (intestinal obstruction), malabsorption in infancy (pancreatic duct obstruction), biliary cirrhosis (biliary ductule obstruction), or persistent chronic bronchial infections (bronchial obstruction). Fat malabsorption and steatorrhoea occur in 80% of cases. Heterozygotes (carriers) are clinically normal.

Bile salt deficiency. In this situation the lack of conjugated bile salts inhibits fat digestion and absorption (defective micelle formation). Deficiency may be caused by:

1 impaired hepatic synthesis and secretion of bile salts in severe chronic liver disease (e.g., obstructive jaundice, chronic hepatitis)

2 interruption of the enterohepatic circulation of bile salts due to (a) bile duct obstruction, (b) ileal disease (e.g., Crohn's disease) or resection of the terminal ileum, and (c) bacterial overgrowth in the small bowel, causing deconjugation, hydroxylation and precipitation of the bile salts.

Bacterial overgrowth. Bacteria such as *E. coli* are able to deconjugate bile salts and render them ineffective in micellar solubilisation (Figure 15.3) --

bile salt activity depends on the detergent properties of the conjugated compound. Overgrowth may occur where there is stagnation of bowel contents such as in:

1 Altered bowel motility (denervation as in diabetes mellitus, infiltrations as in amyloidosis, and strictures);
2 Fistula between small and large bowel;
3 Blind loops (small bowel diverticula, surgical loops).

Small gut mucosal disease. Insufficient or defective mucosae resulting in an inadequate absorptive surface occurs in coeliac disease, tropical sprue, gut resections, and infiltrations of the gut wall. The commonest cause is coeliac disease.

Coeliac disease. This disease, which occurs in both children and adults, is due to sensitivity to the wheat protein gluten (gluten-sensitive enteropathy) and is characterised by flattened villi and villous atrophy. It presents as a generalised malabsorption syndrome with steatorrhoea and responds to removal of wheat protein from the diet. The definitive diagnosis depends on demonstration of the characteristic villi morphology (biopsy) and the response to therapy.

Specific defects

Disaccharidase deficiency. Any of the three disaccharidases, lactase, maltase, and sucrase may be congenitally deficient, or the defect may be associated with disease processes such as coeliac disease and Crohn's disease. The commonest disorder is lactase deficiency which results in milk intolerance. The characteristic features are abdominal cramps and distension, borborygmus (increased bowel sounds), and frequent frothy diarrhoea following milk ingestion. The diarrhoea is due to an increased osmotic load of undigested lactose and its degradation products such as lactic acid.

Diagnosis is confirmed by identification of the deficiency enzyme in a small gut biopsy. There are two available screening tests:

(1) hydrogen breath test (the most reliable), and

(2) a glucose-tolerance type test using the appropriate disaccharide instead of glucose (e.g., lactose tolerance test).

220

LABORATORY EVALUATION OF MALABSORPTION SYNDROMES

The selection of laboratory tests (Figure 15.5) will depend on the organ or function that is (or appears to be) disordered. A faecal fat estimation is the usual screening procedure for fat malabsorption (the ^{14}C-triolein breath test may also be used), a xylose absorption test for upper small bowel dysfunction, and the Schilling test for lower small bowel dysfunction. Disorders of the small bowel mucosa (e.g., coeliac disease) should always be confirmed by a mucosal biopsy. Pancreatic insufficiency can also be assessed by the NBT-PABA (Bentiromide) test or the secretin-cholecystokinin test; whilst the bile salt or hydrogen breath tests are used to evaluate a provisional diagnosis of bacterial overgrowth in the small bowel.

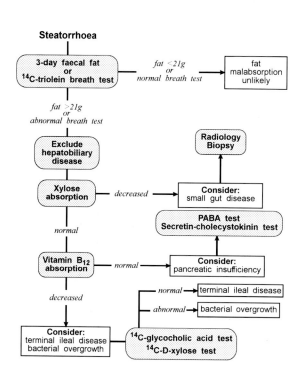

Figure 15.5. Laboratory evaluation of steatorrhoea.

Faecal fat. Normally less than 7 g are excreted daily. The estimation should be performed on a 3-day sample because of inconsistent bowel action.

^{14}C-triolein breath test. Because of the unpleasant nature of the faecal fat estimation a number of screening tests for fat malabsorption have been devised, e.g., serum carotene estimation, serum optical density after a fat load. The most reliable of these screening tests is the estimation of ^{14}CO$_2$ in the breath after an oral dose of glycerol tri[1-^{14}C]oleate. In the absence of malabsorption the labelled triglyceride is hydrolysed by pancreatic lipase and the free labelled oleic acid is absorbed and metabolised, producing radioactive ^{14}CO$_2$ which is excreted by the lungs. The percentage excretion of the dose administered is calculated from the ^{14}CO$_2$ trapped from the exhaled breath over several hours. The best test protocol incorporates a repeat test done on a separate day with an equimolar dose of labelled oleic acid (which is absorbed and metabolised independently of pancreatic exocrine function). The ratio of ^{14}CO$_2$ exhaled using the free and the esterified fatty acids gives an estimate of pancreatic exocrine function.

Xylose absorption. D-xylose is absorbed in the small intestine, undergoes very little metabolic change *in vivo*, and is excreted in the urine. The urinary excretion after an oral dose can be used to evaluate intestinal absorptive function. If the liver and renal functions are normal and there is no delay in gastric emptying, about 23% of the oral dose should appear in the urine within 5 hours of ingestion (with a dose of 5 g, 1.2 g or more should appear in the urine).

Abnormal results are obtained in over 90% of patients with intestinal malabsorption caused by diffuse mucosal disease (e.g., coeliac disease, tropical sprue). In contrast, normal results are obtained in 95% of patients with chronic pancreatitis -- pancreatic insufficiency or bile salt deficiency causing intra-luminal maldigestion and subsequent malabsorption.

Schilling test. The absorption of vitamin B$_{12}$ is tested by giving radioactive (^{57}Co-)B$_{12}$ (cyano-cobalamin) and measuring its excretion in the urine. If the radioactivity excreted in the urine over the next 24 hours is less than 8% of that administered, cyano-cobalamin malabsorption is present. The absorption is decreased in ileal disease, intrinsic factor deficiency (pernicious anaemia), and bacterial overgrowth. Repeating the test with the addition of intrinsic factor will differentiate between pernicious anaemia (normal absorption) and ileal disease (abnormal result). Repeating the test with an anaerobicidal antibiotic will provide further differential between ileal disease (absorption remains abnormally low) and bacterial overgrowth (normal absorption is recovered).

Secretin-cholecystokinin test. In this test the duodenum is intubated and the juice is collected for the estimation of volume, bicarbonate, and trypsin activity before and after the administration of the two hormones. It is time consuming and costly and has been generally replaced by the NBT-PABA test.

NBT-PABA test. N-benzoyl-tyrosyl-*p*-aminobenzoic acid (NBT-PABA) is administered orally after an overnight fast, together with a protein load (e.g., 25 g casein). In the presence of chymotrypsin free *p*-aminobenzoic acid (PABA) is liberated. The PABA is absorbed, metabolised by the liver, and then excreted in the urine. Thus the urinary recovery can be used as an index of pancreatic chymotrypsin activity.

To eliminate extrapancreatic factors a small quantity of ^{14}C-PABA is given with the NBT-PABA and the amounts of PABA and ^{14}C-PABA excreted are measured and expressed as a fraction of the respective dose given. The results may also be expressed as a PABA excretion index, calculated as follows:

$$\frac{\text{mole fraction of PABA excreted}}{\text{fraction of } ^{14}\text{C-PABA excreted}} \times 100\%$$

Values less than 50% would be considered abnormal, suggesting pancreatic exocrine insufficiency. An oral dose of 500 mg and a 6-hour urine collection have been shown to provide optimal test sensitivity.

Bile salt breath test. In this test cholyl-1-^{14}C-glycine is administrated orally. If bacteria are present in the small gut the bile acid is deconjugated and the released ^{14}C-glycine is absorbed and metabolised. The amount of glycine released is reflected by the amount of ^{14}CO$_2$ appearing in the expired air. Normally only less than 5% of the bile salts is not reabsorbed (and recirculated to the liver) and thus enters the colon where they are deconjugated. Bacterial overgrowth causes an interruption of the enterohepatic circulation of the bile salts resulting in increased deconjugation, fat malabsorption and steatorrhoea.

Hydrogen breath test. Most of the small amount of hydrogen in the breath is derived from the fermentation of ingested carbohydrates by intestinal bacterial. Thus bacterial overgrowth in the small bowel and malabsorbed carbohydrates reaching the large bowel (disaccharidase deficiency) will result in increased amounts of hydrogen expired.

Pancreatic disorders

Disorders of the pancreas include diabetes mellitus, haemochromatosis, tumours (carcinoma and functioning adenomas), which are dealt with elsewhere in this text, and acute and chronic pancreatitis.

Acute pancreatitis

This common cause of acute abdominal pain is classically associated with high plasma levels of amylase and lipase. The exact cause is unclear but most cases are associated with either acute alcoholism or biliary tract disease; it can also be associated with hypocalcaemia, hyperlipidaemia, trauma, and some drugs (thiazides, furosemide, azathioprin, glucocorticoids). The initial lesion appears to be the release of digestive enzymes into the peritoneal cavity which sets up a vicious cycle by digesting the pancreas and causing the release of more enzymes. The characteristic biochemical features are elevated plasma levels of amylase (page 181) and lipase, and hypocalcaemia (page 97).

Chronic pancreatitis

Like acute pancreatitis, the cause of chronic pancreatitis is obscure. It is most often associated with alcoholism, recurrent attacks of acute pancreatitis, and calcification of the pancreatic tissue. The clinical features, in addition to steatorrhoea, include abdominal pain and weight loss.

GIT hormone-secreting tumours

Many of the hormone-secreting tumours of the APUD cells (page 287) occur in the GI tract and pancreas; the amine-precursor-secreting carcinoid tumours also mainly occur in the intestine.

Gastrinoma. The Zollinger-Ellison syndrome, due to excessive circulating gastrin, presents with gastric hyperacidity, recurrent peptic ulceration, and often persistent diarrhoea. It may be due to a gastrinoma or, more rarely, hyperplasia of the G-cells of the gastric antrum. The gastrinomas are usually located in the pancreas (80% are malignant).

Glucagonoma. These rare tumours of the pancreatic islets produce a characteristic necrosis of the epidermis (necrolytic migratory erythema) and mild diabetes. Ninety per cent occur in women and 60% are malignant.

VIPoma. These tumours which secrete VIP are located in the pancreas and produce the Verner-Morrison or WDHA (watery diarrhoea, hypokalaemia, and achlorhydria) syndrome. They are rare but potentially fatal if unattended to urgently.

- Flushing, often paroxysmal
- Diarrhoea, often very severe
- Bronchospasm
- Fibrotic lesions of the right side of the heart
- Urinary excretion of 5-hydroxyindole acetic acid (5-HIAA)

It is due to a tumour of the APUD cells (see page 287, the argentaffin cells), which synthesise serotonin (5-hydroxytryptamine) from tryptophan (Figure 15.6).

The syndrome usually only appears after the tumour metastasises to the liver (this allows serotonin to escape into the peripheral circulation without being metabolised by the liver). These tumours most often occur in the ileocaecal region but can occur in any tissue derived from the embryonic gut (stomach, rectum, bronchus, pancreas).

The diarrhoea and heart lesions may be due to the circulating serotonin but the causes of the other symptoms are unclear; they may be due to histamine or peptides (e.g., substance P) secreted by the tumour. The diagnosis is made by demonstrating excessive amounts of the serotonin metabolite, 5-HIAA, in the urine.

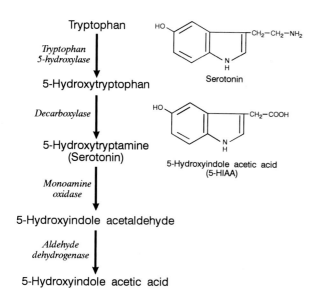

Figure 15.6. Serotonin metabolism. **Inset:** Structures of serotonin and 5-hydroxyindole acetic acid.

Carcinoid syndrome. The carcinoid syndrome is characterised by:

REFERENCES/FURTHER READING

Epstein M, Pusch AL. Watery diarrhoea and stool osmolality. Clin Chem 1983;29:211

Go VLW, DiMango EP. Assessment of exocrine pancreatic function by duodenal intubation. Clinics Gastroenterol 1984;13:701-715.

King CE, Toskes PP. The use of breath tests in the study of malabsorption. Clinics Gastroenterol 1983; 12:591-610.

Lawson N, Chestner I. Tests of exocrine pancreatic function. Ann Clin Biochem 1994;31:305-314.

Shiau Y-F. Clinical and laboratory approaches to evaluate diarrheal disorders. CRC Crit Rev Clin Lab Sci 1987;25:43-63.

Theodossi A, Gazzard BG. Have chemical tests a value in diagnosing malabsorption? Ann Clin Biochem 1984;21:153-165.

West PS, *et al.* Comparison of screening tests for fat malabsorption. Br Med J 1981;282:1501-1504.

Chapter 16

The Hypothalamus and Pituitary Gland

The hypothalamus, forming the floor and part of the lateral walls of the third ventricle, and the pituitary gland, located at the base of the brain below the optic chiasma, play a pivotal role in metabolism through their influence, via hormones, on a number of other endocrine glands and tissues. Pituitary function depends on hypothalamic neurosecretion. The anterior pituitary gland is regulated by hormones originating in the hypothalamus which generally stimulate the gland, with the exception of dopamine which inhibits prolactin secretion, and somatostatin which inhibits growth hormone. The posterior lobe of the pituitary is involved with arginine vasopressin (AVP) and oxytocin secretion and is discussed elsewhere (page 4).

The hypothalamus

Neuronal cell bodies or nuclei, located in the hypothalamus, synthesise specific hormones which are transported along the cell axons to the median eminence. At this terminus the hormones are released into the capillaries of the hypothalamic-hypophyseal portal system and carried to the anterior pituitary where they stimulate or inhibit hormone production by specific cells.

To date seven hypothalamic hormones (excluding AVP and oxytocin) have been characterised (Table 16.1). All are peptides with the notable exception of dopamine, the principal prolactin release-inhibitory factor, and all are now commercially available for human investigational and clinical use. Whilst control of their synthesis and secretion is as yet generally unclear, the hypothalamic nuclei where they are synthesised are known to be closely related to many neurosecretory neurones and obviously receive input from various parts of the central nervous system (e.g., influences such as light, darkness, sleep, stress, etc).

The gonadotrophin releasing hormone-secreting peptidergic neuronal cells, for example, are capable of responding to both nervous and chemically transmitted stimuli, and the arcuate nucleus, where they are located, thus acts as a neuroendocrine interface by translating the frequency of neuronal signals into changes in circulating hormone levels. In addition, some hypothalamic nuclei partake in negative feedback from (a) their related anterior pituitary hormone (short loop) and (b) the target organ secretions (long loop).

Thyrotrophin-releasing hormone (TRH)

TRH is a tripeptide (pyroGlu-His-ProNH$_2$), an intact amide group and the cyclised glutamic acid residue being essential for its biological activity. TRH induces thyroid stimulating hormone (TSH) secretion and release by the pituitary thyrotroph. It acts by binding to specific receptors on the plasma membrane of the pituitary cell. Its action is mediated mainly through hydrolysis of phosphatidylinositol, with phosphorylation of key protein kinases. The stimulatory effect of TRH is inhibited by the negative feedback effect of the thyroid hormones; the latter reduce the number of TRH receptors on the thyrotroph. TRH is also a potent prolactin-releasing factor, although the exact role of TRH as a physiological regulator of prolactin secretion is not established.

Gonadotrophin-releasing hormone (GnRH)

GnRH controls both luteinising hormone (LH) and follicle-stimulating hormone (FSH) secretion and release. GnRH, like other neuropeptides, are released in pulses, the frequency of which can alter the pattern of LH and FSH secretion. Sustained high levels of GnRH suppress secretion of both gonadotrophins; normal secretion is restored by intermittent pulses of the right frequencies. In patients with hypothalamic GnRH deficiency, complete restoration of gonadal function (in both males and females) has been achieved by administering GnRH in appropriate doses in a pulsatile manner. High doses of GnRH (LHRH) analogues are used to suppress gonadal hyperactivity in patients with precocious puberty.

Corticotrophin-releasing hormone (CRH)

CRH is a relatively large peptide (41 amino acids) which is synthesised, as with other neuropeptides, as part of a larger prohormone and undergoes enzymatic cleavage and modification. Release of CRH, which

224

Table 16.1. The hypothalamic hormones.

Hypothalamic hormone	Structure	Target cell	Effect
Corticotrophin-releasing hormone (CRH)	41 aa* peptide	Corticotroph	Stimulates ACTH secretion
Thyrotrophin-releasing hormone (TRH)	Tripeptide	Thyrotroph	Stimulates TSH secretion
Gonadotrophin-releasing hormone (GnRH)	Decapeptide	Gonadotroph	Stimulates LH, FSH secretion
Growth hormone-releasing hormone (GHRH)	44 aa peptide	Somatotroph	Stimulates GH secretion
Somatostatin	14 aa peptide	Somatotroph	Inhibits GHRH action
Dopamine	Amine	Lactotroph	Inhibits prolactin release

* aa, amino acid residues (Tables 16.1 and 16.2)

occurs episodically, causes a prompt increase in the secretion of ACTH, and of cortisol, both in similar episodic patterns. The effect occurs only in the presence of calcium ions and is inhibited by glucocorticoids.

Growth hormone (GH)-regulating factors

GH secretion is regulated by a dual control system, one stimulatory (GH-releasing factor or GHRH) and the other inhibitory (somatostatin). GHRH, like GnRH, depends on pulsatile secretion for its physiological effect, as evidenced by the decrease in GH levels with sustained infusions of GHRH over several hours in individuals with normal pituitaries. The term somatostatin is used to describe a family of related molecules which inhibit not only GH secretion but also TSH secretion in the pituitary. They are not only widely distributed in cells throughout the nervous system but are present in many extraneural tissues. Their inhibitory effects have been demonstrated in virtually all endocrine and exocrine secretions of the pancreas, gut and gallbladder.

Prolactin-regulating factors

The predominant hypothalamic influence on prolactin

secretion is an inhibitory one. Dopamine is the most important prolactin-inhibiting factor (PIF); another putative PIF is γ-aminobutyric acid (GABA). PRL levels drop sharply upon administra-tion of dopamine or dopamine agonists such as bromocriptine and this action accounts for the therapeutic effect of the latter in patients with hyperprolactinaemia, including prolactinoma. Several putative prolactin-releasing factors (PRFs), including TRH and AVP (arginine vasopressin), appear to bring about PRL release.

The pituitary gland

The pituitary gland is located at the base of the brain in a bony pocket called the sella turcica and is connected to the hypothalamus by the pituitary stalk. The anterior and posterior lobes have different embryological origins (the posterior lobe is an outgrowth of the hypothalamus and the anterior lobe is derived from the buccal cavity) and they function independently. The anterior lobe contains five known cell types each of which synthesise and secrete specific polypeptide hormones in response to the appropriate hypothalamic factors (Tables 16.1 and 16.2).

Table 16.2. The anterior pituitary hormones.   *aa, amino acids

Anterior pituitary hormone	Structure	Target tissue
Adrenocorticotropic hormone(ACTH)	Polypeptide 39 aa*	Adrenal cortex
Thyroid-stimulating hormone (TSH)	Glycopeptide, α-subunit 89 aa β-subunit 112 aa	Thyroid gland
Luteinising hormone (LH)	Glycopeptide, α-subunit 89 aa β-subunit 115 aa	Gonads (steroid-producing cells)
Follicle-stimulating hormone (FSH)	Glycopeptide, α-subunit 89 aa β-subunit 115 aa	Gonads (gamete-producing cells)
Growth hormone (GH)	Polypeptide 191 aa	Bone, soft tissue
Prolactin (PRL)	Polypeptide 198 aa	Breast

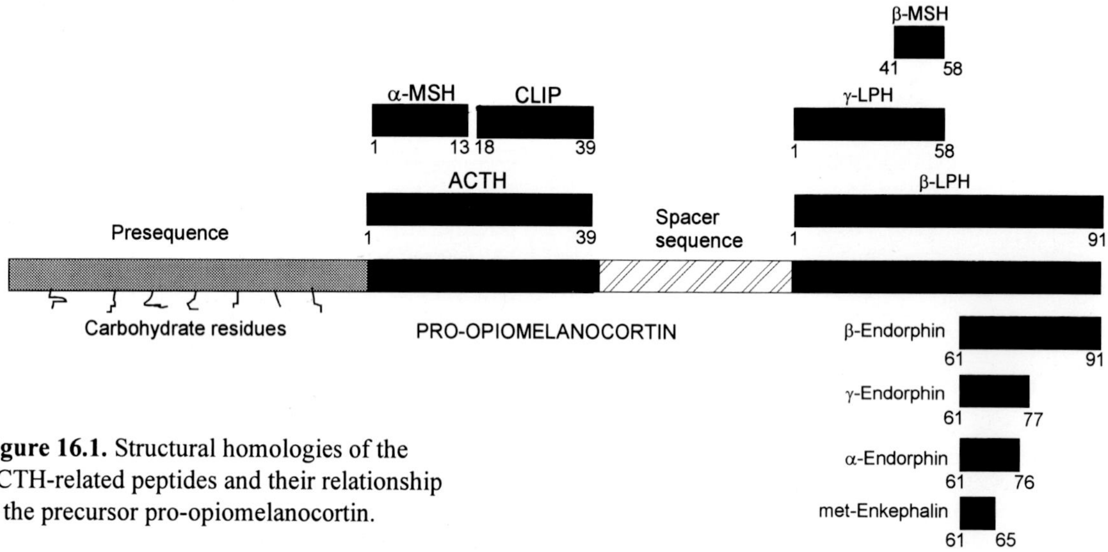

Figure 16.1. Structural homologies of the ACTH-related peptides and their relationship to the precursor pro-opiomelanocortin.

Adrenocorticotropic hormone (ACTH)

The corticotrophs synthesise a large, 241-amino-acid precursor peptide, proopiomelanocortin (POMC), which is then split into a number of bioactive peptides which include ACTH (39 amino acids), β-lipotrophin, β-endorphins, and enkephalins (Figure 16.1). The ACTH molecule also includes the 13 amino acid sequence of melanocyte-stimulating hormone -- high circulating levels of ACTH are often associated with excess pigmentation as in primary hypoadrenalism.

ACTH stimulates the adrenal cortex to produce principally cortisol , with adrenal androgens as minor,

secondary products (Figure 18.1, page 248). It is in turn regulated, in a synergistic manner, by CRH, AVP and adrenaline, which stimulate production. Gluco-corticoids, principally cortisol, act at multiple sites within the corticotrophs by inhibiting the ACTH response to CRH and by inhibiting ACTH synthesis via blockade of POMC gene transcription and synthesis. At the hypothalamus, cortisol inhibits CRH and AVP synthesis and release. In addition, ACTH inhibits its own secretion (ultra-short loop), primarily by suppressing CRH release (Figure 16.2).

ACTH is released in a pulsatile fashion, with most of the pulses occurring in the early morning hours and hence higher circulating levels ensue during this period. This characteristic circadian rhythm reflects the pattern of CRH release and is in turn mirrored by the pattern of cortisol release. Another major factor influencing CRH release (and ACTH and cortisol secretion) is stress, both psychological and physical, which can be associated with very high circulating cortisol levels. Stress factors include trauma, major surgery, fever, hypoglycaemia, and burn injury.

Synthetic ACTH (1-24) analogues (eg, Synacthen), containing the essential first 18 amino acid residues at the amino terminal in which its biological activity resides, are commercially available. Synthetic ACTH has a longer half-life than native ACTH (1-18) and are used in the ACTH stimulation test (page 255).

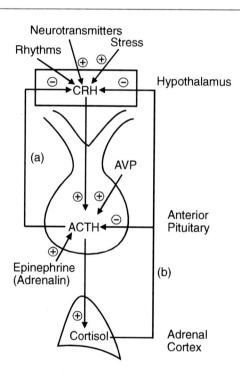

Figure 16.2. Control of ACTH secretion.
CRH, corticotrophin-releasing hormone; AVP, arginine vasopressin (a) short feedback loop; (b) long feedback loop; ⊕ stimulatory action; ⊖ inhibitory action.

Thyroid-stimulating hormone (TSH)

TSH, released in response to TRH by the pituitary thyrotroph cells, stimulates the thyroid gland to produce thyroxine and tri-iodothyronine. The stimulatory effect of TRH is inhibited by the negative feedback effect of the thyroid hormones, and also by high levels of cortisol, dopamine, and somatostatin (Figure 16.3).

TSH is a glycopeptide consisting of two polypeptide subunits -- an α-subunit of 89 amino acids, which is identical to the α-subunits of the pituitary gonadotrophins and human chorionic gonadotrophin, and a β-subunit of 112 amino acids which confers specificity.

Gonadotrophins

The gonadotrophins, LH and FSH, are similar-sized glycopeptides containing identical α-subunits (shared with TSH and HCG) and different β-subunits which confer specificity to each of them. They both target the gonads, with LH stimulating steroid synthesis and

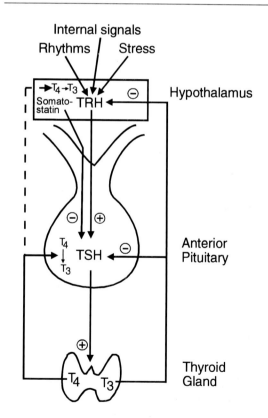

Figure 16.3. Control of TSH secretion.
TRH, thyrotrophin-releasing hormone; T_4, thyroxine; T_3, tri-iodothyronine; ⊕ stimulatory action; ⊖ inhibitory action.

FSH promoting follicle development in the ovary and spermatogenesis in the testes.

Both hormones are released in a pulsatile fashion in response to GnRH (Figure 16.4), which in turn is moderated via negative feedback by the gonadal steroids (oestradiol in the female and testosterone in the male), in addition, oestradiol also acts as a positive stimulator to produce the midcycle LH surge. GnRH control of gonadotrophin secretion is obligatorily intermittent (consequent to its own intermittent release into the hypophyseal portal veins). Continuous exposure of the pituitary gonadotrophs to GnRH leads to the desensitisation phenomenon ('down regulation' of its receptors), whereby persistently elevated GnRH levels flood the GnRH receptors on the cell membranes, preventing their regeneration. Another controlling factor is the negative feedback exerted by the gonadal peptide inhibin, which is produced by the Sertoli cells (male) and the granulosa cells of the follicle (female).

Prolactin and endogenous opioids inhibit GnRH and gonadotrophin release -- high circulating prolactin levels, as occurs with prolactinomas, is an important cause of infertility in the female.

Growth hormone (GH) (see Figure 16.5)

Growth hormone is a single-chain, nonglycosylated polypeptide of 191 amino acid residues (Table 16.2). It is produced by the anterior pituitary somatotrophs and circulates in the plasma bound to two specific carrier proteins (growth hormone-binding proteins) which protect it from renal degradation. Its biological effects are wide-ranging and include:

- increased cell uptake of amino acids
- decreased glucose metabolism (by its counter-regulatory action to insulin)
- increased fat mobilisation
- inhibition of protein catabolism
- promotion of epiphyseal bone growth.

Most of these effects are mediated through another group of hormones, the insulin-like growth factors (IGF), previously called somatomedins, which are produced by the liver and other peripheral tissues in response to GH stimulation. The most important is IGF-1 (also known as somatomedin-C) which has a negative feedback on GH secretion at the pituitary and hypothalamic levels.

GH is released in pulsatile volleys (with the major peaks occurring during sleep) and is under the control of two hypothalamic factors, GH-releasing hormone GHRH) and GH-inhibiting hormone (or somatostatin, see Table 16.1). Between bursts of GH release, which are probably induced by multiple bursts of GHRH secretion into the hypophyseal-portal blood during periods of reduced somatostatin secretion, serum GH concentrations are undetectable. The secretion of these two control agents is influenced by a number of factors including neural, hormonal, and metabolic stimuli, the more important being:

GH inhibition: hyperglycaemia, IGF-1
GH stimulation: sleep, stress, hypoglycaemia, exercise, arginine

Most of these factors appear to act on somatostatin rather than GHRH (Figure 16.5). Knowledge of their effects on GH secretion is applied in dynamic testing to assess pituitary reserve for GH secretion in patients with suspected GH deficiency or excess (page 231).

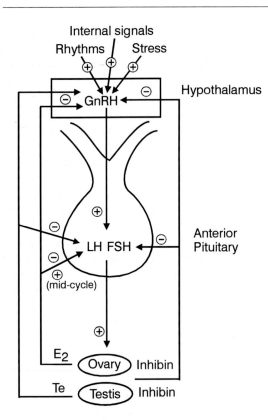

Figure 16.4. Control of FSH and LH secretion.
GnRH, gonadotrophin-releasing hormone; E_2 oestradiol; Te, testosterone; ⊕ stimulatory action; ⊖ inhibitory action.

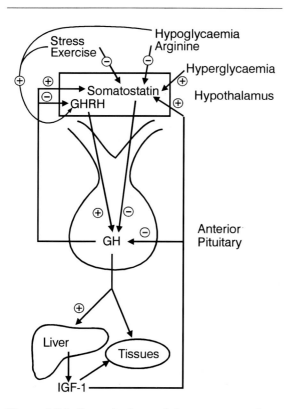

Figure 16.5. Control of growth hormone secretion. GHRH, GH-releasing hormone; IGF-1, Insulin-like growth factor-1; ⊕ stimulatory action; ⊖ inhibitory action.

Prolactin (PRL) (see Tables 16.1 and 16.2)

Prolactin is a 199-amino-acid polypeptide whose major role is to initiate and maintain milk production by breast tissue already 'primed' by oestrogens. Like the other pituitary hormones, it is released in a pulsatile manner, with maximum pulses occurring just after sleep commences; increased secretion also occurs during stress. Secretion increases markedly during pregnancy (from a normal of <20 ng/mL to over 600 ng/mL) and remains high in the postpartum period during lactation (suckling causes a 5-10 fold increase). PRL secretion is unique in that it is under tonic inhibition by the neurotransmitter dopamine (PRL-inhibiting hormone) and hence destruction or resection of the hypothalamus or the pituitary stalk will result in increased secretion. Drugs which block dopamine receptors, e.g., chlorpromazine, metochlorpramide and haloperidol, or which deplete neural tissues of dopamine, e.g., α-methyldopa and

reserpine, elevate PRL levels; dopamine agonists (e.g., bromocriptine) decrease PRL secretion. A PRL-releasing hormone has not been identified -- although pharmacological doses of TRH result in increased PRL secretion (e.g., during the TRH stimulation test, see page 244), the clinical significance of this in homeostatic control is uncertain. The acute bursts of prolactin secretion during suckling is not accompanied by a parallel increase in TSH secretion and patients with primary hypothyroidism may not have concomittant hyperprolactinaemia.

PRL deficiency in the female causes an inability to lactate but has no known ill effects in the male. High circulating levels inhibit GnRH and gonadotrophin release, which may account for the temporary infertility of lactating mothers during suckling and the chronic infertility associated with prolactinomas.

Disturbed function

Disease of the hypothalamic-pituitary complex is proclaimed by variable degrees of isolated or multiple pituitary hormone excess or deficiency and, depending on the pathological process, local non-pituitary manifestations. Hypothalamic injury may result in various anterior pituitary hormone deficiencies, hyperprolactinaemia and, if the disease is extensive, antidiuretic hormone deficiency, causing diabetes insipidus. Pituitary tumours can present with systemic symptoms of hormone deficiency or excess and local symptoms of a mass lesion such as headache, visual field defects (involvement of the optic nerve), and cranial nerve III palsy.

From a hormone point of view these diseases can result in (a) excess production of individual hormones, (b) isolated deficiency of individual hormones, and (c) deficiency of two or more hormones. The following discussion will look at lesions involving the individual hormones and at general or (pan)hypopituitarism.

ACTH

Excessive secretion of ACTH leads to cortisol excess and Cushing's syndrome (page 257) and is due to a pituitary adenoma (in 90% of cases) or hyperplasia (? consequent to CRH excess). Nelson's syndrome is a specific ACTH excess syndrome caused by a pituitary tumour (originally diagnosed as Cushing's disease) that has become exceedingly aggressive, following treatment by bilateral adrenalectomy.

Isolated ACTH deficiency due to local disease is a rare finding but is common in patients treated with glucocorticoids. ACTH deficiency is more usually associated with other pituitary hormone deficiencies, as in panhypopituitarism. The resulting secondary adrenal insufficiency affects only adrenal steroid synthesis under predominant ACTH regulation, i.e., cortisol and adrenal androgens. These patients usually do not experience an adrenal crisis, due to preservation of mineralocorticoid secretion. A relatively trivial illness, however, may precipitate vascular collapse, hypoglycaemia, seizures or coma. Thus adrenal insufficiency, regardless of the cause, should be treated promptly and monitored closely. These disorders and their evaluation are further discussed in Chapter 18.

TSH

Primary hypothyroidism is associated with high circulating levels of TSH and, often though not invariably, with high circulating levels of prolactin, consequent to increased TRH release due to the low thyroid hormone titres. Excessive autonomous production of TSH is very rare; only a small number of TSH-producing tumours have been described in the literature. Deficiency of TSH due to pituitary (or hypothalamic) disease leads to secondary (or tertiary) hypothyroidism, and is commonly associated with other hormone deficiencies in patients with pituitary (or hypothalamic) tumours or panhypopituitarism; it rarely occurs as an isolated deficiency. These disorders are discussed in the next chapter on Thyroid Function.

LH and FSH

LH and FSH deficiency usually occur together, producing hypogonadism and may be due to:

(a) destructive or infiltrative lesions of the pituitary or hypothalamus,
(b) excessive prolactin production,
(c) systemic disturbances such as anorexia nervosa, severe weight loss, stress, and intense physical training or exercise,
(d) congenital deficiency of gonadotrophin-producing cells (Kallman's syndrome).

In adolescents, it causes delayed or arrested puberty. In women, it causes infertility, menstrual irregularities, or amenorrhoea, and low serum oestrogen levels. In men, it results in prepubertal serum testosterone levels, and decrease in testicular size.

Excess production of gonadotrophins by pituitary tumours (mainly macroadenomas) is rare and usually clinically silent. In the polycystic ovarian syndrome (page 269) serum LH is increased but FSH is normal (the significance and cause of this abnormal LH to FSH ratio is unclear).

The most useful investigations in hypogonadism are estimations of the serum gonadotrophin levels. Elevated values indicate primary hypogonadism (the result of absence of sex-hormone feedback on the pituitary), and low or undetectable levels point to a pituitary or hypothalamic problem.

GH

Growth hormone excess results in acromegaly in adults and giantism in children; GH deficiency is clinically significant only in children where it is associated with short stature and stunted growth. Neonatal GH deficiency is characterised by hypoglycaemia, which is particularly dangerous in this group of patients.

GH excess. Chronic hypersecretion of GH is usually due to an adenoma of the pituitary somatotrophs (these make up about 10% of all pituitary tumours) and results in acromegaly in the adult and giantism in children. The characteristic features of acromegaly are:

- coarsening of facial features
- enlargement of hands, feet, and jaw
- muscle weakness
- degenerative joint disease
- visual field defects
- thickening and coarseness of the skin
- hirsutism

Up to a third of GH-producing tumours also produce prolactin which can result in galactorrhoea. The secretion of GH is sustained in some patients and episodic in others but the clinical effects are the same and are the result of increased circulating levels of insulin-like growth factor-1 (IGF-1), the measurement of which is a useful diagnostic tool.

230

Evaluation: Serum GH levels in the normal subject fluctuate throughout the day and the estimation of random levels can be misleading when evaluating the possibility of excessive production. The usual diagnostic approach is to estimate the serum GH value one hour following a 75 g glucose load (a glucose load suppresses GH secretion); values in excess of 10 mU/L in a patient with the clinical manifestations of acromegaly sustains the diagnosis, values less than 2 mU/L essentially rules out the diagnosis. Serum IGF-1 (increased in acromegaly) can serve either as a useful confirmatory test or as a screening procedure.

Growth hormone deficiency. This is the commonest anterior pituitary hormone deficiency but is only of clinical significance in children where it results in short stature. It is usually an isolated congenital defect due to deficient production of hypothalamic GHRH; however, it can also occur in hypothalamic or pituitary disease (e.g., pituitary tumours) as part of a general acquired deficiency.

Evaluation: As in many hormone-deficient states the definitive diagnosis usually involves demonstrating the inability of the hormone level to rise in response to an appropriate stimulus. In the investigation of suspected GH deficiency there are many stimuli to choose from including hypoglycaemia, arginine infusion, L-dopa administration, exercise, and sleep. The safest and most commonly used tests are exercise provocation, multiple sampling during sleep (with an indwelling venous catheter), and serum IGF-1 estimations.

In the *'sleep' procedure* blood samples are collected at 30-minute intervals for 3-4 hours after the onset of sleep; a peak value of at least 10 mU/L occurs in the normal subject but not in the GH-deficient patient. In the *exercise test* the patient is subjected to very hard physical exercise (such as running up and down a flight of stairs or use of a bicycle ergometer so as to generate a pulse rate of >150/min), and blood is collected at 0, 2, and 20 minutes after cessation. A normal response is a GH rise to above 20 mU/L or to >10-fold the basal level.

PROLACTIN

The commonest disorder of prolactin secretion is one of excess which is often due to a pituitary tumour; prolactin deficiency is uncommon and clinically unimportant but there have been reports of lactation failure due to this abnormality.

Table 16.3. Causes of hyperprolactinaemia.

Physiological
  Exercise, Stress, Sleep,
  Suckling, Pregnancy
Pharmacological
  Oestrogens, α-methyldopa,
  Narcotics, Phenothiazines,
  Reserpine, Tricyclic antidepressants,
  Nicotine, Cimetidine
Pathological
  Prolactin-secreting tumours,
  Acromegaly, Hypothyroidism,
  Hypothalamic disease,
  Section of pituitary stalk,
  Cirrhosis, Renal failure

Prolactin excess. This is a common disorder which may be due to a large variety of causes including tumours, medications, hypothyroidism, acromegaly, renal failure (Table 16.3). Excessive circulating prolactin inhibits FSH and LH release leading to secondary gonadal failure which presents as infertility and amenorrhoea in women, and as impotence, infertility and signs of hypogonadism in men. In addition, there may be gynaecomastia and galactorrhoea. Some 30% of women with non-gestational amenorrhoea have hyperprolactinaemia; if galactorrhoea also occurs, the fraction rises to 70%.

Whilst not all patients with hyperprolactinaemia will have a tumour (Table 16.3), the most important cause of hyperprolactinaemia is a pituitary tumour and up to 65% of pituitary tumours may be associated with increased prolactin secretion.

Evaluation. The plasma PRL level can give some indication of the cause, e.g., tumours usually give values in excess of 100 ng/mL. Values in excess of 200 ng/mL, in the absence of renal failure, are strongly indicative of a PRL-secreting tumour (PRL levels increase in renal failure because of decreased clearance). A raised plasma prolactin level should always be confirmed by a repeat analysis on a fresh specimen, collected without stasis or stress.

Stimulation and suppression tests have not been found to be useful in differentiating the causes of hyperprolactinaemia; diagnosis is made either by demonstrating the presence of a tumour using techniques such as magnetic resonance imaging (MRI) or by a process of diagnostic elimination. In many cases of microadenomas, such tumours may be too small to be identified by neuroradiological techniques.

Hypopituitarism

Subjects with hypopituitarism may have single or multiple hormone deficiencies; in some cases all hormones may be deficient but there is great variation in the severity of the lesions.

Causes: The aetiology includes large lesions such as pituitary tumours (functional and non-functional), brain tumours, metastatic carcinoma, granulomas, pituitary abscess, and aneurisms; and smaller lesions due to trauma (head injury), surgery, irradiation, and haemochromatosis. Other possibilities are postpartum pituitary necrosis (Sheehan's syndrome) and auto-immune disease, both of which are rare. Pituitary tumours can also be part of the multiple endocrine adenosis type I (MEA I) syndrome with associated tumours in the parathyroid glands and pancreatic islet cells (page 287).

Clinical aspects: The clinical features are variable depending on the type of lesion and the severity of the hormone deficiencies. Fatigue, weakness, sexual dysfunction, and regression of secondary sex characteristics are the most common presenting symptoms. Amenorrhoea and galactorrhoea may be present indicating a pituitary tumour. In long-standing cases there is sparseness of axillary and pubic hair. Large lesions may produce local effects such as visual defects due to involvement of the optic nerve. Polyuria will occur if the posterior pituitary lobe is involved (diabetes insipidus).

Laboratory findings: Hypoglycaemia and hyponatraemia are common. The endocrine defects will depend on the number of pituitary hormones involved, i.e., low serum TSH and thyroid hormones, low serum ACTH and cortisol levels, low serum FSH and LH concentrations (and low serum testosterone in men), GH deficiency, or a combination thereof. The classic finding is progressive loss of pituitary hormone secretion in the following order: gonadotrophins, GH, TSH, ACTH; however, this pattern may not be followed. Prolactin deficiency is uncommon and is usually caused by pituitary infarction (e.g., Sheehan's syndrome). In the case of tumours there may be hyperprolactinaemia.

Evaluation: The demonstration of a low target hormone level in the presence of a low trophic hormone is suggestive of the disease and should be followed up by appropriate stimulation tests, e.g., GH response to exercise, TSH response to TRH administration, cortisol response to stress such as hypoglycaemia. A common procedure in use is the so called *triple function test* where the patient is administered GnRH to stimulate LH/FSH, TRH to stimulate TSH and prolactin, and insulin to produce hypoglycaemia which will stimulate ACTH and GH production (measurement of the aforementioned hormones after stimulation will produce a picture of the pituitary hormone deficiencies). However, this can be a risky procedure and should only be carried out in specialised units under close clinical supervision.

REFERENCES AND FURTHER READING

Devesa J, Lima L, Tresgurres JAF. Neuroendocrine control of growth hormone secretion. Trends in Endocrinol Metab 1992;3:175-182.

Lechnan RM. Neuroendocrinology of pituitary hormone regulation. Endocrinol Metab Clinics N Am 1987;16:475-489.

Molich MG. Pathological hyperprolactinaemia. Endocrinol Metab Clinics N Am 1992;21:877-901.

Thorner MO, Vance ML, Horvath E, Kovacs. The anterior pituitary. In Wilson JD and Foster DW (eds). *Williams' Textbook of Endocrinology, 8th edn.* Philadelphia: WB Saunders, 1992:221-310.

Chapter 17

The Thyroid Gland

The thyroid gland is composed of two lateral lobes, one on either side of the trachea joined by a thin isthmus. The basic functional unit is the follicle consisting of a colloid-filled central lumen surrounded by a single layer of cuboidal epithelial cells. Scattered throughout the gland in the interfollicular connective tissue and, in lesser numbers, within thyroid follicles, are parafollicular or C-cells. The follicular cells produce two hormones, thyroxine (T_4) and tri-iodothyronine (T_3) which influence many of the metabolic processes of the body; the C-cells secrete calcitonin, a calcium-lowering hormone.

Normal Metabolism

The thyroid gland, under the influence of the pituitary-derived thyroid stimulating hormone (TSH, page 227), synthesises the thyroid hormones from iodine and tyrosine residues, stores them in the follicular colloid, and releases them to the peripheral circulation when required. In addition to T_3 and T_4 there is an inactive product of T_4 metabolism, reverse T_3 (rT_3), found in the blood (Figure 17.2).

IODINE AND THYROID HORMONE METABOLISM

The minimum daily requirement of iodide is about 50 µg; many times this quantity may be taken in depending on its availability in the environment, principally in the diet or in pharmaceuticals. About 200-600 µg of iodide are absorbed by the gut daily and distributed in the extracellular fluid; ~70% is excreted by the kidneys whilst the remaining 30% (80-200 µg) is taken up by the thyroid gland for thyroid hormone synthesis. Besides dietary sources, iodide is released back to the ECF pool from the thyroid (~50 µg) and from peripheral iodothyronine deiodination.

The conversion of iodide into circulating thyroid hormones (iodinated thyronines) involves five distinct processes (Figure 17.1):

1. Trapping of iodide by the gland
2. Oxidation of iodide to iodine
3. Incorporation of iodine on to tyrosine residues (Organification)
4. Coupling of iodinated tyrosine residues to form thyroid hormones
5. Secretion of thyroid hormones into the peripheral circulation

Iodide trapping: Iodide in the circulation is taken into the gland by an energy-dependent process which is capable of producing a cell-to-plasma iodide gradient of 20-100:1; the process requires oxidative metabolism and phosphorylation. The salivary and mammary glands can also trap iodide but 90-95% of the body's iodide (~8000 µg under normal circumstances) is sequestered in the thyroid gland. The transport process is not specific for iodide, with anions such as pertechnetate, thiocyanate and perchlorate also being transported, and can be blocked by these competitive inhibitors of iodide transport. It is enhanced by TSH.

Oxidation and organification: The trapped iodide is rapidly oxidised to molecular iodine by peroxidases and then incorporated into the tyrosine residues of thyroglobulin, a viscid glycoprotein (MW 660,00) forming the bulk of the follicular colloid. Two types of iodinated tyrosine are formed (Figure 17.2): monoiodotyrosine (MIT) and diiodotyrosine (DIT). The organification step, which is also catalysed by peroxidase, can be blocked by the antithyroid drug carbimazole and by excessive iodine, and is enhanced by TSH stimulation. The peroxidase enzyme is a haem protein and requires molecular oxygen for its activity and is inhibited by cyanide and azide.

Coupling: The iodotyrosines can be enzymatically coupled in two ways: one molecule each of MIT and DIT produces tri-iodothyronine (T_3); two molecules of DIT produces tetra-iodothyronine (thyroxine, T_4). These reactions, of which T_4 production predominates, are also catalysed by peroxidase and are inhibited by virtually the same compounds that inhibit organification. Both hormones are stored in the colloid and released when required.

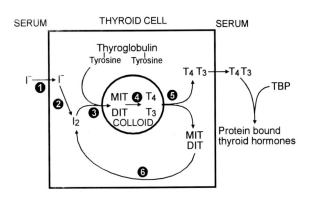

Figure 17.1. Iodine metabolism. (1) Iodide uptake and trapping, (2) Iodide oxidation, (3) Organification, (4) Coupling, (5) Pinocytosis, proteolysis and secretion of thyroid hormones, (6) Iodine salvage.

Secretion: During thyroid hormone secretion small amounts of thyroglobulin are taken up by the follicular cells (pinocytosis), and digested by proteases (after fusion with lysosomes) to release T_3 and T_4 to the circulation in the ratio of 1:5. Uncoupled MIT and DIT are also released from thyroglobulin but they are catabolised within the gland and the iodine is partly re-utilised (salvage pathway) and partly lost from the gland (the iodide leak). High intrathyroidal concentrations of iodine decrease the rate of iodide uptake and the response to TSH.

T_4 is the principal hormone synthesised and secreted by the gland (Figure 17.2). At the peripheral tissue level, particularly in the liver and kidney, about 20-30% of the secreted T_4 is converted to T_3 by β-deiodination (~80% of the circulating T_3 is produced in this manner). In many illnesses, including trauma and stress, α-deiodination occurs which has the effect of lowering the production of T_3 and producing the biologically inactive r-T_3.

CIRCULATING THYROID HORMONES

In the blood almost all of the thyroid hormones (99.95% of T_4 and 99.5% of T_3) are bound to plasma proteins (thyroid-binding proteins, TBP) which include albumin, thyroxine-binding prealbumin (TBPA), and thyroid-binding globulin (TBG). Binding of T_4 to these three carrier proteins is normally in the

ratio 10:15:75. It is the free hormones which can diffuse into the cells that are metabolically active; their concentrations are defended by homeostatic mechanisms. The bound forms act as a metabolically inert reservoir. Because the bulk of the thyroid hormones in circulation is bound, changes in the carrier protein levels (which bear no relation to thyroid function) affect the total T_3 and T_4 levels but not those of the free hormones.

T_3 is biologically more active than T_4; it is also more rapidly degraded, with a daily turnover rate of ~75%. The relative metabolic potencies and plasma half-lives of T_4 and T_3 are 0.3 and 1.0, and 6-7 days and 18-24 hours, respectively.

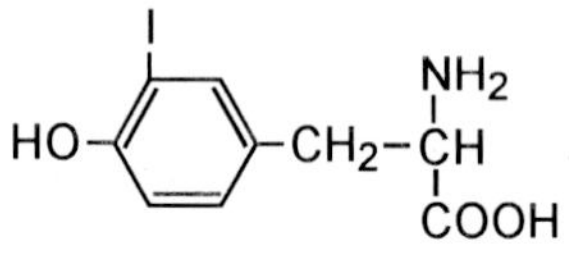

Mono-iodotyrosine (MIT)

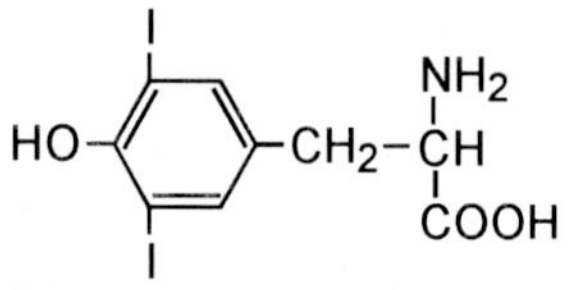

Di-iodotyrosine (DIT)

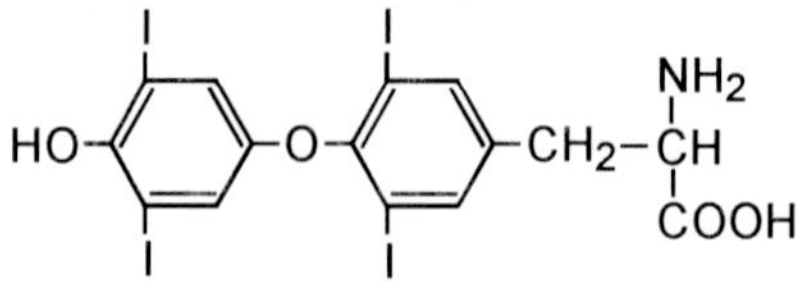

Thyroxine (T₄)

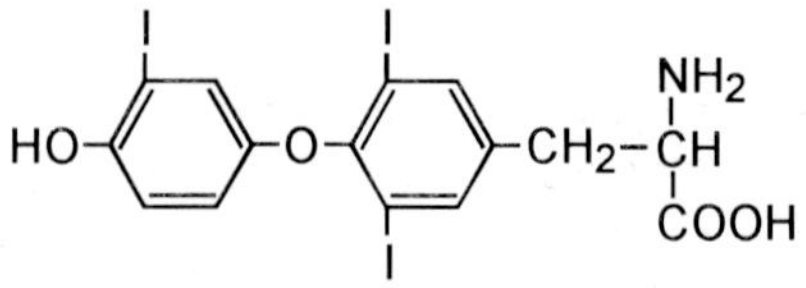

Tri-iodothyronine (T₃)

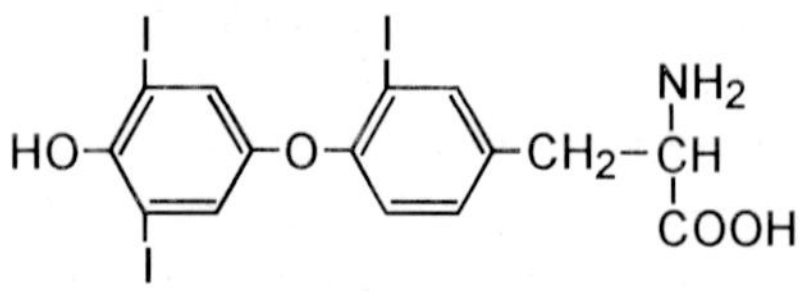

Reverse T₃ (rT₃)

Figure 17.2 Structures of iodinated tyrosine and thyronine compounds .

CONTROL OF SECRETION

Regulatory mechanisms serve to defend the near constancy of the rate of thyroid hormone synthesis over the short term (see Figure 16.3, page 227). Their secretion by the thyroid gland is stimulated by TSH which is released from the anterior pituitary in response to thyrotropin-releasing hormone (TRH, page 224). The free hormones in turn suppress both the synthesis and release of TSH by negative feedback. Several other factors, such as somatostatin, dopamine, and glucocorticoids, also reduce basal TSH secretion and inhibit TSH response to TRH, although the overall importance of their effects in regulating TSH secretion and activity is probably small.

ACTION AND METABOLISM

The thyroid hormones stimulate and speed up may metabolic activities including the metabolism of carbohydrates, lipids, and proteins. They are necessary for normal growth and development, and they increase the sensitivity of the α-receptors to circulating catecholamines. Many of the features of hyperthyroidism reflect this increased adrenergic activity.

Degradation of the thyroid hormones takes place in the liver. They are mostly deiodinated, the released iodine being returned to the extrathyroidal iodine pool and the thyronine residues further metabolised. Small amounts are conjugated with glucuronic acid and excreted in the urine and bile.

Thyrometabolic Disorders

There are two thyrometabolic disorders, hypothyroidism and thyrotoxicosis, which are characterised by low and high circulating levels of thyroid hormones, respectively. The term thyrotoxicosis is often used synonymously with hyperthyroidism but there is a subtle difference between the two. Thyrotoxicosis refers to the biochemical and physiological complex that results when the tissues are exposed to excessive circulating levels of thyroid hormones. It is the more appropriate term as the syndrome need not always originate in the thyroid gland, which is implied by the term hyperthyroidism. The latter term is best reserved for disorders in which thyrotoxicosis results from overproduction of hormones by the thyroid itself, Graves' disease being the archetype and the most common.

Disorders associated with thyrotoxicosis but without ongoing overproduction of thyroid hormones fall into two categories:

- those in which the high circulating hormone concentrations originate from non-thyroid sources, e.g., thyrotoxicosis factitia (exogenous thyroid hormone administration) and metastatic thyroid carcinoma (ectopic hyperfunctioning thyroid tissue)

- those in which inflammatory disease of the thyroid leads to leakage and loss of stored hormones into the blood, e.g., subacute thyroiditis.

Both thyrotoxicosis and hypothyroidism produce characteristic but non-specific signs and symptoms which are also common in 'normal' subjects, e.g., anxiety in thyrotoxic patients and tiredness in hypothyroid patients. Hence the necessity for, and the common performance of, thyroid function tests for the evaluation of suspected thyrometabolic disease.

A significant number of patients with thyroid disease have an autoimmune basis for their disorder and the evaluation of thyroid antibodies is a useful procedure; these will be considered first.

AUTOIMMUNE ANTIBODIES AND THYROID DISEASE

Patients with the two autoimmune thyroid disorders, Graves' disease and Hashimoto's disease (autoimmune thyroiditis), have a high frequency of antibodies against one or another thyroid antigen. The major autoimmune antibodies found in association with these disorders are those directed against thyroglobulin (TgAb), thyroid microsomal peroxidase (TMAb), and the TSH receptor (TRAb). The first two are commonly associated with autoimmune thyroiditis (Hashimoto's disease); the third, with Graves' disease.

Autoimmune thyroiditis is characterised by a goitre with diffuse lymphoid infiltration. The precise antigens and antibodies involved have not been clearly established but thyroid peroxidase and thyroglobulin antibodies are the likely candidates. Of the two, TMAb is present more frequently and usually in higher titres, particularly in younger patients (less than 20 years of age). Titres and frequency increase with age, particularly in women. TMAb is present in about 95-99%, and TgAb in about 55-85% of patients, depending on the age group.

These antibodies are not specific for Hashimoto's disease as 2-17% of normal subjects have moderately increased circulating levels of either one or both antibodies, as do subjects with Graves' disease (about 80% are TMAb-positive and 30% are TgAb-positive). They may also be associated with other autoimmune disorders such as pernicious anaemia, systemic lupus erythrematosus, and rheumatoid arthritis. However, very high serum values (e.g., titres >1: 25600) strongly support a diagnosis of autoimmune thyroiditis.

Graves' disease, a common cause of thyrotoxicosis, is now considered as an organ-specific autoimmune disorder. It is characterised by the presence of antibodies directed against the TSH receptor (TRAb). These are IgG antibodies that bind to the antigenic (TSH receptor) region of the thyroid cell membrane and activate adenylate cyclase which promotes thyroid growth and hypersecretion. As stated above Graves' disease is also often associated with high titres of TMAb and TgAb.

Thyrotoxicosis

High plasma levels of total T_4 and T_3 (Table 17.1) are not always associated with thyrotoxicosis because the plasma levels of the biologically active free hormones can be normal in disorders associated with high levels of thyroxine-binding proteins. In cases of peripheral resistance to thyroid hormones, the high plasma levels of free thyroid hormones are ineffective.

The effects of an excess of thyroid hormones on organ systems are common to thyrotoxic states regardless of their underlying causes. Increased thyroid hormone activity affects many metabolic processes and results in numerous non-specific *clinical features* including:

- Increased appetite, weight loss, diarrhoea
- Emotional lability, heat intolerance
- Increased adrenergic activity: tachycardia, fine finger tremor, warm moist skin.
- Eye signs: exophthalmos, lid lag
- Goitre (often with a bruit due to increased vascularity)

The *biochemical features* of thyrotoxic states include:

- High plasma levels of free T_4 and T_3 (and usually increased total T_4 and T_3 levels)
- Low plasma concentration of TSH (negative feedback on thyroid and pituitary by thyroid hormones)
- Flat TSH response to TRH stimulation
- Hypocholesterolaemia (increased cholesterol metabolism) -- not present in all case
- Increased metabolic rate

The three most common hyperthyroid disorders are Graves' disease (70-80%), multinodular goitre (~10%), and toxic adenoma (~5%).

Table 17.1. Causes of high plasma levels of thyroid hormones.

Thyrotoxicosis
 Thyroid overactivity
  Graves' disease, toxic multinodular goitre, toxic adenoma, TSH-secreting tumour (rare)
 Thyroid destruction (with release of hormone)
  Subacute thyroiditis, Hashimoto's thyroiditis
 Ectopic thyroid hormone production (rare)
  Struma ovarii, metastatic thyroid carcinoma
 Exogenous thyroxine
  Thyrotoxicosis factitia, iatrogenic

Euthyroid hyperthyroxinaemia
 Increased thyroxine-binding proteins
  Congenital, pregnancy, oestrogen therapy, familial dysalbuminaemic hyperthyroxinaemia
 Peripheral resistance to thyroid hormones

Graves' disease

This is due to an autoimmune process whereby an IgG antibody (TRAb) attaches to the TSH receptor and stimulates gland growth (goitre) and hypersecretion. The autoimmune process may also result in swelling of tissues behind the eye causing exophthalmos and pretibial swelling (infiltrative dermopathy, pretibial myxoedema). In some cases the infiltrative eye problem may be of a much greater extent than the thyroid problem; in any one case, the ophthalmopathy may or may not manifest together with the thyrotoxic component.

It is the most common cause of spontaneous hyperthyroidism in patients less than 40 years old. There appears to be a genetic predisposition to the disease in people with certain histocompatibility antigens (HLA) and the prevalence is higher in women than in men (approximately 8:1). In women, it tends to become manifest during puberty, pregnancy, and the menopause. This implies an influence by physiological factors related to reproductive function. In men, the disease occurs at a later age and tends to be more severe. There is an increased incidence of other autoimmune disorders, such as Hashimoto's disease, pernicious anaemia, rheumatoid arthritis, etc.

Laboratory evaluation. The patient who displays all the major manifestations of the disease (thyrotoxicosis, goitre, and infiltrative opthalmology) does not pose a diagnostic problem. It is in the borderline case of thyrotoxicosis that the laboratory tests are of greatest utility, in particular, the tests of thyroregulatory mechanisms. There is an override of normal regulatory control by the action of abnormal stimulatory immunoglobulins. The serum TSH level is suppressed and there is no response to TRH stimulation. The presence of TRAb in the serum strongly suggests Graves' disease.

Two notable points regarding TRAb titres in relation to Graves' disease deserve mention.

- In the pregnant patient with Graves' disease, an elevated titre of TRAb raise the likelihood of neonatal thyrotoxicosis in the offspring.

- In patients with established disease completing a course of antithyroidal drug therapy, absence or suppression of TRAb augurs well for a long-term remission after withdrawal of therapy.

Toxic multinodular goitre

This occurs in patients of an older age group and predominantly in women. It is probably caused by the development of autonomous hypersecretion in localised areas of a long-standing non-toxic goitre, or stimulation by TRAb, which is detectable in about 20% of cases. The disorder emerges slowly and insidiously from its forerunner, a non-toxic multinodular goitre. The two hallmarks of the disease, reflecting its natural history of development, are structural and functional heterogeneity and functional autonomy.

Laboratory evaluation. The main clinical problem is to determine whether the patient with a multinodular goitre is thyrotoxic. The most appropriate laboratory test to use for resolving the issue is the serum TSH concentration (supersensitive assay, see page 244). If this is suppressed (to less than 0.1 mU/L), and especially if free T_4 is elevated as well hyperthyroidism is confirmed. Serum TSH levels between 0.1 and 0.4 mU/L suggest thyroid autonomy but no frank thyrotoxicosis. The increase in serum T_4 and T_3 are only marginal and the clinical manifestations are not as marked compared to Graves' disease. The two hallmarks of the condition produce characteristic patterns in scintiscans and autoradiographs of excised tissues, and serve as good diagnostic tools.

Toxic adenoma

This far less common form of hyperthyroidism is produced by one or (rarely) more adenomas in an otherwise intrinsically normal thyroid gland. The adenoma is usually solitary, palpable, and autonomous in function. The natural course is one of slow, progressive growth and increasing hypersecretion over many years. Some time may elapse before the patient manifests overt thyrotoxicosis. As toxic adenomas are autonomously functional, serum TSH concentrations are not raised (see below). The extranodular tissue, which becomes increasingly suppressed, generally retains its capacity to function if TSH is provided, and does so on ablation of the nodule, with or without exogenous TSH administration. The disease occurs in a younger age group than does toxic multinodular goitre.

Laboratory evaluation. Results of laboratory tests depend on the stage of the disorder. In the early stages, all indices may be normal, with the exception of a borderline suppression of the serum TSH in some cases. At a later stage, TSH secretion becomes subnormal, with elevated serum thyroid hormone concentrations and abnormal metabolic indices. Occassionally, serum T_3 concentration alone is increased (T_3 toxicosis). The toxic adenoma may be detectable in the scintiscan as a localised zone of increased radioiodine accumulation ("hot" nodule). The availability of supersensitive TSH assays in recent years has made laboratory diagnosis of the disease less dependant on scintiscanning techniques.

T_3 toxicosis

In some cases of thyrotoxicosis, the only biochemical abnormality, other than a suppressed serum TSH, is a

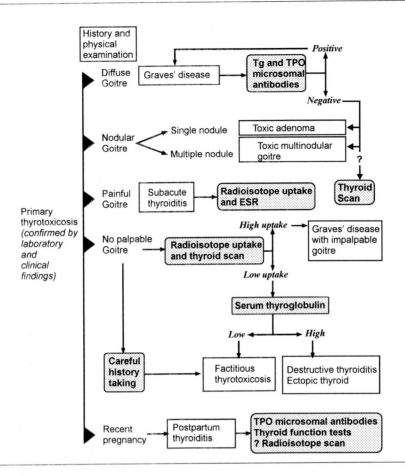

Figure 17.3. A check-list for the evaluation of the thyrotoxic patient.

high circulating T_3. It probably represents an early stage in thyrotoxicosis (before there is an increased T_4). The T_3 appears to be secreted by the gland rather than originating in increased peripheral conversion of T_4. This disease is more common in geographical areas associated with iodine deficiency.

TSH-secreting tumours

A TSH-secreting pituitary adenoma is a rare occurrence and treatment usually requires surgical resection.

Laboratory evaluation. A mass lesion in the pituitary may be detectable. Serum TSH concentrations are invariably raised. Together with cases of thyroid hormone resistance, this is the only other thyrotoxic condition in which serum TSH concentrations are not suppressed in the face of elevated free T_4 and/or T_3 concentrations. An unusual feature is the finding of

elevated levels of free alpha subunits of TSH in the patients' sera.

Thyroiditis

In the early stages of subacute thyroiditis (de Quervain's disease) and Hashimoto's disease (see below), the destruction of the gland is associated with release of some of its contents including thyroid hormones. This can result in thyrotoxicosis, with many of the clinical and biochemical features described above (page 236).

Thyrotoxicosis factitia

This form of thyrotoxicosis arises from ingestion, often surrepticious, at times iatrogenic (usually as part of a regimen for weight reduction), of excessive quantities of thyroid hormone. Diagnosis may be made difficult by the patients not admitting to taking the hormone supplement. Such patients are often women with a background of psychiatric disease, or those for whom thyroid hormone supplement was prescribed previously. Typical thyrotoxic manifestations, often severe, are found together with evidence of thyroid atrophy and hypofunction.

Laboratory evaluation. Increased serum T_3 and T_4 concentrations (note: the latter is not raised in those taking T_3), and *low* serum thyroglobulin concentrations suggest that thyrotoxicosis results from exogenous rather than endogenous hormone sources. Subnormal values of the radioiodine uptake test, which can be increased by administration of TSH, are characteristic.

Binding protein abnormalities

High plasma levels of total T_4 associated with euthyroidism are generally due to increased circulating levels of thyroxine-binding proteins. The plasma free hormone and TSH levels are normal. Increased binding proteins are generally due to increased liver synthesis consequent to oestrogen excess (therapy, pregnancy, oral contraceptives). Congenital excess may also occur. An unusual condition is *familial dysalbuminaemic hyperthyroxaemia* (FDH) in which there is an increase in an albumin fraction, which is present in normal sera, that has an unusually high affinity for T_4. It is inherited as an autosomal dominant trait and presents with a high total T_4 but normal free T_4 values. T_3 levels remain normal as albumin has a low afinity for T_3.

Thyroid hormone resistance

This condition, in its severest form, presents with deaf-mutism, skeletal abnormalities, goitre, and a euthyroid state. The serum free T_4 and T_3 levels are increased, the latter more so than the former, and the serum TSH is normal or slightly raised. This is due to preferential synthesis of T_3 by residual functioning thyroid tissue under stimulation by TSH. Increased T_4-to-T_3 conversion with falling serum T_4 levels may be a contributing factor. There are two types of the disorder:

1. General resistance to thyroid hormones presenting with goitre and high serum thyroid hormone levels. The subjects are euthyroid but can be slightly hypothyroid.

2. Isolated pituitary resistance producing hyperthyroidism and varying degrees of inappropriately raised TSH levels.

Hypothyroidism

Low levels of circulating thyroid hormones (Table 17.2) may be due to decreased synthesis associated with hypothyroidism or due to transport protein deficiency and associated with euthyroidism. A convenient classification of the causes of hypothyroidism divides them into three categories:

1. Loss or atrophy of thyroid tissue (thyroprivic hypothyroidism)
2. Compensatory goitrogenesis as a result of defective hormone synthesis (goitrous hypothyroidism)
3. Inadequate stimulation of an intrinsically normal gland due to hypothalamic or pituitary disease (trophoprivic hypothyroidism)

The first two categories account for ~95% of cases and are subgroups of primary hypothyroidism.

As in hyperthyroidism the **clinical features** of hypothyroidism are legion and non-specific, some of which are listed below. The extent of the clinical manifestations is more dependant on the degree of thyroid hormone deficiency rather than the underlying disorder, a decrease in secretion of the thyroid hormones being common to all types of hypothyroidism, irrespective of the underlying cause. Hypothyroid patients often present with:

- Loss of appetite, weight gain, constipation
- Mental slowness, cold intolerance
- Dry skin and hair, facial puffiness
- Bradycardia

The **biochemical features,** reflected in the laboratory test results, include:

- Low plasma levels of total and free T_4 (total and free T_3 are often normal).
- High serum TSH levels in primary hypothyroidism (loss of negative feedback regulation) and low TSH levels in disorders secondary to pituitary failure.

239

- Elevated TMAb and TgAb antibodies (common in Hashimoto's thyroiditis)
- Raised serum cholesterol (decreased metabolism)
- Raised serum prolactin levels in primary hypothyroidism (TRH-driven, see page 228)
- Often raised serum creatine kinase levels (? decreased plasma clearance)

Table 17.2. Causes of low circulating thyroid hormones.

Hypothyroidism
Loss of thyroid tissue (high TSH)
    Thyroidectomy, radioactive iodine therapy, dyshormonogenesis, congenital thyroid agenesis, idiopathic
Goitrous (high TSH)
    Synthesis defect: in organification, coupling, etc
    Autoimmune: Hashimoto's disease
    Drugs: carbimazole, propylthiouracil, lithium
    Dietary: severe iodine deficiency
Hypothalamic-pituitary disease
    Tumours, abscess, granuloma, etc
    Panhypopituitarism (Sheehan's syndrome)
    Isolated TSH deficiency

Euthyroidism
Thyroxine-binding protein deficiency
    Congenital, androgen or glucocorticoid therapy, severe liver disease, protein-losing states
Miscellaneous
    Sick euthyroid syndrome, inadequate replacement therapy, drug displacement of T_4 from proteins (penicillin, salicylates)

PRIMARY HYPOTHYROIDISM

In primary hypothyroidism, the thyroid gland is at fault (not secondary to pituitary or hypothalamic disease). It may be due to destruction of the gland (Hashimoto's disease, thyroid ablation by surgery or radioactive iodine), in which case it may not be palpable. On the other hand, if there is no structural problem and the thyroid can respond to TSH it will be enlarged (goitre). This can occur in dyshormono-genesis (enzyme deficiencies), antithyroid drug therapy, and in very severe iodine deficiency.

Hashimoto's (autoimmune) thyroiditis

This autoimmune disease includes a group of overlapping varieties with differing degrees of severity. There is diffuse infiltration of the thyroid tissue by lymphocytes and plasma cells, a variable degree of destruction of thyroid architecture, and fibrosis. Initially there is usually a brief period of thyrotoxicosis due to destruction of follicles, with release of their contents including preformed thyroid hormones. As destruction progresses, hypothyroidism develops.

Laboratory diagnosis. High titres of antiperoxidase antibodies (TMAb) are found in most cases whereas high titres of antithyroglobulin antibodies (TgAb) are less common. Plasma T_4 levels are low during the hypothyroid phase but the plasma T_3 levels are often normal; the serum TSH level is elevated (e.g., to >20 mU/L). Serum cholesterol is usually increased.

Postablative hypothyroidism

Hypothyroidism invariably develops after total thyroidectomy. It is also common (>30% frequency) following subtotal resection of the diffuse goitre in Graves' disease. The severity of hypothyroidism is related to the amount of tissue removed and the patient usually becomes hypothyroid within the first year after surgery. The incidence of post-radioiodine hypo-thyroidism increases progressively with time. Some of the milder cases may go into remission.

Congenital and developmental defects

Development defects of the thyroid are responsible for most cases of congenital hypothyroidism in the neonate (1 in every 4000-5000 births). They include:

- the complete absence of thyroid tissue
- failure of the gland to descend to its normal site during embryological development
- biosynthetic defects (less frequent cause)

Failure to treat promptly results in development of full-blown cretinism. Neonatal screening programmes are set up to avert this problem. Whilst costly, the benefits derived from such programmes are enormous.

SUBCLINICAL HYPOTHYROIDISM

This label describes the patient with: (a) no clinical evidence of thyroid disease (euthyroid), (b) normal, or sometimes slightly depressed, serum free T_4 values, and (c) a mildly elevated TSH in the range of 4-15 mU/L (see below). The inference is that the patient is at an early stage of thyroid failure and has diminished thyroid reserve. Studies have shown that the progression to overt hypothyroidism is at a rate of less than 5% per year and that this progress is more likely if the subject has high serum levels of antiperoxidase antibody (TMAb).

TROPHOPRIVIC HYPOTHYROIDISM

Pituitary (secondary) hypothyroidism

Decreased thyroid hormone secretion and thyroid atrophy is consequent to TSH deficiency, and this type of hypothyroidism is much less common than thyroidal (primary) hypothyroidism. It may be caused by destruction of the pituitary thyrotrophs by space-encroaching macroadenomas; from postpartum pituitary necrosis (Sheehan's syndrome), trauma and infiltrative processes. TSH deficiency may occur as an isolated deficiency (rarely) or in conjunction with deficiencies of other tropic hormones (panhypopituitarism). The differentiation of secondary hypothyroidism from primary hypothyroidism is important from the therapeutic viewpoint. Failure to recognise the former may lead to disastrous consequences for the patient when thyroid replacement is given without coverage for the concomitant adrenal cortical insufficiency that may accompany the hypothyroidism.

Laboratory evaluation. Conclusive differentiation depends on the results of laboratory tests, with measurement of either serum TSH (if the super-sensitive immunometric assay is available), and/or the TRH stimulation test. Serum TSH levels are usually suppressed and may be undetectable, and there is little, if any, increment in TSH secretion following TRH administration. In intrinsic thyroid failure, the basal serum TSH is invariably high, and often very much so, obviating the need for a TRH stimulation test in this situation (Figure 17.4).

As stated above, the availability of supersensitive

TSH assays that are capable of measuring low levels of TSH accurately (down to 0.1 mU/L) has superceded the use of TRH stimulation for diagnosing pituitary hypothyroidism. However, the TSH response to exogenous TRH may provide useful information for distinguishing between hypothalamic hypothyroidism (normal but somewhat delayed response) and pituitary hypothyroidism (blunted response). Figure 17.4 depicts an ideal differentiation but in practice, the results may also be equivocal and thus may not be too helpful.

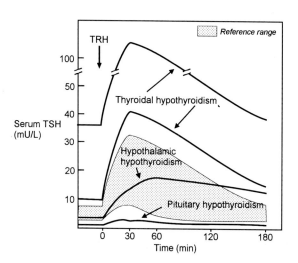

Figure 17.4. Typical serum TSH responses to TRH in patients with thyroidal (primary), pituitary (secondary) and hypothalamic (tertiary) hypothyroidism.
Modified from Utiger RD. In: Ingbar SH, Braverman LE (eds). *The Thyroid*, 5th edn., J.B. Lippincott, Philadelphia, 1986, p 515.

HYPOTHALAMIC (TERTIARY) HYPOTHYROIDISM

TRH deficiency also causes hypothyroidism, although more rarely. As with TSH deficiency, TRH deficiency may be isolated or may occur in association with other hypothalamic hormone deficiencies. It may arise as a result of trauma to, or infiltration or malignancy of, hypothalamic tissue; hypothalamic stalk resection; or lesions interrupting the hypothalamic-pituitary portal circulation.

Laboratory evaluation. Basal serum TSH levels are low or normal. A more diagnostic feature is a serum TSH response to TRH administration which is of normal magnitude but delayed in time (Figure 17.4), perhaps the last vestige of the usefulness of this dynamic test.

Binding protein abnormalities

A decrease in the amount of serum protein-bound T_4 (but not serum free T_4) may occur in two situations:

- *Decreased levels of TBG:* congenital deficiency; decreased synthesis (anabolic steroids, glucocorticoids); protein-losing states

- *Displacement of T_4 from TBG:* drugs (salicylate, penicillin, phenytoin)

In these cases the serum free T_4 and TSH levels are normal and the patient is euthyroid.

The sick euthyroid syndrome

Varying abnormalities of thyroid function, some profound, can occur in patients with non-thyroidal illness. Most reflect abnormalities in transport and peripheral metabolism of the thyroid hormones and are characterised by low levels of total and free hormones in the serum. Common to all is a decline in the conversion of T_4 to T_3 with increased metabolism of T_4 to reverse T_3 (rT_3). The serum thyroid hormone levels are variable and may include:

- Low levels of free and total T_3
- Increased levels of rT_3
- Low normal to low levels of total and free T_4; these parameters may rarely be increased
- TSH usually normal but may be suppressed during the illness and slightly elevated during recovery

The associated clinical disorders include:

1 Acute disorders: febrile illness, myocardial infarction, respiratory failure, major surgery

2 Chronic diseases: cirrhosis, renal failure
3 Starvation/calorie deprivation

It is important to recognise the effects of nonthyroidal illnesses on thyroid function parameters and that no further investigation or specific treatment in relation to thyroid function are required.

DRUGS AND THE THYROID

A large variety of drugs can affect thyroid function (some severely), serum TBG levels, and the peripheral metabolism of thyroxine. Only the more common ones will be discussed.

Antithyroid drugs

Iodine: Small doses have little or no effect but as the dose increases organic binding and production of iodothyronines are depressed; hence its use in the emergency treatment of severe thyrotoxicosis (thyroid storm).

Thiocyanate & Perchlorate: These monovalent ions inhibit iodide transport into the thyroid cell and decreases thyroxine production. They are too toxic to be used as therapeutic agents.

Carbimazole & Propylthiouracil (PTU): These agents are used in the treatment of thyrotoxicosis and act by inhibiting the organic binding and coupling reactions.

Drugs affecting TBG levels

Androgens, glucocorticoids: Decreased synthesis
Oestrogen preparations: Increased synthesis

Miscellaneous

Lithium: Interferes with TSH action at the adenylate cyclase level and can result in hypothyroidism in chronic users. It accentuates any predisposition to goitre.

Phenytoin: May result in a low circulating T_4 without any increase in the serum TSH. The precise cause is unclear but appears to be part of a complex drug interaction with the pituitary-thyroid axis.

Amiodarone: This drug produces symptomatic hyperthyroidism in up to 2.5% of users (? related to release of iodine during metabolism of the drug). High serum levels of total T_4 and free T_4 are normally seen in subjects on the drug which is due to inhibition of 5-monodeiodinase (conversion of T_4 to T_3).; thus in diagnosing amiodarone-related hyperthyroidism it is essential to demonstrate a depressed serum TSH. The drug may also be associated with hypothyroidism, particularly if thyroid antiperoxidase antibodies (TMAb) are present.

Propranolol: This agent inhibits 5-monodeiodinase activity resulting in a decreased T_3 level and an increased reverse T_3 concentration.

Cholecystographic agents: A number of the agents used in radiological examination of the gall bladder, such as iopanoic acid and sodium ipodipate, inhibit the peripheral conversion of T_4 to T_3 in similar manner to amiodarone and propranolol.

THYROID FUNCTION TESTS

In most medical units the front-line thyroid function tests include an estimation of the serum TSH and the circulating free T_4 (direct or indirect estimation, see below). However, there have been recent moves to 'screen' patients with suspected thyrometabolic disease by estimating the serum TSH only and proceeding onto a T_4 estimation if the TSH is either suppressed or elevated. Estimations of the serum T_3 are not routinely used but are useful in certain situations (see below).

Serum total and free T_4

Reference range levels of total (free plus protein-bound) T_4 is of the order of 60 to160 nmol/L. Levels are increased in thyrotoxicosis and decreased in hypothyroidism; however, because of protein binding abnormalities it is possible to have normal total hormone values in thyrometabolic disease and high and low values in euthyroid subjects. Before the advent of improved free hormone assays, a derived index which includes an estimation of the circulating bound hormone, the Free Thyroxine Index (FTI), was developed to overcome this problem of varying protein binding.

Free thyroxine index (FTI)

Free protein binding sites are estimated by measuring the T_3 resin uptake (T_3RU): Patient's plasma is equilibrated with a known quantity of radioactive T_3 which binds to the unoccupied thyroxine binding sites. The unbound radioactive T_3 is 'mopped-up' by adding a resin. This resin (+ unbound T_3) is separated from the mixture and the amount of radioactivity it contains is measured and reported as a proportion of the total added radioactivity. Normally the T_3RU is of the order of 25-35%, varying with the assay. Higher values indicate low numbers of binding sites (as occurs in thyrotoxicosis and decreased binding protein levels) and low values indicate increased number of binding sites (hypothyroidism and increased binding proteins). The FTI is then determined by multiplying the total T_4 by the T_3RU. Low FTI values occur in hypothyroidism, high values indicate hyperthyroidism, and normal values will occur in euthyroid subjects with binding protein abnormalities.

Free T_4

Although a useful test, the FTI has been replaced by methods which estimate the free T_4 and are not influenced by binding protein abnormalities. These methods are in wide use and are generally reliable; however, there are still some technical problems to overcome, e.g., interference by circulating antibodies.

The normal serum level of free T_4 is around 12-20 pmol/L. High values occur in thyrotoxicosis and low values in hypothyroidism. In the sick euthyroid syndrome the values are generally normal but a number will have low values, and a smaller percentage will have high values.

Serum T_3

Both serum total and free T_3 are readily measured in the laboratory and are useful in the following two situations:

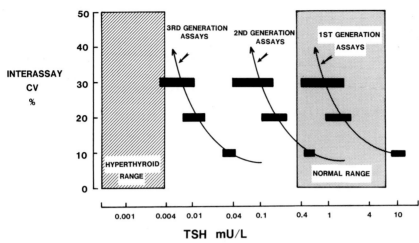

Figure 17.5. The development of TSH assays with greater sensitivity.

With the 2nd and 3rd generation TSH assays, it is possible to distinguish between normal TSH concentrations and the suppressed concentrations in hyperthyroidism. Each generation of assays represents a ten-fold improvement in diagnostic sensitivity, at the 20% interassay coefficient of variation level. The black bars denote the 95% confidence limits of measurement of different TSH concentrations. (From Nicoloff JT, Spencer CA. The use and misuse of the sensitive thyrotropin assays. J Clin Endocrinol Metab 1990; 71:553-558. ©The Endocrine Society)

- T_3-*toxicosis* where a clinically thyrotoxic patient presents with a normal free T_4 and a suppressed serum TSH.

- *Thyrotoxicosis factitia* where the offending medication is tri-iodothyronine and the subject's thyroid function tests exhibit suppression of both T_4 and TSH.

Thyroid stimulating hormone (TSH)

Reference values for TSH depend on the population studied and more importantly on the type of assay performed. Prior to the recent development of the 'supersensitive' TSH (sTSH) assays the lower limit of the assay's working range was of the order of 1.0 mU/L. The second generation sTSH assays were able to measure down to 0.1 mU/L and the more recent third generation assays down to 0.01 mU/L (Figure 17.5). With the sTSH assay a reference range of around 0.15-3.0 mU/L is applicable. Levels <0.15 mU/L are considered to be suppressed and levels above ~4.0 units represent elevation.

Suppressed values (<0.15 mU/L) are characteristic of thyrotoxicosis (suppression by thyroid hormone feedback on the anterior pituitary and hypothalamus). However, there are a number of non-thyrotoxic conditions that may be associated with suppressed TSH levels (see below). In one recent study 17% of subjects with suppressed serum TSH values had non-thyroidal causes.

- Pituitary failure (associated with low serum free T_4).
- During the first trimester of pregnancy
- Glucocorticoid and dopamine administration
- Acute psychiatric illness (acute depression, acute paranoid psychosis, hyperemesis gravidarum)
- Sick euthyroid syndrome
- 3-5% of 'normal' subjects over the age of 60 years

Elevated serum TSH values indicate primary hypothyroidism (except for the rare TSH-secreting tumour). Values in excess of 20 mU/L are generally found in subjects with overt clinical features of hypothyroidism (and low serum free T_4 values). Values in the area 4.0-15 mU/L (generally associated with a 'normal' serum free T_4 level) indicate subclinical hypothyroidism (see above).

There have been recent moves, cost-initiated, to screen suspected thyrometabolic disease with a single serum TSH estimation; Figures 17.6 and 17.7 outline this approach to the laboratory diagnosis of thyroid disease using the serum TSH as a first-line test.

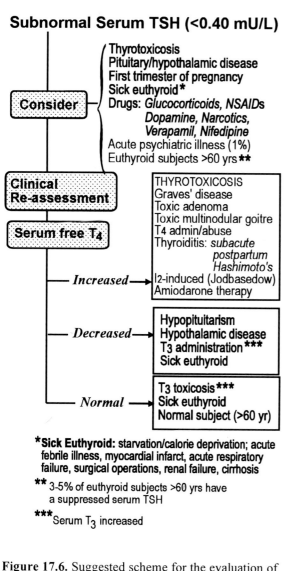

Subnormal Serum TSH (<0.40 mU/L)

Consider —
Thyrotoxicosis
Pituitary/hypothalamic disease
First trimester of pregnancy
Sick euthyroid*
Drugs: *Glucocorticoids, NSAIDs*
Dopamine, Narcotics,
Verapamil, Nifedipine
Acute psychiatric illness (1%)
Euthyroid subjects >60 yrs **

Clinical Re-assessment

Serum free T₄

Increased — THYROTOXICOSIS
Graves' disease
Toxic adenoma
Toxic multinodular goitre
T4 admin/abuse
Thyroiditis: *subacute*
postpartum
Hashimoto's
I2-induced (Jodbasedow)
Amiodarone therapy

Decreased — Hypopituitarism
Hypothalamic disease
T3 administration ***
Sick euthyroid

Normal — T3 toxicosis ***
Sick euthyroid
Normal subject (>60 yr)

*Sick Euthyroid: starvation/calorie deprivation; acute febrile illness, myocardial infarct, acute respiratory failure, surgical operations, renal failure, cirrhosis

** 3-5% of euthyroid subjects >60 yrs have a suppressed serum TSH

*** Serum T3 increased

Figure 17.6. Suggested scheme for the evaluation of a suppressed TSH

TRH stimulation test

This test was initially used to assess TSH reserve by using exogenous TRH (200 μg in 2 mL saline, iv) to amplify the TSH signal, and to assess the feedback inhibition by circulating thyroid hormones. Three blood samples are drawn for TSH measurement -- at 0 min (basal TSH specimen), and at 20 min and 60 min after TRH administration. Thyrotoxic patients will not exhibit any response to the TRH injection, due to the

negative feedback inhibition. The need to use this test to exclude hyperthyroidism has been erased with the development of the sTSH assays, as discussed above.

However, it is still useful in two situations:

* to distinguish between pituitary (secondary) and hypothalamic (tertiary) hypothyroidism in both of which the serum T₄ level is low and the TSH is either low or within the reference range (see page 241 for this use)

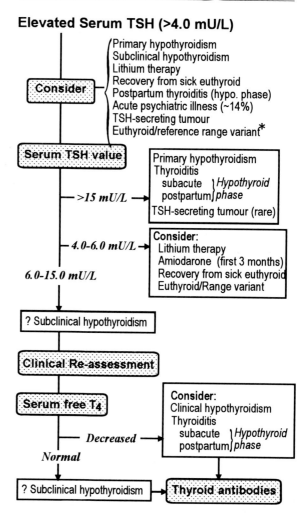

Elevated Serum TSH (>4.0 mU/L)

Consider —
Primary hypothyroidism
Subclinical hypothyroidism
Lithium therapy
Recovery from sick euthyroid
Postpartum thyroiditis (hypo. phase)
Acute psychiatric illness (~14%)
TSH-secreting tumour
Euthyroid/reference range variant*

Serum TSH value

>15 mU/L → Primary hypothyroidism
Thyroiditis
subacute |*Hypothyroid*
postpartum |*phase*
TSH-secreting tumour (rare)

4.0-6.0 mU/L → Consider:
Lithium therapy
Amiodarone (first 3 months)
Recovery from sick euthyroid
Euthyroid/Range variant

6.0-15.0 mU/L
↓
? Subclinical hypothyroidism
↓
Clinical Re-assessment
↓
Serum free T₄

Decreased → Consider:
Clinical hypothyroidism
Thyroiditis
subacute |*Hypothyroid*
postpartum |*phase*

Normal
↓
? Subclinical hypothyroidism → **Thyroid antibodies**

*Around 2% of elderly have an elevated TSH. Upper reference limit is difficult to define--skewed distribution and outliers are common--value lies between 3.0-6.0 mU/L.

Figure 17.7. Suggested scheme for the evaluation of an increased TSH.

- as an aid in the differential diagnosis of a patient with elevated serum thyroid hormone levels and 'normal' serum TSH. The absence of a TSH response could be compatible with either hyperthyroidism or an adenoma of the pituitary thyrotrophs (rare). An adequate response, on the other hand, suggest possible pituitary resistance to thyroid hormones.

REFERENCES/FURTHER READING

Cavlieri RR and Gerard SK. Unusual types of thyrotoxicosis. Adv Intern Med 1991;36:272-286.

Cooper DS. Subclinical hypothyroidism (editorial) JAMA 1987;258:246-247.

Docter R, Krenning EP, de Jong M. The sick euthyroid syndrome: Changes in thyroid hormone serum parameters and hormone metabolism. Clin Endocrinol 1993;39:499-518.

Jordan RM. Myxedema coma. Pathophysiology, therapy, and factors affecting prognosis. Med Clinics North Am 1995;79:185-194.

McDougall IR. Graves' disease: Current concepts. Med Clinics North Am 1991;75:79-84

Nicoloff JT, Spenser CA. The use and misuse of sensitive thyrotropin assays. J Clin Endocrinol Metab 1990;71:553-557.

Tietgens ST, Leinung MC. Thyroid storm. Med Clinics North Am 1995;79:169-184.

Chapter 18

The Adrenal Cortex

The adrenal glands are located behind the peritoneum immediately above and posteromedial to the kidneys. Each gland weighs 4-5 g and consists of an outer cortex (90%) which is of mesodermal origin and an inner medulla derived from ectodermal tissue (page 295). The cortex produces mineralocorticoids (aldosterone, page 62), glucocorticoids (cortisol), and androgens (testosterone, androstenedione, dehydroepi-androsterone), and some oestrogens. These hormones are all steroids which are lipid soluble; thus they can readily enter cells where they bind to specific receptors to produce their effects.

Normal physiology

The adult adrenal cortex is composed of three distinct anatomical zones: an outer glomerulosa (15%), a mid fasciculata (~70%), and an inner reticularis (~15%). Aldosterone is produced in the zona glomerulosa (but not cortisol or androgens as this area lacks the enzyme 17α-hydroxylase, see below). Cortisol is produced in both the zona fasciculata and the zona reticularis. The zona fasciculata is also the site of androgen production; it is prominent during foetal life producing large amounts of dehydroepiandrosterone sulphate (DHEAS) which is converted by placental sulphatases to DHEA, the precursor of maternal oestrogens.

The common precursor of all adrenal steroids is cholesterol (Figure 18.1) which is derived either from *de novo* synthesis or from uptake of plasma LDL cholesterol, the latter predominating. The cholesterol is transported to the inner mitochondrial membrane where the cholesterol side-chain cleavage enzyme (P-450scc, page 63) converts it to pregnenolone which then leaves the mitochondria for the smooth endoplasmic reticulum. A series of further enzymatic steps converts pregnenolone into steroids with glucocorticoid, mineralocorticoid, or androgen activity. Specific inherited enzyme defects result in the aberrant synthesis of one or more of these three classes of adrenal steroids. Because pregnenolone is a common precursor for all three classes, relative or absolute blockade of one pathway results in overflow synthesis of the other adrenal steroids.

CORTISOL SYNTHESIS

In the endoplasmic reticulum pregnenolone is converted to 11-deoxycortisol by two pathways:

Major path

Pregnenolone → 17α-OH Pregnenolone *(17α-hydroxylase)* → 17α-OH Progesterone *(3β-HSD)* → 11-deoxycortisol *(21-hydroxylase)*

Minor path

Pregnenolone → Progesterone *(3β-HSD)*
→ 17α-OH Progesterone *(17α-hydroxylase)*
→ 11-deoxycortisol *(21-hydroxylase)*

The intermediate metabolite 11-deoxycortisol is then converted to cortisol by the mitochondrial enzyme, *11β-hydroxylase*.

Note. (1) The first and last steps of the biosynthetic pathways occur in the mitochondria, the remainder in the endoplasmic reticulum. (2) All enzymes, except *3β-hydroxysteroid dehydrogenase (Δ^5-oxysteroid isomerase)*, are members of the cytochrome P450 group of mixed oxidases (Table 4.1, page 63).

PLASMA CORTISOL

Cortisol circulates in the plasma largely bound to two carrier proteins, cortisol-binding globulin (CBG) and albumin. The bound fraction constitutes 90-98% of the total (CBG~85%, albumin 5-10%); only the free or unbound cortisol fraction is physiologically active. Albumin has a low affinity but a high capacity for the hormone and is the most important carrier when supra-physiological amounts of cortisol are present. One function of the binding proteins, and perhaps the major one, is to act as a reservoir to ensure uniform hormone distribution among all the target cells; another function is perhaps to protect the hormone from inactivation by the tissues.

CBG is a glycoprotein synthesised primarily in the liver. It has a single steroid-binding site which has equal affinity for cortisol and progesterone. Oestrogen

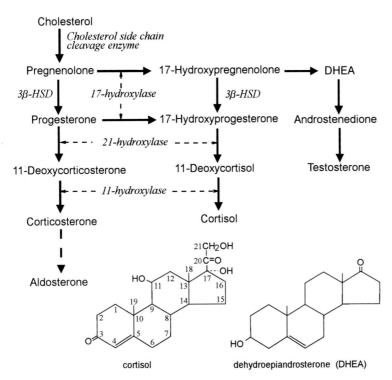

Figure 18.1. Adrenal steroidogenesis. See text for details.

3β-HSD 3β-hydroxysteroid dehydrogenase, Δ5-isomerase

excess, such as during pregnancy and in subjects on exogenous oestrogen therapy, are associated with increased CBG production; this may result in up to a two-fold increase in the plasma CBG level causing high bound and total plasma cortisol values, but the free hormone levels are not affected and remain within normal limits.

The plasma cortisol level exhibits a 'circadian' rhythm, being high in the morning (5 am to 10 am) and falling to low values at night, with a nadir occurring between midnight and 4 am (this is an important point to keep in mind when evaluating plasma values). This rhythm is sleep-related and reverses in shift workers and such like.

METABOLISM

Intra-adrenal cortisol storage is minimal. In the adult the cortisol production rate is of the order of 15-25 mg/24 hours. Less than 1% of this is excreted by the kidney in the pure form. Most of the cortisol is

metabolised by the liver where there is reduction to tetrahydro metabolites, cortols, and cortolones. These reduction products are made more water soluble by conjugation to glucuronic acid or sulfate and then excreted in the urine. The half-life of plasma cortisol is approximately 80 minutes.

CONTROL OF SYNTHESIS

Adrenocortical activity and cortisol production is under the control of the anterior pituitary hormone adrenocorticotropic hormone (ACTH). The synthesis and secretion of ACTH are in turn regulated by corticotropin releasing hormone (CRH) and arginine vasopressin (AVP) which promote production and release, and by plasma cortisol (negative feedback), which directly inhibits production and release. In addition, plasma ACTH may also exert an effect on CRH activity via the short feedback loop(Figure 18.2). Both ACTH and cortisol secretion display a distinct diurnal pattern which are very similar.

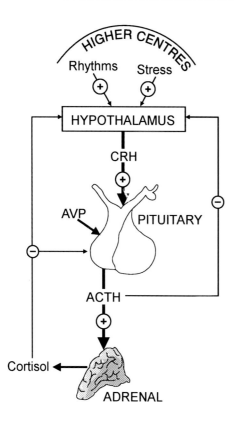

Figure 18.2. Regulation of cortisol synthesis. See text for details.

ACTH

ACTH is a 39-amino-acid peptide hormone produced in the anterior pituitary corticotrophs by cleavage of a large polypeptide, pro-opiomelanocortin (POMC); biogical activity resides in the first 18 amino terminal residues. In the adrenal cortex ACTH binds to specific cell-surface receptors to increase production of low density lipoprotein (LDL) receptors and stimulate steroidogenesis through the adenyl cyclase system.

Corticotropin releasing hormone (CRH)

CRH is a 41-amino-acid residue polypeptide produced in the hypothalamus. It is transported down neuronal axons to the median eminence and released into the hypophyseal portal venous system. In the anterior pituitary it stimulates the corticotrophs to synthesise and release ACTH. CRH release is influenced by the

higher brain centres, e.g., physical, psychological, or emotional stress stimulates production, and the sleep-wake cycle initiates the circadian rhythm (low in afternoon and night, high during early morning and day, see above). It is inhibited by cortisol and ACTH.

ACTIONS OF STEROIDS

Cortisol

Intracellularly cortisol acts via a specific cytoplasmic glucocorticoid receptor although recent evidence suggests that this is the same as, or similar to, the mineralocorticoid receptor . Its multiple physiological actions on intermediary metabolism include:

1   An anti-insulin effect whereby it raises the blood glucose level by:

   (a) promoting gluconeogenesis via mobilisation of amino acids from tissue proteins
   (b) promoting glycogenesis
   (c) depressing glucose utilisation in muscle and fat tissue
   (d) increasing fatty acid mobilisation from adipose tissue and promoting a shift from glucose to fatty acid catabolism by muscle tissue.

Cortisol production is increased during exercise making more glucose and fatty acids available for energy.

2   An as yet undefined protective role in stress: It is responsive, within minutes, to a variety of physical and psychological stresses (other stress-related hormones include the catecholamines and arginine vasopressin).

3   Anti-inflammatory effects: In pharmacological doses it dampens defence mechanisms helping to prevent their dangerous overactivity.

4   Mild mineralocorticoid activity: There is evidence that the aldosterone receptor cannot distinguish between cortisol and aldosterone and reacts to both equally. However, aldosterone-sensitive tissues contain the enzyme 11β-hydroxysteroid dehydro-genase (11β-HSD) which converts cortisol to the inactive cortisone. Hence 11β-HSD allows unimpeded aldosterone action on the receptor. The mineralocorticoid effects of high circulating levels of cortisol (as in the ectopic ACTH syndrome, see

below) may reflect the overwhelming of this enzyme by a massive local concentration of cortisol.

5 An increase in renal free water clearance: Brought about by increasing the renal blood flow.

Androgens

As noted above, the foetal adrenal produces massive amounts of DHEAS; after birth the foetal tissue atrophies but the adrenal still produces DHEAS and DHEA which have no known significance during adult life (they are only mildly androgenic). The major adrenal androgens are testosterone and androstenedione. In the child these cause adrenarche which precedes gonadal androgen secretion and they also stimulate the first sexual hair of puberty.

The androgens are C_{19} steroids which promote male secondary sexual characteristics through inhibition of the female characteristics (defeminisation) and accentuation of the male ones (masculinisation). In the female excessive androgen activity produces hirsutism and virilism (page 250).

Diseases of the adrenal cortex

Congenital adrenal hyperplasia

Congenital adrenal hyperplasia (CAH) describes a number of conditions, presenting at birth, characterised by bilateral adrenal hyperplasia. This is due to excessive production of ACTH secondary to cortisol deficiency, which in turn reflects an enzyme defect affecting steroidogenesis. Defects of all five enzymes necessary for cortisol synthesis (Figure 18.1) have been described but they are rare; defects of 21-hydroxylase and 11β-hydroxylase are the most common, with the 21-hydroxylase defect accounting for more than 90% of cases.

21-hydroxylase deficiency

21-hydroxylase converts 17-hydroxyprogesterone to 11-deoxycortisol and progesterone to 11-deoxy corticosterone. Thus a deficiency will result in decreased synthesis of cortisol and all mineralocorticoids and increased synthesis of precursors

proximal to the block (including the androgens), and increased synthesis of renin.

Pathogenesis. Deficient 21β-hydroxylase → ↓cortisol synthesis → ↑ACTH

- ↑ACTH → ↑progesterone and ↑17-OH-progesterone

- ↑17-OH-progesterone → ↑androstenedione → ↑testosterone → virilisation

- ↓ aldosterone synthesis → salt wasting, dehydration and hypotension, and hyperkalaemia (mineralocorticoid-deficient syndrome).

Biochemistry. Increased levels of ACTH, cortisol precursors (progesterone and 17-OH-progesterone), and adrenal androgens (androstenedione and testosterone) ensue. DHEA is moderately increased. Basal and ACTH-stimulated plasma levels of 17-OH-progesterone are useful for screening purposes and for following the efficacy of therapy.

Clinical features: May present as three forms:

1. Mild deficiency of enzyme: simple virilism at birth or during the neonatal period and salt wasting not a feature.

2. Severe deficiency of enzyme: salt wasting, hypotension, and virilism at birth.

3. Late onset with premature adrenarche, hirsutism, and infertility in later life.

11β-hydroxylase deficiency

Deficiency of 11β-hydroxylase activity causes decreased conversion of 11-deoxycortisol to cortisol and of 11-deoxycorticosterone (11-DOC) to corticosterone and aldosterone. This results in:

- Virilisation (↑testosterone) in the female.

- ACTH-dependent hypertension (mineralocorticoid excess syndrome due to ↑11-DOC which has significant mineralocorticoid activity).

250

- Increased plasma levels of ACTH, adrenal androgen and cortisol precursors, especially 11-deoxycortisol and 11-DOC, and increased urinary excretion of the tetrahydro derivatives of the last two compounds, which are normally excreted in only trace amounts.

- Low cortisol and aldosterone levels.

- Suppressed plasma renin levels (negative feedback effect of increased 11-DOC).

- Hypokalaemia (effect of 11-DOC excess) in most cases.

3β-hydroxysteroid dehydrogenase (3β-HSD) deficiency

In this defect there is, in addition to low cortisol and mineralocorticoid production, increased synthesis of steroid precursors with the Δ^5-3-hydroxy configuration, i.e., pregnenolone, 17-OH-pregnenolone, and DHEA (because of the inability to convert any of these steroids into the respective Δ^4-3-ketosteroids in the absence of 3β-HSD). Diagnosis is established by demonstrating a greatly increased ratio of Δ^5-Δ^4 steroids in plasma or urine. Patients present with severe adrenal insufficiency and ambiguous genitalia.

Cholesterol side chain cleavage defect

This defect, caused by deficiency of the P450scc enzyme which is responsible for the rate-limiting step in adrenal steroidogenesis, results in the absence of steroidogenesis and the accumulation of cholesterol in adrenal cells (congenital lipoid adrenal hyperplasia). It is incompatible with life but some subjects with partial deficiency of the enzyme have survived.

17α-hydroxylase deficiency

Deficiency of 17α-hydroxylase, a rare form of CAH, results in:

(a) Hypertension (effect of mineralocorticoid excess syndrome due to ↑11-deoxycorticosterone) in most cases. The hypertensive trait is what distinguishes deficiency of 17α-hydroxylase from that of 21-hydroxylase.

(b) Failure of sexual maturation (deficiency of C_{18} and C_{19} steroids), causing amenorrhoea in female patients and pseudohermaphroditism in the male patients.

(c) Increased plasma levels of pregnenolone, progesterone (immediate precursors to the block), 11-DOC and corticosterone.

(d) Low levels of plasma renin activity and aldosterone (mineralocorticoid excess due to 11-DOC).

(e) Deficient cortisol synthesis

Hypocortisolism

Hypocortisolism is defined as decreased cortisol secretion (adrenal insufficiency) with its associated clinical and biochemical consequences. It is related to, but not synonymous with, the term hypocortisolaemia. Hypocortisolaemia refers to low plasma levels of *total* cortisol, i.e., both bound and free fractions (see page 247).

Although hypocortisolism is usually associated with hypocortisolaemia, this is not always so; in some cases, e.g., in high oestrogen states, it may occur in conjunction with plasma cortisol levels falling within the reference values. Additionally, low plasma (total) cortisol levels can occur in the absence of hypocortisolism (e.g., in people with low CBG levels). Hence a random plasma (total) cortisol estimation can be at times misleading in the evaluation of patients with suspected hypocortisolism.

The most common acute presentation of adrenal insufficiency is Addison's disease but the most common cause is excessive or prolonged exogenous cortisol administration which produces "atrophy of disuse".

CAUSES/PATHOPHYSIOLOGY

The causes of hypocortisolism (adrenal insufficiency) are listed in Table 18.1; also included are the causes of hypocortisolaemia in otherwise normal patients, i.e., those with decreased cortisol-binding globulin levels. Patients with hypocortisolism may present clinically in one of three ways:

- Acute adrenal failure (see below)
- Chronic adrenal failure (see below)
- At birth, with congenital adrenal hyperplasia

From the viewpoint of pathophysiology the disorder may be primary, where the adrenal gland is at fault, or secondary, where the problem resides in the pituitary or hypothalamus and is directly related to deficient ACTH secretion.

Note: In some medical textbooks, adrenal insufficiency resulting from insufficient CRH or other hypothalamic ACTH secretagogues is referred to as tertiary adrenal insufficiency. We prefer the former terminology (see Table 18.1).

Table 18.1. Causes of hypocortisolism and hypocortisolaemia.

PRIMARY (increased plasma ACTH)
Adrenocortical deficiency
    Addison's disease: autoimmune, tuberculosis,
      metastatic carcinoma
    Acute deficiency: Waterhouse-Friderichsen
      syndrome
    Iatrogenic: adrenalectomy
Congenital adrenal hyperplasia
    Specific enzyme defects in steroidogenesis:
      21-hydroxylase, 11β-hydroxylase,
      17α-hydroxylase,
      3β-hydroxysteroid dehydrogenase

SECONDARY (decreased plasma ACTH)
    CRH deficiency: hypothalamic disease
    ACTH deficiency: pituitary disease
    Prolonged steroid administration

DECREASED CBG (normal plasma ACTH)
    Congenital
    Androgen therapy
    Protein-losing states: nephrotic syndrome,
      protein-losing enteropathy

Primary adrenal failure

Primary adrenal failure denotes that the disease process is localised to the adrenal and that the remainder of the hypothalamic-pituitary-adrenal axis is normal, i.e., the cardinal problem is a defect in glucocorticoid (and also in mineralocorticoid and adrenal androgen) production and this results in the characteristic high circulating levels of ACTH. All three zones of the adrenal cortex are usually affected by the destructive process.

Addison's disease is a general term describing primary adrenal failure. The causes include disorders of steroidogenesis (CAH, see above) as well as destruction of the adrenal cortex, for example, by granulomatous diseases (tuberculosis, histoplasmosis), autoimmune insult, infarction, and metastatic carcinoma (breast, lungs). Previously the commonest cause was bilateral adrenal tuberculosis but now autoimmune adrenalitis is more common; adrenal haemorrhage and infarction associated with meningococcaemia (Waterhouse-Friderichsen syndrome), although rare, has the most dramatic presentation.

Autoimmune Addison's disease. In this condition the cortex shows atrophy associated with lymphocytic infiltration; some 70-80% also have circulating autoantibodies against the adrenal cortex. It may be an isolated process or part of the polyglandular autoimmune syndrome (PGA) of which there are two types:

Type I PGA: This begins with chronic mucocutaneous candidiasis in early childhood followed by hypoparathyroidism and Addison's disease by the age of 9-13 years.

Type II PGA: This consists of Addison's disease, thyroid disease (hyper- or hypo-thyroidism), and diabetes mellitus. The combination of Addison's disease and hypothyroidism is referred to as Schmidt's syndrome.

Other autoimmune associations are common and include ovarian failure, pernicious anaemia, vitiligo, and alopecia. The full syndrome consisting of adrenal failure, hypothyroidism, hypoparathyroidism, diabetes mellitus, premature menopause (ovarian failure), alopecia, and mucocutaneous candidiasis, is called the *candida-endocrinopathy syndrome;* it is very uncommon.

Waterhouse-Friderichsen syndrome. This term describes acute adrenal failure due to bilateral adrenal infarction associated with meningococcal septicaemia. Infarction can also occur in other conditions such as birth injury and haemorrhagic disorders (e.g., following anticoagulant therapy); it is not uncommon as a terminal event in dying patients.

Secondary adrenal failure

In secondary adrenal failure the adrenal cortex is intact and non-diseased and the primary problem is an ACTH deficiency due either to pituitary or hypothalamic disease (page 229). It is most often due to prolonged exogenous steroid therapy which suppresses the hypothalamic-pituitary part of the adrenal axis. Three points are worth emphasizing:

- Prolonged ACTH deficiency will result in atrophy (of disuse) of the adrenal cortex but the suppressed glands will eventually overcome the inertia after prolonged ACTH administration, a feature that is used to distinguish primary from secondary adrenal insufficiency (see ACTH stimulation test, page 254).

- Mineralocorticoid synthesis, which is not ACTH dependent, remains intact so these subjects do not present with the characteristic electrolyte abnormalities (hyperkalaemia, etc, see below) associated with primary Addison's disease.

- Glucocorticoids are necessary for normal renal free water clearance and hence cortisol deficiency can be associated with water retention and dilutional hyponatremia.

CONSEQUENCES OF ADRENAL FAILURE

Chronic deficiency (Addison's disease)

The onset of manifestations of adrenal insufficiency is usually insidious and the disorder may go undetected until an intercurrent illness or stress precipitates a crisis. In the subject with slowly developing adrenal failure some or all of the following may be present:

1 Pigmentation of exposed areas, palmar grooves, buccal mucosa, pressure areas, genital areas. This is associated with the high ACTH but not due to it (ACTH, along with β-lipotropin, is split off from the precursor proopiomelanocortin molecule. β-lipotropin contains the β-MSH sequence which probably causes the pigmentation.)

2 Vomiting, muscle weakness, general debility

3 Hypotension due to mineralocorticoid deficiency (page 69)

4 Hyponatraemia, hyperkalaemia, and mild normal anion gap metabolic acidosis, reflecting aldosterone deficiency (page 69)

5 Hypoglycaemia (page 133) and hypercalcaemia (page 92)

In addition to the electrolyte abnormalities, the characteristic biochemical features are:

- Elevated plasma ACTH levels
- Low, or more usually, low normal plasma cortisol levels that do not rise after ACTH administration.

Acute deficiency (Adrenal crisis)

This is an acute medical emergency which presents with severe hypotension (shock), hyponatraemia, and hyperkalaemia. It may occur in patients with characteristic Addisonian features, including pigmentation, as described above, or there may be no overt evidence of chronic adrenal insufficiency. It can occur in the following situations:

- Withdrawal of glucocorticoid or ACTH therapy, or loss of medication following persistent vomiting

- Stress, e.g., trauma, surgical operation, infections, in patients with latent adrenal deficiency

- Bilateral adrenalectomy, e.g., for tumours

- Adrenal injury, e.g., trauma, haemorrhage (anticoagulant therapy), sepsis

Subjects presenting with hypotension, hyponatraemia, and hyperkalaemia, whether pigmented or not, should be considered to have an acute adrenal problem until proven otherwise (see below), i.e., they should be given immediate steroid cover (hydrocortisone) and appropriate iv fluid therapy before considering any endocrinological diagnostic procedures.

The severe abdominal pain and fever which are often seen in such patients, especially in those with sudden bilateral adrenal infarction, may lead to erroneous diagnosis of an acute surgical abdomen. A surgical exploration without adequate adrenal steroid coverage would be potentially catastrophic under these situations.

Adrenal crisis is uncommon in patients with secondary adrenal insufficiency; mineralocorticoid deficiency, the major factor precipitating the crisis, is not a feature.

LABORATORY EVALUATION

The most useful investigations in patients with suspected adrenocortical deficiency are the plasma ACTH level and the plasma cortisol response to ACTH or Synacthen stimulation of the adrenal, the latter being the most important. Two other useful dynamic tests of the residual adrenocortical function, which may be used in the differential diagnosis, are the insulin-induced hypoglycaemia stress test and the metyrapone blockade test (see below and Figure 18.3).

Plasma ACTH

When Addison's disease is first considered it is useful to take a blood sample for measurement of ACTH and cortisol levels before giving any steroid therapy. A low plasma cortisol associated with a high plasma ACTH is characteristic of primary Addison's disease. A very high ACTH associated with a very high cortisol value in a patient with 'Addisonian pigmentation' is characteristic of the ectopic-ACTH syndrome (page 258).

ACTH stimulation

It is important to remember that adrenal failure (primary and secondary) can be associated with a 'normal' plasma cortisol level and this generally invalidates the usefulness of random plasma cortisol measurements in the evaluation of suspected adrenal failure. The appropriate investigation is to stimulate the gland with exogenous ACTH and evaluate the plasma cortisol response. The usual preparation is tetracosactrin, a synthetic formulation of the amino-terminal 24 amino acid residues of the ACTH molecule (e.g., Synacthen, Ciba-Geigy). Should the patient require steroid cover, Dexamethasone, which will not interfere with the plasma cortisol assay, can be substituted for hydrocortisone. The front-line test is the *short Synacthen test* which may be supplemented by the *prolonged Synacthen test* if necessary.

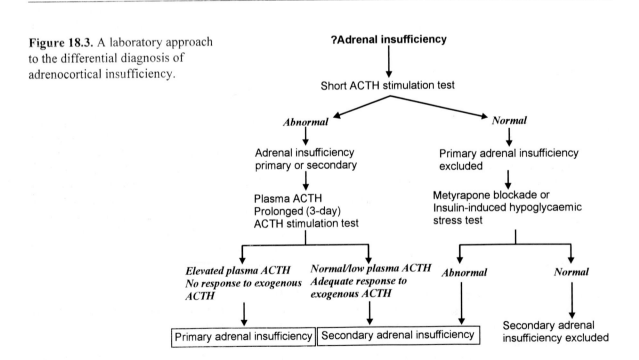

Figure 18.3. A laboratory approach to the differential diagnosis of adrenocortical insufficiency.

Short Synacthen test: Obtain a blood specimen for a baseline plasma cortisol level. Administer 250 μg of Synacthen by deep intramuscular injection. Take further blood specimens for cortisol estimations 30 and 60 minutes later.

Interpretation: The response may be *normal, nil,* or *sluggish.*

- *Normal response:* The plasma cortisol increases by at least 200 nmol/L to a level in excess of 550 nmol/L, with the 30 minute value being greater than the 60 minute value.

- *Nil response:* In this case there is no increase in the cortisol at both 30 and 60 minutes which is characteristic of primary Addison's disease. It should be noted that the cortisol assay may only have a precision (CV) of around 10% so 'increases' of less than 20% (2xCV) should be disregarded.

- *Sluggish response:* This is defined as an increase of more than 20% but less than 200 nmol/L over the baseline level, with the 60-minute level exceeding the 30-minute level. This is suggestive of secondary adrenal dysfunction and should be followed by a prolonged stimulation test.

Prolonged Synacthen test: In this test 1 mg of depot slow-release Synacthen is given im at 0900h daily for 3 days. Blood specimens are collected at 1400h each day with a short Synacthen test performed at 1400 h on day 3.

Interpretation: In subjects on long-term steroid therapy and in patients with secondary adrenal dysfunction there will be an 'awakening' of the adrenal gland with a stepwise increase in the plasma cortisol each day and an improvement in the short Synacthen response on day 3.

The hypoglycaemia stress test

The test is used to assess the hypothalamic-pituitary response to hypoglycaemia, a reproducible form of chemical stress. Increases in plasma ACTH, cortisol, GH, and prolactin and activation of the adrenergic system is the normal stress response elicited. Because the magnitude of the response depends on the degree of hypoglycaemia, stringent criteria of adequate hypoglycaemia must be applied to ensure a maximal stress response. Adequate hypoglycaemia is defined as a blood glucose concentration of 2.2 mmol/L (40 mg/dL) or less, with neuroglycopaenic symptoms (a profuse cold sweat, nausea, drowsiness, anxiety). It is usually achieved 30 to 45 min after insulin injection. A second booster dose of insulin is given if adequate hypoglycaemia is not achieved with the initial dose.

Blood is obtained for plasma glucose and cortisol assays immediately before insulin is injected and 30 and 60 min thereafter (an additional sample drawn at 45 min is recommended in some protocols). The important point to grasp is that the final, definitive sample should be obtained 5 to 10 min after the patient develops adequate hypoglycaemia, as defined above.

Some additional procedural measures which must be strictly adhered to in order to ensure accurate and meaningful results are:

- The patient should fast for at least 8 h before the test and must remain supine during the test duration, with an IV line established.

- A physician must be present during the entire procedure.

- The patient should be closely monitored for development of any serious complications such as seizures, chest pain, disorientation, and confusion, and emergency measures to correct the overwrought hypoglycaemia must be available at the bedside. The usual practice is to keep a 30-mL syringe containing hypertonic (50%) glucose solution on standby.

- The usual insulin dose (0.15 U/kg body weight, iv) should be reduced to 0.1 U/kg body weight for patients suspected of having hypopituitarism or primary adrenal insufficiency. Conversely, it should be increased to 0.25 U/kg body weight for obese patients or those with diabetes mellitus or suspected acromegaly, because of probable insulin resistance. These options are usually exercised with extreme caution and after careful review of patient history.

- The blood glucose levels must be confirmed by an established method, if a bedside monitoring device is used to give an initial rapid result.

- The test should be terminated briskly, after achieving adequate hypoglycaemia, by infusing

10% glucose solution or giving a sweetened drink, as patients with primary or secondary adrenal insufficiency or long-standing diabetes mellitus have impaired compensatory response to hypoglycaemia.

- A patent IV line must be maintained for collection of multiple blood samples and injection of either repeat insulin doses or hypertonic glucose solution.

Interpretation: Plasma cortisol level (using an immunoassay with minimal interference from cross-reacting compounds) should reach 550 nmol/L at some point during the test. Failure to reach this level indicates a subnormal response, provided adequate hypoglycaemia was attained. An inadequate response can be due to hypopituitarism of any aetiology, including partial or panhypopituitarism, isolated ACTH deficiency, CRH deficiency, acute or chronic ingestion of synthetic glucocorticoids.

If plasma ACTH levels are also measured, at least one value should exceed 150 pg/mL (or $\geq$ 33 pmol/L). Simultaneous measurement of plasma GH levels can provide another index of anterior pituitary function.

Note: This test is certainly unpleasant to the patient and not without risk, and should only be carried out if there are strong indications for its use. Otherwise, it can be substituted by the relatively simple, less expensive and less risky ACTH stimulation test, which provides essentially the same information. It is most often performed as part of the triple (combined) anterior pituitary function test (page 232), together with TRH and GnRH stimulation.

Metyrapone test

The test assesses the pituitary response to (induced) hypocortisolaemia. The drug metyrapone is a competitive inhibitor of P-450$_{C11}$, the enzyme that catalyses the conversion of 11β-deoxycortisol to cortisol, the last step in the biosynthetic pathway from cholesterol to cortisol (Figure 18.1). Unlike cortisol, 11-deoxycortisol does not inhibit ACTH secretion by negative feedback. Its buildup, coupled with falling cortisol levels, as a consequence of the metabolic blockade, results in increased ACTH secretion, enhanced adrenal steroidogenesis, and further buildup of cortisol presursors, especially 11-deoxycortisol. Measurement of the latter, either in blood or in urine

(as 17-hydroxycorticosteroids), provides an index of the pituitary's response to hypocortisolaemia. There are two variations of the test.

Standard 3-day metyrapone test: This involves three 24-h urine collections, one before taking metyrapone, and two, on the day of the drug administration and the day after (6 doses of 750 mg metyrapone every 4 h taken orally). Urinary 17-OHCS and creatinine excretion are measured. A two- to threefold increase above the baseline value on either the day of, or the day after the drug dose, constitutes a normal response.

Overnight metyrapone test: A single-dose metyrapone (30 mg/kg body weight) at midnight, followed by blood sampling at 0800 h the next morning for plasma 11-deoxycortisol and cortisol (and ACTH) measurement. The plasma 11-deoxycortisol concentration should be greater than 210 nmol/L; plasma ACTH concentration should exceed 75 pg/mL (or 17 pmol/L).

Interpretation: The metyrapone test is the most sensitive test of pituitary ACTH secretory reserve (hypocortisolaemia is a much less powerful stimulus than hypoglycaemia or other stresses). An individual with a normal response, as discussed above, has an intact hypothalamic-pituitary-adrenal axis and requires no further investigation. A subnormal response can be due to primary or secondary adrenal insufficiency or ingestion of synthetic glucocorticoids.

CRH stimulation test

The differentiation between secondary adrenal insufficiency due to pituitary or hypothalamic disease can be made using the CRH stimulation test. CRH is injected iv and the basal plasma ACTH (at 0 min) and CRH-stimulated plasma ACTH concentrations at 30 min and 60 min measured.

Pituitary disease will produce a blunted or nil response whereas in patients with hypothalamic lesions, a positive response will be observed. However, the test is infrequently used, as the distinction sought is rarely important from the therapeutic standpoint.

Hypercortisolism

Hypercortisolism infers excessive cortisol production. It may be appropriate, as in the case of stress where it is a normal physiological response, or inappropriate, as in Cushing's disease. It may result in a high circulating plasma (total) cortisol level (hypercortisolaemia) but this does not *always* ensue because of the episodic nature of cortisol secretion which may occur even in the inappropriate variety. On the other hand, a high plasma (total) cortisol level need not indicate increased cortisol secretion, e.g., high levels of CBG in otherwise normal subjects can result in plasma (total) cortisol values that exceed the upper reference value.

CAUSES/PATHOPHYSIOLOGY

The common causes of hypercortisolism are listed in Table 18.2. The clinical features and biochemical consequences of hypercortisolism are discussed below but it is important to point out that prolonged exposure to high plasma levels of cortisol (due to any cause) produces a symptom complex called Cushing's syndrome; the term Cushing's disease describes a specific entity in which Cushing's syndrome is due to excessive production of ACTH by the pituitary.

Table 18.2. Causes of hypercortisolism and hypercortisolaemia

Physiological (appropriate) hypercortisolism
   Stress, obesity, depression

Inappropriate hypercortisolism
Excess ACTH production
   Pituitary: Cushing's disease
   Extrapituitary: Ectopic ACTH syndrome
   Alcoholism
Suppressed ACTH
   Adrenal tumour: adenoma, carcinoma
   Iatrogenic: steroid therapy

Excess cortisol-binding globulin
   Oestrogen therapy
   Oral contraceptives
   Pregnancy

Stress

Stress increases ACTH secretion which results in increased cortisol secretion. Increased plasma cortisol levels are characteristic of the stress reaction whether it be of physical, mental, or emotional origin. In some cases, such as severe endogenous depression, it may be a prolonged process and may present with Cushingoid features.

Obesity

Although the cortisol secretion rate may be increased in obese subjects, the plasma total cortisol and urinary free cortisol levels (see below) are within normal limits.

Alcoholism

Alcohol-induced *pseudo-Cushing's syndrome* is a rare consequence of chronic alcoholism. It may be difficult to distinguish both clinically and biochemically from Cushing's syndrome due to other causes, e.g., plasma and urinary cortisol levels are raised and the plasma ACTH is inappropriately high. The exact cause is unclear but there seems to be direct activation of the hypothalamic-pituitary-adrenal axis by alcohol. Diagnosis depends on demonstrating the relationship to alcohol -- the changes rapidly return to normal when drinking is ceased.

Cushing's disease

Cushing's disease is the commonest cause of Cushing's syndrome (70-80% of cases) and is due to pituitary ACTH hypersecretion. It is also called pituitary-dependant Cushing's syndrome to distinguish it from extra-pituitary causes of the syndrome -- adrenal tumours (10-15% of cases) and ectopic-ACTH syndrome (5-15% of cases). About 90% of subjects with Cushing's disease have a pituitary adenoma, the remainder, hyperplasia. The chronic hypercortisolaemia suppresses hypothalamic CRH secretion and inhibits ACTH secretion by the normal, non-adenomatous pituitary corticotrophs, which subsequently atrophy. The cells of the pituitary adenoma or the hyperplastic cells appear to function at a higher than normal set point for cortisol feedback.

Adrenal tumours

About 15% of patients with Cushing's syndrome have functioning adrenal tumours, with benign adenomas and malignant carcinomas occurring in equal numbers. Non-functioning benign adenomas are common (1-9% of autopsies) but the incidence of non-functioning carcinomas is very low (<5 per million). The majority of carcinomas produce some hormonal products including cortisol and androgens and in women functioning adrenal carcinomas are often associated with virilisation consequent to androgen as well as cortisol excess. The chronic autonomous hyper-cortisolaemia suppresses both CRH and ACTH synthesis and secretion. Pituitary corticotrophs atrophy, as do the non-tumour adrenocortical tissue.

Ectopic ACTH syndrome

In the ectopic ACTH syndrome the non-pituitary tumour secretes ACTH which causes bilateral adrenal hyperplasia and excessive cortisol production. The commonest tumour associated with this disorder is the oat cell carcinoma of the lung; others have included carcinomas of the thymus, pancreas, ovary and breast, medullary carcinoma of the thyroid, and phaeo-chromocytoma. Characteristically the patients are pigmented (? elevated lipotropin), have very high plasma ACTH levels, have high plasma total and urinary free cortisol levels, and present with hypokalaemic metabolic alkalosis (? mineralocorticoid effect of 11-deoxycorticosterone). They rarely develop Cushing's syndrome because survival time is short. In some of these cases tumour production of corticotrophin releasing hormone has been implicated rather than tumour production of ACTH.

CONSEQUENCES OF HYPERCORTISOLISM

The increased cortisol production rate may express itself as :

- High plasma (total) cortisol levels
- Loss of circadian rhythm
- Increased urinary excretion of free cortisol

Although these hormonal features are characteristic of inappropriate hypercortisolism they cannot always be demonstrated in all proven cases of Cushing's syndrome. This reflects the episodic nature of the disease, particularly in the early stages. Prolonged

hypercortisolism produces the clinical and biochemical features of Cushing's syndrome. The characteristic features include some or all of the following:

Fat metabolism. There is a characteristic redistribution of fat to the central location with a plethoric "moon face", supraclavicular fat pads, "buffalo hump", a protuberant abdomen, and thin extremities (often described as resembling a lemon with tooth picks for limbs).

Protein metabolism. There is excessive protein catabolism with loss of protein from bone (osteoporosis, backache), muscle (atrophy, weakness), blood vessel walls (bruising), and subdermal areas (striae, stretch marks).

Carbohydrate metabolism. Increased gluconeo-genesis (there is increased amino acid substrates from stepped-up protein catabolism) results in hyperglycae-mia and diabetes mellitus in 40-50% of cases.

Electrolytes. There is often evidence of mineralo-corticoid excess (?11-deoxycorticosterone, ? mineralo-corticoid effect of cortisol), but hypokalaemia and metabolic alkalosis is uncommon except in the ectopic-ACTH syndrome.

Androgens. Evidence of androgen excess in women is common and can vary from frank virilism to mild hirsutism and acne.

Miscellaneous. Other features include hypertension, poor wound healing, steroid psychosis, susceptibility to infection, and polyuria.

LABORATORY INVESTIGATION

Many of the features of hypercortisolism such as obesity, hypertension, and diabetes mellitus are common clinical findings in non-Cushingoid individuals; the main problem is to differentiate between these subjects and those with Cushing's syndrome. Thus the initial approach in the laboratory investigation of suspected Cushing's syndrome should be a screening procedure to identify those subjects with inappropriate hypercortisolism. If this proves positive the next step is to determine the aetiology, i.e., pituitary-dependant, adrenal tumour, or ectopic ACTH syndrome. Two schemes for a diagnostic laboratory approach to confirming the existence of Cushing's syndrome and determining its cause are shown in Figures 18.4 and 18.5.

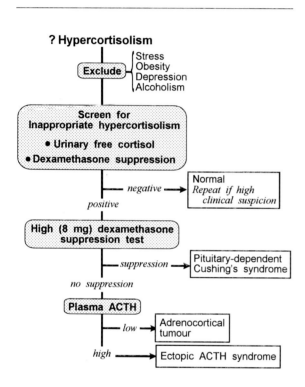

Figure 18.4. Laboratory evaluation of Cushing's syndrome.

Screening tests

Random plasma (total) cortisol estimations are of little use because often the level in hypercortisolism is normal. Three screening tests have been described:

(1) assessment of the circadian rhythm in cortisol secretion,

(2) 24-hour urinary free cortisol secretion, and

(3) low-dose Dexamethasone suppression of ACTH secretion.

Midnight plasma cortisol. A characteristic feature of Cushing's syndrome is loss or abolition of the circadian rhythm. Two approaches have been used to establish this:

(1) Estimate the plasma cortisol levels at 11-12 pm and at 8-9 am. A night (trough) value greater than 50% of the morning (peak) value suggests loss of diurnal variation.

(2) Estimate the plasma cortisol level (single estimation) at midnight. Values in excess of 300 nmol/L suggest loss of circadian rhythm.

The above screening test, whilst simple, is unreliable because (a) in the early stages of Cushing's syndrome the circadian rhythm may be normal, and (b) elevated midnight values may be found in stress, pregnancy, and oral contraceptive therapy.

24-hour urinary free cortisol. 5-10% of the circulating cortisol is unbound and can be filtered by the glomerulus; some of this appears in the urine and the excretion rate reflects the biologically active fraction in the plasma. In Cushing's syndrome values usually exceed 280 nmol/day; levels less than this virtually exclude the diagnosis. However the excretion rate may be raised by up to 50% in obese subjects.

Dexamethasone suppression. Dexamethasone is a synthetic glucocorticoid with 50-100-fold cortisol activity. Hence it can be administered in small doses in an attempt to suppress pituitary ACTH release. Two low-dose dexamethasone suppression test protocols are in current use for the screening of Cushing's disease.

(1) *Overnight screening test.* This is a quick and reliable test. 1 mg of dexamethasone is taken orally between 11 pm and 12 midnight and blood is collected for cortisol estimation at 8 am the next morning. The normal response is a plasma cortisol less than 140 nmol/L and if this is found, Cushing's syndrome is virtually excluded. Levels between 140 and 280 nmol/L are equivocal, and values in excess of 280 nmol/L are highly suggestive of Cushing's syndrome.

(2) *Two-day low dose test.* A baseline 24-hour urine is collected for free urinary cortisol estimation and over

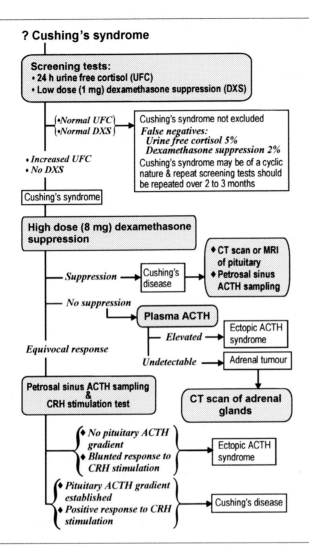

Figure 18.5. A more elaborate diagnostic approach to confirming Cushing's syndrome and determining its aetiology.

the next two days 0.5 mg of dexamethasone is taken 6-hourly -- the daily urine collections are continued, the last urine being collected 6 hours after the last dose. Blood can also be taken at 8.00 am for cortisol estimation. The normal response is a fall in the 24-hour cortisol excretion rate to less than 55 nmol/day. The morning plasma cortisol level should fall to below 140 nmol/L. In Cushing's syndrome there should be no suppression of the urinary or plasma cortisol levels.

The above dexamethasone suppression tests are relatively reliable screening tests (false positive rate of 12-15%). Non-suppression may occur in the following situations:

- Cushing's syndrome
- Pseudo-Cushing's syndrome due to alcohol abuse
- Severe depression and other stress situations
- Inadequate serum levels of dexamethasone due to non-compliance or accelerated metabolism by drugs (phenytoin, phenobarbitone, primidone, etc)
- Pregnancy and oestrogen therapy

Tests to determine aetiology

There are a number of tests available for the determination of the cause of Cushing's syndrome. The two that have been found to be the most useful are the plasma ACTH level and the high-dose dexamethasone suppression test.

Plasma ACTH. A plasma ACTH which is undetectable or below the reference range suggests an adrenal tumour whereas normal or high values are associated with pituitary and ectopic tumours. The ACTH level is not always useful in differentiating between pituitary and ectopic sources but very high values usually indicate the ectopic ACTH syndrome.

The specimen should be taken in the morning (~8.00 am) and transported on ice as it is very unstable at room temperature and is destroyed by enzymes from cells and platelets. The manner of collection must be standardised, e.g., indwelling needle, and stress to the patient must be kept to a minimum because of its effects on ACTH secretion.

Differentiation between pituitary and ectopic origins can be resolved by sampling the inferior petrosal sinus (for ACTH) after CRH stimulation. This, however, is not routinely practised.

High-dose Dexamethasone suppression. The rationale for this procedure is that ACTH secretion in Cushing's disease (pituitary-dependent) is not completely resistant to glucocorticoid suppression. Hence large doses of Dexamethasone can cause some ACTH suppression in Cushing's disease; it does not interfere with ectopic ACTH secretion and adrenal tumours are of course ACTH-independent.

The test is conducted over two days following a baseline 24-hour urine collection for free cortisol estimation. 2 mg of dexamethasone are taken 6-hourly (8 mg per day) for two days during which the urine collections are continued. Patients with Cushing's disease show significant suppression of the cortisol excretion rate (by 50% or more). Patients with the ectopic ACTH syndrome and adrenal tumours show no suppression. However, it should be noted that the patients with adrenal tumours and the ectopic ACTH syndrome may exhibit day-to-day variation in cortisol secretion which may present as a false suppression. In addition to the above laboratory tests the diagnostic process can be improved by radiological scans (CAT, MRI) of the pituitary and ultrasound studies of the adrenals searching for neoplasms.

FURTHER READING

Grua JR, Nelson DH. ACTH-producing tumours. Endocrinol Metab Clinics N Am 1991;20:319-362.

Miller WL. Congenital adrenal hyperplasias. Endocrinol Metab Clinics N Am 1991;20:721-749.

Sheaves R. Adrenal profiles. Br J Hosp Med 1994;51: 357-360.

Trainer PJ, Grossman A. The diagnosis and differential diagnosis of Cushing's syndrome. Clin Endocrinol 1991;34:317-330.

Vallotton MB. Endocrine emergencies: Disorders of the adrenal cortex. Baillieres' Clinics Endocrinol Metab 1992;6:41-54.

Wallace AM. Analytical support for the detection and treatment of congenital adrenal hyperplasia. Ann Clin Biochem 1995;32:9-27.

Chapter 19

Reproductive Endocrinology

Various parts of the brain, the anterior pituitary gland, and the gonads form an integrated system to periodically produce gametes and hormones. Familiarity with the factors involved in the neural and endocrine regulation of reproduction and their interrelationships is essential for the interpretation of diagnostic investigations and the clinical management of reproductive disorders. This chapter provides a basic outline of the hormonal relationships associated with the menstrual cycle and with reproductive processes in the male and considers the approach to the evaluation of patients with abnormalities of the menstrual cycle and some of the commoner disorders associated with reproduction. For a more detailed treatment of these subjects the reader is referred to the references given on page 270.

Normal Physiology

The functions of, and hormone secretion by, the ovary and the testis are controlled by the pituitary gonadotrophins, luteinising hormone (LH) and follicle-stimulating hormone (FSH). These are in turn controlled by gonadotrophin-releasing hormone (GnRH), alternatively known as LH-releasing hormone (LHRH), produced in the hypothalamus (see pages 224, 227). A patent hypothalamo-pituitary-gonadal axis is thus a prerequisite for normal reproductive function (compare adrenal and thyroid function in the previous chapters).

The central nervous system is now recognised as the primary site of functional disturbances which lead to disordered reproduction. The cerebral cortex is involved in the control not only of sexual activity, but also of sexual function, in as much as a disturbed psychological state may lead to abnormal function, e.g., secondary amenorrhoea associated with severe psychological stress. In addition, destructive lesions or damage to specific regions of the hypothalamus may result in regression of sexual function or produce disorders such as precocious puberty, presumably by influencing the release of GnRH.

These influences are mediated through GnRH-secreting peptidergic neural cells located in the arcuate nucleus of the hypothalamus, which are capable of responding to both nervous and chemically transmitted stimuli (page 224).

Gonadotrophin-releasing hormone (GnRH)

GnRH release into the hypophyseal-portal veins is characterised by intermittent pulses; GnRH control of gonadotrophin secretion is thus obligatorily intermittent. Continuous pituitary exposure to GnRH leads to "down regulation" of the GnRH receptors (desensitisation of the gonadotrophs), preventing their regeneration and resulting in decreased gonadotrophin secretion. GnRH secretion and release is also subject to negative feedback by the pituitary gonadotrophins, and possibly by its own circulating levels.

Pituitary gonadotrophins (LH and FSH)

Both hormones are secreted in pulses by the same basophilic pituitary gonadotrophs under GnRH stimulation. Their secretion is, however, not always in tandem. This variable response to GnRH stimulation is probably modulated by feedback influences of circulating oestrogens, androgens and gonadal peptides such as inhibin.

In the female, FSH stimulates follicular growth and oestrogen production; LH initiates ovulation and, in synergism with FSH, promotes luteinisation of the follicle and production of progesterone. The feedback control by oestrogens on LH secretion is complex -- the initial effect of oestrogens is to inhibit secretion (negative feedback) but exposure to oestrogens for a longer duration (e.g., the period of the pre-ovulation oestrogen peak) produces a paradoxical increase in circulating LH (positive feedback), giving rise to the mid-cycle LH surge which is essential for ovulation induction.

In the male, LH (more appropriately known as interstitial cell-stimulating hormone or ICSH) stimulates testosterone synthesis by the interstitial cells of the testis, maintaining optimal androgen concentrations necessary for spermatogenesis. Repleted titres of testosterone, through feedback modulation at both the hypothalamic and pituitary, inhibit further LH secretion. FSH secretion is inhibited by the *inhibin* factor produced by the Sertoli cells within the seminiferous tubules, the site of spermatogenesis.

Prolactin

The anterior pituitary also produces prolactin, which augments the sex hormone milieu, particularly during pregnancy and lactation. Prolactin secretion is inhibited by the hypothalamic neurotransmitter, *dopamine*, which is now generally thought to be the *prolactin inhibitory factor (PIF)* initially discovered to have the same function.

Impairment of this natural hypothalamic control causes hyperprolactinaemia (page 231). Excess prolactin production interferes with normal pituitary-gonadal function during the menstrual cycle and may be associated with amenorrhoea (page 268) and infertility (page 269).

Prolactin, acting synergistically with other hormones, promotes mammary tissue development and milk secretion during pregnancy and lactation. The lower amounts of prolactin found in the non-pregnant state helps to maintain follicular luteinisation and progesterone production. Plasma concentrations of prolactin are slightly higher in non-pregnant women than in men, due to the positive stimulatory effect of oestrogens on prolactin synthesis and release.

Gonadal hormones

During the menstrual cycle the developing ovarian follicles, especially the dominant follicle destined to undergo ovulation, secrete both oestrogens and androgens. The feedback control of GnRH, FSH and LH by gonadal hormones is discussed above.

Oestrogens

The oestrogens are derived from androgens produced locally in the theca cells, after aromatisation of the A-ring of the steroid nucleus. Only the granulosa cells contain the aromatase enzyme that brings about the conversion (Figure 19.1). Oestradiol is the most potent of the oestrogens; oestriol, a relatively inactive secretory product, and oestrone is converted mainly from adrenal androgens in the liver and adipose tissue.

Progesterone

Progesterone is produced by the corpus luteum in a

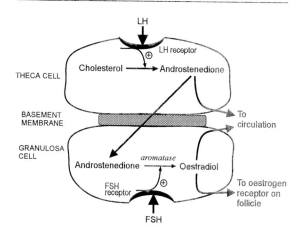

Figure 19.1. Gonadotrophic and cellular interactions in ovarian oestrogen biosynthesis -- the two-cell, two-gonadotrophin hypothesis.

synthetic fashion similar to that in the adrenal cortex (see Chapter 18, page 247).

The granulosa cells, before luteinisation (i.e., prior to corpus luteum formation), have limited ability to produce progesterone. Due to their avascularity, they do not have ready access to circulating low density lipoproteins (LDL), which is the prime source of intracellular cholesterol for steroidogenesis, and are thus limited by substrate availability. Extensive postovulatory neovascularisation of the follicle increases the availability of LDL to the granulosa-lutein cells, and hence their increased secretion of progesterone during the luteal phase of the menstrual cycle (Figure 19.2).

The presence of a mid-luteal progesterone peak (Figure 19.3) verifies the occurrence of ovulation and the subsequent development of the corpus luteum from the ruptured Graaffian follicle. This is one of the first-line tests normally performed in the assessment of probable infertility in the female (see page 266 for a more extensive discussion of its clinical usefulness).

Testosterone

Testosterone is the predominant androgen secreted by the Leydig cells of the testis while the ovary secretes a smaller titre of both testosterone and androstenedione (page 269).

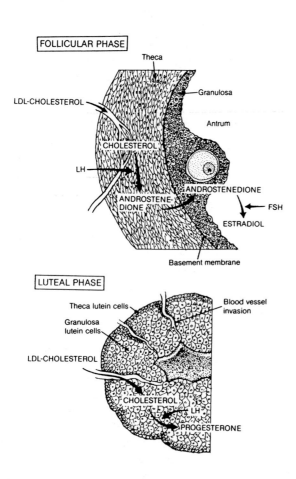

Figure 19.2. Cellular interactions in relation to steroidogenesis in the ovary during the follicular phase (top) and luteal phase (bottom). Adapted from Carr BR, MacDonald PC, Simpson ER. The role of lipoproteins in the regulation of progesterone secretion by the human corpus luteum. Fertil Steril 1982;38:303-311. Reproduced with permission of the publisher, the American Society for Reproductive Medicine (The American Fertility Society).

Foetal sexual development

At birth, a female infant possesses within her immature ovaries the full complement of several million primordial follicles or oocytes, all of which have entered the first stage of meiosis. From thence their numbers decline due to natural growth and atrophy; the span of reproductive viability is limited by this finite number of oocytes which are not replenishable.

At about the seventh week of foetal life the primitive gonads start to differentiate to fo rm either the testes or the ovaries. If the Y chromosome is present in the karyotype the gonads develop into the testes; its absence results in the development of ovaries. The differentiated gonads then influence the development of the internal genitalia from either of two sets of structures, present in both sexes. From about the eighth to tenth week, one set starts to develop rapidly while the other regresses. In the male foetus the Wolffian ducts develop into the epididymis, vas deferens, seminal vesicles, ejaculatory ducts and prostate. In the female foetus the Müllerian ducts develop into the fallopian tubes, uterus and vagina.

The development of female structures is spontaneous and independent of ovarian endocrine function. In contrast, the testis actively secretes two essential hormones, i.e., an anti-Müllerian hormone which prevents the inherent trend towards development of female genitalia, and testosterone which actively stimulates development of male internal genitalia. Conversion of testosterone to dihydro-testosterone by the enzyme 5-α-reductase enables normal development of male external genitalia.

Exposure of female foetuses to androgens will 'masculinise' their external genitalia as occurs in the adrenogenital syndrome (page 250), whilst deficiency of 5-α-reductase or insensitivity of the gonadal tissues to androgen action in the male result in 'feminised' external genitalia, e.g., in male pseudohermaphroditism and testicular feminisation.

Puberty

Prepubertal plasma levels of gonadotrophins are low due to depressed hypothalamic production of GnRH. At puberty a switch occurs wherein GnRH begins to be produced in pulses of greater magnitude and frequency and this in turn stimulates increased secretion of FSH and LH by the pituitary gonadotrophs. The trigger for this functional switch remains unresolved.

In the male, the pubertal spike in LH production causes a marked increase in testicular size and a sharp rise in testosterone production which stimulates development of secondary sexual characteristics; a similar increase in FSH stimulates spermatogenesis.

In the female, LH and FSH bring about the changes that characterise the menarche, i.e., development of the breast and other secondary sexual characteristics and the onset of ovulation and menstruation.

oocyte (ovulation). These phases are defined by characteristic morphological and functional changes of the "dominant" follicle.

The follicular phase prior to ovulation is dominated by the rising output of oestrogen (oestradiol) associated with the growing follicle whereas in the luteal phase after ovulation, progesterone, produced by the evolved corpus luteum, predominates. Ovulation itself is marked by the LH surge and if fertilisation of the ovum and implantation of the fertilised egg does not take place, luteal function regresses and menstruation occurs. This is accompanied by the return of higher levels of gonadotrophins (suppression of negative feedback) which are needed to initiate a new cycle.

Changes influenced by the hormonal milieu and characteristic of the chronologic stage of the menstrual cycle also occur in the uterine endometrium.

The follicle (Figure 19.4)

The initial growth of the primordial follicle is independent of any external control and occurs spontaneously at all ages from the late intrauterine period into the menopause, presenting a continuous trickle of preantral (primary and secondary) follicles within the ovary at any point of time. The granulosa cells of these follicles develop receptors for oestrogen and FSH and their theca cells develop LH receptors; subsequent follicle development is critically dependent upon pituitary gonadotrophin stimulation. Most of the follicles undergo atresia and oocyte death. Atresia is prevented only if adequate tonic plasma levels of FSH and LH coincide with the development of these receptors.

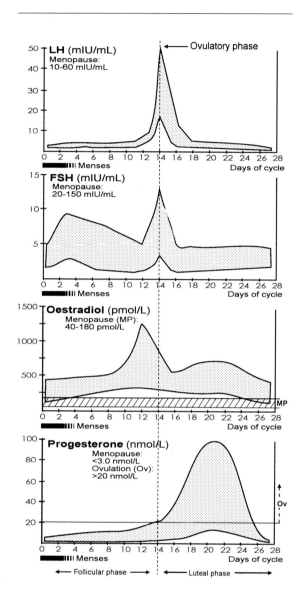

Figure 19.3. Serum hormone levels during the normal menstrual cycle and the values seen after menopause. *The values relate to the Author's laboratory and should not be used with results from other laboratories.*

Normal ovarian function: The menstrual cycle

The complex sequence of events that comprise the menstrual cycle (Figure 19.3) is orchestrated by the sex hormones produced by the follicle that is destined to ovulate. This cyclic ovarian activity shows two distinct phases separated by the release of the mature

Pre-ovulatory (follicular) phase: During menstruation the plasma oestrogen level is low (the immature preantral follicles do not produce much oestrogen). The diminished negative feedback on the hypothalamus stimulates the production of LH and FSH which in turn promotes the growth and development of a group of preantral follicles into tertiary follicles. The tertiary follicle is characterised by further hypertrophy of the theca and the appearance of the antrum, a fluid-filled space among the granulosa cells (Figure 19.4). Normally, only one of these mature to the antral stage whilst the others atrophy.

The dominant follicle produces increasing amounts of oestradiol as it matures, stimulating a surge of LH release by positive feedback and regenerating the previously shed endometrium. There is a coincidental appearance of additional LH receptors on the outer granulosa cells at this time, a critical development that enables both the granulosa and theca cells to engage the large increase in circulating LH. Under the influence of LH, the dominant follicle rapidly increases in size to form the mature Graafian follicle. At this stage, it is ready to release the ovum by the process of ovulation.

Ovulation: Ovulation occurs about 12-18 hours after the LH surge. The average time from recruitment and subsequent development of the primordial follicles

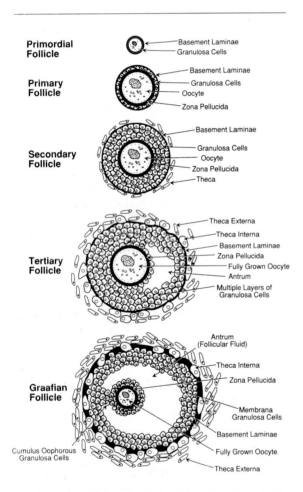

Figure 19.4. The structure and classification of the ovarian follicle during growth and development. (Reprinted from Erickson GF, Magoffin DA, Dyer CA. The ovarian androgen producing cells: a review of structure/function relationships. Endocr Rev 1985;6:371-9. © by The Endocrine Society, with permission..)

through the various stages discussed above until ovulation is about 10 to 14 days.

Luteal (post-ovulation, secretory) phase: During this stage LH stimulates further development of the corpus luteum and the secretion of progesterone and oestradiol from it. An appropriately high mid-luteal progesterone level indicates that ovulation had taken place -- a useful diagnostic feature in the investigation of infertility in women. Progesterone prepares the endometrium for transplantation of the fertilised ovum, and provides luteal support during early pregnancy. If conception does not occur, the corpus luteum aborts and oestrogen production falls, causing endometrial sloughing and rising LH and FSH levels which begin a new cycle.

From the foregoing description of hormonal changes in the menstrual cycle, it follows that interpretation of sex hormone levels must take into account the stage of the cycle at the time of specimen collection.

Pregnancy

If pregnancy ensues, the fertilised ovum normally implants in the endometrium, and the chorion and developing placenta begin production of human chorionic gonadotrophin (HCG), which has a remarkable structural similarity to LH. This additional luteotrophic stimulus supplements the low endogenous pituitary gonadotrophin levels during the luteal phase and overcomes any luteolytic tendencies that may arise from endogenous ovarian oestrogen and prostaglandin production. The corpus luteum is kept patent for the next 10 to 12 weeks, continuing its secretion of oestrogen and progesterone.

At about 13 weeks placental secretion of HCG falls and the placenta and foetus, as a unit, take over the production of oestradiol and progesterone, which are essential for maintaining the pregnancy. Plasma levels of these hormones and their metabolites increase with gestational age. The production of oestriol from oestradiol requires a normally functioning placenta as well as a normal foetus (Figure 26.2, page 323). Its 24 hour urinary excretion rate and plasma levels may be used as an indicator of foeto-placental function.

Another hormone derived from the placenta is *human placental lactogen* (HPL). This peptide hormone, whose significance is unclear, begins to appear in the plasma at about the eighth week of pregnancy, rises to a concentration plateau at 35-38 weeks, and then falls slightly. Its estimation in plasma has been used as a "placental function test" but it is rarely used in this manner now.

Lactation

After about the tenth week of pregnancy prolactin levels progressively increase (possibly oestrogen-induced) until term when they may be 20-times the levels of the non-pregnant state. This prolactin together with HPL, oestrogens and progesterone, prepare the breasts for lactation. They are usually sufficiently developed to begin mild secretion by the fourth month of pregnancy but do not do so until after parturition. It is now known that oestrogens and progesterone prevent milk secretion and thus lactation can only start some time after delivery of the placenta.

Lactation is dependent on sustained prolactin levels. Despite stimulation of prolactin secretion by suckling, its postpartum level progressively falls over the next 3 to 5 months; lactation ceases when "non-pregnant" titres are reached. The level of prolactin during lactation suppresses the function of the pituitary-gonadal axis producing a period of infertility (as does high prolactin values associated with pituitary adenomas, see below).

Menopause

The term menopause refers to the actual cessation of menses and marks definitively the termination of the reproductive phase in the woman. Ovarian "failure" and decreased ovarian production of oestrogens removes the feedback on the hypothalamus and pituitary, and secretion of FSH and LH continues unopposed; thus, the menopause is characterised by low oestrogen levels and high gonadotrophin levels (Figure 19.3).

Menopause is often preceded by the climacteric, a symptom complex which occurs during the transitional stage between the reproductive and non-reproductive phases and may last up to 5 years.

Reproductive disorders

Reproductive disorders may emanate from multiple aetiologies and are difficult to classify in both clinical presentation and circulating hormone abnormalities. Only the more common ones wiil be discussed.

Hypogonadism

Hypogonadism may be due to hypothalamic/pituitary disease resulting in deficient gonadotrophin secretion (*hypogonadotrophic hypogonadism*) or to gonadal dysfunction (*hypergonadotrophic hypogonadism*) -- the rise in gonadotrophins in the latter being due to lack of the normal feedback inhibition by the suppressed gonadal steroids. Infertility in both sexes may be due to hyperprolactinaemia.

Hypogonadism implies, and often presents as, a lack of sexual development and infertility in both sexes. Primary gonadal dysfunction in women can present with amenorrhoea, infertility, hirsutism and virilism. Testicular dysfunction may present as delayed puberty or infertility; there may be only failure of spermatogenesis (seminiferous tubular failure) with normal levels of LH and testosterone (and high levels of FSH).

Hypogonadotrophic hypogonadism: This disorder arises from hypothalamic and pituitary abnormalities and may be idiopathic, genetic, or organic, and may result from isolated deficiency of gonadotrophin secretion, or may be associated with multiple pituitary hormone defects. Isolated gonadotrophin deficiency is associated with anosmia or hyposmia (a midline developmental defect) in about 80% of patients with Kallman's syndrome, as well as other mid-line abnormalities, such as hare lip and cleft palate. These patients are often very tall, sexually immature and with eunuchoidal proportions.

Hypergonadotrophic hypogonadism: Gonadal failure can occur at any age; it is accompanied by amenorrhoea, hypoestrogenism, and elevated gonado-trophins. It can result from multiple causes, including gonadal dysgenesis (e.g., Turner's syndrome), ovarian enzyme deficiency (e.g., that of 17,20-lyase), polycystic ovarian syndrome, and ovarian tumours.

Investigations: In primary gonadal disorders the plasma testosterone (male) or oestradiol (female) will be low and LH and FSH levels elevated (in women this is the picture of the menopause which is, after all, ovarian failure, see Figure 19.5). In pituitary or hypothalamic disease the FSH, LH, and gonadal steroids will all be low. Stimulation of the pituitary with exogenous GnRH will not result in an increased secretion of the gonadotropins (see page 227).

In children with delayed puberty the ability of the

gonads to respond to stimuli can be assessed by ultra-sound examination of the ovaries after FSH administration and by serum testosterone measurement in boys before and after HCG administration -- this normally increases testosterone production in the male; failure to do so suggests primary gonadal failure.

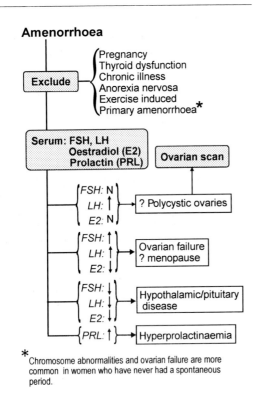

Amenorrhoea

* Chromosome abnormalities and ovarian failure are more common in women who have never had a spontaneous period.

Figure 19.5. Suggested approach to the evaluation of amenorrhoea.

Amenorrhoea

If the subject has failed to menstruate by the age of 16 years, then the amenorrhoea is primary; if she previously had periods which have then ceased it is secondary.

Primary: This is most commonly due to delayed puberty but it may also be due to such disorders as congenital abnormalities of the reproductive tract and Turner's syndrome (chromosomal abnormality with the pattern XO and absence of normal ovaries). Any of the causes of secondary amenorrhoea can also cause primary amenorrhoea.

Secondary: The commonest causes are pregnancy and menopause. Other causes include (a) primary ovarian failure, e.g., autoimmune destruction of ovary, polycystic ovarian syndrome (see below) and (b) secondary ovarian failure due to pituitary or hypothalamic dysfunction. Causes of the latter include: hyperprolactinaemia and gonadotrophin suppression due to chronic illness, thyroid dysfunction, anorexia nervosa, severe long-term exercise.

Investigations: This is outlined in Figure 19.5 and should involve a close clinical examination, estimation of the plasma levels of HCG (to exclude or confirm pregnancy), LH, FSH, oestradiol, and prolactin. If polycystic ovaries are suspected an ultrasound examination of the ovaries will be useful.

Hyperprolactinaemia should always be considered as prolactin-secreting tumours are a fairly common cause of amenorrhoea and infertility (common causes of hyperprolactinaemia are listed in Figure 19.6).

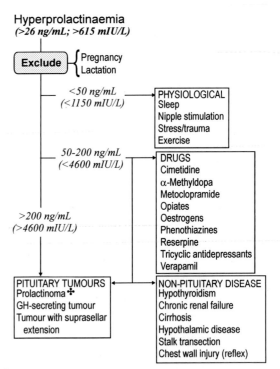

✛ Usually >150 ng/mL (3450 mIU/L) & generally >200 ng/mL (4600 mIU/L). Small microadenomas can have values <150 ng/mL (3450 mIU/L).

Figure 19.6. Check list of causes of hyperprolactinaemia. *Values relate to Author's laboratory.*

Hypergonadism

Primary hypergonadism may be caused by excessive androgen production from a testicular tumour (Leydig cell or interstitial cell tumour), or elevated oestrogen levels produced by an oestrogen-producing tumour. In children this may result in precocious puberty. Sexual precocity from pituitary stimulation of the gonads *(secondary hypergonadism)* is often familial in males and idiopathic in origin in females. It is distinguished from primary hypergonadism by increased levels of gonadotrophins, in contrast to the suppressed levels found in the primary variety.

Polycystic ovarian syndrome (PCOS): This condition of uncertain aetiology (? hormonal imbalance) is characterised by infertility and anovulation, menstrual abnormalities, mild androgen excess (usually hirsutism), a tendency to obesity, and characteristic cystic ovaries which can be visualised by ultrasonography. The hormonal abnormalities are moderately increased serum testosterone levels and a high LH:FSH ratio (LH usually raised, FSH normal).

Infertility

This is a complex subject and the appropriate specialised texts should be consulted for detailed information. In the female subject the causes are legion varying from local pelvic diseases such as endometriosis, tubal disorders, and pelvic infections to ovarian failure (including polycystic ovaries), and hypothalamic or pituitary disease including hyperprolactinaemia. In some 45% of cases the cause can be traced to the male partner in whom there may be psychogenic problems, genital tract disorders such as congenital defects, testicular lesions such as Klinefelter's syndrome, and hypothalamic-pituitary problems such as hyperprolactinaemia. Investigation of infertility is discussed at greater length in Chapter 26.

Hirsutism and virilism

These disorders in the female are due to increased circulating androgen levels or increased tissue sensitivity to these hormones.

Androgen metabolism: (see page 63 for synthetic pathway) In the female the important androgens include testosterone, androstenedione, and dehydroepiandrosterone sulphate (DHEA-S).

Testosterone is derived from the ovary (~60%) and from the peripheral conversion of androstenedione (~40%). Androstenedione is secreted in equal amounts by both the ovary and the adrenal cortex. In the skin testosterone is converted by the enzyme 5-α-reductase to dihydrotestosterone (DHT) which stimulates the hair follicle (Figure 19.7). DHEA-S is secreted only by the adrenal cortex.

In the plasma testosterone is bound to protein (~65% to sex hormone-binding globulin, SHBG, and ~33% to albumin) with about 2% remaining free; only the free testosterone can enter cells and exercise its androgen effect. The concentration of SHBG is variable: increased levels are associated with oestrogen therapy, pregnancy, cirrhosis, phenytoin therapy, and anorexia nervosa, and low values occur in obesity, hyperinsulinism, androgenisation, hyperprolactinaemia, and the menopause. Hence the estimation of total serum testosterone may not reflect the free, biologically active, level. To overcome this problem both testosterone and SHBG should be measured and some allowance made for the SHBG concentration. The usual manipulation is to calculate the total testosterone to SHBG ratio and to consider the result proportional to the free testosterone (see Figure 19.7)

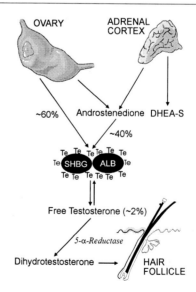

Figure 19.7. Metabolism of testosterone. Te, testosterone; SHBG, sex hormone-binding globulin; DHEA-S, dehydroepiandrosterone sulphate. ~60% of testosterone is derived from the ovary (direct secretion) and ~40% is from androstenedione (ovarian and adrenal).

Causes of androgen excess: Excessive production of androgens as evidenced by high serum testosterone, androstenedione, or DHEA-S levels may be due to:

a. Polycystic ovarian syndrome
b. Ovarian tumours: arrhenoblastoma, hilus-cell tumours
c. Adrenal disorders: adrenal tumours (usually carcinoma), adrenogenital syndrome, Cushing's syndrome
d. Androgen (testosterone) administration
e. Drugs: Phenytoin, Danazol, glucocorticoids.

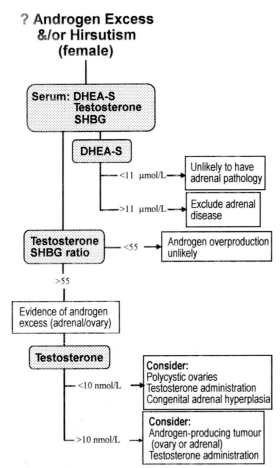

SHBG: sex hormone-binding globulin
DHEA-S: dehydroepiandrosterone sulfate

Figure 19.8. Suggested scheme for the evaluation of suspected hyperandrogenism. *The concentrations refer to the Author's laboratory and should not be applied elsewhere.*

Hirsutism: In the context of female endocrinology this term defines increased production of sexual hair, i.e., on the face, chest, abdomen, and inner thighs. It may be familial or racial (normal circulating androgens), related to increased activity of 5–α-reductase, associated with minor increases in circulating androgens, or associated with androgen excess and menstrual irregularities such as in the polycystic ovarian syndrome.

Virilism: This condition is less common than simple hirsutism (which is a part of the disorder) and has more sinister implications. It is always associated with increased circulating androgen levels and with other evidence of excess androgen activity, e.g., growth of hair in a male distribution, receding temporal hair line, deepening of the voice, breast atrophy, and enlargement of the clitoris. Such a picture should always institute a search for a tumour.

Laboratory evaluation: The laboratory investigation of hirsutism and suspected androgen excess is shown in Figure 19.8. Three points worth emphasising are:

1. A high DHEA-S suggests an adrenal cause.
2. A normal testosterone/SHBG ratio suggests androgen overproduction is unlikely.
3. A very high serum testosterone (e.g., >10 nmol/L) suggests an androgen-producing tumour.

REFERENCES AND FURTHER READING

Beastall GH. Role of endocrine biochemistry laboratories in the investigation of infertility. J Clin Pathol 1993;46:790-794.

Blackwell RE. Hyperprolactinaemia: evaluation and management. Endocrinol Metab Clinics North Am 1992;21:105-124.

Handelsman DJ, Swerdloff RS. Male gonadal dysfunction. Clinics Endocrinol Metabol 1985;14:89-121.

Morris DV, Adams J, Jacobs HS. The investigation of female gonadal function. Clinics Endocrinol Metab 1985;14:125-143.

Chapter 20

Iron

Iron plays a central role in oxygen transport and an important part in energy metabolism. It forms part of the haem molecules of haemoglobin and myoglobin and is an important constituent of flavoproteins, cytochromes and most oxidases. Free iron is highly toxic; this probably relates to inhibition of certain enzymes (e.g., those with thiol groups) and initiation and catalysing of free radical-mediated reactions.

Normal homeostasis

The toxicity of free iron is overcome in the body by its attachment to proteins. It is transported in the plasma attached to the protein transferrin, incorporated into the red cells as part of haemoglobin, and stored as the protein complexes, ferritin and haemosiderin.

DISTRIBUTION

The total body iron content is about 3 to 4 grams, most of which is in the form of haemoglobin (60-70%); the stores, in the form of ferritin and haemosiderin, constitute 20 to 30%. Smaller amounts are incorporated into myoglobin and only a minute portion (<0.1%) is found in plasma, where it is bound to transferrin. The approximate distribution is shown in Table 20.1.

INTAKE/ABSORPTION

Iron is absorbed in the duodenum, then attached to transferrin and transported throughout the body where it can be taken up by most cells. The cellular uptake is dependant on receptors for transferrin which are found on all cells but particularly the erythron (erythropoiesis), hepatocytes (stores), and macrophages of the spleen, bone marrow, and liver (stores).

The daily intake is about 20-30 mg of which 5-10% (1-2 mg) is absorbed in the upper small intestine, mainly the duodenum, by an active process. Dietary iron is in two forms, *haem* molecules (haemoglobin, myoglobin) and *uncomplexed ferric iron* (Fe^{3+}) attached to proteins.

- **Haem iron:** The haem molecule is detached from its apoprotein by the gastric acids and then absorbed intact by the small gut.

- **Uncomplexed iron:** Ferric iron is split from its associated proteins by gastric HCl, reduced to the ferrous state (Fe^{2+}) by dietary reducing substances (e.g., vitamin C), and absorbed in this form. After absorption it is oxidised back to the ferric state.

Table 20.1. Iron distribution.

	mg	% of total
Haem proteins:		
haemoglobin	2500	60-70
myoglobin	150	3-5
Enzymes: cytochromes, etc	8	0.2
Plasma: transferrin	4	0.1
Stores: ferritin, haemosiderin	1000	20-30

In the mucosal cells the iron is either transferred across the cell and attached to transferrin for further distribution, or it is attached to apoferritin molecules to form ferritin and stored in the cells as such.

Iron requirements are increased in women (menstruation and pregnancy), during childhood, and during adolescence. This increased need can be met by increased absorption of up to five-fold from a normal diet. Factors which influence the rate of absorption are:

- **Dietary iron content:** Increased intake can be associated with increased absorption.

- **Gastric acidity:** Proteases in the gastric juice liberates the haem from its apoprotein and HCl solubilises the iron, making it more available for absorption. Achlorhydria is associated with decreased absorption.

- *Reducing substances:* Dietary vitamin C and other reducing substances increase the ferrous fraction and hence encourage absorption.

- *Alcohol:* Alcohol consumption is associated with increased iron absorption which may be a non-specific effect or related to alcohol-induced stimulation of gastric acid secretion.

- *Pancreatic bicarbonate:* Bicarbonate encourages production of poorly absorbed ferric hydroxide. In chronic pancreatic disease increased iron absorption is associated with the decreased pancreatic bicarbonate secretion.

TRANSPORT

Iron is transported in the plasma attached to liver-derived transferrin, a 80 000 molecular weight protein which binds two atoms of ferric iron per molecule (and is normally about 30% saturated). Transferrin conveys iron to either the bone marrow (developing erythrocytes) for haem synthesis, or to the iron stores, depending on requirements. When iron stores are low, transferrin levels increase and the now relatively unsaturated protein preferentially delivers iron to the bone marrow. Conversely, if stores are increased (iron overload), the transferrin level falls and iron is preferentially transported to the stores.

IRON STORES

About 1 gram of iron is stored in the reticulo-endothelial cells (bone marrow, spleen, liver) and the hepatic parenchymal cells as ferritin and haemosiderin. The stores in women are less than in males (women ~5 mg/kg, men ~10 mg/kg).

Ferritin: This is a large molecule (MW ~460 000) comprising an outer protein shell (apoferritin) and an inner core of ferric hydroxide phosphate; it is synthesised and found in all cells where it protects against iron toxicity. When fully saturated, its iron content is about 50% dry weight (usually ~25%). This storage iron is readily available and can be quickly released when needed for haemoglobin synthesis. A small amount of ferritin circulates in the plasma, the level of which is directly proportional to the iron stores (each 1 µg/L of plasma ferritin represents ~8 mg of stored iron).

Haemosiderin: This is derived from ferritin (possibly a ferritin aggregate), is water insoluble, and less available as a source of iron.

IRON TURNOVER

The metabolism of iron is dominated by its role in haemoglobin synthesis. Erythrocytes, at the end of their life-span (~120 days), are engulfed by macrophages of the reticuloendothelial cell system. These cells release the iron from haem for reutilisation in the synthesis of new haemoglobin, the remainder of the porphyrin molecules being converted to bilirubin (page 143). Some of the released iron enters the blood stream and is transported to the stores by transferrin. About 20 mg of iron, derived from 8-10 g of haemoglobin, is recycled daily in this manner. A smaller fraction (1-2 mg) leaves the plasma and is taken up by the liver and other tissues where it is utilised for synthesis of other haemoproteins such as cytochromes and myoglobin.

Excretion

Iron is an unusual metabolite in that there is no specific mechanism for its excretion, homeostasis being maintained by the rate of absorption. Each day, in the adult male, about 1-2 mg of iron is lost via the following routes.

Skin: cell loss (0.3 mg)
Gut: epithelial cell desquamation (0.7 mg)
       blood loss (1.0-1.5 mg)
Urine: shedded cells (0.1 mg)

In the female the loss is slightly more because of menstruation, an extra 20 to 30 mg being lost monthly. Losses during pregnancy are an extra 800 to 1200 mg and during lactation, an extra 150 mg in six months.

Control of homeostasis

Iron balance is controlled by the rate of gut absorption, there being no control over excretion.

A simplistic view of the control mechanism is as follows. The absorbed iron is either transported across the mucosa for further distribution about the body, or it is attached within the cell to apoferritin and stored. The mucosal cells have a lifespan of 2 to 3 days after which they, with their stored iron, are shed into the gut and lost to the body. This continual turnover of mucosal cells constitutes the "excretion" of iron, the rate being increased or decreased by the cell iron content. This content varies with the total body iron stores: if stores are high the apoferritin content of the mucosa is increased (more iron stored and excreted, and less transported to the plasma); when stores are low, less apoferritin appears in the mucosa and thus more iron is absorbed and less "excreted".

PLASMA IRON

The total plasma iron content is about 4 mg (15-30 μmol/L) all of which is attached to transferrin (20-50% saturated). In any individual, the plasma iron concentration may vary greatly even under physiological conditions. The causes of these changes (often rapid and probably involving shifts between plasma and stores) are poorly understood.

The *physiological factors* affecting plasma iron levels include:

- Age: Lower levels during first two years of life.

- Sex: Levels 10-20% lower in females.

- *Time of day:* The circadian rhythm may vary up to 50% (high in morning between 8 to 10 am, lowest at 9 pm).

- *Pregnancy:* Elevated during first trimester

- *Menses:* Levels fall just before and during first day of menses.

- *Diet:* A diet high in iron (or iron-containing medication) results in transient high values.

Note: Blood for iron studies should be taken in the morning (8 -10 am) and the subject should be fasting.

The *pathological conditions* (Table 20.2) affecting the plasma iron levels are:

- Iron deficiency and iron over load, usually associated with low and high levels, respectively.

- Any acute or chronic illness, regardless of state of stores, will lower the plasma iron level.

- Increased plasma levels are found in any condition associated with impaired utilisation of iron for haem synthesis, e.g., marrow hypoplasia, vitamin B_{12} deficiency.

- In haemolytic anaemias the plasma iron is often high during the haemolytic episodes.

- Hepatocellular damage releases iron from stores causing a transient rise in the plasma level.

Note: The lack of a tight control over the plasma iron concentration, coupled with the fact that it represents only a very small proportion (0.1%) of the total body iron content, makes plasma iron measurements of limited clinical value when assayed as a single parameter. They are best interpreted with other relevant biochemical and haematological data (see below).

TRANSFERRIN & IRON-BINDING CAPACITY

The plasma transferrin levels, either measured directly or more usually, measured indirectly as the total iron-binding capacity (TIBC), are less labile than plasma iron levels. In most situations, the diagnostic precision is improved by measuring and evaluating both the plasma iron and the plasma TIBC (plus an estimation of the % saturation of transferrin).

Plasma transferrin levels vary with the iron stores: increasing when iron stores are low and decreasing when they are high. However, there are a number of other factors which cause variations (Table 20.2):

Increased: Oestrogen excess (pregnancy, oestrogen therapy, oral contraceptives)
Decreased: Chronic illness, malignancy
Protein-losing states

The iron saturation of transferrin, which is normally 20-50%, is decreased in iron deficiency, and increased in iron overload.

PLASMA FERRITIN

Only a small amount of ferritin circulates in the blood

Table 20.2. Iron parameters in various clinical conditions.

	Plasma iron	Transferrin	% saturation	Plasma ferritin	Marrow stores
Low iron states					
Iron deficiency	↓	↑	↓↓	usually↓	absent/↓↓
Acute illness	↓	N	N or ↓	N or ↑	N
Chronic illness	↓	↓	N or ↓	N or ↑	N or ↓
High iron states					
Iron overload	↑	↓	↑↑	↑	↑
Early pregnancy	↑	N	N	N	N
Late pregnancy	N or ↑	↑	N	N	N
O/C therapy	variable	↑	N	N	N
Impaired marrow utilisation	↑	N or ↓	N or ↑	↑	↑
Haemolysis	↑	N or ↓	N or ↑	↑	↑
Liver disease	↑	↓	↑	↑	N or ↑

O/C, oral contraceptives

(10-200 mg/L), but it is a valuable diagnostic tool (Table 20.2) because it is directly related to the subject's iron stores (approximately 1 μg/L is equivalent to 8 mg of storage iron). However, high plasma ferritin levels also occur in liver disease, inflammatory conditions, and malignant disease, regardless of the level of the stores.

Disorders of iron metabolism

Iron deficiency, which characteristically presents as a hypochromic microcytic anaemia, is a common condition said to affect 500 to 1000 million people globally; iron overload is less common, for example, the haemochromatosis gene is present in 3 to 5% of the population, with 1 in 400 to 1000 at risk of developing the disease.

Iron deficiency

The classical presentation of iron deficiency is hypochromic, microcytic anaemia but this represents a late stage in the process and iron stores can be depleted well before anaemia occurs.

CAUSES

Iron deficiency is due to either inadequate intake relative to requirements or blood loss.

Low intake
  nutritional, malabsorption
Increased requirements
  growth, pregnancy, lactation,
  therapy of megaloblastic anaemia
Blood loss
  acute or chronic haemorrhage

In adults dietary deficiency is rare and the commonest cause is blood loss, particularly gastrointestinal, and the finding of iron deficiency should always prompt a search for a gut source of bleeding unless another cause is obvious. The tendency for pregnant women and children to develop iron deficiency reflects the increased iron requirements in these two groups.

274

CONSEQUENCES

As stated above, anaemia is a late presentation in iron deficiency and the classical picture of hypochromia due to subnormal mean cell haemoglobin concentration, microcytosis manifested by a low mean corpuscular volume (MCV), and anaemia, generally does not occur until well after depletion of the iron stores. A characteristic sequence of events is as follows:

1. Depletion of iron stores which can be associated with:

    No anaemia (blood picture may show anisocytosis)
    No decrease in MCV
    Serum ferritin <30 μg/L
    Rise in TIBC (transferrin)

    Followed by:

2. Fall in serum iron
    Fall in transferrin saturation
    Normocytic anaemia

    and finally

3. Fall in MCV (microcytic anaemia)

LABORATORY EVALUATION

Laboratory indices are useful in evaluating the underlying cause of microcytic anaemia in a patient (Figure 20.1); these include the plasma iron parameters (plasma iron, transferrin, transferrin saturation, ferritin) and other tests such as faecal occult blood and haemoglobin electrophoresis.

The definitive diagnosis depends on demonstration of absent bone marrow iron (or low serum ferritin) and the response to iron therapy. A bone marrow biopsy is a procedure not undertaken lightly and diagnosis usually depends on the evaluation of the plasma iron, transferrin, and ferritin levels.

Plasma iron. The serum iron is an unreliable indicator for iron deficiency because it is also low in:

- The anaemia of chronic disease: renal failure, chronic infections, collagen diseases, malignancy
- Protein-losing states
- Late afternoon (see above)
- Just prior to and during early menses

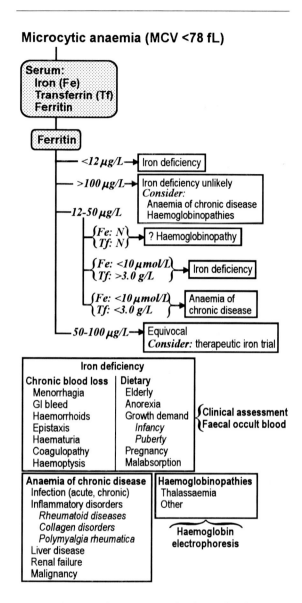

Figure 20.1. Laboratory evaluation of microcytic anaemia.

Plasma transferrin. In iron deficiency this is increased and with this increase the % saturation falls (Note: the % saturation also falls in the anaemia of chronic disease but the transferrin level also falls).

Plasma ferritin. Iron deficiency is the only cause of a low serum ferritin (e.g., <12 μg/L). However, depleted iron stores can be associated with normal serum ferritin values if there is an associated malignancy, chronic infection, collagen disease (see above); in these situations serum values less than 30 µg/L suggest iron deficiency. A serum value in excess of 100 µg/L excludes the diagnosis.

Having made a diagnosis on the basis of the above parameters, the disorder should be confirmed by monitoring the subject's response to iron therapy. With adequate iron replacement the haemoglobin should rise at around 0.15 g/dL/day or around 1 g/dL/week.

Iron overload

In iron overload the excess iron is deposited in the tissues in the form of ferritin and haemosiderin. The term *haemosiderosis* is a histological diagnosis describing increased stainable iron in the cells of the reticuloendothelial system (liver, bone marrow, spleen). If the deposited iron causes cell damage it is called *haemochromatosis.*

CAUSES/PATHOPHYSIOLOGY

Iron overload is always due to increased intake either through the gut, as in idiopathic haemochromatosis, or parenteral as in multiple transfusions.

Primary
    Idiopathic haemochromatosis

Secondary
Increased absorption
    High red cell turnover: haemolytic anaemia
    High dietary iron: African haemosiderosis,
        alcoholic cirrhosis
High parenteral intake
    Excessive iron therapy
    Multiple blood transfusions
Miscellaneous
    Hereditary transferrin deficiency
    Sideroblastic anaemia
    Porphyria cutanea tarda

Idiopathic haemochromatosis. This is an autosomal recessive disorder due to increased gut absorption of iron which results in iron overload (e.g., 10-30 g) and damage to a number of organs. The clinical features depend on the type of organ involved and the extent of damage, e.g.,

Liver: cirrhosis
    (10-20% develop hepatic carcinoma)
Pancreas: diabetes mellitus
Heart: cardiac failure
Adrenal cortex: Addison's disease
Pituitary: secondary gonadal failure

In addition there is a curious pigmentation of the skin due to deposition of increased amounts of melanin. Although the classical triad of *bronze skin, diabetes mellitus, and cirrhosis* does occur, this is a late development and these days the patients usually present with symptoms such as arthralgia (chondrocalcinosis), gonadal failure, and hepatomegaly.

The basis of the disease is a long-term increased absorption of iron by the gut (cause unclear). As the iron build-up is slow the condition is rare before middle age, and women present some 5 to 10 years later than men because of iron loss during menses. It is inherited as an autosomal recessive trait with linkage to HLA-A3 and HLA-B14 or HLA-A3 and HLA-B7 (the gene incidence is around 3 to 5% of the population).

Treatment involves iron-depleting the patient by repeated venesections (1 mL of blood contains 0.5 mg of iron).

LABORATORY EVALUATION

The laboratory findings depend on the severity and the organs involved. They include abnormal liver function tests (elevated AST and ALP), hyperglycaemia if there is severe pancreatic disease, and abnormalities of the serum iron parameters. The definitive diagnosis depends on demonstration of excessive iron in the liver (biopsy).

Serum iron parameters. The serum iron is elevated, the transferrin normal or low, and the saturation greater than 60% (usually greater than 80%). The serum ferritin is greatly increased, with levels in excess of 3000 µg/L not unusual.

Dietary iron overload. This is rare except in the unusual African haemosiderosis where it is due to excessive consumption of iron-containing beer (brewed in iron pots). Usually it only results in haemosiderosis but a small proportion of subjects develop haemochromatosis.

Parenteral iron overload. Multiple transfusions, e.g., treatment of aplastic anaemia, can result in iron overload (500 mL of blood contains 250 mg of iron). The deposition usually occurs in the reticulo-endothelial system (haemosiderosis) but some cases of haemochromatosis have been described.

LABORATORY EVALUATION

The laboratory findings are discussed above and in Table 20.2 but include the following:

Plasma iron: Increased

Plasma transferrin: Decreased with high (>80%) transferrin saturation

Plasma ferritin: Increased

Liver biopsy: Increased iron stores, with or without cirrhotic changes.

Bone marrow: Stainable iron content usually appears normal in haemochromatosis.

Urinary iron excretion: The increased iron stores can be assessed by measuring the urinary excretion of iron after parenteral administration of desferrioxamine which chelates the iron and is excreted by the kidney.

REFERENCES/FURTHER READING

Adams PC, Halliday JW, Powell LW. Early diagnosis and treatment of haemochromatosis. Adv Intern Med 1989;34:111-126.

Adams PC, Halliday JW *et al.* Clinical presentation of haemochromatosis: A changing scene. Am J Med 1991;90:445-449.

Cavill I, Jacobs A, and Wormwood M. Diagnostic methods for iron status. Ann Clin Biochem 1986;23: 168-171.

Jacobs A. (ed) Disorders of iron metabolism. Clin Haematol 1982;11:241-248.

Chapter 21

Porphyrins

Porphyrins, a group of tetrapyrroles differing in the composition of their side chains (Figure 21.1), are intermediate metabolites on the haem synthetic pathway. A number of defects involving specific enzymes catalysing intermediary steps of this pathway, either inherited or acquired, result in the group of disorders collectively known as the porphyrias.

Haem synthesis

This process, which occurs in the liver and the bone marrow, is shown in Figure 21.2.

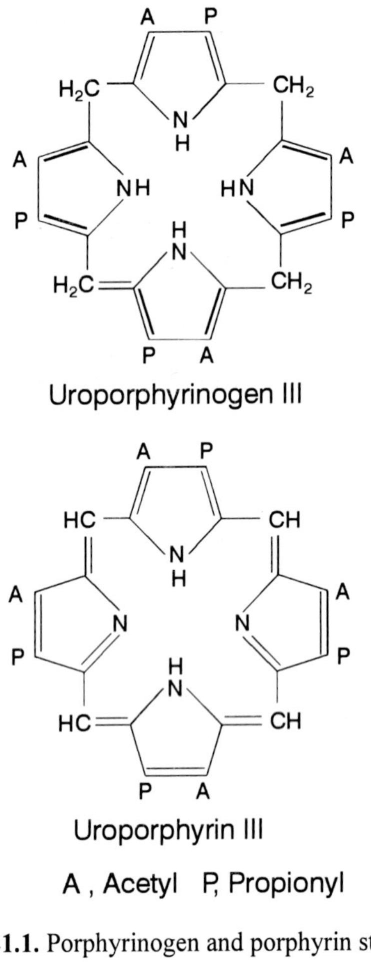

Uroporphyrinogen III

Uroporphyrin III

A , Acetyl   P, Propionyl

Figure 21.1. Porphyrinogen and porphyrin structure.

The first and the last steps in the pathway occur inside the mitochondria; the remaining intermediate steps take place in the cytosolic compartment. The rate-limiting enzyme is *ALA synthetase* which forms δ-aminolaevulinic acid (ALA) from succinyl-CoA and glycine (initial step). This enzyme is subject to end-product negative feedback by the haem molecule. It is repressed by glucose loading and can be induced by a number of compounds including drugs that are microsomal enzyme inducers such as phenobarbital.

Two ALA molecules condense to form the monopyrrole, porphobilinogen (PBG) under the influence of *ALA dehydratase,* an enzyme that is inhibited by lead. In the presence of two enzymes, *uroporphyrinogen I synthetase* (*PBG deaminase*) and *uroporphyrinogen III cosynthetase,* four molecules of PBG are combined to form uroporphyrinogen III (very little uroporphyrinogen I is produced). Uroporphyrinogen I synthetase is deficient in acute intermittent porphyria. Uroporphyrinogen III cosynthetase is deficient in congenital erythropoietic porphyria.

Uroporphyrinogen III is converted to coproporphyrinogen III by *uroporphyrinogen III decarboxylase* which acts on the four acetate (-CH$_2$-COOH) side-chains, converting them to methyl (-CH$_3$) side-chains. The activity of this enzyme is decreased in porphyria cutanea tarda. *Coproporphyrinogen oxidase* converts coproporphyrinogen III to protoporphyrinogen IX, by changing the propionyl (-CH$_2$-CH$_2$-COOH) side-chains into vinyl (-CH=CH$_2$) ones. This enzyme is deficient in hereditary coproporphyria and is inhibited by lead.

Oxidation of protoporphyrinogen IX by *protoporphyrinogen oxidase* converts it to protoporphyrin IX. Ferrous iron (Fe^{2+}) is incorporated into the latter by the enzyme *ferrochelatase* to form haem. Ferrochelatase is deficient in protoporphyria and is also inhibited by lead. Both protoporphyrinogen oxidase and ferrochelatase are deficient in variegate porphyria.

PORPHYRINS

The porphyrins are oxidation products of the various porphyrinogens (Figure 21.1). They do not take part in the haem pathway. The differential solubility of the different porphyrins determine their excretory route;

solubility increases with the number of carboxyl groups.

ALA, PBG, and uroporphyrin are relatively water soluble and appear in the urine. Coproporphyrin and protoporphyrin are relative water insoluble and are excreted in the bile to appear in the faeces. Normally only small amounts of these compounds are excreted, but when excessive amounts are produced, as in the porphyrias, large quantities are excreted.

Disordered haem synthesis (porphyrias)

The porphyrias are a rare group of disorders due to enzyme defects along the porphyrin synthetic pathway. The characteristic clinical and biochemical features are related to reduced activity of a particular enzyme which results in deficient haem production. The low haem concentration in turn stimulates ALA synthetase activity causing increased production of

precursors prior to the block. This increase in intracellular substrate concentration, through operation of the negative feedback control of ALA synthetase activity, appears to be a compensatory adjustment that attempts to maintain the rate of haem synthesis in these patients.

CLASSIFICATION/PATHOPHYSIOLOGY

In all forms of porphyria where inheritance of an enzyme defect has been demonstrated, decreased activity of the enzyme involved has been found in all tissues that have been studied. In contrast, the compensatory changes discussed above are restricted to certain tissues. For example, in acute intermittent porphyria and variegate porphyria, they are evident only in the liver and there is no detectable increase in the concentration of the porphyrin precursors in the erythroid cells. Thus the porphyrias are traditionally divided into hepatic and erythropoietic varieties based on the tissue where the effect of the enzyme defect predominates. In practice, measurement of erythrocyte

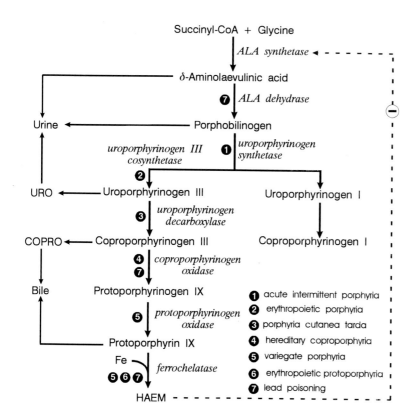

Figure 21.2. Porphyrinogen and haem synthesis.

URO, uroporphyrin;
COPRO, coproporphyrin;
ALA, δ-aminolaevulinic acid.

porphyrin concentration has differentiated the porphyrias falling under these two categories which are accompanied by important clinical differences.

In the following discussion, lead toxicity is included because of its dramatic effect on haem synthesis, particularly in the erythrocyte.

Hepatic porphyrias *(normal red cell porphyrins)*
Acute intermittent porphyria (AIP)
Variegate porphyria (VP)
Hereditary coproporphyria (HCP)
Porphyria cutanea tarda (PCT)

Erythropoietic porphyrias *(increased red cell porphyrins)*
Congenital erythropoietic porphyria (CEP)
Erythropoietic protoporphyria (EP)

Patients with porphyria present in one of three ways:

- with acute attacks (AIP)
- with skin lesions (CEP, EP, PCT)
- with acute attacks and skin lesions (VP, HCP)*

*In VP and HCP, acute attacks are not necessarily accompanied by skin lesions in the same individual, or *vice versa*.

In most affected families, individuals with latent porphyria, who possess the inherited gene but have not developed any clinical features, are more common than those with symptoms.

Acute intermittent porphyria (AIP)

Enzyme defect. Uroporphyrinogen I synthetase.

Transmission. Autosomal dominant.

Chemical pathology. **Urine:** increased ALA and PBG (PBG oxidises to porphobilin under acidic conditions and on exposure to sunlight); urine darkens on standing. **Faeces:** no abnormality.

Clinical. Acute attacks, usually in early adulthood and brought on by drugs (see below). Skin lesions are not a feature.

Varigate porphyria (VP)

Enzyme defect. Protoporphyrinogen oxidase (? ferrochelatase also).

Transmission. Autosomal dominant.

Chemical pathology. **Urine:** increased ALA, PBG, uroporphyrin and coproporphyrin III. **Faeces:** increased coproporphyrin III and protoporphyrin.

Clinical. Acute attacks brought on by drugs as in AIP, and skin lesions (can arise independently).

Hereditary coproporphyria (HCP)

Enzyme defect. Coproporphyrinogen oxidase.

Transmission. Autosomal dominant.

Chemical pathology. **Urine:** increased ALA, PBG, uroporphyrin and coproporphyrin III. **Faeces:** increased coproporphyrin III.

Clinical. Acute attacks as in AIP. Skin lesions in 30% of cases and always associated with acute attacks.

Porphyria cutanea tarda (PCT)

Enzyme defect. Uroporphyrinogen decarboxylase.

Transmission. Usually acquired but many cases have a familial basis, with the defect inherited as an autosomal dominant characteristic.

Chemical pathology. **Urine:** normal PBG, increased uroporphyrins. **Faeces:** occasionally increased porphyrins.

Clinical. Differs from the other hepatic porphyrias in that only the skin lesions occur. It is the most common porphyria and is often associated with liver dysfunction. Predisposing factors are alcoholism and increased hepatic iron stores (haemosiderosis).

Congenital erythropoietic porphyria (CEP)

Enzyme defect. Uroporphyrinogen III cosynthetase (erythrocytes).

Transmission. Autosomal recessive.

Chemical pathology. **Red cells:** increased uroporphyrinogen. **Urine and Faeces:** increased uroporphyrinogen I and coproporphyrin III.

Clinical. Onset in infancy, with bullous skin lesions and red urine. The teeth are brownish-pink and fluoresce under UV light. Afflicted subjects often have haemolytic anaemia and hirsutism.

Erythropoietic protoporphyria (EP)

Enzyme defect. Ferrochelatase.

Transmission. Autosomal dominant.

Chemical pathology. **Red cells:** increased protoporphyrinogen. **Urine:** normal. **Faeces:** increased protoporphyrin.

Clinical. Onset in childhood with photosensitivity (skin lesions). Usually a mild disorder.

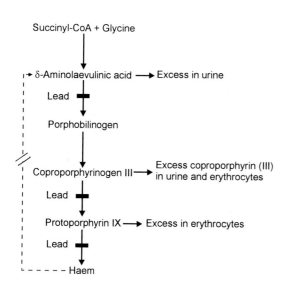

Figure 21.3. Effects of lead on haem synthesis. See also Figure 21.2 for the enzymes involved.

Lead poisoning

Lead inhibits ALA dehydratase, coproporphyrinogen

oxidase, and ferrochelatase (Figure 21.3). The resulting decrease in haem synthesis stimulates ALA synthetase. This can result in:

- Anaemia due to decreased haem synthesis
- Increased ALA synthesis and increased urinary excretion
- Increased coproporphyrinogen synthesis and increased urinary excretion
- Accumulation of protoporphyrin in red cells

CONSEQUENCES/CLINICAL FEATURES OF PORPHYRIAS

Clinically the porphyrias usually present with acute porphyria attacks, often drug-related and reflecting intermittent nervous system dysfunction, or skin lesions due to increased sensitivity to sunlight.

Acute attacks. The acute presentation is probably related to the induction of ALA synthetase. This speeds up the biosynthetic pathway up to the stage blocked by the defective enzyme and results in

(a) accumulation of intermediates prior to the block and
(b) inadequate haem production and further stimulation of ALA synthetase.

Many acute illnesses and the ingestion of apparently unrelated substances, the most common being drugs (particularly barbiturates, Table 21.1), can precipitate the attack. Most of the incriminated drugs are metabolised in the liver by haem-containing microsomal enzyme systems such as cytochrome P-450 (the need to increase production of this enzyme complex requires stimulation of ALA synthetase which becomes sustained due to ineffective production of haem).

The acute attack has a neurological basis related to the accumulation of ALA and PBG and may present as:

- Abdominal symptoms: pain, vomiting, constipation
- Peripheral neuritis: limb pain, muscle weakness
- Psychiatric disturbances: depression, anxiety, psychosis

Episodic acute attacks are the only clinical feature in AIP, but they are accompanied by skin lesions in about 50% of patients with VP and in about a third of those with HCP. They are not a feature of the acquired PCT, nor of the erythropoietic porphyrias.

Table 21.1. Some drugs causing acute porphyria.

Barbiturates	Oestrogens
Carbamazepine	Oxazepam
Chlorpropamide	Phenytoin
Ethanol	Primidone
Griseofulvin	Progesterone
Halothane	Sulphonamides
Methyldopa	Theophylline

Skin lesions. Photosensitivity occurs in those areas of the skin where the high levels of porphyrins circulating in the peripheral veins are exposed to sunlight. Porphyrins absorb energy at around 400 nm and it is thought that the "excited" porphyrins damage lysosomal membranes via lipid peroxidaton (releasing lysozymes and proteases). The lesions, in addition to photosensitivity, include subepidermal bullae, oedema, pigmentation, and hirsutism. Skin lesions may occur in VP, HCP, PCT, and the erythropoietic porphyrias. They do not occur in AIP.

LABORATORY EVALUATION

Most porphyrias can be diagnosed on the basis of the clinical presentation and the results of a few simple screening tests (Figure 21.4). Definitive diagnosis may require the quantitative estimation of urinary and faecal porphyrin levels, which are mostly complex and labour-intensive procedures and perhaps demonstration of the deficient enzyme.

For subjects presenting with a suspected *acute attack,* the screening tests should include at least urinary PBG and urinary and faecal porphyrin estimations.

Urinary PBG. This is positive in all three acute porphyrias (AIP, VP, HCP) during the acute attack. It is often negative in VP and HCP during remission but may be positive in AIP. (The only other condition in which PBG excretion may be increased is severe lead poisoning, see above).

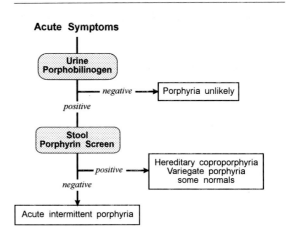

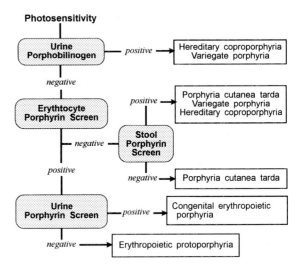

Figure 21.4. Suggested schemes for the evaluation of suspected porphyrias.

Urinary porphyrins. Increased levels occur in all three acute porphyrias. In AIP there is no *in vivo* increased porphyrin synthesis but non-enzymatic polymerisation of PBG in urine left standing produces uroporphyrin.

Faecal porphyrins. Screening tests show increased excretion in VP and HCP (normal in AIP).

In patients with *skin lesions* the useful screening tests are:

Erythrocyte porphyrins. Increased in EP and CEP.

282

Urine porphyrins. Increased in PCT, HCP, CEP, and sometimes in VP (PCT and CEP have normal PBG excretion).

Faecal porphyrins. Increased in VP, HCP, PCT, and the erythropoietic porphyrias.

In the laboratory evaluation of suspected porphyria, the following points warrant emphasis:

- Fresh or adequately preserved samples of urine, faeces, or erythrocytes are essential to minimise false positive or false negative results.

- Failure to investigate faecal excretion of porphyrins is an important source of error by omission.

- Acute attacks of porphyria are always associated with increased urine excretion of PBG, which is an essential test in the laboratory diagnosis of acute porphyrias. The urine samples may be dark reddish-brown (port wine colour) or normal straw-coloured, darkening on standing.

- A negative screening PBG test does not exclude increased PBG excretion, as the test has a sensitivity limit of ~30 μmol/L, which is about 3x the upper limit of the reference values.

- PBG excretion falls rapidly and is negative during remission of HCP and VP, but not in the case of AIP. In these situations, screening for faecal porphyrins is essential, enabling the positive detection of those with HCP and VP who test negative for the urine PBG screening test; their faecal porphyrin screens are usually positive. The test also differentiates AIP cases (negative faecal porphyrins) from the other two conditions.

- Provided the samples are fresh, a positive screening test for urine porphyrins and a negative screening test for PBG in the urine, *in a patient with acute abdominal pain,* is almost always due to one of the causes of secondary coproporphyrinuria (Table 21.2).

- Conditions in which red cell protoporphyrins are

increased include:

(a) erythropoietic protoporphyria (increased protoporphyrins)

(b) iron deficiency, lead poisoning, sideroplastic anaemias, haemolytic anaemias (increased zinc-protoporphrins).

Table 21.2. Causes of coproporphyrinuria.

Primary
  Variegate porphyria
  Hereditary coproporphyria
  Congenital erythropoietic porphyria*

Secondary
  Toxic conditions
    Alcoholism
    Lead poisoning
  Impaired biliary secretion
    Hepatocellular disease
    Cholestasis
    Pregnancy
  Miscellaneous
    Dubin-Johnson syndrome
    Severe infections
    Rheumatic fever

---

*without acute abdominal symptoms

REFERENCES/FURTHER READING

Elder GH, Smith SG, Smyth SJ. Laboratory investigation of the porphyrias. Ann Clin Biochem 1990;27:395-412.

Hindmarsh JT. Clinical disorders of porphyrin metabolism. Clin Biochem 1982;16:209-219.

Magnus IA. Drugs and porphyria. Br Med J 1984;288:1474-1475.

Chapter 22

Biochemical Syndromes of Tumours

Many benign and malignant tumours synthesise and secrete compounds which can be detected in the blood or serous fluids. These include amines, hormones, enzymes, and proteins. Since these compounds are produced within the tumours, whether by malignant or stromal cells, they are said to be tumour-derived and provide evidence of the tumour's existence (tumour markers). In many tumours, tumour-derived antigens are not secreted into the blood (or serous fluids) but are expressed as cell-surface antigens.

There are thus, broadly speaking, two ways of assaying tumour markers produced by solid tumours:

- by measuring their concentrations in the plasma or serum, and
- by detecting their presence on cells or tissues, using immunochemical staining with conjugated monoclonal antibodies.

In this section, we will only discuss the tumour marker assays of the first type.

Aside from measuring tumour markers which are essentially gene products, in situ hybridization with end-labelled nucleic acid probes and other molecular techniques are increasingly being used to identify the genes and genetic defects (deletions, mutations, translocations, etc) associated with malignancy. We will not describe these recent developments which are, by and large, still confined to research and medical oncology laboratories.

Some of the tumour markers, e.g., onco-foetal proteins, certain enzymes, and ectopic hormones, are believed to be produced by the tumour cells as a result of derepression of genes not normally expressed in the non-cancerous tissue. Others are endogenous products of normal cells such as hormones, enzymes, and amines, which are produced at higher rates by the transformed cancer cells, their synthesis not being regulated by the normal homeostatic mechanisms.

Some tumour markers are themselves biologically active products (e.g., hormones, amines) and may cause distressing symptoms, e.g., severe hyper-cortisolism associated with the ectopic production of ACTH (adrenocorticotrophic hormone). Others are biologically inert, but the finding of high plasma concentrations may alert to the presence of an occult malignancy in someone with non-specific symptoms.

CLINICAL USEFULNESS OF TUMOUR MARKERS

The measurement of some of these markers can be useful and may aid in:

- the diagnosis of cancer
- cancer staging and prognosis
- the monitoring of therapeutic response
- the monitoring of disease progression or regression

Regrettably, despite initial high expectations when tumour marker assays first appeared on the scene, only rarely does a tumour marker exhibit sufficient diagnostic specificity and sensitivity (see below) to be of any use in screening for the presence of primary tumours, even among high risk groups, let alone the population at large. One rare exception is the close association between high plasma calcitonin concentrations and medullary carcinoma of the thyroid.

The diagnosis of cancer

It would be ideal if a tumour marker could help in establishing the diagnosis of malignancy in a patient with symptoms, preferably in the early stages of tumour formation. Commonly, tumour marker assays are used in conjunction with radiology and tissue biopsy to establish the disease. The efficacy or predictive accuracy of a tumour marker depends on its diagnostic specificity and sensitivity. Naturally, the higher the diagnostic specificity and sensitivity of a test, the better it is. A brief explanation of these important attributes of a tumour marker assay, as defined by Galen and Gambino (see reference on page 290), follows.

Diagnostic specificity: This is defined as negativity in health. It is calculated by dividing the true negatives (those without the disease and who test negative using the assay) by the total number of subjects without the disease (i.e., true negatives and false positives). A tumour marker is specific to the extent that it identifies (correctly) those who do not have the malignancy, and particularly to the extent that it minimises the number of false positives. A related concept, the negative predictive value of a tumour marker assay (true negatives divided by true negatives plus false negatives), gives the probability that a negative result indicates absence of disease.

Diagnostic sensitivity: This defines the number of true positive results (those with cancer who test positive) divided by the total number of subjects who have cancer (i.e., true positives plus false negatives). From this, it can be appreciated that a negative result cannot be used to exclude malignancy in a patient except in the rare situation where a tumour marker has 100% sensitivity for a specific tumour type. The positive predictive value of a test, which fulfils the more practical need to know the probability that a positive result indicates the presence of malignancy, is given by the true positives divided by true positives plus false positives.

Cancer staging and prognosis

In order to be of value in prognostication, the measured tumour marker concentration should correlate closely with the size and/or activity of the tumour from which it is derived. It stands to reason that if this relationship holds true, then a massive, disseminated tumour or an aggressively growing lesion would produce a much greater increase in concentration than a small, contained or localised tumour. Unfortunately, this assumption is rarely borne out in practice, and tumour markers contribute little to prognosis in cancer patients.

However, there are some specific situations where knowledge of a tumour marker concentration provides a very useful clue to the possibility of tumour recurrence in a patient with a resected primary cancer. For example, in patients who have had malignant teratomas removed by surgery and in whom there are no clinical evidences of metastasis, elevated concentrations of α-fetoprotein in the immediate post-operational period would suggest the likelihood of residual cancerous tissues or probable metastasis. They warn of a high chance of tumour recurrence and stress the need for strict surveillance and intensive followup.

The monitoring of therapeutic response

Whilst the usefulness of tumour markers in screening and diagnosis remain circumspect, they are well established as an invaluable tool in monitoring the efficacy of therapy in diagnosed cases of malignancy. Effective therapeutic measures (whether by surgery, chemotherapy, radiation, or a combination of these), resulting in the successful containment of the malignant process will be indicated by a corresponding fall in the tumour marker concentration.

Following successful therapy, the plasma concentration usually stabilises, often reverting back to normal or even undetectable levels. A significant and sustained rise in the concentration of the tumour marker provides an invaluable early indication of tumour recurrence, prompting the institution of timely and effective second line therapy. The value of such early evidences of tumour recurrence based on tumour marker assay results is greatest for those tumour types where clinical evidence of recurrence is most difficult to obtain.

It is important to ensure that a rise that has been detected in the serial monitoring of a particular patient is a significant one which can be interpreted with confidence as indicative of tumour recurrence. This involves:

(a) the determination of appropriate cut-off or action limits for the tumour marker assay used, and

(b) detailed documentation of its inter-assay (or inter-day) imprecision at an analyte concentration close to the proposed action limit.

A significant rise is one in which the increase over the previous result is more than that which could be attributed to purely analytical variability inherent in the assay.

A second important factor to take into consideration in the interpretation of the tumour marker assay results is the appreciation that the finding of concentrations that fall within the quoted reference range of the assay has little or no relevance in these situations, the key parameter being the *change* in concentration, using the patient's previous level as his or her own referent baseline.

TUMOUR MARKERS IN CURRENT USE

In the following sections, established tumour markers that have gained general acceptance in clinical practice or 'new' markers which are promising and may prove useful will be discussed. They are a structurally and functionally diverse group which includes amines, hormones, enzymes, paraproteins, and tumour-associated antigens. Those that have been discussed elsewhere in this text are mentioned and cross-referenced. Hormone receptors have not been included in our review.

Amines

There are three amine-producing tumours:

- **Carcinoid tumours:** Produce serotonin (5-hydroxytryptamine) and the carcinoid syndrome (page 223).

- **Phaeochromocytomas:** Produce catecholamines (adrenalin, noradrenalin) and hypertension (page 295).

- **Neuroblastomas:** Produce catecholamines and dopamine (page 296).

Hormones

There are two types of hormone-producing tumours:

1. *Tumours of endocrine tissue*
2. *Tumours of non-endocrine tissue which produce hormones* (ectopic hormone production).

Tumours of endocrine tissues

These tumours may be benign or malignant and in some cases there may be more than one hormone-producing tumour in the same patient. Hormone-producing tumours have been described for all of the body's endocrine tissue, although none of them occurs commonly. Hormones produced by tumours of endocrine tissues are referred to as eutopic hormones (appropriate to the tissue of origin). Measurement of the eutopic hormone concentration is essential to the diagnosis of the tumour since most endocrine tumours tend to be small; symptoms arising from the hormone excess is usually evident before the tumour can be detected by basic radiological techniques.

Whilst most hormones are measurable in plasma, the diagnosis of some tumours relies on the measurement of hormone metabolites in the urine or plasma rather than on the plasma concentration of the parent hormones. For example, the use of normetanephrines or vanillyl mandelic acid and of 5-hydroxyindole acetic acid in the diagnosis of phaeochromocytomas and carcinoid tumours, respectively.

- **Anterior pituitary:** Adenomas producing prolactin (page 231), growth hormone (page 230), ACTH (page 257).

- **Thyroid:** Thyroxine-producing adenomas, medullary carcinomas producing calcitonin (see below)

- **Parathyroids:** Adenomas and carcinomas producing PTH (page 93).

- **Adrenal cortex:** Adenomas or carcinomas producing cortisol (page 258), or androgens (page 270) or aldosterone (page 66).

- **Adrenal medulla:** Phaeochromocytomas producing catecholamines (page 295).

- **Pancreatic islets:** Insulinomas (page 134), gastrinomas (page 222), VIPomas (page 223).

- **Trophoblastic tissues:** Choriocarcinomas producing human chorionic gonadotrophin (HCG, see below)

- **Multiple tumours:** Multiple endocrine neoplasia (MEN, see below).

Medullary carcinomas of the thyroid: These tumours are derived from the parafollicular cells (C-cells) of the thyroid gland and secrete large amounts of calcitonin. Although calcitonin is recognised as a calcium-lowering hormone, these tumours do not normally result in hypocalcaemia, probably because there is a concomitant compensatory increase in PTH production. These tumours may also secrete ACTH (ectopic ACTH production), prostaglandins, and serotonin and, in addition, they may be associated with other hormone-producing tumours, e.g., phaeochromocytomas and parathyroid adenomas (see below). The detection of high blood levels of calcitonin is pathognomonic of the condition; hence calcitonin is an excellent diagnostic marker.

Choriocarcinomas: These tumours are derived from trophoblastic tissues. They occur in 5-10% of women with hydatidiform molar pregnancies. Serum HCG concentrations correlate well with tumour mass and allow for the detection of as few as 10^5 cells (1 mg of tissue), making serum HCG one of the most sensitive tests for human tumours. Rising or grossly elevated serum β-HCG concentrations a month or two after evacuation of the molar pregnancy or similar findings associated with persistent uterine bleeding 4-6 months after evacuation are strong indications for chemotherapy, as is an unexpected and sustained rise in β-HCG at any later date.

Multiple endocrine neoplasia (MEN): This rare familial disorder, inherited as an autosomal dominant trait, may present as one of two distinct syndromes. Several of the tumours involve APUD cells, derived from tissues of neuroectodermal origin. APUD (amine precursor uptake and decarboxylation) tumours which may be malignant include insulinoma, gastrinoma, carcinoid tumour, phaeochromocytoma, neuroblastoma, and medullary carcinoma of the thyroid. This common origin partially explains the occurrence of these pleuriglandular syndromes.

Type 1 (MEN₁): This syndrome involves two or more of the following: parathyroid adenoma, pancreatic islet cell tumours (insulinoma, gastrinoma), adenoma of the anterior pituitary gland, adenoma of the adrenal cortex, thyroid adenoma. The clinical presentation is variable and depends on the types of tumour involved.

Type 2 (MEN₂): This syndrome consists of medullary carcinoma of thyroid, phaeochromocytoma (often bilateral), and parathyroid adenoma.

Hormone-producing tumours of non-endocrine tissues

A number of malignant tumours, the best example being bronchial carcinoma, are capable of producing peptide hormones such as ACTH and ADH, which are not normally produced by the non-cancerous tissues. These are termed *ectopic hormones* and have the same biological activities as their native hormone counterparts. There are two main theories to explain this phenomenon:

1. *Gene derepression:* All cells have the potential to synthesise any peptide produced endogenously by the body but most of this activity is repressed during specific tissue development. As a cell undergoes malignant transformation, some genes become derepressed and resume expression.

2. *Arrested differentiation:* This theory suggests that some cells fail to fully differentiate from the primitive level during development. These cells retain functions that are normally present during the developmental stage, expressing them fully under certain circumstances, e.g., malignancy.

However, as good as these theories appear, they do not hold up well upon closer examination and the pathogenesis of ectopic-hormone production is still unclear.

The two commonest ectopic hormones are ACTH and ADH; tumour-related hypercalcaemia, a common condition, was once considered to be due to ectopic PTH production but this is now considered unlikely (see below). Other ectopic hormones that have been described are: calcitonin, growth hormone, prolactin, human chorionic gonadotrophin, human placental lactogen (HPL), insulin, and erythropoietin.

Tumour hypercalcaemia: Ten to 20% of patients with malignancy will develop hypercalcaemia. In many cases the cause is bone metastases, but around 10% have no evidence of bone secondaries. In this latter group the hypercalcaemia is often associated with hypophosphataemia and increased urinary excretion of cyclic-AMP; these are features of hyperparathyroidism and hence the thought that the disorder may be due to ectopic PTH production. However, the plasma level of immunoreactive PTH is generally low in these cases and DNA probe studies suggest that, with rare exceptions, native PTH is not produced by these tumours.

Recent investigations have shown that the mechanism of this so-called humoral hypercalcaemia of malignancy is the production by the tumour of a peptide designated PTH-related protein (PTH-rP). This compound, which binds to PTH receptors, contains 141 amino acids of which 8 of the first 13 (from the amino-terminal) are identical to those of human PTH. This protein enhances osteoclastic activity (bone resorption), enhances renal tubular calcium reabsorption, and causes hypercalcaemia.

Note: A recent survey has shown that up to 10% of patients with malignancy-related hypercalcaemia have primary hyperparathyroidism (Walls *et al*, 1994, see page 290).

Ectopic ADH secretion: The syndrome of inappropriate secretion of ADH (SIADH) which results in hyponatraemia is discussed more fully on page 14. It is commonly associated with oat-cell carcinoma of the bronchus but may also occur in association with tumours of the gut, pancreas, and lymphoid tissue.

Ectopic ACTH syndrome: Ectopic production of ACTH may occur in a variety of tumours including carcinomas of the bronchus, pancreas and thymus. It results in hyperpigmentation (ACTH effect) and hypokalaemic metabolic alkalosis (adrenal steroid effect). The patients generally do not survive long enough for the classical features of Cushing's syndrome to develop (see page 257). The prognosis of this tumour is so poor that the use of any tumour marker is unlikely to alter the clinical outcome once the accompanying distressing symptoms of hypercortisolaemia have been minimised. In these situations, repeated measurement of ACTH is of little use and is not recommended.

Calcitonin: High circulating levels of calcitonin (due to ectopic production) have been reported in patients with carcinoma of the bronchus and breast.

Growth hormone: Ectopic production has been reported in patients with carcinomas of the bronchus and of the stomach. The lung tumour may be associated with hypertrophic osteoarthropathy, a condition that resembles the bone disorder produced in acromegaly.

Prolactin: Breast carcinomas, renal cell carcinomas, and oat cell carcinomas of the bronchus have been reported to be associated with increased plasma levels of immunoreactive prolactin. Galactorrhoea, a common condition in hyperprolactinaemia due to pituitary prolactinomas (page 231), has not been described in patients with the ectopic hormone.

Human chorionic gonadotrophin (HCG): High levels of HCG, which is normally only found in pregnancy, may occur as an ectopic hormone in tumours of the testes and ovaries (particularly teratomas). It has also been described in tumours of the stomach, pancreas and liver. It is essential for assays measuring HCG as a tumour marker to have much lower detection limits than those meant as pregnancy tests, and the improved specificity of β-subunit detection. With appropriate cut-off limits, β-HCG concentrations in serum or urine are elevated in 40-80% of cases of non-seminomatous germ cell testicular carcinoma. The sensitivity of HCG assays for these tumours is improved significantly by the simultaneous measurement of AFP. The production of HCG in choriocarcinomas, tumours derived from trophoblastic tissue, is eutopic and was discussed above.

Human placental lactogen (HPL): This hormone which is normally produced by the placenta has been reported in patients with tumours of the ovary, testes, and lung.

Tumour hypoglycaemia: Hypoglycaemia due to non-pancreatic tumours has been described in mesenchymal tumours (e.g., retroperitoneal fibromas), hepatomas, adrenocortical carcinomas, and carcinomas of the gut. They are not associated with increased circulating insulin levels, as was first thought to be so. The cause is still unclear -- suggestions include the elaboration of an insulin-like substance or substances by the tumour and increased metabolic activity and glucose uptake by the tumour (see also page 133).

Erythropoietin: This hormone, normally produced by the kidney, stimulates red cell production by the bone marrow. Increased circulating levels have been described in patients with hepatomas, bronchogenic carcinomas, and haemangioblastomas.

Enzymes

High plasma levels of a number of enzymes are frequently detected in malignant states. They are released from malignant cells due to cell necrosis or increased production of the enzyme (tumour-derived), or from the tissue damage associated with malignant invasion (tumour-associated), e.g., elevated alkaline phosphatase and transaminases are associated with liver secondaries.

The enzymes derived from malignant cells may be *glycolytic enzymes, organ-specific enzymes, or*

288

"ectopic" enzymes.

Glycolytic enzymes: Malignant cells have high rates of glycolysis and enzymes involved in this pathway, such as lactate dehydrogenase, aldolase, and hexokinase, are often found in the blood in large quantities when the malignant cells break down. This is the reason why an isolated finding of raised lactate dehydrogenase requires further investigation for possible harboring of an occult malignancy.

Organ-specific enzymes: This group includes pancreatic amylase (carcinoma of the pancreas, page 182), prostatic acid phosphatase (carcinoma of the prostate, page181), bone alkaline phosphatase (osteogenic sarcoma, page 178), and neurone-specific enolase.

Neurone specific enolase (NSE): This isoenzyme of enolase is found in high concentrations in nerve cells and cells with neuroendocrine function. Tumours arising from these cell types, such as small cell lung cancers and neuroblastomas, express high levels of this marker. The clinical application of NSE as a tumour marker needs further verification but currently its primary use is in monitoring patients with small cell lung cancers for efficacy of therapy.

Ectopic enzymes: High plasma enzyme levels may occur in patients with neoplasms of tissues not normally associated with that particular enzyme. Such is probably not a true ectopic production; it probable represents an increased production of an enzyme normally present in the tissue in very small amounts.

The isoenzyme of alkaline phosphatase known as the Regan isoenzyme has been described in patients with carcinomas of the lung, ovary, testes, and colon. This enzyme is similar to placental alkaline phosphatase in physical and biochemical properties (page 179). Similarly, increased plasma levels of amylase have occurred in patients with carcinomas of the lung, ovary, and colon.

Proteins

Most patients with malignancy have a low plasma total protein due to hypoalbuminaemia (page 165). In patients with paraproteinaemia (page 170), the increased immunoglobulins may result in hyperproteinaemia. Paraproteins serve as excellent tumour markers, with their concentrations in serum correlating very well with tumour burden. Two other conditions that may be associated with plasma protein abnormalities in malignancy are the acute phase reaction (page 174) and the production of tumour-associated antigens.

Tumour-associated antigens

The tumour-associated antigens are proteins not normally present in significant quantities in the plasma of adult subjects but which may be produced in excess by transformed malignant cells. Amongst those that have been clinically useful are carcinoembryonic antigen, (CEA), alpha-fetoprotein (AFP), prostatic specific antigen (PSA), and cancer antigen 125 (CA-125). A number of other tumour-associated antigens have been described in recent years, but their potential as tumour markers require to be more extensively studied before their place in cancer screening and diagnosis can be established. These include carbohydrate antigen 19-9 (CA 19-9), ovarian cystadenomacarcinoma antigen (OCCA), mucin carcinoma antigen (MCA), mammary specific antigen (MSA), neurone specific enolase (NSE) and carcinoma antigen 50 (CA-50). Also included in this group of antigens is inhibin (page 262).

When using these antigens in screening for cancer it is important to note that the following apply:

- None of the antigens are organ specific.
- They are not generally useful for the early detection of cancer.
- They may be associated with non-malignant disease.

An exception to the above is prostate specific antigen which is organ specific and has an application in the detection and monitoring of prostatic carcinoma.

Carcinoembryonic antigen (CEA): This is a glycoprotein (MW ~200 000) synthesised by foetal intestinal tissue which is present in very small amounts in adult plasma (<2 µg/L). High plasma levels may be found in patients with carcinoma of the gut (70-80%) and those with lung and breast cancer (10-20%). Non-tumour elevations may occur in pancreatitis, ulcerative colitis, heavy smokers, alcoholic liver disease, and colonic polyps (these elevations tend to be moderate: 2.5-10 µg/L). The main application of this antigen is in the monitoring of cancer therapy in patients with elevated pretreatment levels, e.g., after removal of the primary tumour the plasma CEA value should return to normal within six weeks, failure to do so suggests secondaries.

Alpha-fetoprotein (AFP): In the foetus this protein is synthesised initially by the yolk sac cells and later by the liver and probably assumes the role of albumin (shows 30% structural homology with albumin). Its synthesis ceases at birth and it is almost undetectable in the blood of adults. Raised plasma levels occur in patients with hepatomas (70-90%), teratomas and other germ cell tumours. Non-tumour elevations may be seen in hepatitis, cirrhosis of the liver, and ulcerative colitis (and pregnancy). A major use is in monitoring testicular teratocarcinoma, where it is used in combination with HCG.

Prostatic specific antigen (PSA): This is a glycoprotein enzyme (serine protease) which is prostate specific, being found in prostatic tissue (normal and malignant), seminal fluid, and plasma (small amounts, <4.0 mg/L). It is elevated in ~85% of patients with carcinoma of the prostate but also in up to 15% of subjects with benign prostatic hypertrophy (levels usually less than 10 mg/L). It is considered a useful screening test for prostatic cancer in patients 50 years and above and is very useful for following therapy of prostatic malignancy (page 181).

Cancer antigen 125 (CA-125): CA-125 is present in trace amounts in the serum of normal adults and high values are found in some 80% of subjects with non-mucinous epithelial ovarian cancers. It has also been described in some patients with pancreatic, colonic, lung, and breast cancers. Non-tumour elevations can occur in patients with endometriosis, peritonitis, pelvic inflammation, liver failure, acute pancreatitis, and ectopic pregnancy. Its most useful application is in the monitoring of ovarian carcinoma therapy (providing the pretreatment level is raised).

Carbohydrate antigen 19-9 (CA 19-9): This is a high molecular weight carbohydrate-rich glycoprotein which is frequently elevated in patients with intra-abdominal carcinomas, particularly malignancy of the pancreas (~80%). It has also been described in patients with carcinomas of the lung, bile ducts, and gastro-intestinal tract (20-30% of colorectal cancers).

Mammary specific antigen (MSA): This antigen is elevated in breast cancer (70% of patients with stage I/II and 80% with stage III/IV) and, rarely, in carcinoma of the ovary, lung and pancreas. Non-tumour elevations have been noted in benign breast disease, cirrhosis, and hepatitis.

Inhibin: This is a peptide normally produced by ovarian granulosa cells (page 262). High levels have been detected in the sera of patients with granulosa cell tumours of the ovary. The routine assay for this peptide is not yet generally available.

REFERENCES/FURTHER READING

Ambruster DA. Prostate specific antigen: Biochemistry, analytical methods, and clinical application. Clin Chem 1993;39:181-195.

Beastall GH, Cook B, Rustin GJS, Jennings J. A review of the role of established tumour markers. Ann Clin Biochem 199;28:5-18.

Bone HG. Diagnosis of the multiglandular endocrine neoplasias. Clin Chem 1990;36:711-718.

Clark AJL. Ectopic hormone production. Bailliere's Clinics Endocrinol Metab 1988;2:967-983

Duffy MH. New cancer markers. Ann Clin Biochem 1989;26:379-397.

Galen RS, Gambino SR. *Beyond Normality: the Predictive Value and Efficiency of Medical Diagnostics.* New York: Wiley, 1975.

Heath DA. Parathyroid hormone related protein. Clin Endocrinol 1993;38:135-136.

Walls J, Ratcliffe WA, Howell A, Bundred NJ. Parathyroid hormone and parathyroid hormone related protein in the investigation of hypercalcaemia in two hospital populations. Clin Endocrinol Oxf 1994;41: 407-13.

Chapter 23

Biochemical Aspects of Hypertension

The blood pressure is the balance between the force with which blood is pumped from the heart and the peripheral vascular resistance which determines the rate at which blood re-enters the small arteries, capillaries, and veins. An increase in peripheral resistance, due to increased arteriolar vasoconstriction, results in hypertension.

For the purposes of treatment hypertension is usually defined as a diastolic blood pressure in excess of 90 mmHg. The WHO criteria in defining hypertension are a systolic blood pressure of 160 mm Hg or more and/or a diastolic blood pressure of 95 mm Hg or more. Based on the latter criteria, approximately a quarter of the adult population in western countries have hypertension at first screening. In many people a lower pressure is found on rechecking or on subsequent clinic visits, emphasising the need to confirm a single raised blood pressure reading before making a clinical decision to start drug treatment.

Blood pressures tend to rise with advancing age, and patients with higher pressures sustain a faster rise than those with lower pressures. In subjects over the age of 40 years, 40% have a diastolic pressure >90 mmHg, 25% >95 mmHg, and 15% >100 mmHg. Some clinicians treat (with antihypertensive drugs) all patients with a diastolic pressure >90 mmHg whilst others use 100 mmHg as the cut-off point. Patients with borderline values are usually managed initially with simple non-pharmacological measures such as dietary control (in obese patients), moderation of alcohol intake, and lowering of dietary salt (NaCl) intake. In most populations, about 10% are in need of drug therapy.

CAUSES/PATHOPHYSIOLOGY

The majority of hypertensive subjects, variously put as 70 to 95%, have idiopathic or *essential* hypertension, i.e., no cause can be found after intensive evaluation. In these subjects there appears to be no primary biochemical abnormality other than alterations in sodium transport across cell membranes. In patients with non-essential hypertension the most common cause is renal disease (parenchymal and renovascular); endocrine disorders such as Conn's syndrome and phaeochromocytomas are uncommon (<1% of all hypertensives).

A convenient classification is as follows:

Primary (essential) hypertension

Non-essential hypertension **secondary** to:

Renal disease:
Parenchymal disease (glomerulonephritis, diabetic renal disease, analgesic nephropathy, pyelonephropathy)
Renovascular disease (renal artery stenosis, atheroma)

Endocrine disease:
Pancreas: diabetes mellitus
Adrenal medulla: phaeochromocytoma
Adrenal cortex: primary hyperaldosteronism; Cushing's syndrome, enzyme defects
Thyroid: thyrotoxicosis
Parathyroid: hyperparathyroidism (part of multiple endocrine neoplasia (page 287)
Pituitary: acromegaly

Drugs
oral contraceptives, hormone replacement therapy, nephrotoxic drugs, liquorice and carbenoxolone, sympathomimetic amines, non-steroidal anti-inflammatory drugs

Miscellaneous:
Renin secreting tumour, toxaemia of pregnancy, coarctation of aorta, systemic lupus erythematosus

Renal disease and hypertension. Renal insufficiency is often a complication of hypertension (hypertensive nephropathy) and renal disease is a cause of hypertension. The latter may be due to parenchymal disease or to renovascular disease.

Parenchymal renal disease. Acute and chronic renal failure are often accompanied by hypertension. This may be due to sodium and water retention (usual cause), failure to inactivate circulating vasopressor agents, activation of the renin-angiotensin system, or failure to produce the necessary vasodilators (e.g., prostaglandins, bradykinin).

Renovascular hypertension. Stenosis of the main renal artery or one of its major branches stimulates renin secretion by that kidney (decreased renal blood flow, decreased perfusion pressure). This results in high circulating levels of angiotensin II which in turn causes vasoconstriction, increased aldosterone secretion, and stimulation of the adrenergic nervous system; hence hypertension. There may also be hypokalaemia due to the hyper-aldosteronism an d the condition can be confused with Conn's syndrome (page 66).

Whilst surgical correction is possible, this is usually carried out on younger patients. Renovascular hypertension, however, mainly afflicts older patients (>40 years of age), and may be the consequence of hypertension due to some other cause and aggravating it.

Drug-induced hypertension. Taken together, this is an important cause of hypertension and an evaluation of a hypertensive patient should always include a careful drug history. Various drugs are implicated:

- About 5% of women on oral contraceptives, and perhaps a smaller percentage of those on hormone replacement therapy, will develop hypertension, usually a mild or moderate form.

- Excessive habitual ingestion of liquorice-containing sweets, lozenges or mixtures and treatment with carbenoxolone for peptic ulceration may lead to a mineralocorticoid-like hypertension.

- Non-steroidal anti-inflammatory drugs and sympathomimetic amines (often found in cold cures and nasal decongesants) may cause a mild elevation of the blood pressure; their use may also interfere with the action of anti-hypertensive drugs.

- Prolonged glucocorticoid and ACTH therapy may lead to Cushingoid features, including hypertension.

- The use of drugs with known nephrotoxic effects should be carefully monitored as their indiscriminate or overenthusiastic usage will result in acute or chronic renal failure, which may be accompanied by hypertension.

CONSEQUENCES

Hypertension may cause cardiac failure, retinopathy, encephalopathy and other non-specific clinical disorders but from a biochemical point of view the major complication is renal failure. A number of metabolic abnormalities have a high association with hypertension but a causal relationship is sometimes difficult to prove; these include:

- Diabetes mellitus
- Primary hyperparathyroidism
- Hyperuricaemia
- Hyperlipidaemia

The identification of hypertensive patients who are at higher risk on the basis of hyperlipidaemia, renal impairment or glucose intolerance substantially influences their management.

LABORATORY EVALUATION

The careful investigation of hypertensive patients at the time of diagnosis must be seen in the light of their lifelong need for constant vigilance of their blood pressures and antihypertensive therapy. The majority of patients with hypertension have the essential or idiopathic variety for which the treatment is symptomatic. Extensive laboratory investigation is unwarranted in most cases and is usually limited to the evaluation of renal function and lipid metabolism.

If the hypertension is of sudden onset or occurs in a young age group (<40 years), a secondary (and perhaps curable) cause is possible and appropriate investigations should be performed (Figure 23.1). The line of investigation will be directed by the clinical picture, e.g., catecholamines measurement in paroxysmal hypertension, and the results of the routine laboratory tests, e.g., evaluation of plasma renin and aldosterone secretion if hypokalaemia is present. Failure to detect the hypokalaemia due to renal potassium loss may result in subjecting a patient with a resectable aldosterone-producing adenoma (and thus curable hypertension) to years of unnecessary expense of inappropriate and ineffective drug therapy.

The aims of laboratory investigation of hypertensive patients may be summarised as follows:

- To exclude the rare identifiable causes of hypertension secondary to renal, adrenal or other endocrinological disorders which are potentially curable.

- To assess the extent of involvement and damage to target organs, e.g., renal impairment.

- To determine the presence of hyperlipidaemia and glucose intolerance, factors that will aggravate the relative risks of morbidity and mortality in any hypertensive patient, and which may influence the subsequent management.

The laboratory investigations may include:

- Urinalysis
- Evaluation of renal function, lipid metabolism and glucose tolerance
- Evaluation of catecholamine metabolism (page 293)
- Evaluation of renin-aldosterone system (page 68)
- Evaluation of cortisol status (page 258)
- Radiological examination of the kidney (? renovascular disease)

Urinalysis

This is usually performed by using dipstick technology to detect proteinuria, haematuria and glycosuria.

- Proteinuria, when present in hypertensive patients, suggests a poorer prognosis for both renal and non-renal disease. It may be due to hypertensive nephrosclerosis (a consequence of hypertension) or to intrinsic renal disease (a cause of hypertension), or to urinary tract infection.

- Haematuria may also be present in any of the above mentioned situations, but it may also indicate the presence of renal or bladder carcinoma.

- Glycosuria suggests diabetes mellitus. If this is confirmed by random or fasting blood glucose concentrations (see below), the use of thiazide diuretics (for the hypertension) should be discontinued or avoided, as these drugs are diabetogenic. Glycosuria and hypertension may also both be secondary to other endocrine disorders such as Cushing's syndrome, phaeochromocytoma, or acromegaly.

First-line "routine" biochemical tests

These include the renal function tests (serum sodium, potassium, bicarbonate, creatinine), blood or plasma glucose, serum calcium and phosphate, and serum cholesterol, triglycerides, and HDL cholesterol. At the time of diagnosis, every patient must be evaluated for any abnormalities in these basic parameters. Selective screening may be repeated on follow-up visits. Although a fasting specimen of blood is preferred, a non-fasting sample may be acceptable.

Glucose. Hyperglycaemia confirms diabetes mellitus or hyperglycaemia secondary to endocrine abnormalities. About 50% of both insulin-dependant and non-insulin-dependant diabetics have hypertension; and diabetes is a frequent disorder among hypertensive patients (up to 10%). The incidence of glucose intolerance increases with advancing age and the degree of obesity.

Potassium. Marked hypokalaemia is associated with primary hyperaldosteronism (Conn's syndrome). Common causes of hypokalaemia such as diuretics therapy, purgative or laxative abuse, or treatment with carbenoxolone, should be excluded, e.g., the hypo-kalaemia should be confirmed with a second specimen after cessation of diuretics for at least a month. The hypokalaemia, if present, is less severe in secondary hyperaldosteronism. Patients with acute renal failure may present with hyperkalaemia, especially if they are on potassium supplements or potassium-sparing diuretics.

Creatinine. Renal disease, both parenchymal or renovascular disease, may cause hypertension. Persistently raised blood pressures may also lead to renal impairment. The latter carries an exceedingly poor prognosis. Serial measurement of serum creatinine is usually sufficient for tracking the course of hypertensive renal disease (by plotting the reciprocal of the serum creatinine against time) and estimations of creatinine clearance are not necessary in most cases.

Cholesterol and triglycerides. As mentioned earlier, the presence of hyperlipidaemia in a hypertensive patient substantially worsens the prognosis, and should be aggressively treated. Both beta blockers and thiazide diuretics (the most commonly prescribed anti-hypertensive drugs) may adversely affect existent hyperlipidaemia and should be discontinued or avoided in patients with overt hyperlipidaemia.

Calcium and phosphate. Hypertension is found in about 50% of patients with primary hyper-parathyroidism (raised serum calcium and low or low normal serum phosphate). Thiazide diuretics may also cause hypercalcaemia (albeit rarely) and these drugs should be stopped for a few weeks before rechecking to confirm or exclude primary hyperparathyroidism. Parathyroidectomy, however, rarely results in any amelioration of the blood pressure, unless there is concurrent renal failure.

Gamma-glutamyl transferase. About 10-20% of hypertension may be related to a high alcohol intake, and this increasingly common cause of hypertension appears to be readily reversible on abstinence or moderation of alcohol intake. A raised serum gamma glutamyl transferase indicates this as a probable cause (page 154).

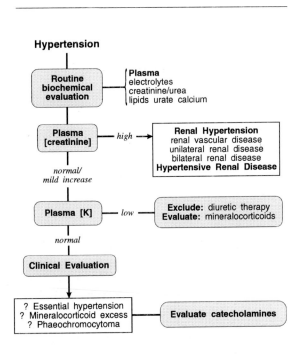

Figure 23.1. Laboratory evaluation of hypertension. Plasma [K], plasma potassium concentration.

Further investigations

The next line of investigations depends on the clinical picture, the results of the first-line routine tests described above, and the cause suspected (Figure 23.1). As the majority of secondary non-essential hypertension is associated with renal impairment, the most frequently requested tests are an estimation of the 24 h urinary protein excretion, a creatinine clearance test, an intravenous pyelogram (IVP) or other radiological investigations (especially for renovascular disease), and possibly a renal biopsy.

The clinical features and the laboratory evaluation of patients suspected of several of the endocrine-related disorders have been dealt with elsewhere in the book and the reader is referred to these sections for further clarification -- Conn's syndrome and its non-tumorous varieties (page 258), Cushing's syndrome (page 68), primary hyperparathyroidism (page 93), and acromegaly (page 230). Further evaluation of the patients with renovascular hypertension and those with phaeochromocytoma are discussed in the next sections.

Renovascular hypertension

In cases of suspected renal artery stenosis, the investigation is mainly radiological and biochemical tests, when employed, are based on estimations of plasma renin activities. Basal activities of the enzymes in peripheral blood are of very limited value, and may be high or normal. Renal vein sampling from both the affected side and the contralateral side, together with a sample from the inferior vena cava provide much more useful renin activity data, but these difficult procedures are only resorted to if surgical treatment is to be considered. The rational of the test is that the narrowed renal artery will supply less blood to the kidney and the reduced renal blood flow stimulates renin secretion resulting in a higher renin activity on the affected side.

The fractional renin secretion [i.e., (RV-IVC)/IVC] from each kidney can be calculated, where RV is the renal vein renin concentration and IVC, the inferior vena cava renin concentration.

Normally the calculated value which represents the fractional increase in renin concentration in the renal veins as compared to that in the peripheral circulation is about 0.24. In cases with significant renal artery stenosis and in which surgical reconstruction or angioplasty is likely to be successful in correcting the defect, the value may be doubled on the affected side

angioplasty is likely to be successful in correcting the defect, the value may be doubled on the affected side and considerably suppressed (close to zero) on the contralateral side.

Catecholamines and phaeochromocytomas

The catecholamines are a group of compounds which include adrenaline, noradrenaline, and dopamine, released from nerve endings of the sympathetic nervous system and the adrenal medulla. They have important effects on the blood pressure and are the cause of hypertension in patients with phaeochromocytomas.

NORMAL METABOLISM

Synthesis and metabolism

Noradrenaline and adrenaline are synthesised from tyrosine and converted to normetadrenaline, metadrenaline, and 4-hydroxy 3-methoxy mandelic acid (HMMA, or vanillylmandelic acid, VMA) prior to excretion in the urine (Figure 23.2). Noradrenaline is produced in sympathetic nerve endings and in the adrenal medulla. Adrenaline is produced in the adrenal medulla, and dopamine, a precursor of adrenaline and noradrenaline, is produced in large quantities in the central nervous system.

The main excretory product of dopamine is homovanillic acid (HVA), which is excreted in the urine in significant amounts by patients with neuroblastomas and by some patients with malignant and poorly differentiated phaeochromocytomas.

Actions of catecholamines

The principal actions of the three main catecholamines are:

Noradrenaline: Increases blood pressure
                            Decreases heart rate
                            Induces sweating

Adrenaline: Increases heart rate
                            Increases plasma glucose

Decreases blood pressure

Dopamine: Increases blood pressure
                          Decreases prolactin production by the anterior pituitary gland

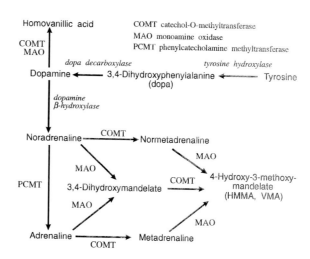

Figure 23.2. Metabolism of the catecholamines.

DISORDERS OF CATECHOLAMINE METABOLISM

Disordered catecholamine metabolism occurs in two rare tumours, phaeochromocytoma and neuroblastoma.

Phaeochromocytoma

This tumour, a rare cause of hypertension (<0.5% of cases), is derived most often from the adrenal medulla and secretes large amounts of noradrenaline and lesser quantities of adrenaline. Over 90% of the tumours are located in the abdomen and 90% of these are in the adrenal (the others can occur any where along the sympathetic nerve chain). Some 10% are bilateral, 10% are malignant, and 10% are not associated with hypertension.

The mode of presentation varies. It classically occurs in the 20 to 50-year age group with paroxysmal hypertension associated with adrenergic symptoms (anxiety, tachycardia, profuse sweating, palpitations). More commonly it presents with sustained hypertension and periodic bouts of further increases in the blood pressure. Hyperglycaemia due to excess adrenaline may also occur.

Biochemically they are characterised by increased plasma and urinary levels of noradrenaline and adrenaline, and increased urinary excretion of metadrenaline, normetadrenaline, and HMMA.

There is a close association between phaeochromocytomas and neurofibromatosis and between phaeochromocytomas and MEN_1 (the Type I multiple endocrine neoplasia which includes parathyroid adenoma, medullary carcinoma of thyroid, and phaeochromocytoma, page 287).

Neuroblastoma

This very malignant neoplasm, like the phaeochromocytoma, originates in tissues derived from the embryonic neural crest. They may occur anywhere along the sympathetic chain and in the adrenal gland. Most present during the first decade of life.

They are associated with increased catecholamine metabolism, but not always with hypertension. There is increased secretion of (a) noradrenaline (but not adrenaline), HMMA, and normetadrenaline, and (b) dopamine and its metabolite homovanillic acid, which is characteristic of the tumour. The lack of adrenaline and the high levels of dopamine probably reflect the poorly differentiated nature of the tumour.

LABORATORY EVALUATION

The tests available for the evaluation of the patient with suspected phaeochromocytoma are urinary HMMA (VMA), urinary metanephrines (metadrenalin, normetadrenaline), and plasma and urinary catecholamines (adrenaline and noradrenaline).

Many drugs, such as ephedrine, isoprenaline, L-dopa, and methyldopa, as well as vanilla-containing foods such as bananas, ice-cream, chocolate, and coffee interfere with the estimation of VMA which limits its diagnostic usefulness.

The most reliable screening test is the urinary metanephrines estimation but this is subject to interference by the monamine oxidase inhibitor group of drugs. The most sensitive diagnostic test is the 24-hour excretion rate of urinary catecholamines (adrenaline and noradrenaline).

As most phaeochromocytomas secrete catecholamines in an episodic manner it is advisable to collect urine over at least three consecutive days for any of the above estimations. Assays should be limited to symptomatic patients and cases of severe or malignant hypertensives, and those who have proved resistant to conventional antihypertensive drugs, even if they do not exhibit the characteristic paroxysmal symptoms.

REFERENCES AND FURTHER READING

Bonowitz NL. Pheochromocytoma. Adv Intern Med 1990;35:195-220.

Bravo EL, Gifford RW. Phaeochromocytoma. Endocrinol Metab Clinics N Am 1993;22:329-343.

Harvey JM, Beevers DG. Biochemical investigation of hypertension. Ann Clin Biochem 1990;27:287-296.

Vaughn ED. Renovascular hypertension. Kidney Internl 1985;27:811-827.

Werbel SS, Ober KP. Pheochromocytoma. Update on diagnosis, localization, and management. Med Clinics North Am 1995;79:131-153.

Chapter 24

Inherited Metabolic Diseases

The clinical and biochemical abnormalities observed in a given inherited metabolic disease reflect the mutation of a specific gene. Most of the inherited metabolic disorders (inborn errors of metabolism) are due to the defective synthesis of a single protein or peptide which normally functions as an enzyme or as a transport system. An enzyme which is defective or absent will manifest itself in one or more of the following ways (Figure 24.1):

1. Accumulation of the enzyme substrate, e.g., phenylalanine in phenylketonuria, glycogen in glucose-6-phosphatase deficiency.

2. Conversion of the enzyme substrate to other metabolites by an alternative pathway, e.g., phenylalanine to phenylpyruvic acid in phenylketonuria.

3. Lack of formation of end products subsequent to the block, e.g., melanin in phenylketonuria, cortisol in congenital adrenal hyperplasia.

If the accumulated products are soluble they will accumulate in the body fluids and be excreted in the urine (e.g., phenylpyruvic acid in phenylketonuria); if insoluble they may be stored in cells (e.g., glycogen in glycogen storage diseases) or excreted in the faeces via the bile (e.g., coproporphyrins and protoporphyrins in certain porphyrias).

TYPES OF INHERITANCE

Inherited characteristics are determined by a pair of genes on homologous chromosomes (one from each parent). The different genes governing the same characteristic are called alleles. If two alleles are identical the subject is said to be homozygous for that gene; and heterozygous if the alleles differ. The chromosomes carrying the genes may be similar in both sexes; these are known as autosomes. If the genes are carried on the sex chromosomes (X, Y) then they are said to be sex-linked genes (X-linked if on the X chromosome). Autosomal and sex-linked genes exhibit different patterns of inheritance.

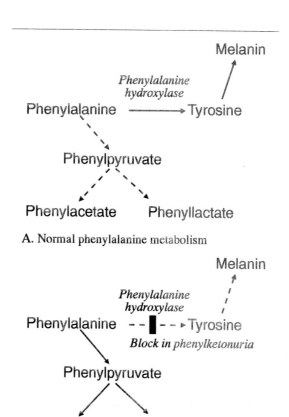

A. Normal phenylalanine metabolism

B. phenylalanine metabolism in phenylketonuria

·········· *Minor pathway* ———— *Major pathway*

Figure 24.1. Example of the consequences of an enzyme deficiency. A. normal phenylalanine metabolism. B. metabolism in phenylketonuria.

Autosomal inheritance

Autosomal inheritance may show the following permutations:

- If one parent is heterozygous for an abnormal gene and the other is homozygous for the normal gene, it is possible for 50% of the offspring to receive the abnormal gene and be heterozygous for it.

- If both parents are heterozygous then the statistical possibilities are that 25% of the offspring will be

- homozygous and 50% heterozygous for the abnormal gene, the remaining 25% will be homozygous for the normal gene.

- If one parent is homozygous for the abnormal gene ant the other homozygous for the normal gene then all offspring will be heterozygous.

The expression of the gene depends on its potency. *Dominant* genes will produce effects in both homozygous and heterozygous individuals; *recessive* genes only produce effects in homozygous subjects. However, the terms are relative and dominance may not be absolute. For example, a dominant gene may show *incomplete penetrance* in that it may skip a generation, or it may vary in its degree of potency and produce a lesser effect. Sometimes a recessive gene which normally only produces its effect in the homozygous patient may be of sufficient potency to produce minor effects in the heterozygote.

Sex-linked inheritance

Some abnormal genes are carried on the sex chromosomes (XX in females, XY in males), mostly on the X chromosome.

X-linked recessive. A recessive gene on an X chromosome will manifest itself if:

a it is combined with a Y chromosome, i.e., in the male, or
b the female is homozygous for it, having inherited one abnormal gene from her father and one from her mother.

The best known X-linked recessive disorder is haemophilia.

X-linked dominant. In this situation both males and females will be affected. One such disorder is familial hypophosphataemia.

Inherited metabolic diseases

The inborn errors of metabolism are legion but fairly rare. For example, even the most common of them (in Caucasian populations), cystic fibrosis and congenital hypothyroidism, occur in 1:3000-4000 and 1:3000-5000 live births, respectively. Phenylketonuria, cystinuria, and Hartnup disease have incidences of 1 in 10000 to 1 in 25000, galactosaemia, 1 in 50000-100000, and maple syrup disease, 1 in 200000-400000. The majority are inherited as autosomal recessive traits and relative few as X-linked or autosomal dominant traits. Thus consanguinity and a family history of similarly affected individuals, increased neonatal deaths, or an increased incidence of miscarriage are strong indications that the disease may be of genetic origin.

In the following discussion some of the better known disorders will be listed but only a few will be discussed (others are discussed elsewhere in this text and the appropriate page numbers are appended). For a full coverage the reader should consult the text by Stanbury JB *et al*, referenced at the end of the chapter.

CLASSIFICATION

Carbohydrate metabolism

Glycogen storage disease, galactosaemia, hereditary fructose intolerance, diabetes mellitus (page 126), red cell glucose-6-phosphate dehydrogenase deficiency and red cell pyruvate kinase deficiency (page 189).

Lipid metabolism

Hyperlipoproteinaemia and hypolipoproteinaemia (Chapter 14)

Plasma proteins

Immunoglobulin deficiencies (page 167), α_1-antitrypsin deficiency (page 166), carrier protein deficiencies -- transferrin, thyroxine binding globulin (page 242), albumin (page 165).

Metal metabolism

Haemochromatosis (page 276), Wilson's disease (page 159).

Porphyrin metabolism

Porphyrias (Chapter 21).

Bilirubin metabolism

Congenital hyperbilirubinaemias (page 146).

Steroid metabolism

Congenital adrenal hyperplasia (page 250).

Iodine metabolism

Congenital goitre, dyshormonogenesis (page 233).

Purine metabolism

Primary gout (page 118), Lesch-Nyhan syndrome (page 116), xanthinuria (page 121).

Amino acid metabolism

Phenylketonuria, alkaptonuria, cystinosis, homocystinuria, maple syrup disease, disorders of the urea cycle (page 341).

Organic acidaemias

Maple syrup disease, methylmalonic aciduria and other causes (see Figure 24.4).

Digestion

Cystic fibrosis (page 220), disaccharidase deficiency (page 220).

Precipitation by drugs

Suxamethonium sensitivity (page 187), porphyrias (page 278).

Cellular transport

Amino acids: cystinuria, Hartnup disease
Glucose: renal glycosuria (page 80)
Potassium: familial periodic paralysis (page 31)
Calcium: pseudohypoparathyroidism (page 98)
Hydrogen ion: renal tubular acidosis (page 81)

Bilirubin: Gilbert's disease, Dubin-Johnson syndrome (page 146)
Multiple defects: Fanconi syndrome (page 80).

Lysosomal storage disease

Mucopolysaccharidoses: Hurler, Hunter, Morquio syndromes
Lipoidoses: Gaucher's, Niemann-Pick, Fabry, Tay-Sachs diseases.

CLINICAL ASPECTS

Early recognition of any inborn error of metabolism is an important part of clinical medicine because, although many are completely harmless, a number of them are potentially dangerous but may be successfully treated if recognised early. Others may express themselves later in life in response to some precipitating factor and knowledge of their existence is thus vital. Yet others, which are completely harmless, may be misdiagnosed and lead to inappropriate management.

- Early diagnosis and treatment may prevent irreversible damage in:

  a phenylketonuria
  b galactosaemia
  c maple syrup disease
  d congenital hypothyroidism

- Disorders that respond to some precipitating factor and thus should be sought amongst blood relatives of an affected individuals are:

  a cholinesterase variants (page 187)
  b Wilson's disease
  c haemochromatosis
  d cystinuria
  e porphyrias

- Disorders that are harmless but may be confused for more serious conditions are:

  a Gilbert's syndrome
  b renal glycosuria (page 80)
  c alkaptonuria

- Some clinical features that can suggest an inherited disorder in infants are (see page 306 for evaluation):

  a failure to thrive, poor feeding, persistent vomiting
  b hypoglycaemia
  c persistent jaundice
  d hepatosplenomegaly
  e neurological problems (convulsions, spasticity, lethargy)
  f mental retardation
  g unexplained metabolic acidosis, ketosis

Amino acid disorders

Disorders of amino acid metabolism are usually expressed biochemically as aminoaciduria (page 81). This can be due to a transport defect as in cystinuria and Hartnup disease, or it may be an overflow type of disorder resulting from excess production of amino acids or their metabolites due to an enzyme deficiency, e.g., phenylketonuria, maple syrup disease. In the first type of aminoaciduria, the serum levels of one or more amino acids affected by the transport (reabsorption) defect are normal or decreased, whereas urine levels are high. Both serum and urine amino acids will be increased in the overflow aminoacidurias (Figure 24.2).

A variant of the overflow aminoacidurias is caused by a congenital enzyme block in the biochemical processing of an amino acid that leads to accumulation in the urine of an intermediate amino acid not normally seen in the urine. If these intermediates compete with the amino acid for reabsorption by the same transport mechanism, it will also create a relative "leak" for the latter. The problem is in the *normal* lack of a physiological mechanism for the reabsorption by the tubules of the intermediate metabolites.

In addition to the primary aminoacidurias discussed above, secondary aminoaciduria may be caused by other diseases or toxins that result in liver necrosis or damage of the tubular transport mechanisms. In these diseases, a non-specific aminoaciduria involving many or all the amino acids occurs. More than 50 hereditary diseases leading to aminoaciduria have been identified; most have a very low incidence. Only a few of the more common ones are briefly discussed.

Cystinuria. This is the commonest inborn error of amino acid transport and is due to failure of the renal tubular and gut transport mechanisms concerned with absorption of the basic amino acids cystine, ornithine, arginine, and lysine. This results in cystinuria and often the formation of cystine renal stones. There are two recognised phenotypes:

Type 1 or recessive cystinuria where there is increased renal excretion of all four dibasic amino acids and commonly associated with stone formation.

Type 2 which is incompletely recessive and associated with increased urinary levels of cystine and lysine only (stone formation is rare).

Diagnosis is made by demonstrating excessive urinary excretion of these amino acids. A useful screening test is the cyanide-nitroprusside reaction with cystine. Since these diabasic amino acids are not essential amino acids, nutritional deficiency does not occur despite the reduced absorption from dietary sources. The disorder is usually asymptomatic but the development of urinary cystine stones can occur and is the main clinical problem. Cystine is relatively insoluble and treatment is aimed at preventing stone formation by reducing its urinary concentration. This is usually achieved by simply increasing fluid intake or making the urine alkaline (cystine precipitates out readily at a pH below 7 but only sparingly at a pH above 7.5).

Hartnup disease. This is a rare recessive disorder where there is a renal and gut transport defect involving the neutral amino acids (monoamine-monocarboxylic) including tryptophan, an essential amino acid. It may present with a pellagra-type rash, mental confusion, and ataxia which may be due to tryptophan deficiency (tryptophan is a precursor of nicotinic acid, or vitamin B_2, which causes pellagra when deficient). The metabolic defect is diagnosed by demonstrating the characteristic excess of neutral amino acids in the urine.

Phenylketonuria (PKU). PKU is an autosomal recessive disorder caused primarily by a deficiency of *phenylalanine hydroxylase* activity (Figure 24.1) which converts phenylalanine to tyrosine. In a small proportion of cases (~3%), the biochemical lesion resides in enzymes that synthesise cofactors for phenylalanine hydroxylase (phenylalanine hydroxy-

300

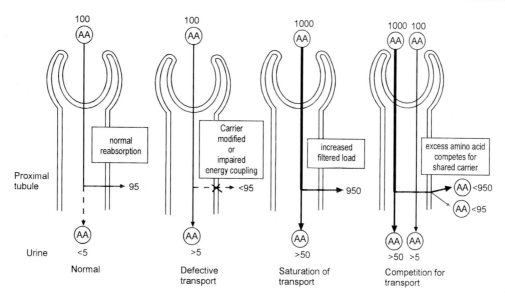

Figure 24.2. Normal amino acid excretion and mechanistic defects in the primary aminoacidurias. Redrawn, with permission of W.B. Saunders, from: Scriver CR. Hyperaminoaciduria. In: Wyngaarden JB and Smith LH (eds), *Cecil Textbook of Medicine, 18th edn.* W.B. Saunders, Philadelphia, 1988.

-lase requires tetrahydrobiopterin as a cofactor which in turn depends on the enzymes *dihydropteridine reductase* and *dihydropteridine synthetase* for maintenance -- deficiency of either enzyme will cause the disorder). In addition, there are two minor disorders of phenylalanine hydroxylase resulting in hyperphenylalaninaemia: a benign variety due to minor deficiency of the enzyme and a transient type due to delayed maturation. There is accumulation of phenylalanine in the blood (and urine) and reduced tyrosine formation. Activation of alternate pathways of metabolism leads to formation of phenylalanine derivatives such as phenyllactate, phenylacetate, and phenylpyruvate which are produced in excess and appear in the urine.

The clinical features are irritability, vomiting, seizures, and a tendency to reduced melanin formation which may result in a pale skin, fair hair, and blue eyes (tyrosine is a precursor of melanin). Mental retardation develops at a later date, e.g., 3-6 months of age; hence the importance of early diagnosis and therapy. Diagnosis is based on the finding of high plasma phenylalanine levels and there are a number of screening tests to detect the abnormality (e.g., Guthrie test). Urinary phenylpyruvate can also be detected by the ferric chloride reaction, e.g., Phenistix.

PKU patients are treated by maintenance on a special diet in which the bulk of protein is replaced by an artificial amino acid mixture low in phenylalanine.

Alkaptonuria. Alkaptonuria results from an abnormal enzyme block along the same metabolic pathway as PKU and tyrosinosis. Deficiency in the enzyme *homogentisic acid oxidase* leads to a build-up of homogentisic acid (HGA), an intermediate compound in the metabolism of tyrosine.

In infancy and childhood, the only symptom is darkening of the urine, which occurs when the urine stands in an alkaline pH or is exposed to air. The disease is usually detected by mothers who notice dark stains on diapers. Clinical symptoms begin in adulthood and include degenerative arthritis and dark pigmentation of cartilage caused by binding of HGA and its metabolites to collagen in the connective tissues and cartilage.

No completely satisfactory treatment for alkaptonuria has yet been found. If detected early, dietary restriction of tyrosine and phenylalanine may be beneficial. Vitamin C therapy is also often used, as it has been shown that the vitamin is required for maximal activity of HGA oxidase.

Reye's syndrome

Homocystinuria. Homocysteine is an intermediate in the metabolism of methionine to cystine. The main intermediate in this pathway is cystathionine, formed from homocysteine and serine by *cystathionine-β-synthase*. Homocysteine may also be reconverted to methionine by N^5-*methyltetrahydrofolate reductase*. Normally, there is very little homocysteine in either the serum or urine (it is relatively unstable in aqueous solutions and is converted to homocystine when present).

The most common cause of homocystinuria is a partial or complete lack of cystathionine-β-synthase, resulting in increased levels of methionine, homocystine, and other sulphur-containing amino acids in body fluids. By age five, nearly all patients present with impaired vision from dislocated optic lenses, which can result in glaucoma. Vascular complications caused by damaged vascular endothelium, are the most serious clinical manifestation. Arterial occlusion can be fatal before age ten. Mental retardation and osteoporosis may also be present in a few cases.

A much rarer cause of homocystinuria is N^5-methyltetrahydrofolate reductase deficiency due to defects in folate metabolism or to a genetic defect in the enzyme synthesis. These conditions present with milder symptoms and are easier to manage.

Cystinosis. The disease is characterised by the lysosomal accumulation of cystine leading to crystal formation in the cornea, bone marrow, kidney, leucocytes and other tissues. It is inherited in an autosomal recessive manner and has an incidence of 1 in 300000. The defect responsible for cystinosis has yet to be identified.

The most severe form is nephropathic cystinosis with impaired renal function and the Fanconi syndrome. Growth may be retarded and vitamin D-resistant rickets may develop. The only treatment is renal transplantation -- cystine does not accumulate in the transplant.

Organic acidaemias

This is a diverse group of disorders which result in the accumulation of organic acids in the blood and urine. They occur in a wide variety of diseases affecting intermediary metabolism (see below), particularly that of the branched-chain amino acids, the fatty acids, and pyruvate. The incidence is around 1 in 3000 live births. The disorder presents early in life with an acute onset of metabolic acidosis, vomiting, convulsions, or coma. There may also be varying combinations of ketosis, hypoglycaemia, and hyperammonaemia.

The possibility of organic acidaemia should be considered when an acutely ill child presents with one or more of the following features:

- vomiting, convulsions, coma of uncertain aetiology
- unexplained metabolic acidosis
- hypoglycaemia or ketosis of dubious origin
- unexplained hyperammonaemia
- unresolved CNS disorders

The more common causes of organic acidaemia are those involving the branched-chain amino acids (leucine, isoleucine, valine), methionine and threonine (see Figures 24.3 and 24.4). The commonest or best known of these disorders, methylmalonic aciduria and maple syrup disease, are briefly discussed below.

Maple syrup disease. This is caused by a deficiency of the enzyme which decarboxylates the deaminase products (the 2-oxoacids, see Figure 24.3) of the branched chain amino acids (leucine, isoleucine, valine). The amino acids and their oxoacid derivatives accumulate in the blood and are excreted in the urine producing the characteristic maple syrup odour. Affected subjects develop cortical atrophy due to defective myelinisation and present with a severe neonatal illness which includes convulsions, vomiting, and often hypoglycaemia and ketosis. Early treatment by a diet low in branched chain amino acids prevents the development of serious neurological problems.

Methylmalonic aciduria. (Figure 24.4). This autosomal recessive disorder, the commonest of the organic acidaemias, is due to either a deficiency of the enzyme, methylmalonyl CoA mutase, or a defect in the metabolism of adenosylcobalamin, a cofactor for the enzyme. The disorder also occurs in severe vitamin B_{12} deficiency. The characteristic features include metabolic acidosis, ketosis, hypoglycaemia and hyperammonaemia. Those with the cofactor defect may also have homocystinuria (methylcobalamin is required in homocystine metabolism) and may not have overt ketosis.

Carbohydrate disorders

The two commonest disorders of carbohydrate metabolism, other than diabetes mellitus, are galactos-

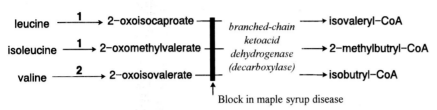

Figure 24.3. Branched-chain amino acid metabolism and the block in maple syrup disease.

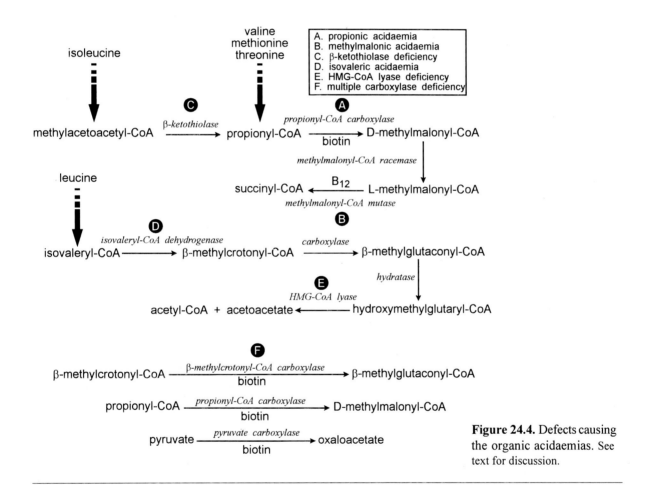

Figure 24.4. Defects causing the organic acidaemias. See text for discussion.

aemia and von Gierke's disease (Type I glycogen storage disease), both of which may be associated with hypoglycaemia. Less common inherited disorders of this group include the inborn errors of gluconeogenesis, hereditary fructose intolerance, and the other glycogen storage diseases (Types II–X).

Galactosaemia. This name refers to either of two inborn errors of galactose metabolism: *galactose-1-phosphate uridyl transferase* deficiency and *galacto-kinase* deficiency (Figure 24.5). These enzymes, together with UDP-galactose 4-epimerase, catalyse the conversion of galactose to glucose-1-phosphate. Both

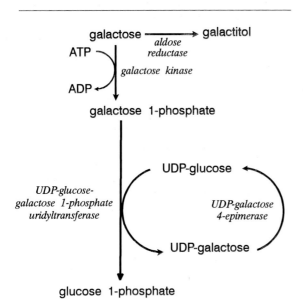

Figure 24.5. Galactose metabolism. See text for details.

deficiencies are transmitted as autosomal recessive traits. Heterozygotes have half-normal enzyme activities but are asymptomatic. Diagnosis is made by demonstrating the deficiency of the relevant enzyme in red cells, the clinical picture, and the finding of galactose (reducing sugar) in the urine.

Deficiency of galactose-1-phosphate uridyl transferase, which converts galactose-1-phosphate to glucose-1-phosphate, is the cause of the classical type of galactosaemia. The clinical syndrome, which only occurs after milk has been added to the diet, is due to toxic effects of accumulated galactose-1-phosphate. In addition to galactosaemia and galactosuria, infants afflicted with this disorder develop diarrhoea and vomiting and hypoglycaemia after meals containing galactose. The accumulation of galactose in tissues results in liver damage with jaundice, the Fanconi syndrome, and hepatomegaly. If treatment with a galactose-free diet is not instituted early on, mental deficiency and cataracts will develop. The latter is due to the accumulating galactitol in the lens of the eye which results in the ingress of water and swelling.

Galactose kinase deficiency leads primarily to

cataract formation. In this condition galactose accumulates in the blood and tissues; in the optic lens galactose is reduced to galactitol, a sugar to which the lens is impermeable and this causes cataract formation.

Hereditary fructose intolerance. This is caused by a deficiency in *fructose bisphosphate aldolase*, a key enzyme in fructose metabolism (Figure 24.6). Normally, the two triose phosphates, dihydroxy-acetone phosphate and glyceraldehyde 3-phosphate, can be converted to glucose (gluconeogenesis) or to pyruvate (glycolysis). Fructose bisphosphate aldolase appears to have eqipotent cleavage activity towards both its physiological substrates, fructose 1-phosphate and fructose 1,6-bisphosphate.

The disorder is characterised by hypoglycaemia and vomiting following a fructose-rich feed. The clinical manifestations are due to the accumulation of fructose1-phosphate, the immediate precursor of the enzyme blockade, and include hepatomegaly, jaundice, and aminoaciduria. The hypoglycaemia is consequent to depression of glycogenolysis (inhibition of liver phosphorylase) and gluconeogenesis (the causal enzyme deficiency). Generally the affected individuals learn to avoid fructose-containing foods, and thus limit the adverse effects. Diagnosis is based on the clinical picture, the finding of fructose (reducing sugar) in the urine, and estimation of the aldolase activity in liver biopsy material.

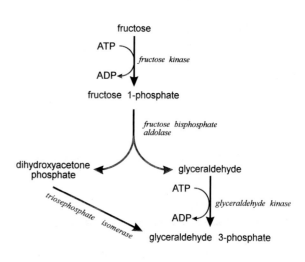

Figure 24.6. Fructose metabolism.

304

Glycogen storage disease

The glycogen storage diseases are disorders of glycogen mobilisation associated with enzyme defects of the glycogenolysis. They have been classified according to the particular enzyme deficiency involved:

- Type I: *glucose 6-phosphatase* deficiency in the liver (von Gierke's)
- Type II: *lysosomal-±-1,4-glucosidase* deficiency (Pompe's)
- Type III: *amylo-1,6-glucosidase* deficiency (Cori's, Forbes', limit dextrinosis)
- Type IV: *amylo-1,6-glucosyltransferase* deficiency (Anderson's, amylopectinosis)
- Type V: *muscle phosphorylase* deficiency (McArdle's)
- Type VI: *liver phosphorylase* deficiency (Hers)
- Type VII: *muscle phosphofructokinase* deficiency
- Types VIII, IX, X: variants of Type VI.

Pathogenesis. The breakdown of glycogen (glycogenolysis) is brought about by the coordinated activities of several glycogenolytic enzymes: glycogen phosphorylase, debrancher enzyme (with dual catalytic activities -- a glucosyltransferase activity and an amylo-1,6-glucosidase activity). The end-products of their combined action are glucose-1-phosphate (~90%) and free glucose residues (7-10%). In the liver, glucose-1-phosphate is converted to glucose-6-phosphate (phosphoglucomutase) and then to glucose (glucose-6-phosphatase). Muscle tissue does not have glucose-6-phosphatase activity and hence is unable to produce free glucose from glycogen. Deficiency in any of these enzymes will lead to glycogen storage disease. Only the most common type, von Gierke's disease, will be discussed. The reader is referred to more specialised texts for information about the other types.

von Gierke's disease. This is a glycogen storage disease (Type I, the most common variety) due to deficiency of the enzyme glucose-6-phosphatase, which is responsible for the conversion of glycogen, through glucose-6-phosphate, to glucose (hence fasting hypoglycaemia). There are two subtypes: Type IA in which the glucose-6-phosphatase activity is deficient, and Type IB in which the phosphatase activity is normal but there is a deficiency of a translocase (required in the transport of glucose-6-

phosphate from the cytosol to the cisterna of the endoplasmic reticulum where glucose-6-phosphatase resides).

In addition to liver glycogen accumulation (hepatomegaly) and hypoglycaemia, these patients present with ketosis and hypertriglyceridaemia (increased lipolysis to compensate for glucose deficiency), lactic acidosis and hyperuricaemia. Excess lactate production is due to diversion of glucose-6-phosphate to glycolysis; the hyperuricaemia is due to lactate-induced inhibition of renal urate excretion and increased urate synthesis (increased availability of phosphoribosylpyrophosphate as a result of stepped-up activity of the hexose monophosphate shunt, page 316).

Diagnosis is based on the clinical picture and biochemical features and the response to glucagon (no increase in plasma glucose concentration). Treatment consists of frequent feeding to maintain the blood glucose level.

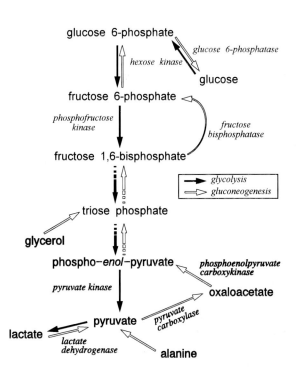

Figure 24.7. Gluconeogenesis.

305

Inborn errors of gluconeogenesis

Gluconeogenesis is the formation of glucose from non-carbohydrate precursors which include lactate, pyruvate, glycerol and amino acids. It occurs exclusively in the liver and the kidney. The gluconeogenic pathway is a partial reversal of the glycolytic pathway, sharing all but three of the reactions of glycolysis (Figure 24.7). The three irreversible (non-equilibrium) reactions are catalysed by hexokinase, phosphofructokinase, and pyruvate kinase. To circumvent these unidirectional steps, four novel gluconeogenic enzymes are required (the enzymes catalysing the corresponding reaction or reactions in glycolysis are placed in parenthesis):

- *glucose 6-phosphatase* (hexokinase)
- *fructose 1,6-bisphosphatase* (phosphofructokinase)
- *phosphoenolpyruvate carboxykinase* and *pyruvate carboxylase* (pyruvate kinase)

Deficiencies of all the above enzymes have been documented. Affected subjects present with fasting hypoglycaemia, lactic acidosis, ketosis, and hyper-alaninaemia. Glucose 6-phosphatase deficiency also results in liver glycogen accumulation (the reaction it catalyses is common to both glycolysis and glycogenolysis). Pyruvate carboxylase deficiency produces severe mental retardation and causes early death.

EVALUATION OF SUSPECTED INHERITED DISEASES

Inborn errors are rare and it is not justified in terms of cost and labour to fully investigate all subjects suspected of having such a disorder. The best that can be done is to screen "at risk" subjects and follow up on those in whom there is a suspicion of some abnormality. In general screening procedures are (or can be) carried out in the following groups:

- All newborns. This group can now be screened effectively and relatively cheaply for congenital hypothyroidism, phenylketonuria, and galactos-aemia using a sample of blood collected on a piece of filter paper (Guthrie test). These programs are widely available and mandatory in some countries.

- Neonates and infants who are very ill or who present with one or more of the following: failure to thrive, persistent vomiting, poor feeding, unexplained jaundice, unexplained hypoglycaemia, ketosis, lactic acidosis, convulsions, onset of illness related to particular foods.

- 'Carriers' in diseases where the heterozygote shows some expression of the gene, e.g., α_1-antitrypsin deficiency, galactosaemia.

- Siblings of patients with proven disease, e.g., α_1-antitrypsin deficiency, suxamethonium sensitivity, porphyrias.

- Expectant mothers with confirmed cases of previous affected offspring. The antenatal diagnosis is usually made by performing the appropriate enzyme assays on cultured fibroblasts obtained form the amniotic fluid, e.g., glucosyl-ceramidase for Gaucher's disease, sphingomyelin phosphodiesterase for Niemann-Pick disease, hypoxanthine-guanine phosphoribosyl transferase for Lesch-Nyhan syndrome.

LABORATORY INVESTIGATION

In clinical practice, the evaluation of possible metabolic disorders is carried out on two groups of patients: the ill patient and the normal (screening programs). As most of these disorders present in the neonate or during infancy only these age groups will be considered below. The presenting illness in the neonate or infant may be acute or of a more chronic nature and these will be discussed separately.

Acute onset

The metabolic disease may present in the neonate or infant with an acute severe illness or with the early onset of symptoms such as lethargy, coma, convulsions, poor feeding, vomiting, hypotonia, and hyperventilation. In these cases the approach should be to perform the routinely available plasma and urinary tests as an initial 'screen', and, depending on the findings, follow up with more specific tests.

Initial screen

Plasma: blood gases, electrolytes, anion gap, glucose, liver function tests, magnesium, calcium
Urine: reducing substances, glucose, ketones

Follow-up

Hypoglycaemia

Consider: glycogen storage disease, disorders of gluconeogenesis, amino acid disorders, organic acidaemias

Perform: Plasma: lactate, ketones, insulin, cortisol
Urine: amino acids, organic acids

Metabolic acidosis (high anion gap)

Consider: organic acidaemias, congenital lactic acidosis

Perform: Plasma: lactate, ketones, ammonia
Urine: amino acids, organic acids

Respiratory alkalosis

Consider: urea cycle defects

Perform: Plasma: ammonia
Urine: amino acids

Abnormal liver function tests

Consider: galactosaemia, fructose intolerance, tyrosinaemia, glycogen storage disease, disorders of gluconeogenesis

Perform: Plasma: lactate, ketones, alpha-1-antitrypsin
Urine: sugars, amino acids, organic acids

In the case of acute onset of neurological dysfunction such as depressed consciousness and convulsions, consider hypoglycaemia, urea cycle deficiencies, and the organic acidaemias but the performance of some or all of the above tests may be necessary to resolve the problem.

Non-acute onset

The evaluation of patients with non-acute illness is more difficult than that of those described above. A reasonable approach would be as follows.

Failure to thrive: Although failure to thrive is a feature of many metabolic disorders there are many other and more common causes, e.g., feeding problems, malabsorption. However, in the context of inborn errors consider amino acid, organic acid, and urea cycle disorders; thus, in addition to routine tests an estimation of the plasma ammonia and evaluation of the urinary amino acids and organic acids would be appropriate.

Liver disease: Abnormal liver function tests can indicate the presence of the conditions described above.

Mental retardation: This is a difficult problem to investigate as there are many causes including the inborn errors. Investigation will depend on the clinical picture and the family history.

Prenatal diagnosis and carrier status assessment

If there had been a previous affected offspring, expectant mothers can be subjected to antenatal diagnosis. This may be done by performing the appropriate enzyme assay on cultured fibroblasts obtained from the amniotic fluid. Examples are glucosylceramidase for Gaucher's disease, sphingomyelin phosphodiesterases for Niemann-Pick disease, hypoxanthine-guanine phosphoribosyl transferase for Lesch-Nyhan syndrome.

With the advances in molecular genetics in recent years and the adaptation of many of the techniques developed in research laboratories to clinical diagnosis (see below), DNA linkage analysis and direct mutation analyses can be used for prenatal diagnosis of certain inherited disorders. For example, DNA linkage analysis using linked markers on chromosome 7 has been used to detect cystic fibrosis (CF) prenatally for couples who have had a CF child, by testing foetal DNA from amniotic cells or chorionic villi along with blood samples from both the parents and the previous affected offspring (see example in Figure 24.8). The accuracy of the information gained from linkage analysis is related to the distance between the marker loci and the CF gene.

The same technology has also been successfully applied to the assessment of CF carrier status in subjects who have a prior history of the disease in the family, but who have no clinically recognizable symptoms. Blood samples from several family members (including one with CF) have to be analysed for the presence of specific DNA markers that are sufficiently close to the CF gene to permit tracking of the gene in the family. More precise and direct mutation analyses (see section on Molecular Testing below) are not handicapped by this prerequisite, and have largely supplanted the use of linkage analysis in the investigation of CF mutations.

Molecular testing

Investigators have been able to define the molecular basis for an increasing number of inherited disorders. This has largely emanated from the revolutionary progress in DNA technology, the most significant of which include the discovery of enzymes such as restriction endonucleases, reverse transcriptase, and thermostable DNA polymerases, the development of microbiological vectors capable of accepting and propagating DNA of varying lengths (genetic cloning), and the introduction of restriction fragment length polymorphisms (RFLP, Figure 24.9), the polymerase chain reaction (PCR, Figure 24.10), and chromosome "walking" and chromosome "hopping" techniques.

These advances (and others) at the molecular level have been used to map where the defect resides in the DNA blueprint and to identify the genes responsible for many genetic disorders. Cystic fibrosis will be used as a paradigm to discuss the evolution of molecular testing for inherited diseases.

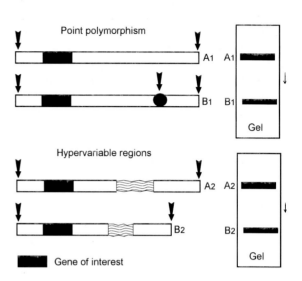

Figure 24.9. The principle of restriction fragment length polymorphism (RFLP) in relation to DNA linkage analysis. A. Point polymorphism. B. Hypervariable region polymorphism.

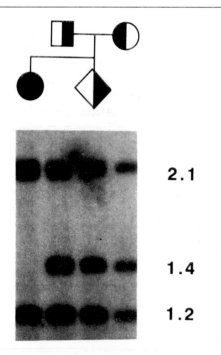

Figure 24.8. DNA linkage (restriction fragment length polymorphism) analysis of a cystic fibrosis-affected family. The pedigree shows father (lane 2 from left), mother (lane 4), affected daughter (lane 1), and foetus of undetermined sex (lane 3). See text for interpretation of results and page 310 for full acknowledgement of source.

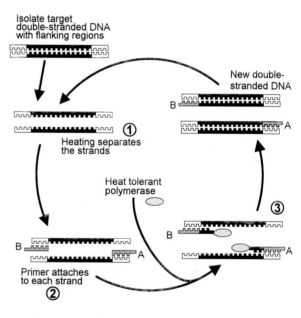

Figure 24.10. The polymerase chain reaction. See text for details. A and B are primers.

The polymerase chain reaction (PCR)

The double stranded specific DNA sequence to be

amplified is heated (Denaturation: step 1) and the primers are allowed to bind to the separated strands (Annealing: step 2). The latter acts as the initiation sequence for the formation of two new chains complementary to the originals (Extension: step 3, carried out by a thermostable DNA polymerase). This series of events is repeated 20-30 times, with each cycling giving a doubling of the DNA. Each cycle of three steps usually takes about 5 minutes or less.

Molecular testing as applied to cystic fibrosis

Cystic fibrosis is the most common hereditary lethal disease amongst Causasians, with an incidence of approximately 1 in 2500 live births and a carrier rate as high as 1 in 20 to 25 adults. The gene responsible has been identified and mapped to the long arm of chromosome 7, and transmission occurs as an auto-somal recessive trait. It spans ~250,000 nucleotides, contains 27 exons, makes an ~6.5 kb mRNA transcript, and encodes a 1480 amino acid protein called the cystic fibrosis transmembrane conductance regulator (CFTR). To date, more than 350 CFTR mutations have been identified. The most common of these, the ɔF508 mutation, accounts for >70% of the mutations, with another 10-40 additional mutations making up the bulk of the remainder.

Besides the DNA-RFLP linkage analysis mentioned above, the molecular techniques that have been applied to the evaluation of CF patients and susceptible family members include:

- *allele-specific hybridisation* for a specific mutation (Figure 24.11)
- *reverse dot-blot hybridisation* for multiple mutations (Figure 24.12)

DNA linkage analysis

This type of analysis is usually used as the initial step in finding the gene and in prenatal diagnosis of an inherited disorder. Probes known to detect sequences located on particular chromosomes, the "linked markers", are used. Any mutation in the DNA nucleotide sequence within that region of the genome produces polymorphism, and the probes used must be able to detect these polymorphic markers.

Markers used initially to search for CF (and other) disorders detected RFLPs caused by a single nucleotide change that either creates or abolishes a recognition sequence for a restriction endonuclease

(Figure 24.8). These specific palindromic stretches of DNA are comprised of 4-8 bases and contains the specific cleavage sites for various restriction endonucleases. The creation of an extra restriction site will result in shorter DNA fragments which migrate further on gel electrophoresis, compared to the unrestricted fragment.

In the example shown in Figure 24.8, the marker linked to the CF locus has two alleles of 2.1 and 1.4 kb (the constant band of 1.2 kb has no bearing on the linkage analysis). The mutant locus is associated to the chromosome bearing the 2.1 allele (the mutation abolishes an extra Taq 1 restriction site near the CF locus). Both the mother and the father, as expected, are heterozygous for the 2.1 and 1.4 alleles. The affected daughter has inherited two mutant alleles, but the unborn foetus has inherited only one and is therefore a heterozygous carrier for the disease, like the parents.

Allele-specific oligonucleotide (ASO) hybridisation

Other mutations that do not produce convenient changes in restriction enzyme sites may be detected by ASO hybridisation (Figure 24.11). This is a precise assay in which different labelled oligonucleotides (15- to 25-base residues) that differ by a single nucleotide defining normal and mutant alleles are hybridised to separate patient DNA samples spotted on a solid support (usually nylon-reinforced paper).

In Figure 24.11, the PCR-amplification products of six patient DNA samples, after denaturation to single-strand forms are hybridised to such a pair of end-labelled oligonucleotides. The one applied to the strip on top is complementary to the normal sequence, and the other (bottom strip) to the mutant sequence. Patients 1, 4, and 5 have only normal alleles (homo-zygous); patients 2 and 6 are heterozygous for normal and mutant sequences; lane 3 is a negative control.

Note: In a deviation from using CF mutations, the example shown in Figure 24.11 is that of a mutation causing the common variety of ʋ⁺ thalassaemia in Mediterranean populations. The mutation is due to a G→A (guanine →adenine) change at position 110 in the first intervening sequence of the ʋ-globin gene. The region of DNA studied is part of a 1.8 kb restriction enzyme fragment, as indicated.

The same principle would of course apply to mutations of the cystic fibrosis gene or those of other diseases which involves a single nucleotide change that does not create or abolish restriction sites.

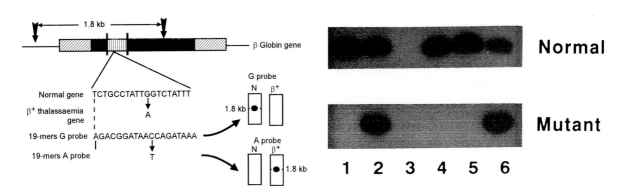

Figure 24.11. Allele-specific hybridisation and the use of oligonucleotide probes for prenatal diagnosis. See text for details. See below for acknowledgement for reprinting the results of the six patient samples shown on the right (24.11R).

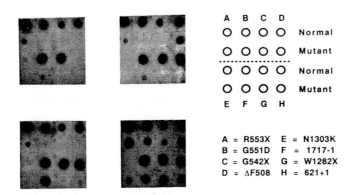

A	B	C	D	
O	O	O	O	Normal
O	O	O	O	Mutant
O	O	O	O	Normal
O	O	O	O	Mutant
E	F	G	H	

A = R553X   E = N1303K
B = G551D   F = 1717-1
C = G542X   G = W1282X
D = ΔF508   H = 621+1

Figure 24.12. Reverse dot-blot hybridisation for multiple cystic fibrosis mutations. Three patient samples (top two and lower left) and a heterozygous control (lower right) are shown. See text for details. **Acknowledgement:** *Figures 24.8, 24.11R, 24.12.* Reprinted with permission from: Kant, JA. The evolution of molecular testing for inherited disorders: cystic fibrosis as a paradigm. *Endocrinology and Metabolism In-Service Training and Continuing Education* 1993;11(11):303-311. ©1993, American Association for Clinical Chemistry, Inc.

Reverse dot-blot hybridisation assay

This is related to the ASO hybridisation technique, and uses the same strategy with one variation -- the patient sample, rather than the oligonucleotide probe, is labelled and hybridised to spots on paper supports containing the affixed oligonucleotides that recognise specific mutations. This technique enables screening of multiple mutations on a single blot; the patient DNA samples are PCR-amplified for specific mutations.

CF mutations are shown in Figure 24.12. The results show that the first patient (upper left) is normal, the second (upper right) is heterozygous for the ΔF508 mutation, and the third (lower left) is heterozygous for the 1717-1 mutation. Non-specific hybridisation with certain oligonucleotide probes occurred in some samples, and the normal N1303K sequence did not work (no signal seen in control sample).

FURTHER READING

Applegarth DA, Dimmick JE, Toone JR. Laboratory detection of metabolic disease. Pediatric Clinics North Am 1989;36:49-65.

Green A. Guide to diagnosis of inborn errors of metabolism in district general hospitals. J Clin Pathol 1989;42:84-91.

Stanbury JB, Wyngaarden JB, Fredrickson DS, Goldstein JL, Brown MS. (eds). *The Metabolic Basis of Inherited Disease, 5th edn.* New York: McGraw-Hill, 1983.

Weatherall DJ. *The New Genetics and Clinical Practice, 3rd edn.* Oxford: Oxford University Press, 1991.

Chapter 25

Nutrition, Vitamins, Trace Elements

A normal nutritional state requires the supply of some 40 essential nutrients (essential in that they can not be synthesised by the body). Deficiency or excess of these substances can result in characteristic clinical and biochemical abnormalities. The major essential nutrients are:

- Water (page 2)
- Energy in the form of carbohydrates, lipids, and proteins
- Amino acids (9 essential)
- Electrolytes: sodium and chloride (page 4), potassium (page 25), magnesium (page 108), calcium and phosphate (page 88)
- Trace minerals: iron (page 271), copper (page 318), zinc (page 318), molybdenum, manganese, selenium (page 319), chromium (page 318), iodine (page 233), fluoride
- Vitamins (page 314)

ASSESSMENT OF NUTRITIONAL STATUS

A common nutritional problem is obesity but in this section only the nutritional deficiencies (malnutrition, undernutrition, etc) will be discussed. The detrimental effects malnutrition can have on the morbidity and mortality of the sick are well recognised and clinical decisions about treatment and prognosis are in part based on the assessment of the nutritional status. Currently in most hospitals, the evaluation of the nutritional state depends much on the dietary history and the clinical assessments including anthropometric measurements -- weight loss, skinfold thickness, mid-arm circumference, response to intradermal injections of common skin antigens, etc. Nevertheless, laboratory investigation plays an important, albeit supplementary, part and should include a wide range of haemato-logical and biochemical tests, as outlined below.

Haematological tests

The haemoglobin and peripheral blood picture will provide information about anaemia which may reflect such conditions as protein starvation, iron deficiency, and folic acid and vitamin B_{12} deficiency. The total lymphocyte count, if low, may indicate depression of the immune system which occurs in severe protein undernutrition. Vitamin K deficiency is associated with a prolonged prothrombin time.

Biochemical tests

The biochemical investigation should include the following tests:

Serum iron studies (serum iron, transferrin and ferritin, page 275): to exclude iron deficiency; serum transferrin concentration is also used to assess visceral protein status and it may be low in severe protein deficiency (page 313).

Serum alkaline phosphatase: high values are seen in vitamin D deficiency (rickets, osteomalacia) and a low value may be associated with zinc deficiency.

Serum calcium and phosphate: both low in vitamin D deficiency. Severely malnourished individuals are susceptible to rapid vascular depletion of phosphate during refeeding -- this is one of the causes of severe hypophosphataemia and this eventuality should be covered by phosphate supplements.

Serum transaminases: The transaminases (alanine aminotransferase and aspartate aminotransferase) are pyridoxine-dependant and may be low in deficiency of this vitamin.

Serum albumin: This is the single most important indicator of visceral protein status. During periods of protein deprivation, albumin synthesis falls by about 50% within 24 hours and this reduced level of produc-tion persists for as long as the reduced protein intake is maintained. However, it suffers from a number of drawbacks and generally is not the protein of choice for short-term nutritional assessment (see below).

Serum osmolality: Indicative of hydration status.

Zinc protoporphyrin haem ratio. Sensitive indicator of subclinical iron deficiency.

Serum and red cell folate. A common nutrient deficiency in alcoholics.

Energy

The human organism requires energy for normal function, activity, growth, and tissue repair. The amount necessary varies with age, sex, and activity but ranges from ~40 Kcal/day in young adults to ~30 Kcal/day in persons over the age of 50 years. Physical activity increases requirements, e.g., sleeping uses about 100 Kcal/hour and strenuous exercise may utilise up to 900 Kcal/hour. Deficiency produces the state known as protein-energy (protein-calorie) malnutrition.

Carbohydrates

Carbohydrates are not essential nutrients providing there is an adequate calorie intake from other sources (fats, proteins). Complete absence from the diet, however, will result in moderate ketosis but an intake as little as 100 g/day will prevent this. Generally the carbohydrate intake constitutes 40 to 50% of the energy intake and current recommendations are that this should be increased to 55-60%.

Fats

Dietary fat is only essential in that linoleic acid is an essential nutrient, being required for the synthesis of arachidonic acid (major precursor of prostaglandins). Deficiency of this fatty acid will result in hair loss, dermatitis, and impaired wound healing (about 5 g is required daily).

Fats are the most concentrated source of energy with the average diet contributing sufficient fat to provide about 40% of body calorie requirements. Current recommendations are that this figure should be lowered to less than 30%. Fats are also needed as a carrier for fat-soluble vitamins.

Proteins

Proteins are essential nutrients because nitrogen is necessary for protein synthesis, and nine amino acids can not be synthesised by the body (leucine, isoleucine, valine, lysine, histidine, phenylalanine, tryptophan, methionine, threonine). On a protein-free diet the adult male loses about 4 grams of nitrogen a day which is approximately equivalent to 25 grams of protein. The recommended intake is 56 g/day for men and 45 g/day for women.

Protein deficiency is associated with inadequate intake (protein-energy malnutrition, marasmus, kwashiorkor), alcoholism, malabsorption, burns, protein-losing enteropathy, and the nephrotic syndrome. It presents with growth retardation in children, oedema, head hair depigmentation, and flaking skin.

Visceral protein status. In the laboratory, visceral protein status can be determined to a limited extent by estimation of the rapidly turning-over plasma proteins (Table 25.1) such as transferrin, prealbumin (transthyretin), and retinol-binding protein. As discussed below, albumin, with a longer half-life, is less useful in the acute state. The alternate protein markers all have shorter half-lives than albumin and are thus more useful in short-term nutritional surveillance. However, their serum levels are also influenced by factors other than protein and energy deficiencies, such as illness, stress, injury, and drug interactions. In the clinical situation, it is often not possible to distinguish between the effects of malnutrition and the effects of illness and injury on serum protein levels and considerable caution must be exercised when ascribing low serum protein levels to malnutrition.

Ideally, the protein of choice should have:

- a short biological half-life
- the ability to reflect closely the protein (and nutritional) status by quantifiable serum concentration changes
- a small total body pool
- a rapid rate of synthesis
- a constant metabolic rate
- Its metabolism (and hence serum concentration) should be responsive only to protein and energy restrictions.

None of the proteins in Table 25.1 is thus an ideal choice in this context (see below). Their respective drawbacks are briefly discussed below.

Table 25.1. Serum proteins useful in the evaluation of protein deficiency.

	half-life (days)	Low serum levels in
Albumin	20	liver disease nephrotic syndrome pregnancy overhydration acute-phase reaction
Transferrin	8.0	chronic inflammation iron overload nephrotic syndrome liver disease
Transthyretin	2.0	liver disease nephrotic syndrome inflammations surgical stress
Retinol-binding protein	0.5	liver disease hyperthyroidism nephrotic syndrome zinc deficiency

Albumin: It may take weeks for the albumin levels in the serum to fall because of its long half-life, a shift of extravascular albumin into the serum, and a reduction in catabolic rate. Normally, only about 30% of the body's total exchangeable albumin resides in the intravascular space. During starvation, the extra-vascular albumin serves as a reservoir to 'top up' the decreasing intravascular pool, and the serum albumin level only begins to fall when the extravascular pool becomes depleted. In addition, its use as a marker of visceral protein status may also be compromised because it is low in a number of other disease states such as the nephrotic syndrome, and it is affected by changes in the volume and distribution of body fluids.

Transferrin: Iron nutriture strongly influences its serum level (increased in iron deficiency, suppressed in iron overload); increased during pregnancy, oestrogen therapy, and acute hepatitis; reduced in protein-losing enteropathy and nephropathy, chronic infections, renal failure, and acute catabolic states.

Prealbumin (transthyretin): Its serum level is very sensitive to stress -- reduced in acute catabolic states, post-surgery, hyperthyroidism. Measurement is less readily available.

Retinol-binding protein (RBP): This protein is catabolised in the renal proximal tubular cell; with renal disease, serum RBP level increases (decreased clearance). Also susceptible to the influence of stress (as prealbumin).

Protein-energy malnutrition

Protein-energy malnutrition is the result of a relative or absolute deficiency of calories and proteins.

1 In developing nations, it classically occurs as two distinct syndromes: *marasmus,* caused by protein and calorie deficiency, and *kwashiorkor,* which is due to protein deficiency in the presence of an adequate calorie intake.

2 In developed nations, the disorder is usually secondary to other diseases such as malabsorption, alcoholism, malignancy, and so on.

It results in pathophysiological changes that can affect every organ. The obvious features are weight loss, loss of fat stores, and loss of muscle mass. As the disorder progresses, the following may occur:

- hepatic synthesis of proteins decreased (low plasma levels of albumin, transferrin, etc)
- cardiac output and contractility are decreased
- lungs are affected by weakness and atrophy of the muscles of respiration
- mucosal atrophy and loss of villi of the GIT resulting in decreased absorptive capacity
- pancreatic insufficiency
- immunological dysfunction (decreased total lymphocyte count, depressed T-cell function, anergic response to common skin antigens)
- decreased serum albumin levels producing oedema

Vitamins

The vitamins are essential nutrients required in small quantities for normal metabolism. With the exception

313

of vitamins D and E, they act as cofactors or cofactor precursors for enzyme systems. They are not produced in the body and thus have to be taken in the diet. The exceptions are vitamin D which can be synthesised in the skin, and nicotinamide, which is produced in small quantities from tryptophan.

A normal balanced diet would provide sufficient supplies of vitamins; thus vitamin supplementation is usually unnecessary. Unprescribed or prolonged supplementation especially of vitamin A and D results in their accumulation in tissues and may produce toxic effects. Vitamin deficiencies are more common than hypervitaminosis. Causes of vitamin deficiency can be categorised under inadequate dietary intake, decreased assimilation, defective utilisation, increased destruction, enhanced excretion and increased requirements.

Vitamins are classified into two groups on the basis of their solubilities.

1   The fat-soluble vitamins, which require normal fat absorption for proper absorption, are transported in the blood attached to proteins and stored in the liver and other tissues. Deficiency thus takes time to develop and increased intake can result in toxicity.

2   The water-soluble vitamins appear in the urine soon after ingestion and are not stored to any degree, thus deficiency can occur in the short-term and toxicity due to overdose is uncommon.

FAT-SOLUBLE VITAMINS

The fat-soluble vitamins are vitamin A, vitamin D, vitamin E, and vitamin K. As stated above, their absorption is dependant on normal fat absorption, and toxicity can occur because of storage in the body and the lack of a route for excretion.

Vitamin A (Retinol)

There are a number of different molecular forms of this compound, the term vitamin A being a collective term. The biologically active forms include retinol, retinal, and retinoic acid, the alcohol, aldehyde, and acid moieties, respectively. Dietary sources provide either preformed vitamin A or precursors, primarily β-carotene.

Sources. Carotenes are found in yellow and green vegetables, carrots being an especially rich source. Milk products and eggs also contain significant amounts.

Metabolism.   Dietary carotenes and preformed vitamin A, as retinal, are first hydrolysed to retinol and esterified in the intestinal mucosal cell before absorption into the circulation via the lymphatic system; any excess retinol esters are temporarily stored in the liver. In blood retinol is transported bound to retinol-binding protein. Retinoic acid is absorbed unchanged. Dietary retinoic acid, as well as that formed endogenously as a normal metabolite of retinol and retinal, is not stored in the body and is readily excreted through the bile as a glucuronide conjugate.

Functions.   Vitamin A is required for the preservation of vision, especially at night. Dim light vision is dependant on the retinal pigment rhodopsin (opsin, a protein, combined with vitamin A). It is also involved in mucus secretion and mucopolysaccharide synthesis.

Deficiency. Clinical effects include night blindness, drying and metaplasia of ectodermal tissue (xerosis conjunctivae, xerophthalmia, keratomalacia), and anaemia. The regulation of retinol concentration in plasma is influenced by the rates of production and turnover of retinol-binding protein. Any condition that affects normal protein synthesis, such as parenchymal liver disease and protein-calorie malnutrition, will result in low plasma retinol levels despite normal liver stores.

Toxicity. Hypervitaminosis A results in nausea, vomiting and abdominal pain. In the long-term there is fatigue, insomnia, hair loss, bone pain, and discolouration of the skin. Hypercalcaemia has also been described. The toxicity is usually caused by indiscriminate excessive intake of vitamin A preparations.

Laboratory evaluation. Measurement of serum retinol is part of the assessment of vitamin A status. Very low plasma vitamin A levels usually confirm deficiency if the diagnosis has been made on clinical criteria. On their own, plasma retinol levels are unlikely to provide sufficient information about the total body stores.

Most of the methods for plasma retinol utilise its

property as a fat-soluble vitamin. Plasma proteins are first precipitated with ethanol and the vitamin is then extracted into an organic solvent. Both fluorimetric assays as well as reverse-phase HPLC separations provide precise, sensitive, and specific measurements, with HPLC techniques being superior in these aspects.

Vitamin D

Vitamin D is discussed in Chapter 6 in association with calcium metabolism and metabolic bone disease.

Vitamin K

Sources. Within the body vitamin K is synthesised not by the human host but by the bacterial flora of the colon. In infants the full complement of the gut bacterial colony develops gradually and they may be vitamin K-deficient. Dietary sources are green leafy vegetables, meats, and dairy produce.

Functions. It is necessary for the synthesis of the clotting factors, prothrombin and Factors VII, IX, and X by the liver. Warfarin, developed as a rat poison, is a vitamin K antagonist and is used therapeutically as an anticoagulant.

Clinical effects of deficiency. Prolonged clotting and bleed tendency, which is particularly severe in newborn infants.

Laboratory evaluation. The prothrombin time estimates the plasma levels of the clotting factors II, VII, IX, and X which are dependant on normal vitamin K activity.

Vitamin E (Tocopherols)

Sources. Vegetable seed oils, wheat germ.

Functions. Vitamin E acts as an antioxidant which is important for scavenging the free radicals arising from peroxidation of unsaturated fatty acids. These free radicals damage cells by increasing their fragility. Vitamin E probably also functions as a component of a number of enzyme systems.

Deficiency. This may occur in premature babies due to inadequate stores where it can cause haemolytic anaemia, thrombocytosis, and oedema. It is not known if deficiency in the adult is important.

Toxicity. High doses can cause clotting abnormalities due to their antagonistic effect to vitamin K.

Laboratory evaluation. The plasma levels of vitamin E can be estimated directly by quantitation, and can be measured simultaneously with vitamin A in fluorimetric assays on extracts into organic solvents. The reference method is a reverse phase HPLC method for the simultaneous determination of both these fat-soluble vitamins. Measurements are useful in the evaluation of the premature baby whose immature red cells are highly susceptible to lysis by the oxygen free radicals.

WATER-SOLUBLE VITAMINS

These include vitamin C and the B complex: thiamine (B_1), riboflavin (B_2), nicotinamide, pyridoxine (B_6), biotin, folate, cobalamins (B_{12}). As they are water-soluble, any excess absorbed is excreted in the urine and toxicity due to increased intake is rare. Stores are not high and short-term deficiency can occur.

Vitamin C (Ascorbate)

Sources. Citrus and other fruits, vegetables. Ascorbate is often used as a food preservative.

Functions. The metabolic functions are not yet well defined. It may act as a hydrogen carrier, and appears necessary for normal collagen formation (hydroxylation of lysine and proline).

Deficiency. The clinical condition is scurvy. There is poor collagen formation resulting in gingivitis, petechial haemorrhages and bruising, poor healing of wounds, haemarthrosis, and subperiosteal bleeding. Elderly people who do not have a diet rich in fruits and vegetables and who eat mainly processed food are particularly vulnerable to ascorbate deficiency.

315

Laboratory evaluation. To assess vitamin C status, the vitamin has been measured in serum, urine and leucocytes. Plasma ascorbate levels give some indication of the dietary intake and are easy to perform. Urine levels are dependant on intake and are only meaningful in nutritional studies where intake is controlled. Leucocyte ascorbate levels provide a better index of tissue stores but require a more elaborate analytical procedure. Chemical and enzymatic assays have been used most often in routine vitamin C estimations, but highly sensitive and specific HPLC methods for plasma and leucocyte ascorbic acid are also available.

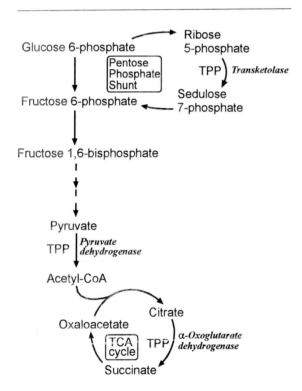

Figure 25.1. Thiamine pyrophosphate (TPP) as a cofactor of various enzymes involved in carbohydrate metabolism.

Thiamine (B₁)

Source. Most dietary components, yeast, wheat germ.

Functions. Thiamine pyrophosphate is an essential

cofactor for enzymatic decarboxylation of oxoacids, e.g., conversion of pyruvate to acetyl-CoA, transketolase reactions of the pentose phosphate pathway (see Figure 25.1).

Deficiency. The clinical condition is beriberi which is classified into the 'dry' (neurological lesions, Wernicke's encephalopathy) and 'wet' (oedema, cardiac failure) forms.

Laboratory evaluation. There are three possible approaches:

1 urinary thiamine excretion rate (useful but influenced by recent intake),
2 red cell transketolase activity (good indicator of body stores),
3 blood pyruvate levels after a glucose load (not specific as increases have also been observed in diabetes mellitus, congestive heart failure, severe liver disease and some infections).

Riboflavin (B₂)

Source. Yeast, peas, beans, meat.

Functions. Riboflavin is a component of flavoproteins (flavin mononucleotide, FMN; flavin adenine dinucleotide, FAD) which are important cofactors in biological oxidative systems.

Deficiency/ariboflavinosis. This causes rough scaling of the skin, angular stomatitis and cheilosis, similar lesions of other mucous membranes, red swollen tongue, and ocular symptoms. The prevalence is notably high, ranging from 5% to 40% in some reports. The classical candidate is the pregnant adolescent living in socioeconomically deprived conditions in whom the increased requirements of pregnancy are not met). A variety of diseases such as cancer, diabetes mellitus, infections, and cardiac disease can precipitate the deficiency.

Laboratory evaluation. FAD is required for the activity of glutathione reductase; the FAD test involves measuring the activity of red cell glutathione reductase before and after the addition of FAD

316

(increased activity after FAD addition suggests deficiency).

Nicotinamide (Niacin)

Source. Nicotinamide is formed in the body from nicotinic acid which is freely available in animal and plant foods. A small amount is synthesised *in vivo* from tryptophan.

Function. It is the active component of the nicotinamide adenine nucleotides (NAD, NADP). These important cofactors in oxidation-reduction reactions are essential for glycolysis and oxidative phosphorylation.

Deficiency. This results in the pellagra syndrome characterised by diarrhoea, dermatitis, and dementia. A similar picture occurs in Hartnup disease (impaired tryptophan absorption, page 300) and in the carcinoid syndrome (accelerated tryptophan metabolism, page 223); hence the endogenous production of nicotinamide from tryptophan is important in supplementing the dietary source.

Laboratory evaluation. Deficiency is detected by estimation of the urinary metabolites of nicotinic acid (N-methylnicotinamide, N-methyl-3-carboxamide-6-pyridone).

Pyridoxine (B$_6$)

Source. Widely distributed in food.

Functions. As pyridoxyl phosphate, it is an important cofactor for the transaminase group of enzymes and for decarboxylation of amino acids.

Deficiency. This may produce a rough skin, peripheral neuropathy, and a sore tongue. Prolonged deficiency may result in similar lesions to those of riboflavin deficiency (see above). Use or overdose of the following drugs may result in classical B$_6$ deficiency: amiodarone, L-dopa, isoniazid, D-penecillamine, tricyclic antidepressants (amitriptyline).

Laboratory evaluation. Measurement of plasma pyridoxal-5-phosphate is the most sensitive parameter but it is not readily performed in most laboratories. Deficiency can be detected by measuring the activity of erythrocyte aspartate aminotransaminase (AST) before and after the addition of pyridoxyl phosphate.

A number of the enzymes involved in tryptophan metabolism require pyridoxyl phosphate and the estimation of the tryptophan metabolites, kynurenine and xanthurenic acid, in the urine after an oral dose of tryptophan gives an indirect indication of the liver stores of B$_6$.

Folate

Source. Folates are a naturally occurring group of substances, found in green vegetables and meat, that are structural derivatives of the parent compound folic acid (pteroylglutamic acid).

Function. The different folate compounds are involved in the transfer of one-carbon groups, primarily as methyl or formyl moieties; hence their importance in metabolic pathways involving one-carbon transfers such as the synthesis of methionine, purines, and thymidylate monophosphate (component of DNA).

Deficiency. The characteristic clinical presentation is megaloblastic anaemia. The causes are manifold including malabsorption, dietary deficiency, and increased requirements (growth, pregnancy, lactation).

Laboratory evaluation. Serum and red cell folate estimations are available in most routine laboratories.

Vitamin B$_{12}$ (Cobalamins)

Sources. Vitamin B$_{12}$ is a group term for several structurally related cobalamins (e.g., cyanocobalamin) found in animal products. It requires gastric-produced intrinsic factor to facilitate absorption in the lower ileum (page 215).

Function. Vitamin B$_{12}$ acts as a coenzyme in nucleic acid synthesis and is an important component of DNA and RNA metabolism.

Deficiency. Deficiency results in megaloblastic anaemia and subacute degeneration of the spinal cord (Addisonian pernicious anaemia). Deficiency is usually due to lack of intrinsic factor, but the malabsorption syndromes including bacterial overgrowth are also important causes (page 220).

Laboratory evaluation. Serum B_{12} estimations are freely available. The Schilling test (page 221) is used to determine the absorptive status of B_{12}.

Trace metals

Trace elements, like vitamins, play an important role in enzyme activity as integral components of metalloenzymes or as essential cofactors. Most are toxic in the elemental form and are transported in plasma attached to proteins, e.g., albumin and transferrin can bind iron, chromium, copper, manganese and zinc.

All the trace elements are absorbed throughout the small intestine and are excreted either in the urine (chromium, iodine, copper, cobalt) or in the faeces via the bile (copper, manganese) or via desquamated mucosal cells (iron, zinc). In man deficiencies have been established with iron (page 271), iodine (page 233), chromium, copper, and zinc.

Copper

This metal plays an important role in many enzyme systems and is involved in the transport and metabolism of iron. It is absorbed from the small intestine and carried in the blood in two major forms. About 90% is incorporated in caeruloplasmin, and α_2-globulin with oxidase activity; the remainder is loosely bound to albumin. Excretion occurs via the bile; a very small amount, representing the plasma non-caeruloplasmin copper, is excreted in the urine.

Abnormal copper metabolism. Abnormalities include deficiency, Wilson's disease, and Menke's syndrome.

Copper deficiency may produce resistant hypochromic anaemia and neutropenia and may occur in patients on long term parenteral nutrition.

Wilson's disease is an inborn error of copper metabolism characterised by deposition of copper in, and damage to, the liver (cirrhosis), brain basal ganglia, proximal renal tubule (Fanconi syndrome), and the cornea of the eye (Kayser-Fleischer rings). The plasma caeruloplasmin level is usually low and the urinary copper level high, reflecting the high level of plasma free copper. The definitive diagnosis depends on demonstration of excess copper in the liver.

Menke's syndrome presents in infancy with growth retardation, seizures, and kinky hair (defective keratinisation). It is caused by an X-linked genetic defect in copper transport.

The method of choice for the estimation of serum and urine copper is atomic absorption spectrophotometry, preferably with graphite furnace facility. Caeruloplasmin is usually determined by immunochemical methods.

Zinc

Zinc is essential in protein and nucleic acid synthesis and is an important component of more than 90 enzymes including RNA polymerase, carbonic anhydrase, and ALA dehydratase. Deficiency may be associated with chronic parenteral nutrition, malnutrition, malabsorption syndromes, and cirrhosis. It results in delayed wound healing, diarrhoea, and dermatitis. Pregnant women are at a relatively high risk for suboptimal levels of zinc which can adversely affect foetal outcome. An inborn error due to defective synthesis of a mucosal zinc-binding protein has been described (acrodermatitis enteropathica). It presents in early infancy with diarrhoea, dermatitis, and alopecia.

In disease states associated with decreased zinc levels the analyst must be able to measure zinc concentrations of the order of <0.5 mg/L. The most specific method is atomic absorption spectrophotometry (AAS) which is sensitive, precise, and accurate.

Chromium

There is a link between glucose metabolism and chromium: glucose tolerance is improved in the elderly subject if chromium supplements are given. Inorganic chromium compounds are converted *in vivo* to an organochromium complex termed the 'glucose tolerance factor', which is believed to enhance the action of insulin, perhaps by facilitating its reaction with its receptor site.

Chromium has toxic properties that most frequently manifest themselves as a result of repeated occupational exposure. Such chromium pollution leads to inflammation and necrosis of the skin and nasal passages, dermatitis, lung cancer, and kidney failure.

Levels of chromium in normal serum are very low and can only be measured accurately by very sensitive methods (neutron activation). Urine chromium levels are within the range of graphite furnace AAS instruments. It is essential to avoid contamination from containers and glassware.

Selenium

Selenium deficiency, which may accompany protein-energy malnutrition, is associated with cardiomyopathy and a deforming arthritic bone disease. The diagnosis is made by estimating the plasma or red cell levels. Deficiency can also be evaluated by estimating the activity of the red cell (or platelet) selenium-containing enzyme, glutathione peroxidase.

Methods for the determination of selenium by AAS use either graphite furnace or hydride-formation procedures. The former is more sensitive but cannot be applied to the analysis of whole blood because of interference by iron.

Aluminium

With the recent advent of extensive haemodialysis programs, aluminium toxicity has become a well-recognised disorder. The main source of this metal is aluminium-contaminated dialysis fluid. Other sources are aluminium-containing phosphate-binding agents used to lower the plasma phosphate in renal failure and cheap aluminium cooking utensils. The manifestations of toxicity are dialysis encephalopathy or dementia, osteomalacia, and hypochromic anaemia.

In most laboratories, aluminium levels in serum, urine, and dialysis fluids are determined by flameless atomic absorption spetrometric analysis.

FURTHER READING

Briggs MH (ed). *Vitamins in Human Biology and Medicine.* Florida: CRC Press, 1981.

Clayton BE. Clinical chemistry of trace elements. Adv Clin Chem 1980;21:147-176.

Strakey BJ. Aluminium in renal disease: current knowledge and future development. Ann Clin Biochem 1987;24:337-344.

Taylor A (ed) Trace elements in human disease. Clinics Endocrinol Metab 1985;14:513-760.

Woolfson AMJ (ed). Biochemistry of Hospital Nutrition. *Contemporary Issues in Clinical Biochemistry, vol 4.* Edinburgh: Churchill Livingston, 1986.

Chapter 26

Pregnancy, Prenatal Diagnosis and Infertility

The areas that will be covered in this chapter are the metabolic changes of pregnancy which may affect plasma analyte concentrations or their interpretations, the biochemical monitoring of pregnancy, prenatal diagnosis of certain congenital defects, and the laboratory evaluation of infertility.

Pregnancy: metabolic changes

A number of the physiological and metabolic changes associated with pregnancy are important from the clinical chemist's point of view because of their effects on plasma analyte values.

Plasma volume

The plasma volume increases by up to 50% in pregnancy, causing a dilutional fall in the concentration of plasma analytes. The two analytes most affected are albumin (falls of up to about 5 g/L), especially during the first trimester, and urea. The fall in the plasma urea (levels less than 2.5 mmol/L are quite common) is due to several factors, including the dilutional effect of an expanding plasma volume, decreased production (positive nitrogen balance), and increased renal excretion as a consequence of a pregnancy-induced increase in the glomerular filtration rate. This fall in plasma urea is accentuated in the face of a low protein diet.

Plasma electrolytes

The only two electrolytes which are affected by the pregnant state are plasma calcium and bicarbonate; all other plasma electrolytes maintain their pre-pregnancy levels.

Calcium. The total plasma calcium concentration, and more specifically the protein-bound fraction, usually falls in tandem with the fall in the plasma albumin level.

Bicarbonate. During the last trimester of pregnancy, it is not uncommon to find the plasma bicarbonate level falling to around 18 mmol/L, this being in compensation for the hyperventilation which probably follows from stimulation of the respiratory centre by the high progesterone levels in circulation. The fall may be more marked during labour.

Plasma proteins

In addition to the dilutional fall in albumin and the appearance of certain pregnancy-associated proteins such as human placental lactogen (HPL), pregnancy-specific β_1-glycoprotein (SP$_1$), and placental alkaline phosphatase, a number of other plasma proteins show an increase in concentration. This is due to stimulation of their synthesis by oestrogens and include the following:

Carrier proteins. Increased levels of transferrin, caeruloplasmin, thyroxine-binding globulin, cortisol-binding globulin and sex hormone-binding globulin occur, with concomitant rises in the plasma concentrations of compounds bound to these proteins.

Coagulation factors. Increased levels of factors II (fibrinogen), VII and X are common.

Lipoproteins. The increase in apolipoprotein synthesis causes a mild increase in the plasma lipoprotein levels, particularly that of the very low density lipoprotein (VLDL) fraction.

Plasma alkaline phosphatase. In the third trimester of pregnancy, the total plasma alkaline phosphatase activity may increase to about 2-2.5 times the non-pregnant adult activities, due largely to the secretion of the placental isoenzyme (page 179). In a small proportion of women, the increase may be partly of hepatic origin -- jaundice, most likely caused by intrahepatic cholestasis, is an uncommon complication of some pregnancies.

Plasma hormones

There is an increase in the plasma concentrations of those hormones that circulate mainly bound to carrier proteins, e.g., the total T_4, total T_3 and total cortisol levels may show increases of as much as 50%. The important issue is to recognise these changes for what they are, and to be aware that in the investigation of suspected thyroid or adrenal dysfunction in pregnant patients (likewise in women taking oral contraceptives), plasma free T_4 and urinary free cortisol excretion should be measured, as their levels are not affected by changes in the carrier protein levels.

Proteins produced by trophoblast tissues (e.g., human chorionic gonadotrophin and HPL) and those associated with the maintenance of pregnancy (e.g., oestrogens, progesterone, prolactin), register marked increases in plasma concentrations, peaking at various times of the gestation period. They will be discussed in the next section.

Note: Use of oral contraceptives (especially those with a high oestrogen content) and oestrogen therapy also produce many of the biochemical changes discussed above.

Biochemistry of the feto-placental unit

The placenta is an organ that does not exist outside of pregnancy -- it is the earliest fetal tissue to differentiate. It produces a large number of proteins, some of which are specific to the pregnant state, including HCG, HPL, SP_1, and placental alkaline phosphatase. It also produces large amounts of steroid hormones -- after the sixth week of gestation, it is the main source of progesterone and is involved in the production of oestrogens, in conjunction with the fetus.

Human chorionic gonadotrophin (HCG)

HCG is synthesised early in pregnancy by the newly formed trophoblasts and is secreted into the maternal circulation. It can be detected as early as the eighth day after conception and its levels in the maternal blood continue to rise rapidly, reaching peak levels at about 10-12 weeks of gestation. HCG measurements have long been used to confirm pregnancy and many "home-test" kits are widely available. Pregnancy kits detecting urine HCG are not as sensitive as those

measuring plasma or serum HCG levels -- the glycoprotein is rapidly metabolised by the liver and kidneys and only a small fraction is excreted unchanged in the maternal urine. HCG has luteotrophic activity and is responsible for maintaining the viability of the corpus luteum into early pregnancy. It may also be responsible for inducing testosterone secretion by the fetal testes before the fetal pituitary is ready to secrete luteinising hormone.

Serum HCG titres are also used in the investigation of a probable ectopic pregnancy -- high titres suggest it as the cause of acute abdominal pain, which is usually the presenting symptom. HCG is also produced by tumours of the trophoblast and thus can occur in males (e.g., testicular teratocarcinoma) and non-pregnant females (e.g., hydatidiform mole and choriocarcinoma). Its use as a tumour marker was discussed on page 288.

Human placental lactogen

This hormone, produced by the syncytiotrophoblasts of the placenta, can be detected in the maternal blood at about the sixth week of gestation. The HPL levels in the maternal circulation increases progessively, up to about 32-34 weeks of gestation; thereafter the levels plateau off until parturition occurs. Maternal serum HPL levels have, in the past, found some use in the assessment of placental function, as they correlate fairly well with placental mass (very high levels are found in multiple pregnancies). However, their use in this context have largely been replaced by techniques such as antepartum cardiotocography which monitors fetal heart beats. The physiological role of HPL is still not well defined. As a result of its anti-insulin activity, HPL may be responsible in part for the development of gestational diabetes.

Oestrogens

Oestrogens (oestrone, oestradiol and oestriol) are produced in much larger amounts in pregnancy (up to 800-900 times as much) compared to the amounts found in non-pregnant women. Oestriol is the major oestrogen produced during pregnancy. Its synthesis involves the interaction of both the fetal adrenal gland and the fetal liver enzymes with those of the placenta (Figure 26.1). The hydroxylation of C16 on the steroid skeleton (e.g., DHEAS → 16α-hydroxy DHEAS) is catalysed by a 16α-hydroxylase enzyme found in the fetal adrenals and liver but not in the placenta; the

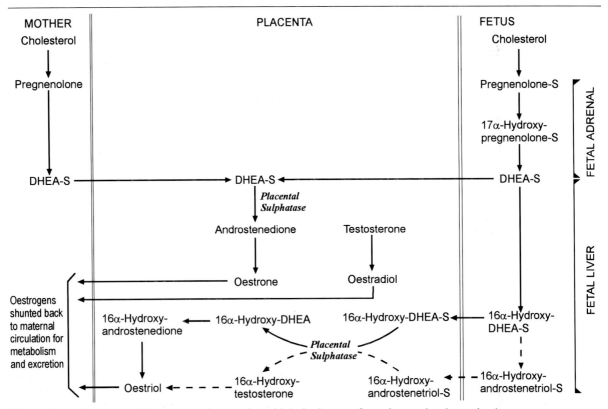

Figure 26.1. Summary of the principal routes by which the human feto-placental unit synthesises oestrogens.
----- minor routes; DHEA, dehydroepiandrosterone; -S, sulphate moiety

removal of the sulphate moiety from 16α-hydroxy-DHEAS, a step that facilitates transfer of all three oestrogens back to the maternal circulation for excretion, requires the placental sulphatase enzyme. This enzyme is not found in fetal tissues. The discovery and recognition of this interplay and interdependance in steroid metabolism as well as other functions led to the concept of the feto-placental unit.

Serial measurement of oestriol output, either in maternal blood or urine, were formerly widely used in monitoring the viability of the feto-placental unit in high-risk pregnancies. An increasing oestriol level is seen with gestational maturity, up to about 34 weeks, after which the rise peters out. Such a trend generally reflects fetal well-being whilst chronically low or declining oestriol levels are a grave prognostic indicator of actual or imminent fetal distress. Single determinations are of little use due to the very broad spread of values at each gestational stage of normal pregnancies. The use of oestriol measurements in this context has now been largely superseded by

ultrasonographic scanning. However, there has been a resurgence of their use in recent years, as part of a prenatal screen for Down's syndrome (see page 326).

Pregnancy-specific β₁-glycoprotein (SP₁)

This protein (function as yet undefined) is also produced by the syncytiotrophoblasts in increasing amounts throughout pregnancy. It is detectable in maternal blood as early as day fourteen after conception. Measurement of circulating SP₁ levels, promulgated as a useful adjunct in the confirmation of the pregnant state in the situations when patients have been treated with HCG, have not been widely adopted.

Placental alkaline phosphatase

This heat-stable isoenzyme of alkaline phosphatase (moderate heating for 10 minutes up to 65° C does not

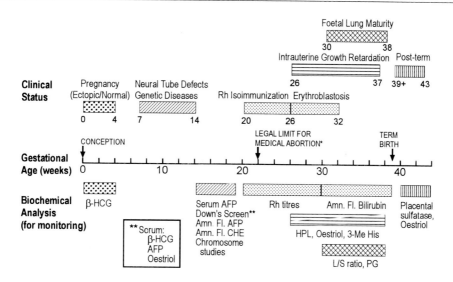

*variable, depending on societal regulations in different countries
**usually includes maternal serum β-HCG, AFP and oestriol
***normally Rh titres are for Rh anti-D antibodies only

Figure 26.2. The use of biochemical tests for maternal and fetal monitoring in pregnancy. See text for details. AFP, alpha-fetoprotein; Amn. Fl., amniotic fluid; CHE, cholinesterase; β-HCG, human chorionic gonadotrophin (β-subunit); HPL, human placental lactogen; L/S ratio, lecithin/sphingomyelin ratio; PG, phosphatidyl glycerol; 3-MeHis, 3-methylhistidine. Adapted with permission from: Pesce AJ and Kaplan LA (ed). *Methods in Clinical Chemistry*, CV Mosby Co, St Louis, 1987.

destroy its activity) is similar in many respects to the Regan isoenzyme found in some malignancies (page 179). As their plasma levels do not correlate well with placental function, its proposed use as a placental function test was rapidly abandoned.

Biochemical monitoring during pregnancy

Biochemical monitoring of the pregnant patient falls into a few related categories: (a) maternal monitoring for pre-existing medical problems, (b) maternal monitoring for assessing feto-placental viability and intrauterine growth, and (c) fetal monitoring for prenatal diagnosis of various types of fetal abnormality. For the tests under (b) and (c), the specific information sought and the natural history of developmental changes in pregnancy dictate the optimal stage of the gestational period when a

particular test is best performed (Figure 26.2). The earliest and most common tests performed are those to confirm pregnancy. They are largely based on the rapid detection of HCG in either urine or serum.

Maternal monitoring

Patients with pre-existing or suspected medical problems may require close monitoring during pregnancy. For example, diabetics who become pregnant have to be stringently controlled to minimise the morbidity to both mother and unborn child. Frequent monitoring of blood glucose and other metabolic indices of diabetic control (serum fructosamine, haemoglobin A_{1c}, serum lipids) is part of good obstetric practice. Likewise, the monitoring of patients with hyper- or hypothyroidism is equally vital and requires the close cooperation of the endocrine laboratory.

At antenatal clinic attendances, urinalysis is a

standard procedure. It is particularly useful in the detection of proteinuria, glycosuria, and possible urinary tract infections. Glycosuria (after allowance is made for the slight decrease in the renal threshold of glucose in pregnancy), may suggest hitherto undiagnosed diabetes and may require appropriate follow-up of the patient (see page 126).

The presence of proteinuria may be an early sign of pre-eclampsia especially in diabetic or hypertensive patients -- due to its deleterious effect on the outcome of the pregnancy and on maternal health, the diagnosis of pre-eclampsia is of some urgency. Left untreated, the condition leads to severe hypertension, pre-eclampsic toxaemia, and renal failure. In severe cases, there may be a need for early termination of pregnancy (see discussion below for appropriate assessment of fetal maturity). Renal function tests should be performed at regular intervals -- an increase in the plasma urate concentration can be a sensitive indicator of deteriorating renal function, as are abnormal electrolyte concentrations.

In addition, every woman would have her blood group typed and blood screened for Rh and other red cell antibodies at her first antenatal clinic visit (Figure 26.2). Management of pregnancies complicated by Rhesus antigen (Rh) isoimmunisation poses some special problems (see below).

Monitoring feto-placental viability

- In early pregnancy, the common problems are threatened abortion with bleeding and a history of recurrent abortions or miscarriages. Tests to monitor placental function (serum HPL), intrauterine growth and fetal well-being (urinary oestriol, ultrasound), performed on a regular basis, preferably daily, may give an indication of the likely outcome of the pregnancy. Patients with serum HPL concentrations that are inappropriately low for the stage of gestation, and which remain low, tend to abort. Likewise, a sharp drop or a persistently low oestriol output indicate intrauterine growth retardation and in women with poor obstetric histories, an attendant high risk of abortion.

- In other types of high risk pregnancies, complications usually arise in the second or third trimesters; hence monitoring of the functional integrity of the feto-placental unit is usually initiated towards the end of the second trimester (from about 28 weeks onwards). Biophysical methods such as ultrasound scanning have to a considerable extent replaced biochemical tests (maternal serum HPL, maternal urine oestriol excretion, molar ratios of 3-methyl histidine to creatinine in amniotic fluid) for the assessment of feto-placental viability. The dwindling popularity of biochemical tests is due in part to the availability of better technologies, and in part to the numerous problems associated with their use, including the high incidence of false-negative and false-positive results, and the need for accurate gestational age records and multiple (serial) testing for proper interpretation of the data obtained. Nevertheless, a chronically low plasma or urinary oestriol would warn of existent or impending complications; it may be due to intrauterine growth retardation, fetal death, fetal abnormalities, placental sulphatase defect, or over-zealous treatment with steroids.

- Women with post-term pregnancies (assuming accurate gestational age computation) with no evidence of fetal distress may have placental sulphatase deficiency. Such individuals usually fail to go into labour and require induction or surgery. Measurement of the enzyme (low or undetectable), maternal urinary oestriol output (persistently low), or of DHEAS in amniotic fluid, or its 16α-hydroxylated form in the maternal serum (both elevated) may be useful.

Foetal monitoring

Rhesus incompatibility

When the mother has been shown to be Rh-isoimmunised, it is important to evaluate the extent of haemolytic disease and its effects on the fetus to identify the fetus severely affected by erythroblastosis, especially if there is a predisposition towards hydrops development *in utero*, and to be able to predict with considerable accuracy when this will occur. There is a reasonable chance for infant survival if delivery can be delayed to avoid the additional complications of prematurity. Testing involves:

1 Serological determination of Rh titres (usually only against Rh anti-D antibodies and performed either at Haematology Departments or Blood Transfusion Centres)

2 Examination of amniotic fluids (obtained at around 30 weeks of gestation) for presence of unacceptably high bilirubin levels is used to assess the risks involved. Amniocentesis is indicated at 20-21 weeks of gestation in an isoimmunised woman who has had a previous stillbirth or an infant requiring exchange transfusion. Serial amniocentesis are recommended for more accurate risk assessment. Normally very small amounts of bilirubin are detectable in the amniotic fluid. Haemolytic disorders such as Rhesus incompatibility produces a glut of bilirubin, the severity of haemolysis and/or erythroblastosis being reflected by the amniotic fluid bilirubin level.

Fetal lung immaturity

When the question of elective induction of birth in high-risk pregnancies arises, amniocentesis is usually performed to obtain an approximate estimate of fetal maturity, particularly fetal lung maturity. The risk of development of respiratory distress syndrome of the newborn has to be assessed against that of intrauterine death.

From 32 weeks of gestation onwards, the fetal lungs secrete a surface-active material which lowers the surface tension in the alveoli, making the lungs more expandable and preventing them from collapsing at birth. The surfactant, which contains primarily dipalmitoyl lecithin and sphingomyelin, drains from the fetal lungs into the amniotic fluid. During the last few weeks of pregnancy (from about 34 weeks onwards), the production of lecithin increases rapidly, and its concentration correlates well with fetal lung maturity. In contrast to that of lecithin, the amniotic fluid sphingomyelin concentration remains relatively unchanged over the same period, and thus provides a 'constant' denominator in the calculation of the lecithin/sphingomyelin (L/S) ratio in amniotic fluid.

L/S ratios above 2 are considered as acceptable risk to proceed with elective early termination of pregnancy; ratios of 1.8-2.0 are borderline and suboptimal; ratios <1.8 indicate fetal lung immaturity; those <1.5 are downright dangerous.

The original format of the test, using thin-layer chromatography, was fraught with potential errors

unless carried out under stringent quality control. Improved modifications have resulted in better accuracy in risk estimation. Fetal lung maturity can also be assessed by HPLC measurement of plasma lecithin, phosphatidyl glycerol or palmitate concentrations, all of which are superior to the L/S ratio.

Monitoring the fetus at birth

Hypoxia, as occurs during a difficult birth, results in anaerobic glycolysis in the fetus and the production of excessive quantities of lactic acid; thus a fall in blood pH. The most widely used biochemical test is blood pH, measured on samples collected from the fetal scalp (a not-too-difficult procedure in vaginal deliveries with head-first presentations). Blood pH values below 7.2 units are associated with severe fetal hypoxaemia. Another (and more direct) indicator of fetal oxygenation is fetal blood Po_2 which can be continuously monitored using a transcutaneous oxygen electrode, once the cervix is sufficiently dilated; it is also considered a less hazardous procedure.

Prenatal diagnosis of fetal defects

Chemical tests for prenatal diagnosis of fetal abnormalities are arbitrarily subdivided into those that are screening tests routinely performed on all pregnancies, and those which are only carried out in at-risk pregnancies. Some of these tests are non-invasive and their performance carry little or no risk to mother and fetus, e.g., maternal blood sampling or ultrasound scans. Others requiring amniocentesis or chorionic villus sampling are invasive and carries an inherent risk, and their performance is probably only justified in at-risk pregnancies. The prenatal diagnosis of inherited metabolic disorders (discussed on page 307), used to be high-risk procedures as they were mostly performed on amniotic fluids or chorionic villi samples; however, new techniques now make it possible to use DNA extracted from leucocytes or buccal cells in mouth washes. In this section we will confine discussion to the prenatal screening for neural tube defects and Down's syndrome (trisomy 21).

Neural tube defects

Alpha-fetoprotein (AFP) production by the fetal liver

begins from the sixth week of gestation onwards, and increases till about 16-18 weeks, after which it falls progressively at a rapid rate. If the fetus has an open neural tube defect, e.g., anencephaly, open spinal bifida, and ventral wall defects such as omphalacele and gastroschisis, significantly increased levels of AFP are found in the amniotic fluid.at 16 weeks' gestation (about 95% of cases). Concurrently, raised levels of AFP are also detectable in maternal serum in the majority (about 80%) of affected pregnancies (AFP readily crosses the placental barrier).

Although it will result in a higher incidence of false negatives, it is viable to use maternal serum AFP (msAFP) as a non-invasive *screening test* for open neural tube defects. This test should be carried out between 16 to 18 weeks of gestation (in many places it is carried out together with ultrasound scanning) with the aim of identifying those women who should be further investigated, if indicated by the msAFP and ultrasound findings, by the more risky amniocentesis procedure. If the diagnosis is confirmed before the 20th week, termination of pregnancy can be offered as an option (Figure 26.2). Women who have previously had an affected pregnancy carry a higher risk than others.

It is vital to appreciate that there is a considerable overlap between msAFP concentrations in normal pregnancies and in the affected pregnancies. In other words, the msAFP test can offer no more than a relative risk statistic in identifying the "high risk" group of women (all positive results must be repeated). Besides the need to beat the legal limit for approved abortions, the optimal time to perform the screening is at 16-18 weeks of gestation, as it provides the best discriminant between normality and abnormality. Calculation of the gestation age has to be very precise -- underestimation or overestimation will lead to erroneous interpretation of the msAFP result against an inappropriate gestational date, and increase the probability of misses.

As mentioned above, high msAFP levels could be found in certain rare non-neurological ventral wall defects; it is also found in multiple pregnancies. The latter should be easily detected by ultrasound examination.

If amniocentesis is carried out, measurements of both amniotic fluid AFP and acetylcholinesterase activity are recommended. The former test will identify over 95% of affected cases; false-positives may be obtained in blood-stained specimens or when ventral wall defects are present. The latter is a more specific test than msAFP for the diagnosis of neural tube defects. The acetylcholinesterase that leaks out

through an open neural tube defect is different from the non-specific cholinesterase that is normally present in amniotic fluid and in maternal serum. It can be identified by electrophoresis.

Down's syndrome

In clinical investigations, low msAFP levels have been associated with an increased risk for chromosomal abnormalities such as Down's syndrome. However, only about 20-25% of pregnancies with fetuses carrying the trisomy 21 abnormality are detected by msAFP testing. Maternal serum oestriol concentrations are also found to be lower, whilst maternal serum β-HCG levels are higher than in corresponding normal pregnancies. Studies indicate that using all three markers (Triple Test) and interpreting the results in relation to maternal age enhances the potential detection of Down's syndrome to 60-70%.

Down's syndrome is a common chromosomal disorder. As the risk for Down's syndrome increases with advancing maternal age, performing a midtrimester amniocentesis for karyotyping purposes (which identifies the chromosomal abnormality with almost 100% accuracy) for women aged 35 and above is an accepted medical practice in most centres. However, 50-70% of children with Down's syndrome are born to women under age 35, since this group represents a much greater proportion of the child-bearing population. The usefulness of the Triple test in screening for Down's syndrome in the under-35 group remains a viable option.

Since its promulgation by Cuckle *et al* (see reference on page 329), it has been claimed that the usefulness of the Triple test is maximised by the conversion of the AFP, HCG, and oestriol concentrations to multiples of the median (MOM). The observed value is divided by the established median value for normal pregnancies of the same gestational age in order to determine the MOM. The AFP MOM is then adjusted for several factors that are known to influence the value, including maternal weight, race and presence of insulin-dependant diabetes.

A patient-specific risk for Down's syndrome is calculated based on maternal age, the adjusted MOM for msAFP, and MOM values for maternal serum β-HCG and oestriol levels. If the Triple test discriminant analysis for Down's syndrome risk equals or exceeds the risk of a 35-year-old at 16-18 weeks of gestation (i.e., 1 in 270), amniocentesis is a recommended follow-up diagnostic procedure.

Laboratory evaluation of infertility

Childlessness is one of the commonest single complaints encountered by the gynaecologist in practice. Estimates suggest that some 10 per cent of all marriages are associated with infertility, with either or both partners being involved. For practical purposes, infertility is defined as the failure of a couple to achieve a pregnancy after at least a year of regular, unprotected sexual relations. The problem must be approached considering both male and female aspects.

Causes of infertility in either the male or the female partner are many and varied. They could have a genetic or congenital basis (absence of vital reproductive organs), arise from a previous insult or injury (infections, illnesses, venereal disease) or treatment (irradiation, previous vasectomy, abortions, pelvic surgery), derived from structural anomalies (cryptorchidism, tubal blocks), or associated with endocrinopathies (prolonged use of oral contraceptives, hypopituitarism, hypothalamic disorders, late-onset congenital adrenal hyperplasia, etc).

Many strategies have been devised for the investigation of the infertile couple -- all with the aim of reaching the specific diagnosis within the shortest time, at minimum cost, and with the least inconvenience to the patient. The basic tenets of all strategies remain the same -- an initial clinical investigation followed by laboratory evaluation of both partners.

The initial clinical investigation involves a carefully taken clinical history and a thorough physical examination of both partners. The findings of the clinical investigation will determine the selection of the first-line laboratory tests.

In turn, the results from the initial first-line tests will help define the second-line investigations. The range of diagnostic investigations is very wide, and some are listed in Tables 26.1 and 26.2. The second-line laboratory investigations should be restricted to tests that either confirm or clarify an endocrine basis to infertility or monitor the response to treatment.

It is beyond the scope of our brief treatment of the subject to discuss the different types of tests available for infertility testing; in the following section we focus only on the role of the diagnostic biochemistry laboratory (more specifically, the endocrine laboratory) in the investigation of the infertile couple.

The female partner. A laboratory approach to female infertility is laid out in Figure 26.3.

Table 26.1. Diagnostic tests used in the evaluation of the infertile man.

Semen analysis
Antisperm antibody tests (performed on serum/semen)
Cultures:
    Ureaplasma, Chlamydia, Neisseria gonorrhoeae
Hormonal evaluation:
    Gonadotrophins, prolactin, testosterone
Sperm penetration test
Bovine cervical mucus penetration test
Hypo-osmotic swelling test
Hemizona assay

Table 26.2. Diagnostic tests used in the evaluation of the infertile woman.

Documentation of ovulation
    Charting of basal body temperature
    Determination of the midcycle LH surge
    Ultrasound documentation of follicle development
    and of ovulation
    Estimation of luteal phase (day 21) progesterone
Postcoital test
Luteal phase assessment
    Serum progesterone
    Endometrial biopsy
Hysterosalpingogram
Laparoscopy and hysteroscopy
Hormonal assessment
    Gonadotrophins, prolactin, oestrogens,
    progesterone (see above)
    Investigation of hypercortisolaemia
    Investigation of thyroid disease
Cervical cultures
    Chlamydia, Ureaplasma, Neisseria gonorrhoeae
Sperm antibodies in the cervical mucus and in serum

■ In women with amenorrhoea, anovulation is a foregone conclusion. The investigation of these women should be along the same lines as outlined above to find the cause of anovulation and infertility. A pregnancy test should be performed first to exclude pregnancy as a cause of the amenorrhoea before the other hormone tests.

■ In the investigation of subjects with primary amenorrhoea, a karyotyping may be helpful in diagnosis, if primary ovarian failure is indicated by the clinical investigation and the plasma FSH, LH and oestrogen levels.

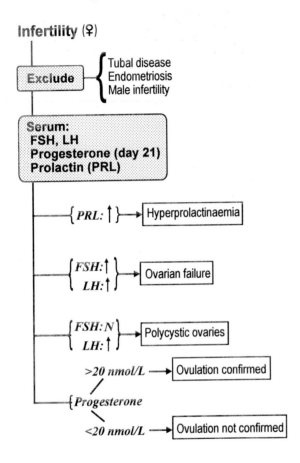

Figure 26.3. Suggested scheme for the evaluation of female infertility.

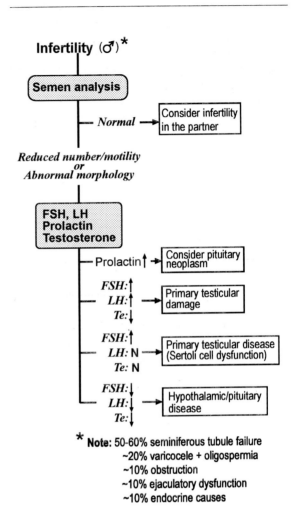

Figure 26.4. Suggested scheme for the evaluation of male infertility.

The male partner. In the laboratory investigation of the male partner (Figure 26.4), the first test should be semen analysis. If the results are normal, no further investigations are required; if abnormal, the serum levels of testosterone, prolactin and gonadotropins should be measured to determine if there is an endocrine problem.

Hyperprolactinaemia is an important cause of infertility in both men and women. Clinically significant hyperprolactinaemia is unlikely unless the serum prolactin concentration is, on two consecutive occasions, more than 1½ times the upper limit of the reference interval (UL) quoted by the issuing laboratory. An initial finding of hyperprolactinaemia should always be confirmed on a repeat specimen taken without stress to the patient. The clinical history should be re-examined and common causes such as pregnancy, lactation, drug-induced hyperprolactinaemia, primary hypothyroidsm, and renal insufficiency should be excluded.

328

The diagnosis of either prolactinoma or other hypothalamic or pituitary disorders causing hyper-prolactinaemia (page 000) requires radiological scans to be performed. Abnormal pituitary radiological findings coupled with a much elevated serum prolactin concentration (>8xUL) suggest a prolactinoma. Non-prolactin secreting tumours (abnormal radiology) are associated with more modest hyperprolactinaemia.

REFERENCES AND FURTHER READING

Butt WR, Blunt SM. The role of the laboratory in the investigation of infertility. Ann Clin Biochem 1988;25:601-9.

Chard T, Mackintosh MCM. Biochemical screening for Down's syndrome. *Progress in Obstetrics and Gynaecology, Vol 11,* pp 39-52, Edinburgh: Churchill Livingston, 1994.

Cuckle HS, Wald NJ, Thompson SG. Estimating a woman's risk of having a pregnancy associated with Down's syndrome using her age and serum alpha-fetoprotein. Br J Obstet Gynae 1987;94:387-402.

Freinkel N, Metzger BE. Metabolic changes in pregnancy. In: Wilson JD, Foster DW (eds). *Williams' Textbook of Endocrinology, 8th edition.* Philadelphia: WB Saunders Company, 1988.

Special report: Maternal serum alpha-fetoprotein screening for neural tube defects: results of a consensus meeting. Prenat Diag 1985;5:77-81.

Swerdloff RS, Wang C, Kandeel FR. Evaluation of the infertile couple. Endocrinol Metab Clinics North Am 1988;17:301-337.

White I, Paphia SS, Magnay D. Improving methods of screening for Down's syndrome. New Engl J Med 1989;320:401-2.

Chapter 27

Paediatric Chemical Pathology

The chemical pathology of the neonate, infant, and child differs from that of the adult in three main areas:

1. Most of the inherited metabolic disorders usually manifest themselves during this period (page 297).

2. Functional immaturity of organs such as the liver and kidney may produce abnormalities peculiar to the neonatal period.

3. The reference intervals of many analytes are age-related.

In this chapter we will deal briefly with the latter two aspects; inherited metabolic disorders are discussed in Chapter 24. A number of age-related reference intervals are quoted, but these are used to illustrate the variations that can be expected and should not be used for diagnostic purposes as reference intervals determined in individual laboratories can differ markedly.

Renal function and electrolytes

At birth the kidney contains the same number of nephrons as it will in later life; the difference is that in the neonate the glomeruli and tubules are immature and this results in some functional differences. However, by the age of two years, all of the kidney functions should be adult-like.

GLOMERULAR FILTRATION RATE (GFR)

The GFR, standardised to the adult surface area of 1.73 m², is low at birth due to immature glomeruli and low renal blood flow (during intrauterine life the placenta receives blood at the expense of the kidneys). There is a rapid increase in the GFR during the first two weeks of life and adult levels are reached at the age of two to three years. The approximate age-related values, adjusted for a surface area of 1.73 m², are:

Birth	0.5-1.0 mL/s
6-12 months	0.8-2.5 mL/s
2-9 years	1.5-2.5 mL/s
Adult	1.5-2.0 mL/s

PLASMA UREA

At birth, during infancy, and during childhood the plasma urea level is significantly less than that of the adult.

Neonate	1.0-2.0 mmol/L
<2 years	1.5-2.0 mmol/L
2-9 years	2.0-5.0 mmol/L
Adult	2.5-7.5 mmol/L

These low levels reflect the avid utilisation of amino acids (nitrogen) to satisfy the protein synthesis necessary for growth. Increased plasma urea levels reflect a decreased GFR, as in prerenal uraemia (dehydration), renal uraemia (renal failure), and postrenal uraemia (obstructive uropathy). However, the plasma urea level is a poor indicator for dehydration because decreased urea production, as may occur with the relative starvation associated with vomiting and diarrhoea, may result in a normal or decreased plasma concentration in the presence of a significantly decreased GFR.

PLASMA CREATININE

Plasma creatinine levels are high at birth, due to contributions across the placenta from the mother and due to a low GFR, but then fall rapidly. During infancy, childhood, and the adolescent period, the values are much lower than those of the adult because of the small muscle mass.

Birth	0.07-0.08 mmol/L
7-days	0.04-0.06 mmol/L
12-months	0.02-0.04 mmol/L
5-years	0.03-0.05 mmol/L
12-years	0.04-0.07 mmol/L
Adult	0.06-0.12 mmol/L

A raised plasma creatinine can reflect:

Decreased GFR: prerenal, renal, and postrenal uraemia.

Ketoacidosis: positive interference with creatinine estimation (Jaffé reaction) by acetoacetate.

Cephalosporin therapy: positive interference with the Jaffé reaction during analysis.

RENAL CONCENTRATING/DILUTING MECHANISMS

At 2 to 3 years of age the infant has the same concentrating ability as the adult, but during the neonatal period the infant can only concentrate the urine to an osmolality of around 600 to 700 mmol/kg. This is due to two factors that reduce the efficiency of the countercurrent mechanism (page 5):

1. *Immaturity of the kidney.* The infantile kidney has a large number of short loops of Henle which do not penetrate deeply into the renal medulla (area of high interstitial tonicity).

2. *Decreased urea production.* A high interstitial urea concentration is necessary for maintenance of the medullary concentraton gradient. On the other hand, infants fed on a high protein diet can increase their concentrating ability to produce urinary osmolalities of around 1000 mmol/kg.

The kidney's ability to dilute urine is well developed at birth, for example, premature infants can dilute their urine to osmolalities as low as 25 mmol/kg. The causes of polyuria and their evaluation are discussed on pages 20-22.

SODIUM HOMEOSTASIS

Proximal tubular sodium reabsorption is inefficient in the neonate because these tubules are relatively shorter than those of adults. However, this disability is balanced by the low GFR in infants and the fractional excretion is maintained at around 1% (page 7). In premature infants of less than 32 weeks gestation, the urinary fractional excretion of sodium is near 5% and hence renal sodium loss can be a problem.

The plasma sodium concentration and plasma osmolality in neonates, infants, and children are similar to adult values (132-144 mmol/L and 270-285 mmol/kg, respectively). The causes of hypernatraemia and hyponatraemia in the child are largely similar to those in the adults, but certain causes are more common in this age group.

Hypernatraemia. This implies a water deficit relative to solute throughout the body. There may be too little water (hypertonic dehydration) or excess solute with normal, or increased, water (salt gain).

Note: Hypernatraemia usually infers an inadequate water intake (page 16).

Hypertonic dehydration. Water depletion greater than salt depletion may occur in:

(a) Decreased water intake in the face of normal losses, e.g., too young or too sick to drink, access to water denied.
(b) Decreased intake in the face of excessive loss of hypotonic fluids (page 17) as occurs in vomiting, diarrhoea and such like.

Salt gain. This may be due to inappropriate IV therapy (with hypertonic solutions), inappropriate feeding (too much salt in foods), sea water ingestion (page 11).

Hyponatraemia. This condition indicates that the extracellular water is relatively greater than the extracellular sodium content (page 18). It may be dilutional where the extracellular volume is increased, or associated with salt and water loss (depletional, hyponatraemic dehydration).

Note: Hyponatraemia, with the exception of pseudohyponatraemia, usually infers inadequate renal water excretion and a positive water balance (page 18).

Dilutional hyponatraemia. Characterised by an absence of clinical or biochemical evidence of dehydration (i.e., with normal serum urea and creatinine, etc), this condition may be due to SIADH (page 14), drug therapy (page 15), and inappropriate infusion of hypotonic fluids.

Hypotonic dehydration. In this situation there has been salt and water depletion (e.g., loss of hypotonic fluids) followed by administration of salt-poor fluids (tap water, 5% glucose). Such may occur in vomiting, diarrhoea, diuretic therapy, and so on. The characteristic feature is clinical evidence of dehydration including such biochemical parameters as high serum urea and creatinine values. The serum urea level, however, may be normal or even low if there is inadequate protein intake (starvation), as can occur in the sick child.

331

POTASSIUM HOMEOSTASIS

Potassium homeostasis in the paediatric age group is similar to that in adults (page 25). The newborn usually has slightly higher (compared to the adult) plasma potassium concentrations (3.5-5.8 mmol/L), presumably due to the hypoxia and acidaemia sustained during birth (or the trauma of blood sampling using the heel prick technique).

Hyperkalaemia. In neonates and infants the commonest causes of hyperkalaemia are pseudohyperkalaemia (haemolysis, heel prick) and inappropriate IV therapy. Less common causes are renal failure, diabetic ketoacidosis, and congenital adrenal hyperplasia.

Hypokalaemia. Potassuim depletion with hypokalaemia may be due to inappropriate IV therapy, prolonged vomiting (pyloric stenosis), severe diarrhoea (commonest cause), renal tubular acidosis, Bartter's syndrome, and diuretic therapy (page 82).

ACID-BASE HOMEOSTASIS

The newborn is often in a state of moderate metabolic acidosis and this can be very pronounced in the premature infant, with serum HCO_3^- levels ranging from 18 to 22 mmol/L. This mild acidosis is due to:

1   A low renal threshold for bicarbonate due to immaturity of the proximal renal tubule (RTA type 2, page 82). In premature infants it is around 18 mmol/L, in the full term infant around 21 mmol/L, and about 23 mmol/L at one year of age.

2   Inability of the immature kidney to excrete a large acid load. The premature infant is unable to lower the urinary pH to less than 6 units; normal values (<5.5) are not realised until after the first month of extrauterine life.

Respiratory acid-base disturbances. These are discussed in the Acid-base Chapter. An important point to recall is that hyperventilation and consequently respiratory alkalosis is associated with a low plasma bicarbonate level and that unless a blood gas evaluation is performed, this may be confused with a hyperchloraemic metabolic acidosis.

Metabolic acidosis. In the neonate and infant a metabolic acidosis is often the first indicator of a serious underlying disorder. From a diagnostic point of view the metabolic acidoses are conveniently divided into high anion gap and normal anion gap (hyperchloraemic) types.

High anion gap metabolic acidosis. This is associated with (1) lactic acidosis (page 140), (2) ketoacidosis (page 136), (3) renal failure, (4) toxin-induced.

Normal anion gap (hyperchloraemic) metabolic acidosis. This group is conveniently divided into the hyperkalaemic and hypokalaemic varieties.

Hyperkalaemic: This type is unusual in infants and usually indicates the adrenogenital syndrome due to 21β-hydroxylase deficiency. The rare 3β-hydroxysteroid dehydrogenase deficiency will also present in a similar manner.

Hypokalaemic: The commonest cause of this variety, and indeed a common cause of metabolic acidosis in children, is *diarrhoea* (loss of bicarbonate and potassium in diarrhoea fluid). Depending on the nutritional (starvation) and volume (poor tissue perfusion) status of the patient, there may also be an underlying ketoacidosis or lactic acidosis. Other possible though infrequent causes of hypokalaemic, normal anion gap metabolic acidosis in children are *renal tubular acidosis* (page 81) and *an imperforated anus*.

Metabolic alkalosis. Severe metabolic alkalosis, except that due to vomiting in pyloric stenosis, is not a common problem in the neonate and infant. The causes and pathogenesis are discussed in Chapter 3; of interest to the paediatrician are congenital chloride diarrhoea and the mineralocorticoid excess syndromes.

Congenital chloride diarrhoea. Severe diarrhoea is usually associated with metabolic acidosis due to intestinal bicarbonate loss (page 218); however, one condition, chloride diarrhoea (so called because of massive amounts of chloride in the diarrhoea fluid), is associated with a metabolic alkalosis. This condition is due to a rare inborn error of intestinal chloride absorption. Sodium and chloride ions are absorbed in the small intestine by a complex exchange process involving hydrogen and bicarbonate ions:

In the absorptive cell hydrogen ions, derived from carbonic acid, are normally secreted in exchange for luminal sodium ions and bicarbonate ions (also derived from carbonic acid) are exchanged for luminal chloride ions. In the lumen the hydrogen and bicarbonate ions combine to form carbonic acid which is converted to carbon dioxide. This carbon dioxide diffuses into the absorptive cell, produces carbonic acid, and thus the whole process is repeated.

In chloride diarrhoea there is defective chloride-bicarbonate exchange but hydrogen-sodium ion exchange proceeds normally; thus chloride remains in the lumen causing an osmotic diarrhoea (page 218) and the cell-generated bicarbonate results in metabolic alkalosis.

Mineralocorticoid excess syndromes. Two mineralocorticoid excess syndromes may occur in infancy and produce a metabolic alkalosis: *Bartter's syndrome* (page 82) and the adrenogenital syndrome due to *11β-hydroxylase deficiency* (page 250).

CALCIUM HOMEOSTASIS

During intrauterine life, the fetus derives its calcium supplies from the placental circulation and the function of the fetal parathyroid glands is of minimal importance. At birth, the supply of maternal calcium is lost and the continual accumulation of calcium in bone associated with immature parathyroid function usually results in hypocalcaemia, with plasma levels falling as low as 1.70 mmol/L. However, the parathyroid glands begin activity at around 48 hours into extrauterine life and by 72 hours the neonate's plasma calcium rises to adult levels (2.15-2.55 mmol/L). The parathyroid response may be delayed in premature and low birth-weight infants, resulting in severe and prolonged hypocalcaemia.

Hypocalcaemia. Neonatal hypocalcaemia may be due to:

- Transient neonatal hypocalcaemia (exaggeration of physiological drop)
- Hypoparathyroidism
- Pseudohypoparathyroidism (page 98)
- Magnesium deficiency
- Inappropriate IV therapy
- Vitamin D deficiency/rickets

In infants and children hypocalcaemia is uncommon but the causes are essentially the same as for adults.

Hypercalcaemia. In the paediatric age group hypercalcaemia is less common than hypocalcaemia but may be due to:

- Infantile idiopathic hypercalcaemia (William's syndrome)
- Familial benign hypercalcaemia (familial hypocalciuric hypocalcaemia, FHH)
- Hyperparathyroidism
- Prolonged immobilisation
- Malignancy
- Vitamin D excess

PHOSPHATE

The plasma phosphate level is high in the newborn and falls throughout childhood and adolescence to reach adult values by the age of 15 to 18 years.

Neonates	1.2-2.8 mmol/L
<7-years	1.3-1.8 mmol/L
>15-years	0.6-1.2 mmol/L

These high values (relative to adult values) are due to renal retention secondary to excessive growth hormone activity.

Hyperphosphataemia usually indicates renal failure or hypoparathyroidism. Infants fed cow's milk may develop a high serum phosphate (high intake) and this may be associated with hypocalcaemia.

Hypophosphataemia. The causes of hypo-phosphataemia in paediatric patients are the same as those for adults, with the commoner causes being low intake (IV therapy), Fanconi syndrome (page 80), familial hypophosphataemia (vitamin D resistant rickets), vitamin D deficiency (secondary hyper-parathyroidism). Phosphate metabolism and its abnormalities are discussed in Chapter 7.

MAGNESIUM

The plasma magnesium values at birth and throughout childhood (0.50-1.00 mmol/L) are slightly lower than those of adults (0.70-1.00 mmol/L). Adult values are reached by 2 to 6 years of age. Hypomagnesaemia is uncommon but may occur in the malabsorption syndromes and in the uncommon specific gut-transport defect. Hypermagnesaemia occurs in severe renal insufficiency and in milder degrees of renal impairment if there is an increased intake.

GLUCOSE HOMEOSTASIS

During fasting, adults can maintain their plasma glucose level between 3.0-5.5 mmol/L for long periods of starvation. On the other hand, children tolerate fasting poorly and the plasma glucose level may fall to below 2.0 mmol/L within 24 hours. This inadequate response, particularly in the neonate, is due mainly to defective glucose production as a consequence of:

1   *Low glycogen stores:* glycogen is laid down over the last 3-4 weeks of intrauterine life and the reserves in the neonate are depleted after 12-18 hours of fasting.

2   *Blunted glycogenolysis:* enzyme immaturity results in inefficient mobilisation of glycogen in the newborn.

3   *Blunted gluconeogenesis:* full activity of the gluconeogenic enzymes is not realised until several days into extrauterine life.

Although hyperglycaemia and diabetes mellitus occur in the paediatric period they are not as common or clinically important as hypoglycaemia, which will be considered in some detail.

Hypoglycaemia

A useful working definition of hypoglycaemia is a plasma glucose level less than 2.0 mmol/L; values greater than 2.5 mmol/L exclude the diagnosis. The symptoms include convulsions, coma, pallor, sweating, hunger, confusion, weakness, bizarre behaviour, irritability, and abdominal pain. In young children convulsions are common whilst in older children symptoms are often vague and non-specific.

CAUSES/PATHOPHYSIOLOGY

There are numerous causes of hypoglycaemia and many classifications have been proposed. The classification used in Table 27.1. is based on age and plasma insulin levels.

Small for gestational dates infants. About 40-50% of newborns, with weights less than the 10th percentile for gestational age, develop transient hypoglycaemia. The delayed growth is often related to placental insufficiency and the hypoglycaemia probably reflects inefficient gluconeogenesis coupled with low liver glycogen reserves.

Transient neonatal hyperinsulinism. This usually occurs in the *infant of a diabetic mother*. These infants have hyperinsulinism due to β-cell hyperplasia, decreased glucagon secretion, and delayed development of the gluconeogenic hormones; all resulting from the sustained maternal hyperglycaemia. Two unusual causes of transient hyperinsulinism due to β-cell hyperplasia are *erythroblastosis foetalis* and the *Beckwith-Widemann syndrome*. The latter is characterised by macroglossia, visceromegaly, exomphalos, and giantism; the hypoglycaemia is usually transient but in some case can be prolonged and severe.

Nesidioblastosis. In this condition there is abnormal differentiation of the β-cells of the pancreas with increased numbers of endocrine cells which appear to arise by budding from the exocrine pancreatic ducts. There is also a decrease in the number of somatostatin cells. The resulting hyper-insulinism can be severe and cause hypoglycaemia which can be difficult to manage.

Leucine sensitivity. Leucine is a potent insulin secretagogue and some infants respond to oral administration (or high protein diets) by developing

Table 27.1. Causes of hypoglycaemia in the paediatric group.

Neonatal

Transient:

↓ Insulin:
1. small for dates babe
2. sepsis/asphyxia/cerebral haemorrhage

↑ Insulin:
1. diabetic mother
2. erythroblastosis foetalis
3. Beckwith-Widemann syndrome

Persistent:

↓ Insulin:
1. enzyme defects (see Table 27.2.)
2. hormone deficiencies: growth hormone, thyroxine, cortisol, glucagon

↑ Insulin:
1. nesidioblastosis
2. islet cell adenoma
3. leucine sensitivity
4. Beckwith-Widemann syndrome

Infancy (first year of life)

As for neonatal persistent

Childhood

↓ Insulin:
1. ketotic hypoglycaemia (accelerated starvation)
2. enzyme defects (see Table 27.2.)
3. hormone deficiencies: thyroxine, growth hormone, cortisol, glucagon
4. Reye's syndrome
5. salicylate overdose
6. ethanol intoxication
7. non-pancreatic tumours (large)

↑ Insulin:
1. islet cell adenoma/hyperplasia
2. exogenous insulin
3. oral hypoglycaemics

hypoglycaemia. The hyperinsulinism in these cases reflects an abnormal β-cell response (due to β-cell hyperplasia or nesidioblastosis) and does not imply a specific aetiology or disease.

Enzyme defects. Although a large number of enzyme deficiencies are associated with hypoglycaemia, their occurrence in practice is rare (Table 27.2). In addition to hypoglycaemia, they are usually associated with moderate to severe metabolic acidosis (lactic acid, ketones, other organic acids). Hyperammonaemia and the presence of non-glucose reducing substances in the urine are also clues to the diagnosis.

Disorders of glycogen metabolism. Hypoglycaemia is usually associated with deficiencies of *glycogen synthetase* and *glucose 6-phosphatase* (Type 1 glycogen storage disease) and, less often, with deficiencies of the *debrancher enzyme* (Type III glycogen storage disease) and liver *glycogen phosphorylase* (Type VI glycogen storage disease). Ketosis is a feature of all of these deficiencies and lactic acidosis is associated with glucose 6-phosphatase deficiency.

Disorders of gluconeogenesis. For gluconeogenesis to proceed it is necessary to have, in addition to the enzymes of glycolysis, four specific enzymes: *pyruvate carboxylase, phosphoenolpyruvate carboxykinase, fructose 1,6-bisphosphatase, and glucose 6-phosphatase.* Deficiency of any of these four enzymes will result in hypoglycaemia, ketosis, and lactic acidosis.

Galactosaemia. This is due to a deficiency of the enzyme *UDP-glucose galactose-1-phosphate uridyl transferase* which results in the accumulation of galactose-1-phosphate after the ingestion of galactose (milk); hypoglycaemia and galactosuria (reducing substance in the urine) also occur. The cause of the hypoglycaemia is uncertain but appears to be due to inhibition of glycogenolysis by galactose-1-phosphate.

Hereditary fructose intolerance. Deficiency of the enzyme *fructose 1,6-bisphosphate aldolase* results in the accumulation of fructose-1-phosphate after ingestion of fructose (fruits, sucrose). The associated hypoglycaemia is probably due to inhibition of glycogenolysis by fructose-1-phosphate. The reducing sugar, fructose, appears in the urine.

Amino acids. Maple syrup disease is due to deficiency of *branched-chain ketoacid decarboxylase* which converts the branched-chain ketoacids to their CoA-derivatives (the ketoacids are derived from transamination of L-leucine, L-isoleucine, and L-

335

valine). Hypoglycaemia, ketosis, lactic acidosis, and hypoalaninaemia may be associated with a high dietary input of branched-chain amino acids or during catabolic illness. The nature of the hypoglycaemia is unclear.

Fatty acids. Several disorders of fatty acid oxidation have been described which are associated with hypoglycaemia. In addition to hypoglycaemia the features include an absence of ketosis, organic aciduria, hyperammonaemia.

Organic acidurias. The organic acidurias are a group of inborn errors of metabolism in which there is accumulation of non-amino organic acids (carboxylic acids) in the tissues and body fluids including the urine. The metabolic pathways involved include those of L- leucine and other branched amino acids, L-lysine and aromatic amino acids, fatty acid oxidation, ketogenesis, pyruvate and carbohydrate metabolism including the TCA cycle.

Table 27.2. Enzyme defects associated with hypoglycaemia.

Carbohydrate
Glycogen: glycogen synthetase, glucose 6-phosphatase debrancher enzyme, liver glycogen phosphorylase
Gluconeogenesis: pyruvate carboxylase, phosphoenol-pyruvate carboxykinase, fructose bisphosphatase, glucose 6-phosphatase
Others: fructose 1,6-bisphosphate aldolase, UDP-glucose galactose-1-phosphate uridyl transferase

Amino acids
branched chain ketoacid dehydrogenase (maple syrup disease)

Fatty acids
carnitine palmityltransferase, acyl-CoA (medium, short & long chain) dehydrogenase, HMG-CoA lyase, carnitine deficiency

Organic acidurias
propionic aciduria, methylmalonic aciduria

Clinically they present acutely in early life with vomiting, convulsions, coma, metabolic acidosis, and ketosis. The biochemical features, in addition to organic aciduria, may include hypoglycaemia, lactic acidosis, ketosis, and hyperammonaemia. The incidence is around 1:3000 live births and diagnosis, in the first instance, is based on the finding of organic acids in the urine (gas chromotography, mass spectroscopy).

Hormone deficiencies. Deficiency of cortisol, growth hormone, and glucagon may be complicated by hypoglycaemia. As intermediary metabolism is intact ketosis, along with appropriate low plasma levels of insulin, is a feature of these disorders. The plasma levels of growth hormone and cortisol should be determined in all cases of ketotic hypoglycaemia but often equivocal results are obtained and the definitive diagnosis can only be made on the basis of stimulation tests, e.g., Synacthen stimulation for cortisol and an exercise test for growth hormone.

Idiopathic ketotic hypoglycaemia. Ketotic hypo-glycaemia occurs in several conditions (see above) but there is a group of children in whom there is no apparent cause. These patients are usually between the ages of 18 months and 7 years and present with ketotic hypoglycaemia during an infection or a period of starvation. The biochemical features include hypogly-caemia, ketosis, low plasma alanine and insulin levels. Plasma lactate levels are usually normal and there is no evidence of endocrine malfunction. Infusion of alanine in these subjects results in a rise in the blood glucose level which suggests (a) gluconeogenesis is intact, and (b) there is some defect in the mobilisation of amino acids by muscle.

The hypoglycaemia may be precipitated by giving a ketotic diet (high fat, hypocaloric) or by starvation (hypoglycaemia occurs within 8-18 hours). This disorder, which is the commonest reported cause of hypoglycaemia in children, probably represents an "accelerated" starvation response. It usually remits spontaneously by the age of 8-9 years.

Reye's syndrome. This condition, which occurs in the 2-7 years age group, appears to be due to some insult to the mitochondria (disordered and swollen mitochondria can be demonstrated by electron microscopy). It usually presents with vomiting, encephalopathy, apnoea, and flaccidity following a mild upper respiratory tract infection (e.g., influenza).

The biochemical features include hypoglycaemia, hyperammonaemia, and increased plasma levels of aminotransferases, free fatty acids, lactate, glutamine, and alanine. Low activities of pyruvate carboxylase, carbamoyl phosphate synthetase, and ornithine carbamoyl transferase have been demonstrated in liver biopsy specimens, indicating defective gluconeogenesis and urea synthesis.

Drugs. Several drugs may cause hypoglycaemia:

- *Insulin and oral hypoglycaemics:* May be due to accidental overdose or malicious administration by parents.

- *Analgesics:* Salicylate and acetaminophen administration have been associated with hypoglycaemia and ketosis in young children. The pathogenesis is unclear.

- *Alcohol:* The administration of ethanol to young infants may be associated with severe hypoglycaemia. The low plasma glucose level is due to defective hepatic gluconeogenesis, possibly a consequence of the high NADH/NAD$^+$ ratio which accompanies ethanol metabolism (page 139).

Laboratory investigation (Figure 27.1)

The direction of investigation depends on the age of the patient, the clinical picture, and a high index of clinical suspicion. At the time of the hypoglycaemia blood should be collected for the estimation of plasma glucose, lactate, ketones, amino acids, insulin, cortisol, and growth hormone.

Plasma

Glucose: Low values confirm hypoglycaemia, e.g. <2.0 mmol/L.
Lactate: increased in defects of the gluconeogenic pathway.
Ketones: indicate activation of lipolysis; increased in hypoinsulin disorders except disorders of fatty acid oxidation; no increase in hyperinsulinism (hypoglycaemia without ketosis suggests hyperinsulinism).

Carnitine: decreased in disorders of fatty acid oxidation.
Ammonia: increased in Reye's syndrome and some of the organic acidaemias.

Urine

Ketones: as for plasma ketones.
Reducing sugars: galactose in galactosaemia, *fructose* in hereditary fructose intolerance.
Organic acids: occur in organic acidaemias and defects of fatty acid oxidation (dicarboxylic acids in acyl-CoA dehydrogenase deficiency), maple syrup disease (branched chain ketoacids)

Hormone studies

Plasma insulin: normally 6-8 mU/L after an overnight fast, levels equal to or greater than this in the presence of hypoglycaemia indicates inappropriate insulin secretion.
Cortisol, growth hormone, thyroxine/TSH: estimate if suspect a hormone deficiency, generally requires a dynamic function test.

Enzyme analysis. The definitive diagnosis of enzyme deficiencies may require enzyme assays on a liver biopsy or on cultured fibroblasts.

LIVER FUNCTON

The plasma total bilirubin concentration of the newborn can vary from 40 μmol/L to over 200 μmol/L without any apparent cause. This disorder, due to unconjugated hyperbilirubinaemia, is termed physiological jaundice and may reflect one or all of the following.

- Immaturity of the hepatocyte and its enzymes
- Overproduction of bilirubin because of a shortened life-span of the erythrocytes
- Reabsorption of unconjugated bilirubin from the gut. The neonate's intestine contains β-glucuronidase which deconjugates bilirubin; if the gut bacteria which convert bilirubin to urobilinogens are absent then some of the unconjugated bilirubin, which is readily absorbed, will be returned to the blood.

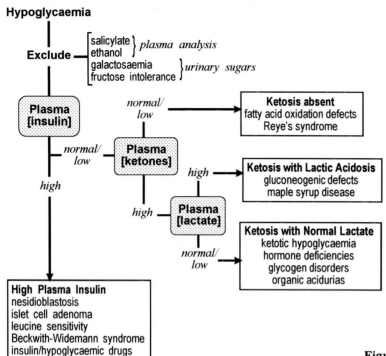

Figure 27.1. Suggested scheme for the evaluation of hypoglycaemia.

Unconjugated bilirubin is lipid-soluble and can cross the blood-brain barrier causing brain damage (kernicterus). However, the plasma albumin can bind up to 340 μmol/L of unconjugated bilirubin and thus prevent it passing across the blood-brain barrier. If the plasma level is in excess of this figure, or if the plasma albumin is low, or if drugs such as sulphonamides or aspirin which compete with bilirubin for albumin-binding sites are present, then kernicterus may occur. Such should be treated by exchange transfusions or by the application of ultraviolet light to the baby which degrades the circulating bilirubin.

Neonatal hyperbilirubinaemia

CAUSES

Some of the commoner causes of hyperbilirubinaemia are listed below. The reader is referred to the review by Fitzgerald J.F. (listed on page 343) for further information.

Unconjugated bilirubin
physiological
breast milk jaundice
haemolytic anaemia (Rh incompatibility)
hypothyroidism
inborn errors of metabolism: Gilbert's disease,
    Crigler-Najjar syndrome

Conjugated bilirubin
inborn errors of metabolism: Dubin-Johnson
    syndrome, Rotor syndrome
'neonatal hepatitis': rubella, toxoplasma,
    cytomegalovirus, herpes, hepatitis B
metabolic: galactosaemia, hereditary fructose
    intolerance, tyrosinaemia,
    α_1-antitrypsin deficiency (page 166)
lipoidoses: Niemann-Pick disease, Gaucher's disease
biliary atresia

Physiological jaundice. Jaundice, due to increased bilirubin production and immaturity of the excretory

338

system (see above), occurs in 60% of full term infants and up to 80% of preterm infants. In full term infants the serum bilirubin level peaks at around 110 μmol/L in two to four days and returns to normal in one to two weeks. In preterm infants the peak occurs in 5 to 7 days with levels reaching up to 220 μmol/L; normality is reached in a month or two. Serum bilirubin in excess of the above figures may occur and require treatment (e.g., exposure to UV light).

Breast milk jaundice. Some 2-4% of full-term, healthy, breast-fed infants develop an unconjugated hyperbilirubinaemia (levels up to 170 μmol/L) during the third week of life. This is rare in infants fed cow's milk and other artificial milks. The cause is unclear but suggested aetiologies include: (a) pregnanediol, a metabolite of progesterone which inhibits glucuronyl transferase *in vitro*, (b) free fatty acids -- found in high concentrations in breast milk of mothers of affected babies and will inhibit glucuronyl transferase *in vitro* (most likely cause), (c) increased enterohepatic circulation of bilirubin. Whatever the cause, the condition is generally harmless.

Hypothyroidism. Protracted neonatal jaundice is a feature of congenital hypothyroidism. It is thought to be due to impaired synthesis of the bilirubin conjugation enzymes.

Neonatal hepatitis. This is a non-specific term inferring inflammation of the liver, associated with patent bile ducts, occurring in the newborn period. It may be due to infective agents such as hepatitis B or to metabolic disease such as galactosaemia.

Biliary atresia. In this disorder the extrahepatic bile ducts are replaced by a fibrous cord. The consequence is progressive obstructive jaundice (cholestasis) resulting in parenchymal damage, and eventually cirrhosis and liver failure, if not treated by bypassing the obstruction (an artificial bile duct is constructed from a loop of jejunum). Characteristically these patients are initially well and then slowly develop jaundice over the next one, two, or three weeks. Hepatocellular damage is reflected in raised plasma transaminase values (usually less than 5-times normal). The main diagnostic problem is differentiation from neonatal hepatitis. The plasma levels of

transaminases, γ-glutamyltransferase, and 5-nucleotidase (see above) can be helpful. Inspection of the stools is a useful diagnostic test (if there is complete biliary obstruction the stools are a pale white colour, in hepatocellular disease at least some bile appears in the gut and the stool colour is a normal brown).

LABORATORY INVESTIGATION

The routine liver function tests are not able to indicate a specific diagnosis but do provide evidence of liver dysfunction and are useful in following the progress of the disease. In certain cases specific tests, such as α_1-antitrypsin assays, will provide a definitive diagnosis but these are rare and the final diagnosis in difficult cases often relies on such laboratory investigations as virology and liver biopsy.

Routine liver function tests. These should include plasma bilirubin (fractions), transaminases (ALT or AST), alkaline phosphatase, γ-glutamyltransferase (or 5-nucleotidase). As mentioned above, the main use of these tests is to determine the presence of liver disease and to follow its progress. In terms of diagnosis the most that can be gained from these tests is the differentiation of hepatocellular disease (e.g., hepatitis) from obstructive or cholestatic disease (e.g., biliary atresia); however, this may not always be clear-cut and overlap between the two disorders often occurs.

Plasma bilirubin: The causes of conjugated and unconjugated hyperbilirubinaemia are listed above. A plasma conjugated value less than 100 μmol/L is probably inconsistent with complete obstruction and indicates hepatocellular disease or incomplete obstruction.

Plasma transaminases: Over the first 6-12 months of life normal plasma transaminase levels are about twice the upper limit of normal of the adult range. In hepatocellular disease values in excess of ten-times normal are found. Obstructive disease (e.g., biliary atresia) may be associated with raised levels but to less than 5 times the upper normal range.

Plasma alkaline phophatase: In infants and children levels up to 2.5-times the adult upper level are normal. Because of this variation this test is generally of little value in the evaluation of liver disease. In the context of neonatal liver disease the plasma γ-glutamyl-transferase (or 5-nucleotidase) activity is probably of more value than the alkaline phosphatase in distinguishing cholestasis from hepatocellular disease.

Gamma-glutamyltransferase: Neonatal values are about 5 times those of the adult; by one year they drop to 50% of adult values and then increase slowly to reach adult levels by 10-12 years. In hepatocellular disease they increase to less than 5 times normal whereas in cholestatic disease (biliary atresia) values are usually in excess of 5 times the upper limit of normal.

ENZYMES

The "liver" enzymes are discussed above.

Alkaline phosphatase. In normal subjects up to the age of 18-20 years the upper reference limit for serum alkaline phosphatase (ALP) is about 2.5 times the adult upper limit. During puberty and periods of rapid growth levels can reach 500 U/L and beyond. Most of this activity is due to the bone ALP isoenzyme.

Hyperphosphatasaemia may be due to:

- Liver or bone disease
- Transient hyperphosphatasaemia of infancy
- Familial benign hyperphosphatasaemia

The latter two conditions occur in the neonatal or early childhood period and present as unexpected isolated elevations of the serum ALP. It is important to recognise them as benign disorders which require no further investigation.

Low serum ALP activitiy is a rare occurrence but occurs in hypophosphatasaemia, an unusual condition associated with vitamin D resistance rickets, skeletal abnormalities, and renal excretion of large amounts of phosphoethanolamine. Artefactually low ALP levels are associated with EDTA-preserved blood samples (EDTA chelates magnesium which is a cofactor necessary for the ALP reaction).

PLASMA PROTEINS

Total protein. Neonatal plasma protein levels (45-65 g/L) are slightly lower than adult values (60-80 g/L), due mainly to low levels of α- and β-globulins. Adult

values (except for immunoglobulins) are acquired by 6 to 12 months of age.

Albumin. At birth the level is similar to that of adults (30-50 g/L) but there may be a slight fall in the few days after birth. Values are usually lower in the premature infant (20-40 g/L). Disturbances of the serum albumin level are discussed on page 165.

α-Fetoprotein (AFP). AFP levels peak at about 20-25 weeks gestation and then decrease progressively reaching adult values by 8-12 months.

Neonates	50-150 mg/L
3-months	10-20 mg/L
8-months	<10 mg/L

This protein is discussed on page 290. Increased serum values during the neonatal period may be due to:

- Neonatal hepatitis (correlates with liver regeneration)
- Congenital biliary atresia
- Embryonal tumours
- Tyrosinosis
- Ataxia telangiectasis.

α$_1$-Antitrypsin. At birth serum values are slightly lower than adult levels which are reached by 6 months of age.

Birth	1.0-1.5 g/L
3-months	0.9-2.1 g/L
6-months/adults	1.0-2.5 g/L

Deficiency is associated with pulmonary emphysema and childhood liver disease (see page 166). Levels are increased in the acute phase reaction (page 174).

Caeruloplasmin. At birth serum levels (0.08-0.25 g/L) are lower than adult values (0.15-0.40 g/L) which are reached by the age of 12 months. Low values are found in Wilson's disease, malnutrition, and nephrosis. High values occur in the acute phase reaction.

Transferrin. Levels at birth (1.5-2.5 g/L) are lower than adult values (2.0-3.5 g/L) which are reached at around 9 months. Low serum values occur in congenital deficiency, malnutrition, malabsorption, and protein-losing states. High values occur in iron deficiency.

Immunoglobulins. These are discussed on page 167.

AMMONIA

Ammonia is derived from the metabolism of amino acids, amines, purines, and pyrimidines. A significant amount originates in the gut where it is produced by urea-splitting organisms and, more importantly, the metabolism of endogenous and exogenous glutamine (glutaminase) by the absorptive cells (Figure 27.2). It is a toxic substance which, in excess, results in vomiting, lethargy, seizures, coma, and eventually death, if it accumulates in large amounts in the tissues. The amount transported in the plasma as free ammonia is low (<50 µmol/L) except in the portal venous system where the level may be ten-fold higher than in other vessels. In the liver ammonia is detoxified by the formation of urea in the ornithine (urea) cycle (Figure 27.3).

$$2HCO_3^- + 2NH_4^+ \rightarrow NH_2\text{-}CO\text{-}NH_2 \text{ (urea)} + CO_2 + 3H_2O$$

Another organ involved in ammonia excretion is the kidney where the process is concerned with acid-base balance (see page 38 and Figure 27.2). However, the amount of ammonia excreted by the kidney is minimal (20-40 mmol/day in the adult) in comparison with that detoxified by the liver (up to 1000 mmol/day in the adult).

Hyperammoniaemia

CAUSES/PATHOPHYSIOLOGY

As mentioned above ammonia is very toxic and can result in encephalopathy and vomiting. Other manifestations are failure to thrive and growth retardation. The causes of hyperammonaemia are listed in Table 27.3.

Inborn errors of urea cycle. These present with vomiting, lethargy, encephalopathy, failure to thrive,

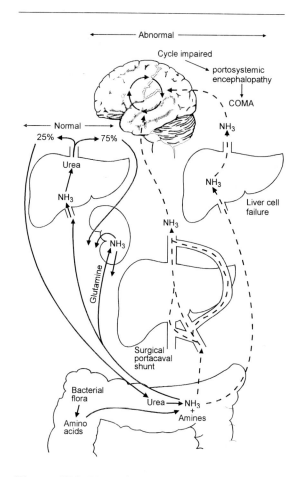

Figure 27.2. Normal and abnormal metabolism of ammonia. See page 159 for acknowledgement of source.

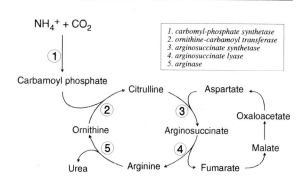

Figure 27.2. Ammonia and the urea cycle.

etc at any period during childhood -- most severe during neonatal period, less severe during infancy and

---

Table 27.3. Causes of hyperammonaemia.

1. **Inborn errors of urea cycle***
   carbamoyl phosphate synthetase deficiency
   ornithine carbamoyl transferase deficiency
   arginosuccinate synthetase deficiency
   (citrullinaemia)
   arginosuccinate lyase deficiency
   (arginosuccinic aciduria)
   arginase deficiency (arginaemia)

2. **Organic acidurias***
   propionic aciduria
   methylmalonic aciduria
   isovaleric acidaemia

3. **Disorders of fatty acid oxidation**
   hydroxymethylglutaryl-CoA deficiency
   acyl-CoA dehydrogenase deficiencies

4. **Liver disorders**
   severe liver dysfunction
   Reye's syndrome
   porto-caval shunt

5. **Miscellaneous**
   transient neonatal hyperammonaemia*
   valproate therapy
   any severe neonatal illness
   urinary tract infections
   ureterosigmoidostomy
   parenteral nutrition

*Three main causes of neonatal hyperammonaemia

---

childhood. Ornithine carbamoyl transferase (OCT) deficiency is the commonest of the disorders whilst arginase deficiency is the least common. All are inherited as autosomal recessive traits except OCT which is X-linked. Diagnosis is based on (a) plasma ammonia levels (values up to 5000 μmol/L may occur), (b) plasma arginine and citrulline levels, (c) urinary arginosuccinate and orotate levels. Definitive diagnosis requires the estimation of enzyme activities in a liver biopsy specimen.

Organic acidurias. These disorders usually present in the neonatal period with severe metabolic acidosis and ketosis (unusual in the urea cycle disorders) and hyperammonaemia (levels up to 1500 μmol/L). The cause of the hyperammonaemia is unclear.

Fatty acid oxidation defects. These disorders may present with hyperammonaemia in addition to hypoglycaemia.

Liver disease. Any severe liver disease will be accompanied by hyperammonaemia. The degree of encephalopathy, however, does not correlate well with the level of the plasma ammonia. Reye's syndrome (page 336) is invariably associated with hyper-ammonaemia which is due to decreased activity of the mitochondrial enzymes carbamoyl phosphate synthetase and ornithine carbamoyl transferase.

Transient neonatal hyperammonaemia. Some preterm babies have been described with a condition indistinguishable from that of the urea cycle disorders -- the difference being that these babies make a complete recovery if the hyperammonaemia is treated rigorously. Other biochemical parameters are unremarkable.

Renal disease. Renal tract infections with urea-splitting organisms may result in the absorption of sufficient ammonia to overwhelm the liver detoxification process. Similarly in ureterosigmoido-stomy, where urine is diverted to the gut, the production of ammonia by the gut bacteria may be of sufficient quantity to produce hyperammonaemia.

Parenteral nutrition. Hyperammonaemia has been described occasionally in intravenous feeding, due probably to an imbalance in the amino acid mixture (e.g., low arginine).

Valproate therapy. Patients on valproate medication have higher plasma ammonia levels than controls (e.g., >60 μmol/L). This is thought to be due to inhibition of carbamoyl phosphate synthetase activity by the breakdown products of this drug. Reye's syndrome has been attributed to this drug.

LABORATORY INVESTIGATION

The laboratory approach to the evaluation of the patient with hyperammonaemia will depend on the clinical picture and the available laboratory facilities. For a definitive diagnosis the laboratory tests would include:

- *Plasma ammonia*
- *Plasma anion gap* (increased in organic aciduria)
- *Liver function tests* (transaminases, etc)
- *Plasma amino acids* especially glutamine, citrulline, arginine
- *Urinary organic acids,* citrulline, arginosuccinic acid, arginine, orotic acid
- *Enzyme analysis on liver biopsy* (urea cycle enzymes)

REFERENCES/FURTHER READING

Evans SE and Durbin GM. Aspects of the physiological and pathological background to neonatal clinical chemistry. Ann Clin Biochem 1983;20: 193-207.

Fitzgerald JF. Cholestatic disorders of infancy. Pediatr Clinics North Am 1988;35:357-370.

Green A. When should we measure plasma ammonia? Ann Clin Biochem 1988;25:199-209.

Snodgrass PP. Biochemical aspects of urea cycle disorders. Pediatrics 1981;68:273-283.

Haymond MW. Hypoglycaemia in infants and children. Endocr Metab Clinics North Am 1989;18: 211-246.

Cole DE, Carpenter TO, and Goltzman D. Calcium homeostasis and disorders of bone and mineral metabolism. In: *Pediatric Endocrinology (2nd Edn)*, Collu R, Ducharme JR, Guyda HJ (eds). New York: Raven Press Ltd, 1989.

Chapter 28

Therapeutic Drug Monitoring and Toxicology

Recent advances in analytical methods and laboratory instrumentation have made it possible to routinely measure accurately and rapidly a large variety of drugs in biological fluids, particularly in serum. These advances in drug monitoring have enabled clinicians to adequately control drug therapy and tailor it to the individual subject, and have contributed to the investigation and management of patients with drug overdose.

Therapeutic drug monitoring

There is no simple relationship between drug dosage, serum drug levels, and drug action. Therapeutic drug monitoring (TDM) is therefore not a panacea and should be regarded not as a substitute for, but rather as an adjunct to, careful clinical assessment and surveillance. In some situations, the intensity of the pharmacologic effects of the drug therapy can be quantitated clinically or by other parameters, e.g., those of antihypertensive drugs, hypoglycaemic agents, and anticoagulants can be assessed on the basis of blood pressure, blood glucose, and prothrombin time measurements, respectively. TDM is also not necessary when the drug dosage need not be individualised, but it is becoming essential, or highly desirable, for an increasing number of drugs.

Conditions which contribute towards the effectiveness of TDM as a practical proposition in clinical medicine include:

- State of the art analytical technology:
  (a) development of specific, sensitive, and accurate methods which measure either the active drug and/or its important metabolites
  (b) ready availability of the service
  (c) quick turnaround times
- No tolerance to the drug at receptor sites
- Concentration of the drug in serum proportional to that at receptor sites
- Reasonably good correlation between serum concentrations and pharmacological effects
- A well defined therapeutic range
- Proper care in interpreting drug levels.

The correct interpretation of a patient's serum drug level requires a knowledge of at least four important factors: pharmacokinetic factors, pharmacodynamic factors, the therapeutic range, and the appropriate time to estimate the serum level (in relation to time of administration). In addition, host factors such as age, sex, body weight, stress, hydration status, and thyroid function also affect the disposition of the administered drug.

PHARMACOKINETIC FACTORS

These are the factors that determine the serum drug level produced by a dose, or doses, of the drug (Figure 28.1) and the pharmacokinetic variation between different subjects accounts for the different responses to the same drug dose in different individuals.

Of most concern to the clinician and the objective of performing TDM is to determine the steady state level produced by chronic (repeated) therapy. This steady state is the level reached after repeated doses when the rate of administration and the rate of elimination approximate each other. It is only a relative term because the serum drug level will vary from hour to hour and minute to minute.

The factors that affect the serum level of a drug are many and varied and only a few will be considered here. For further information about this subject the reader should consult the specialised texts.

Dosage, compliance, absorption and first pass metabolism

It would appear trite to discuss drug dosage in the context of serum levels but it should be remembered that a doubling of the dose does not necessarily result in a doubling of the serum level. The word compliance is self-evident and is one of the most important reasons for monitoring serum drug levels (as patients abuse drugs by overdosage, they also abuse them by underdosage).

Numerous factors can affect the rate of drug absorption from the gut, e.g., gut motility, bioavailability of the drug, stability of the drug at acid pH of stomach, food intake affecting absorption and bioavailability, bowel disease, etc. Furthermore, a

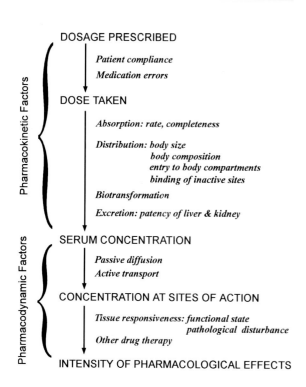

Figure 28.1. Relationship between drug dosage, the serum drug level, and its effect at the tissue level.

to albumin. The activity of a drug will be affected not only by its binding ability but also by the number of available binding sites. The number of sites may be low because of hypoalbuminaemia or because they are occupied by other substances, e.g., phenylbutazone may displace warfarin from protein, causing a lengthening of the prothrombin time. Unfortunately, most TDM methods currently measure the total serum drug concentration rather than the free fraction which is of direct clinical relevance, due to limitations in the technology.

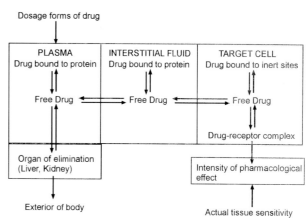

Figure 28.2. Factors influencing the intermediary metabolism and pharmacologic effectiveness of drugs.

number of drugs may be metabolised by enzymatic systems in the gut (e.g., bacterial enzymes), in the gut wall, and during the first passage through the liver.

Biliary recirculation

Some drugs are excreted in high concentrations in the conjugated form in the bile. On re-entering the small intestine there may be deconjugation and reabsorption which can result in two (or more) peaks following a single dose. Erythromycin is such a drug.

Protein binding

Many drugs bind to albumin whilst in circulation and are thus partially inactivated (Figure 28.2); only the free drug is metabolically active. The binding ability varies from drug to drug. For example, about 90% of phenytoin is bound whilst only 20% of digoxin binds

Serum half-life

When a drug is administered, it will reach a peak value in the serum and then decline. The time taken for the serum level to halve is called the serum half-life.

Knowledge of the half-life will determine the dosage, time of dosage, and the number of doses required over a given period. A readily-absorbed formulation will produce high initial peak concentrations, which will then rapidly decay. The slowly-absorbed drug, however, reaches a steady state after a relatively longer time but produces sustained concentrations within the therapeutic range. Serum drug concentrations (and their half-lives) are affected by the rate of absorption, clearance by the liver and kidney, volume of distribution, and binding to proteins and/or tissues at receptor or other non-specific sites (Figures 28.2 and 28.3).

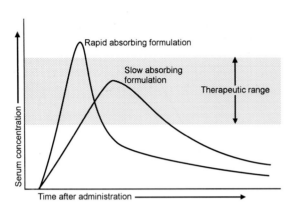

Figure 28.3. Serum concentration/time curve for a rapidly and a slowly absorbed drug.

From a practical point of view the half-life allows the clinician to determine:

i   The interval of administration (usually half-life intervals)
ii When the steady state will be reached (3 to 6 half-lives)
iii When a toxic level will be reduced to a therapeutic level.

Further consideration will be given to the half-lives of drugs in the section on the individual drugs.

Metabolism and excretion

Drugs are usually excreted by the liver or the kidney or both and usually after some modification, e.g., conjugation (Figure 28.2). Thus before embarking on any drug therapy some knowledge of liver and renal function should be acquired. Certain drugs, however, are excreted unchanged in the urine. Generally, slow metabolisers require lower maintenance doses of the drug to achieve optimal therapeutic response, the exception being drugs with pharmacologically active metabolites. In the latter, measurement of only the parent drug would underestimate pharmacological effects.

PHARMACODYNAMIC FACTORS

These are the factors which determine the relationship between the serum drug level and its effect at the tissue level (Figure 28.1). They are poorly understood but generally, for most drugs, the intensity of tissue action relates directly to the serum level, especially if it is the concentration of the free drug or its active metabolite(s) that is being monitored; however, factors such as drug tolerance (e.g., barbiturates, opiates) and the rate of conversion of drugs to active metabolites (e.g., alpha-methyldopa to alpha-methylnoradrenaline) at target sites tend to invalidate this assumption.

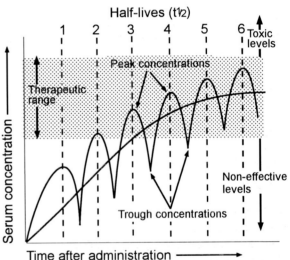

Smooth curve: continuous IV infusion
Peak/trough curve: intermittent oral doses

Figure 28.4. Concept of therapeutic range and steady state.

THERAPEUTIC RANGE

This term implies that there is a serum level below which the drug is ineffective and a level above which the drug produces toxic effects (Figure 28.4). The major problem is how to determine this range; however, a lot of clinically useful information has been gained from prospective and retrospective studies. Maintenance of both the peak and trough levels within the therapeutic range is vital for efficacy and avoidance of toxicity.

Published therapeutic ranges, usually estimated under the ideal conditions of single-drug therapy, underscore the wide interindividual variation in the clinical response to drugs, and thus should only be used to serve as guidelines when applied to individual patients, especially when polypharmacy is practised.

DRUG LEVEL ESTIMATION TIME

All of the above mentioned factors will influence the timing of blood sampling for serum drug monitoring, as does the mode of administration, oral or parenteral. In some cases, where the serum half-life is long (e.g., phenytoin) the timing is not critical; in other cases, particularly if the half-life is short (e.g., digoxin), the timing is crucial. The danger in collecting specimens too soon after starting therapy, before attainment of a steady state, lies in possible misinterpretation and wrongful adjustment of the *apparent* low levels with an increased dosage, thereby leading to toxicity. The timing of samples will be discussed below.

INDICATIONS FOR TDM

Drugs which are commonly monitored by serum estimations are:

Anticonvulsants: carbamazepine, phenobarbital, phenytoin, primidone, ethosuximide.
Antibiotics: gentamicin, chloramphenicol
Bronchodilators: theophylline.
Cardiac agents: digoxin, quinidine, propranolol, procainamide
Analgesics: acetaminophen, acetylsalicylate.
Antineoplastics: methotrexate.
Psychotropics: amitriptyline, lithium carbonate.

TDM is indicated in the following situations:

- Checking for possible non-compliance
- When the drug's toxic and therapeutic levels are close
- When symptoms suggest toxicity
- In multiple drug therapy where there may be interactions
- If there are disorders which affect pharmacokinetic factors, e.g., hepatic, renal, or cardiovascular disease
- Where there is wide interindividual pharmacokinetic variation
- In malabsorption syndromes
- In the aged and in infants where susceptibility may be altered
- When surreptitious drug use is suspected
- In prophylactic drug use, when no other convenient methods of assessing clinical efficacy are available.

ANTICONVULSANTS

Carbamazepine

Toxic effects: diplopia, blurred vision, drowsiness, dizziness, ataxia
Sample collection time: pre-dose
Therapeutic range: 20-50 µmol/L
Half-life: 10-30 hours
Time to reach steady state: 3-5 days
Protein binding: 65-80%
Clearance: hepatic (60-80%), renal (1-10%).

Ethosuximide

Toxic effects: nausea, vomiting, anorexia, drowsiness, lethargy, dizziness, euphoria
Sample collection time: pre-dose
Therapeutic range: 280-700 µmol/L
Half-life: 40-60 hours
Time to reach steady state: 7-14 days
Protein binding: 0%
Clearance: hepatic (80%), renal (20%; unchanged)

Phenobarbital

Toxic effects: confusion, sedation
Sample collection time: pre-dose
Therapeutic range: 60-170 µmol/L
Half-life: 48-120 hours
Time to reach steady state: 10-25 days
Protein binding: 20-40%
Clearance: hepatic (~80%), renal (~20%; mainly unchanged)

Phenytoin

Toxic effects: nystagmus, vertigo, double vision, ataxia, coma, gingival hypertrophy, vitamin D deficiency
Sample collection time: pre-dose
Therapeutic range: 40-80 µmol/L
Half-life: 8-42 hours
Time to reach steady state: 8-12 days
Protein binding: 85-95%
Clearance: hepatic (92%; mainly conjugated), renal (5%; unchanged)

Primidone

Toxic effects: ataxia, vertigo, diplopia, nystagmus, sedation
Sample collection time: pre-dose
Therapeutic range: 25-70 µmol/L
Half-life: 6-8 hours
Time to reach steady state: ~2 days
Protein binding: 0-30%
Clearance: hepatic (50-60%), renal (~40%; mainly unchanged)

Valproate

Toxic effects: nausea, vomiting, sedation, tremors, incoordination, hepatotoxicity
Sample collection time: pre-dose
Therapeutic range: 350-690 µmol/L
Half-life: 8-15 hours
Time to reach steady state: 2-3 days
Protein binding: 85-95%
Clearance: hepatic (60-80%; conjugated), renal (5%,; unchanged)

ANTIBIOTICS

Gentamicin

Toxic effects: nephrotoxicity (renal failure), ototoxicity. This drug is very toxic and should be monitored regularly.
Sample collection time: peak: 0.5-1.0 hours after end of 30 min infusion (1 hour after IM dose); trough: immediately before next dose

Therapeutic range: peak 5-12 mg/L, trough <2 mg/L
Half-life: 2-3 hours
Time to reach steady state: 2.5-15 hours
Protein binding: 0-10%
Clearance: 90% by kidney, unchanged.

CARDIOVASCULAR DRUGS

Digoxin

Toxic effects: anorexia, nausea, vomiting, diarrhoea, ventricular dysrhythmias, A-V block
Sample collection time: 6-8 hours post-dose
Therapeutic range: 1.0-2.6 nmol/L
Half-life: 36 hours
Time to reach steady state: 7-12 days
Protein binding: 25%
Clearance: hepatic (15-25%), kidney (75-85%)

Quinidine

Toxic effects: nausea, vomiting, diarrhoea, hypotension, tachycardia
Sample collection time: pre-dose
Therapeutic range: 10-20 µmol/L
Half-life: 6 hours
Time to reach steady state: 24-36 hours
Protein binding: 80-90%
Clearance: hepatic (60-80%), kidney (10-30%)

PSYCHOTROPIC DRUGS

Lithium

Toxic effects: anxiety, tremors, confusion, sedation, nystagmus, hypothyroidism, hypercalcaemia, diabetes insipidus
Sample collection time: 12 hours after evening dose
Therapeutic range: 0.6-1.2 mmol/L
Half-life: 14-33 hours
Time to reach steady state: 3-7 days
Protein binding: 0%
Clearance: kidney (90-100%)

Amitriptyline

Toxic effects: tachycardia, hypotension, dry mouth, blurred vision, sedation, sweating

Therapeutic Drug Monitoring and Toxicology

Sample collection time: pre-dose
Therapeutic range: 450-900 nmol/L
Half-life: 20-40 hours
Time to reach steady state: 3-8 days
Protein binding: 90%
Clearance: hepatic (95%), kidney (5%)

BRONCHODILATORS

Theophylline

Toxic effects: nausea, vomiting, diarrhoea, irritability, seizures, cardiac arrhythmia, cardiorespiratory collapse
Sample collection time: IV: pre-dose, oral rapid release: 2 hours post-dose, oral sustained release: 4 hours post-dose.
Therapeutic range: 55-100 µmol/L:
Half-life: 3-12 hours
Time to reach steady state: 24-48 hours
Protein binding: 60%
Clearance: hepatic (80%), kidney (10%)

Drug overdose and toxicology

Leaving aside the problems of alcohol and the drugs of abuse, the most frequent causes of overdose are:

• Deliberate overdose with drugs normally prescribed for therapeutic purposes: benzo-diazepine, antidepressants, paracetamol, salicylate, opiates, barbiturates

• Accidental poisoning: organophosphates, paraquat, vitamins (e.g., A and D in food faddists).

• Long-term drug therapy: phenobarbital, phenytoin, lithium, digoxin, carbamazepine.

The commonest result of drug overdose (including alcohol) is impaired consciousness; however, the commoner causes of unconsciousness in patients presenting to the Accident and Emergency Department are head injury, cerebrovascular accidents, and diabetic coma.

EVALUATION OF THE UNCONSCIOUS PATIENT

The problems facing the clinician and the laboratory when dealing with causes of deliberate overdose or poisoning differ from those related to TDM in that it is the clinical condition of the patient and his survival that is paramount, not the serum drug or toxin level. The estimation of the latter is an important part of the diagnostic process but not as important as recognising the condition for what it is and being able to differentiate it from non-toxin-related conditions that present with a similar picture.

Clinical evaluation

In addition to coma, features that may suggest drug overdose include respiratory depression, shock, hypothermia, convulsions, and cardiac arrhythmia. Other factors that should be considered are the possibilities of trauma, cerebrovascular accidents, and epilepsy.

Laboratory investigation

Ideally, an efficient and reliable round-the-clock emergency service in chemical toxicology should be available in every major hospital, in view of the urgency in identifying and treating such patients (although it is not necessary to know the diagnosis to commence supportive therapy and in fact 'overdose' patients can be successfully managed without the clinician being aware of the type or quantity of the offending drug or toxin consumed). The investigations that should be offered by such a service (in an ideal world) are:

(1) the *routine tests* applicable to any unconscious patient and available in any laboratory,
(2) *specific tests* which lead on from the clinical picture and the results of the routine tests,
(3) specialised *toxicological analyses*.

Routine tests should include:

• Plasma electrolytes, anion gap, creatinine, and urea (assess renal function and hydration status)
• Plasma osmolality and osmolar gap
• Plasma glucose (hyper- and hypoglycaemia)
• Blood gases (respiratory acidosis and alkalosis)

- Plasma calcium (hyper- and hypocalcaemia)
- Urinalysis (oxalate crystals in ethylene glycol toxicity, myoglobin in rhabdomyolysis)

Anion gap. This is discussed on page 40. High anion gaps are associated with lactic acidosis, ketoacidosis, and toxicity due to cyanide, carbon monoxide, methanol, ethylene glycol, salicylates.

Osmolar gap. (see page 2) Ethanol is the commonest cause of a high osmolar gap but it also occurs in poisoning with ethylene glycol, methanol, acetone, isopropyl alcohol, and propylene glycol.

Specific tests (depending on the clinical picture) may include:

- Drug screen
- Thyroid function tests (hyper- and hypothyroidism)
- Cortisol status (hyper- and hypocortisolism)
- Liver function tests (hepatic coma, liver damage due to toxins)

Toxicological analysis. The most frequently required blood analyses in emergency toxicology include:

- Paracetamol (acetaminophen)
- Salicylates
- Barbiturates
- Alcohol (ethanol, methanol)
- Lithium
- Paraquat
- Cholinesterase (organophosphate poisoning)
- Carbon monoxide, carboxyhaemoglobin
- Ethylene glycol (component of antifreeze agents)

Only a brief outline of the effects of overdosage/ ingestion of alcohol, paracetamol, salicylates, and herbicides are presented below. The reader should refer to more specialised texts on toxicology for a detailed treatment of the subject.

PARACETAMOL

In small doses paracetamol is fairly harmless but large doses can cause severe liver damage which can result in hepatic failure.

Pathophysiology

The majority of the metabolites of paracetamol are harmless and after conjugation with sulphate and glucuronide are excreted in the urine. With small doses of the drug, a small quantity of the hepatotoxin, N-acetyl-*p*-benzoquinoloneimine, is formed. This is normally detoxified by conjugation with glutathione.

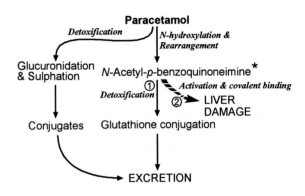

Figure 28.5. Pathophysiology of paracetamol toxicity.

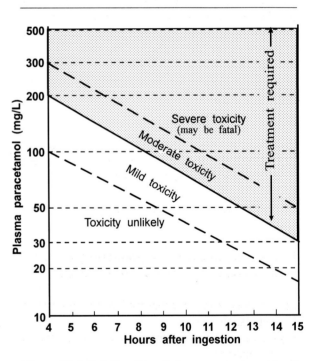

Figure 28.6. Relationship of plasma paracetamol level to severity of liver damage.

If there is a massive dose of the drug, the glucuronide and sulphate conjugation pathways are saturated and large amounts of the hepatotoxin are produced. The amount of glutathione available for conjugation is limited and when this is exceeded liver damage results (Figure 28.5).

Overdose management

The likelihood of liver damage can be predicted from the plasma paracetamol level (Figure 28.6). The available antidotes are N-acetyl cysteine and methionine which promote hepatic glutathione synthesis.

SALICYLATES

Salicylate overdose, producing a plasma level in excess of 2.5-3.0 mmol/L, may result in respiratory alkalosis, metabolic acidosis, and hypo- or hyperglycaemia.

Pathophysiology

Large doses of salicylate affect intermediary metabolism and oxidative phosphorylation and directly stimulate the respiratory centre to produce hyperventilation and respiratory alkalosis.

Intermediary metabolism interference produces a metabolic acidosis and a high anion gap.

(a) Increased lipolysis results in increased ketogenesis
(b) Inhibition of the TCA cycle results in increased pyruvate and lactate production.

   (a) + (b) results in metabolic acidosis

Uncoupling of oxidative phosphorylation will result in a variety of metabolic abnormalities:

(a) Increased oxygen consumption and respiratory stimulation
(b) Increased CO_2 production resulting in respiratory stimulation
(c) Increased ATP demand causing either increased glycolysis and possible hypoglycaemia, or increased gluconeogenesis and hyperglycaemia.

Management of overdose

There is no specific antidote for the salicylates and management rests on increasing the removal of the drug from the body by:

- Alkalinisation of the urine (at high pH salicylate becomes ionised and this inhibits tubular reabsorption)
- Haemodialysis

PESTICIDES/HERBICIDES

Organophosphates (parathion, malathion). These substances inhibit the enzymes acetylcholinesterase and pseudocholinesterase. Diagnosis is made by finding low plasma levels of pseudocholinesterase and low red cell levels of acetylcholinesterase.

Paraquat. This herbicide is particularly toxic to the lungs and kidney. The blood levels are easily estimated in the laboratory.

ETHANOL

Alcohol, particularly the ingestion of excessive amounts, can result in a number of clinical and biochemical abnormalities.

Metabolism

Ethanol is metabolised almost entirely by the liver, a small amount (<10%) being excreted unchanged by the lungs and kidneys. It is oxidised to acetaldehyde by two systems, cytosolic *alcohol dehydrogenase* and the *microsomal alcohol (ethanol) oxidising system* (MEOS). The acetaldehyde is then oxidised by mitochondrial *aldehyde dehydrogenase* to acetate which is eventually converted to acetyl-CoA.

NADH is produced by both the alcohol dehydrogenase and aldehyde dehydrogenase reactions (Figure 28.7) and the consequence, a high NADH:NAD$^+$ ratio, is responsible for many of the biochemical effects of excessive alcohol consumption.

351

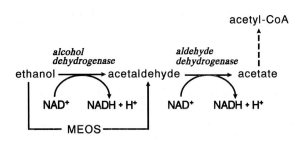

Figure 28.7. Metabolism of ethanol (see text for details)

Biochemical consequences

The metabolic consequences of alcoholism involve seemingly unrelated effects ranging from electrolyte abnormalities to hypoglycaemia to hyperuricaemia. The major abnormalities are listed below; they do not occur in all alcoholic subjects but they are common enough to be markers of alcohol overuse and should be recognised as such.

Increased osmolal gap. The plasma osmolal gap is the difference between the measured osmolality and the calculated osmolality {2 x ([Na] + [K]) + [urea] (mmol/L) + [glucose] (mmol/L)}. It is an estimation of the osmotically active particles in plasma (in this case ethanol) other than electrolytes, glucose, and urea. The presence of alcohol, which is osmotically active, causes a high osmolal gap in alcoholics.

Hypoglycaemia. In the absence of oral carbohydrates and glycogen stores (i.e., starvation), the glucose requirements of organs such as the brain and erythrocytes are derived from gluconeogenesis (lactate, glycerol, amino acids). Inadequate food intake is a not uncommon situation in chronic alcoholics, particularly those on binge-drinking, and if this starvation goes on for a period of time sufficient to deplete the glycogen reserves (18-24 hours) then glucose production will be dependant on gluconeogenesis. However, continued alcohol metabolism depletes the liver cytosol of NAD$^+$ (increased NADH:NAD$^+$ ratio) and this will inhibit gluconeogenesis resulting in hypoglycaemia.

Three of the cytosolic reactions of gluconeogenesis require an adequate supply of NAD$^+$:

(1) lactate ---> pyruvate (lactate dehydrogenase)

(2) glycerol phosphate--> dihydroxyacetone phosphate (glycerolphosphate dehydrogenase)

(3) malate ---> oxaloacetate (malate dehydrogenase)

The amount of nicotinamide adenine nucleotide in the cytosol is limited and present in only small quantities; so if most of it is in the form of NADH the above three reactions will not proceed; hence hypoglycaemia.

Lactic acidosis. Lactate, produced in muscle and other organs, is transported to the liver (and kidney) for conversion, through gluconeogenesis, to glucose. The first stage in this process, lactate to pyruvate, involves lactate dehydrogenase which requires NAD$^+$. If the NAD$^+$ concentration is low in the cytosol, as in excessive alcohol metabolism, then the reaction will not proceed: thus the accumulation of lactate and lactic acidosis.

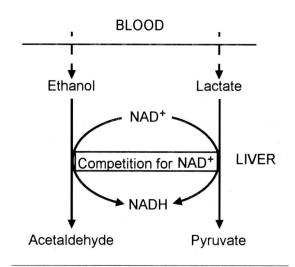

Ketoacidosis. Alcoholic ketosis, which is less common than alcoholic lactic acidosis, reflects starvation. This is described on page 138 but the basic mechanism is as follows:

(1) starvation leads to lowering of the blood glucose → decreased insulin, increased glucagon (and increased catecholamines)

(2) the low insulin:glucagon ratio →

  (a) increased lipolysis and increased production of free fatty acids and subsequent β-oxidation of these acids
  (b) fatty acid oxidation results in increased production of acetyl-CoA by the mitochondria

Under normal circumstances the mitochondrial acetyl-CoA is metabolised in the citric acid cycle. The first reaction here is condensation with oxaloacetate to form citrate (citrate synthetase). If there is insufficient oxaloacetate to clear the acetyl-CoA, as there may well be in the alcoholic (decreased production of pyruvate from lactate, etc), then it will be diverted to ketone formation.

A feature of alcoholic ketosis is the high ratio of β-hydroxybutyrate to acetoacetate (7:1 to 10.:1 in the alcoholics); in diabetic ketoacidosis and uncomplicated starvation the ratio is usually less than 5:1. In the alcoholic this reflects the high $NADH:NAD^+$ ratio in the cytosol because the conversion of acetoacetate to β-hydroxybutyrate by β-hydroxybutyrate dehydrogenase utilises NADH.

Hypophosphataemia. The hypophosphataemia which develops after glucose therapy is due to shift into the cells (page 106). Severe hypophosphataemia may be a causative factor in rhabdomyolysis which could be an explanation for the high plasma creatine kinase activity in these patients although alcoholic myopathy is a more probable cause.

Hypomagnesaemia. This may be due to decreased intake (nutritional, vomiting, diarrhoea) and increased renal excretion as a consequence of alcohol (page 109). Severe magnesium deficiency can result in hypocalcaemia (page 111) and hypokalaemia (page 111), both of which may occur in chronic alcoholics.

Hyperuricaemia. This is common in alcoholics and is due to increased production and decreased renal excretion as a consequence of circulating lactate and ketones which diminish renal tubular urate secretion (page 115).

Abnormal liver enzymes. Increased plasma levels of the transaminases and alkaline phosphatase may reflect alcoholic liver disease (page 154), whilst elevated γ-glutamyltransferase levels may be due to liver disease or enzyme induction (page 158).

Alcoholic pancreatitis. Ethanol abuse is a major cause of acute pancreatitis (page 181).

Plasma lipid abnormalities. Alcoholism is a recognised cause of hypertriglyceridaemia (page 208) due to increased VLDL synthesis.

Endocrine abnormalities. Continued alcohol abuse can, rarely, result in a Cushing's syndrome (page 257). Non-dexamethasone suppressible-hypercortisolaemia, without the clinical manifestations of Cushing's, is common. Hypogonadism and feminisa tion can occur due to impaired synthesis of testosterone (? induction of hepatic enzymes causing inactivation).

REFERENCES/FURTHER READING

Anon. What therapeutic drugs should be monitored? Lancet 1985;i:309-310.

Sabin TD. Coma and the acute confusional state in the emergency room. Med Clin ics North Am 1981;65:15-32.

Widdop B (ed) *Therapeutic Drug Monitoring.* Edinburgh: Churchill Livingstone, 1985.

Wright J, Marks V. Alcohol. *In:* Cohen RD, Lewis B, Alberti KGMM, Denman (eds) *The Metabolic and Molecular Basis of Disease*, London: Balliere Tindall, 1990, pp 602-634.

Abbreviations used in this book

[x]	Concentration of x	CSF	Cerebrospinal fluid
AcAc	Acetoacetic acid	CVD	Cardiovascular disease
ACE	Angiotensin-converting enzyme	DHEA(S)	Dehydroepiandrosterone (sulphate)
ACP	Acid phosphatase	1,25-DHCC	1,25-Dihydroxycholecalciferol
ACTH	Adrenocorticotrophic homone (corticotrophin)	1,25-$(OH)_2$D	1,25-Dihydroxyvitamin D
		DI	Diabetes insipidus
ADH	Antidiuretic hormone	DIT	Diiodotyrosine
AFP	α-Fetoprotein	DKA	Diabetic ketoacidosis
AGap	Anion gap	DNA	Deoxyribonucleic acid
AIP	Acute intermittent porphyria	EABV	Effective arterial blood volume
AKA	Alcoholic ketoacidosis	E_2	Oestradiol 17-β
δ-ALA	δ-Aminolaevulinic acid	ECF	Extracellular fluid
ALP	Alkaline phosphatase	ECV	Extracellular volume
ALT	Alanine aminotranferase	EDTA	Ethylenediamine tetra-acetic acid
AMI	Acute myocardial infarct(ion)	ESR	Erythrocyte sedimentaton rate
ANP	Atrial natriuretic peptide	Fe	Iron
Apo	Apolipoprotein	Fe^{2+}	Ferrous ion
APRT	Adenine phosphoribosyl transferase	Fe^{3+}	Ferric ion
APUD	Amine precursor uptake and decarboxylation	FE_x	Fractional excretion of 'x'
		FPIA	Fluorescence polarisation immunoassay
ARF	Acute renal failure	FSH	Follicle stimulating hormone
AST	Aspartate aminotransferase	fT_3	Free triiodothyronine
ATN	Acute tubular necrosis	fT_4	Free thyroxine
ATP	Adenosine triphosphate	FTI	Free thyroxine index
AVP	Arginine vasopressin	GFR	Glomerular filtration rate
BJP	Bence-Jones protein	γGT	Gamma-glutamyltransferase
BMR	Basal metabolic rate	GH	Growth hormone
BSP	Bromsulphthalein	GHRH	Growth hormone releasing hormone
ca	carbonic anhydrase	GIT	Gastrointestinal tract
Ca	Calcium	GMP	Guanosine monophosphate
Ca^{2+}	Calcium ion (ionised calcium)	G6PD	Glucose-6-phosphate dehydrogenase
CA 19-9	Carbohydrate antigen 19-9	GnRH	Gonadotrophin releasing hormone
CA-125	Cancer antigen 125	GTT	Glucose tolerance test
CA-50	Carcinoma antigen 50	H^+	Hydrogen ion
cAMP	Cyclic adenosine monophosphate	HAGMA	High anion gap metabolic acidosis
CAT	Computerised axial tomography	Hb	Haemoglobin
CBG	Cortisol-binding globulin	HBD	Hydroxybutyrate dehydrogenase
CCF	Congestive cardiac failure	25-HCC	25-Hydroxycholecalciferol
CEA	Carcinoembryonic antigen	25-(OH)D	25-Hydroxyvitamin D
CF	Cystic fibrosis	HCG	Human chorionic gonadotrophin
CHD	Coronary heart disease	HCl	Hydrochloric acid
CK	Creatine kinase	HCO_3	Bicarbonate
Cl	Chloride	HCO_3^-	Bicarbonate ion
Cl^-	Chloride ion	HDL	High density lipoproteins
CNS	Central nervous system	HGPRT	Hypoxanthine guanosine phospho-ribosyl transferase
COAD	Chronic obstructive airway disease		
CO_2	Carbon dioxide		
CRF	Chronic renal failure	5-HIAA	5-Hydroxyindole acetic acid
CRH	Corticotrophin releasing hormone	HLA	Human (histocompatibility) leucocyte antigen
CRP	C reactive protein		

HMMA	4-Hydroxy-3-methoxymandelic acid	PCR	Polymerase chain reaction
HPL	Human placental lactogen	PCT	Porphyria cutanea tarda
HVA	Homovanillic acid	PIF	Prolactin inhibiting factor
ICF	Intracellular fluid	Po_2	Partial pressure of oxygen
IDDM	Insulin-dependent diabetes mellitus	PO_4^{3-}	Inorganic phosphate ion
IDL	Intermediate density lipoproteins	PRA	Plasma renin activity
Ig	Immunoglobulin	PRL	Prolactin
IGF-I	Insulin-like growth factor I	PSA	Prostatic specific antigen
IGT	Impaired glucose tolerance	PTH	Parathyroid hormone
IHD	Ischaemic heart disease	rbc	Red blood cell
IM	Intramuscular	RFLP	Restriction fragment length polymorphism
IMP	Inosine monophosphate		
IV	Intravenous	RIA	Radioimmunoassay
IVV	Intravascular volume	RNA	Ribonucleic acid
K	Potassium	RTA	Renal tubular acidosis
K^+	Potassium ion	sd	Standard deviation
LATS	Long-acting thyroid (receptor) stimulating antibody	SHH	Syndrome of hyporeninaemic hypoaldosteronism
LCAT	Lecithin cholesterol acyltransferase	SI units	Systém Internationale units
LD	Lactate dehydrogenase	SIADH	Syndrome of inappropriate secretion of antidiuretic hormone
LDL	Low density lipoproteins		
LFTs	Liver function tests	$t\frac{1}{2}$	Half-life of a substance
LH	Luteinising hormone	T_3	Triiodothyronine
LHRH	Luteinising hormone releasing hormone	T_4	Thyroxine
		rT_3	Reverse T_3
Lp(a)	Lipoprotein (a)	T_3RU	T_3 resin uptake
L/S ratio	Lecithin:sphingomyelin ratio	TBG	Thyroxine-binding globulin
MCA	Mucin carcinoma antigen	TBP	Thyroxine-binding proteins
MEN	Multiple endocrine neoplasia	TBw	Total body water
Mg	Magnesium	TCA	Tricarboxylic acid (cycle)
Mg^{2+}	Magnesium ion	TDM	Therapeutic drug monitoring
MIT	Monoiodotyrosine	TgAb	Anti-thyroglobulin antibody
mmol/L	millimoles per litre	TIBC	Total iron binding capacity
mosmol/L	milliosmoles per litre	TMAb	Anti-thyroid microsomal peroxidase antibody
MRI	Magnetic resonance imaging		
MSH	Melanocyte stimulating hormone	TRH	Thyrotrophin releasing hormone
Na	Sodium	TSH	Thyroid stimulating hormone
Na^+	Sodium ion	TSI(TSAb)	Thyroid (receptor) stimulating immunoglobulin (antibodies)
NAD^+	Nicotinamide adenine dinucleotide (oxidised form)		
		VIP	Vasoactive intestinal peptide
NADH	Nicotinamide adenine dinucleotide (reduced form)	VLDL	Very low density lipoproteins
		VMA	Vanillyl mandellic acid
NIDDM	Non-insulin dependent diabetes mellitus	WDHA	Watery diarrhoea, hypokalaemia and achlorhydria syndrome
5'-NT	5'-Nucleotidase	↑	Increase
OAF	Osteoclast activating factor	↑↑	Large increase
β-OHB	β-hydroxybutyric acid	s↑	Slight increase
OCCA	Ovarian cystadenoma-carcinoma antigen	↓	Decrease
		↓↓	Large decrease
OH^-	Hydroxyl ion	~	Approximately
PBG	Porphobilinogen	∝	Proportional
Pco_2	Partial pressure of carbon dioxide	N	Normal
PCOS	Polycystic ovarian syndrome	→ N	Approaching normal

INDEX

Aminoglycosides, 79, 348
  gentamicin, 79, 348
    pharmacokinetic parameters of, 348
  renal failure and, 79
Aminoglutethimide,
  vitamin D metabolism and, 98
ρ-Aminohippuric acid,
  renal blood flow and, 75
δ-Aminolaevulinic acid, 79, *F21.2*, 278-80
  lead poisoning and, 281, *F21.3*
Amiodarone, 242, 317
  thyroid hormone metabolism and, 242
Amitriptyline, 348
  γ-glutamyltransferase and, 155
  pharmacokinetic parameters of, 348
Ammonia, 159, 337, 341-3
  hepatic encephalopathy and, 159, 337
  metabolism of,
    abnormal, 341, *F27.2*
    normal, 341
  renal handling of, 341
  urea and, 341, *F27.2*
  urinary buffers and, 38, *F3.1,* 82
Ammonium chloride loading (acidification) test, 82
Ammonium ions, excretion of, 82
Amniocentesis, 325-6
Amniotic fluid, 323-6, *F26.2*
  collection of, 325-6
  fetal lung maturity and, 323, *F26.2,* 325
  α-fetoprotein, 326
  prenatal diagnosis and, 323, *F26.2,* 325-6
  pulmonary surfactants in, 325
  tests done on, 323-6, *F26.2*
Amylase,
  clinical significance of, 181-3, 213-4, *F15.1*
    in pancreatitis, 182, 222
  increased (hyperamylasaemia), causes of, 182
  isoenzymes of, 181
  renal clearance of, 182
Amylase, urine, 182-3
Amyloidosis,
  multiple myeloma and, 171
Amylopectin, 181
Amylopectinosis, 305
Amylose, 181
Anaemia,
  ferritin and, 275-6
  iron and, 215, *T15.2,* 274
  malabsorption and, 215, *T15.2,* 219, 221
  megaloblastic, 215, *T15.2,* 219, 317
  pernicious, 219, 221, 318
Analbuminaemia, 165
Analgesic nephropathy, 76

Anderson's disease, 305
Androgens,
  adrenal, 63, *F4.1,* 65, 250, 258, 269
  congenital adrenal hyperplasia and, 65, 250
  excess (hyperandrogenism), causes of, 258, 270
  evaluation of, 270, *F19.8*
  hirsutism and, 258, 269-70
  metabolism of, 269
  oestrogen synthesis and, 263, *F19.1*
  ovarian secretion of, 263, 269
  Leydig cells and, 264
  sex-hormone binding globulin and, 269
  thyroxine binding globulin and, 242
  tumours and, 270
  virilism and, 270
Androstenedione, 65, 263, 269
Angina pectoris,
  "cardiac enzymes" in, 188
Angiotensin, 64-5
  I, 64
  II, 64, 292
  aldosterone and, 64
  physiological roles, 64
  renin and, 64-5, *F4.2,* 68-9
Angiotensin converting enzyme (ACE), 64, 187
  sarcoidosis and, 187
  inhibitors of, 29, 79
Anion gap, 40
  calculation of, 40
  definition of, 40
  high, metabolic acidosis with, 40
    causes of, 41, 51-2, *F3.11*
  normal, metabolic acidosis with, 40, 42
    causes of, 41-2
Anorexia nervosa, 30
  sex-hormone binding protein and, 269
Anovulatory cycles, 327
  infertility and, 327
  laboratory documentation of, 264-6, *F19.3,* 327
  serum progesterone and, 264, 266, 327
Antacid therapy,
  alkalosis and, 43
Antenatal diagnosis, 307-10, 323-6
Anterior pituitary, *Chapter 16,* 224-32
  disorders of, 229-32, 241, 244, 253, 267, 269
  function of, regulation of, 225-9
  laboratory investigation of, 229-32, 244-5, 254-7, 259-60
  hormones of, 225-9
Antibiotics (see also gentamicin), 343
Antioxidants, 57, 314, 316
  β-carotene, 314
  vitamin E, 315

Antibody(ies),
    anti-insulin, 127
    anti-insulin antibodies, 135
    anti-insulin receptor, 135
    antimicrosomal, 235, 239-41
    antimitochondrial, 152, 161
    antinuclear, 150, 161
    anti-smooth muscle, 150, 161
    anti-thyroglobulin, 235, 239-40
    anti-TSH receptor, 235, 237
    anti-adrenal cortical tissues, 252
    autoimmune diseases and, 127, 150, 152, 161,
      235, 240, 252
α_1-Antichymotrypsin, 174
    as acute phase reactant, 174, *T12.5*
Anticonvulsants, 98, 347
    vitamin D and, 98
Antidepressants (see amitriptylin)
Antidiuretic hormone (ADH),
    ectopic production of, 15, 288
    serum osmolality and, 5
    urine osmolality and, 13-5, 21-2, *F1.11-1.13*
    polyuria and, 21-3
    physiological actions of, 4
    secretion of, inappropriate (SIADH), 15, 288
    secretion of, regulation of, 5
Antilepileptic drugs, 347
Antigen,
    carcinoembryonic (CEA), 289
    cancer, 290
α_1-Antitrypsin, 163, 166, 174, 340
    as acute phase reactant, 174, *T12.5*
    deficiency of, 166
    faecal, protein-losing enteropathy and, 167
    liver disease and, 159, 166, 340
Antrum, 22
Apoferrritin, 272
Apolipoproteins, 195
    apo A, 195-6, *T14.2*, 200, 205, 210
    apo (a), 194, 196, *T14.2, F14.3,* 197, *F14.4,* 202
    apo B, 195-6, *T14.2, F14.3,* 205, 210
    apo B-48, 195-6, 198
    apo B-100, 194-5, 198
    apo C-II, 195-6, 198
    apo E, 195-6, 198, 205
    atherosclerosis and, 196, 202
    distribution of, 196, *T14.2*
    functions of, 195-6, *T14.2,* 198-200
    measurement of, clinical significance of, 205
APUD (argentaffin) cells, 223
    carcinoid syndrome and, 223
    5-hydroxyindole acetic acid and, 223
    serotonin metabolism and, 223

Arginine stimulation test, 228, 231
    growth hormone and, 228
Arginine vasopressin (see antidiuretic hormone)
Ariboflavinosis, 316
Arrhenoblastoma,
    androgens and, 270
Arterial blood gas parameters, 36, 50-3, *F3.11, F3.12*
Arterial hypoxaemia,
    tissue hypoxia and, 53
Arthritis,
    gouty, 119
    rheumatoid, 171
Ascorbate, deficiency of, 315
Aspartate aminotransferase (AST), 147, 149, 151, 183
    in acute viral hepatitis, 147, 183
    in alcoholic liver disease, 155
    in cholestatic liver disease, 147, 151
    in myocardial infarction, 188-9, *F13.6*
Aspirin (see salicylate)
AST:ALT ratio,
    alcoholic liver disease and, 155, 157
Asthma,
    acidosis and, 46
    alkalosis and, 47
    hypoxaemia and, 56
    ventilation perfusion inequality and, 56
Atheroma,
    formation of, 201, *F14.9,* 203, *F14.11*
Atherosclerosis,
    lipoproteins and, 201-3
    lipoprotein (a) and, 202
    oxidised LDL and, 202
Atrial natriuretic peptide,
    sodium homeostasis and, 8
Azotaemia, 76, 78

B lymphocytes, 167
    immunoglobulin synthesis and, 168, *T2.2*
Bacterial meningitis,
    CSF proteins in, 175, *T12.6*
Barbiturates, 349
    antidiuretic hormone and, 15
    γ-glutamyltransferase and, 155
Barium toxicity,
    potassium and, 31
Bartter's syndrome, 31, 52, 80, 82
    aldosterone and, 33, 66, 82
Basal body temperature charts, 327
Base(s), 35
    buffering of, 35
    definition of, 35
    conjugate, of a buffer, 35

Bence-Jones proteins, 170-2
  clinical significance of, 171-2
Bence-Jones proteinuria, 170-2
    benign vs malignant paraproteinaemia and, 170
    in myeloproliferative disorders, 171
    laboratory investigation of, 172
Bentiromide (NBT-PABA) test, 221-2
N-Benzoyl-tyrosyl-ρ-aminobenzoic acid (NBT-PABA), 222
Beri-beri, 316
Bicarbonate,
    alkali ingestion and, 43
    deficit of, 41, 51, *F3.10*
    depletion of, due to buffering, 37
    ingestion of, 43
    filtered, renal reclamation of, 37-9, *F3.2*
    hyperaldosteronism and, 66
    plasma levels of,
        in diabetic ketoacidosis, 129
        in diarrhoea, 32, 219
        in hyperosmolar nonketotic coma, 174
        in metabolic acidosis, 36, 40-1
        in metabolic alkalosis, 36, 40, 43
        in vomiting, 32, *F2.4*, 44, 217-8, *F15.4*
    renal generation of new, 37-8, *F3.1*
    respiratory acidosis and, 36, 45, *F3.7, F3.8*
    respiratory alkalosis and, 36, 47-8, *F3.9*
Bicarbonate/carbonic acid buffer, 35
Biguanides,
    lactic acidosis and, 141, *T10.1*
Bile, 213, *T15.1*
    secretion of, 214
Bile acids, 150, 214
    cholesterol and, 192
    enterohepatic circulation of, 158, *F11.9,* 214
        interruption of, 151, 158, 220
    liver disease and, 151, 158, 220
    metabolism of, 158
    primary, 158
    secondary, 158
    synthesis of, 158
Bile acid (salt) breath test, 222
Bile ducts, impatency of,
    malabsorption of fats and, 219, *T15.3*
Bile pigments,
    urobilinogen in urine, 146, 156
    urobilins (stercobilins) in stools, 145, 151
Bile salts, 158
    fat absorption and, 158, 215, 220
    liver disease and, 151, 158
    micelle formation and, 215-6, *F15.3*
Biliary atresia,
    cholestasis in neonates and, 339

Biliary cirrhosis, primary, 152, 160
Bilirubin(s),
    conjugated, 144-5, *F11.2,*
        increased, causes of, 148, *F11.5*
        diagnosis of jaundice and, 147
        metabolism of, 143-5, *F11.1*
            inborn errors of, 146
        structure and properties of, 144, *F11.2, F11.3*
    increased (hyperbilirubinaemia), 148
        laboratory evaluation of, 147, *F11.5,* 149, 151
        neonates and, 146, 338
        predominantly conjugated, 146, 338
        predominantly unconjugated, 146, 338
    jaundice and, 147, 149, 151, 338
    kernicterus and, 166, 338
    plasma fractions of, 145, *F11.4*
    prematurity and conjugation of, 338
    unconjugated, 144
        albumin and, 144
        inborn errors of, 146
        structure and chemical properties of, 144, *F11.3*
    transport in plasma of, 144
    urine, clinical significance of, 146
Biliverdin, 144
Blind loop syndrome, 220
    vitamin B_{12} and, 221, 318
Blood,
    oxygen in, 53
    oxygen saturation of, 53-4, *F3.13*
    P_{CO_2}, clinical significance of, 36
    pH, clinical significance of, 35-6
    P_{O_2}, clinical significance of, 53
    gases, Henderson-Hasselbalch equation and, 36
Blood pressure, high, 291
Blood volume, 2, 5
    aldosterone and, 65
    dehydration and, 13-4
    effect of, on ADH secretion, 4-5
    organ perfusion and, 13
    renal, renin secretion and, 65
Bohr effect, 55
Bone,
    diseases of, ALP activity in, 100-1, 179-80, *F13.1*
    effect of parathyroid hormone on, 90
    lesions, in primary hyperparathyroidism, 93
    Paget's disease of, 100
Bone marrow,
    immunoglobulin synthesis and, 167, 170
Branched-chain ketoaciduria, 302, *F24.3*
Broad-beta disease (see dysbetalipoproteinaemia and hyperlipidaemia Type III)
Bromocryptine,
    prolactin and, 229

β-Carotene, 314
Catalase, 57
Catecholamines (see also adrenaline and
noradrenaline)
    lactic acidosis and, 141
    magnesium and, 108
    metabolism of, 295
    plasma and urine levels of,
        in phaeochromocytoma, 295
        in neuroblastoma, 296
    potassium and, 25
CEA (see carcinoembryonic antigen)
Cell-mediated immunity,
    in protein-calorie malnutrition, 313
Cellulose acetate electrophoresis,
    for serum proteins, 162-3, *F12.1,* 180, *F13.1*
    for alkaline phosphatase isoenzymes, 180
Central nervous system,
    congenital malformations of, 325-6
    infections, acidosis and, 46
Cephalosporins,
    creatinine estimations and, 75
Cerebral haemorrhage,
    hydration therapy and, 17
    CSF proteins in, 175
Cerebrospinal fluid,
    chloride in, 175
    glucose in, 175
    immunoglobulins of, 175-6
    laboratory findings of,
        in meningitis, 175
        in multiple sclerosis, 176
    oligoclonal banding, 176, *F12.8*
    proteins in, 175, *T12.6*
Cervical cultures, 327
Cervical mucus penetration test, 327
Chenodeoxycholic acid, 158
Chlorambucol,
    cholestasis and, 155
Chloride,
    anion gap calculation and, 40
    acid-base balance and, 40
    in CSF, 175
    uterosigmoidostomy and, 33
Chloride diarrhoea, 333
Chloride shift, 39
Chloride, sweat, 220
Chloride, urine,
    vomiting and, 52
Chlorpromazine,
    cholestasis and, 155
Chlorpropamide,
    antidiuretic hormone and, 15

Chlortetracycline,
    liver disease and, 155
Cholangiocarcinoma, 152
Cholangitis, 156
Cholecalciferol,
    metabolism of, 90
    active metabolite of, 90
Cholecystitis, 146, 156
Cholecystographic agents,
    thyroid hormone synthesis and, 243
Cholecystokinin-pancreozymin, 213
Cholelithiasis, 156
Cholestasis,
    alkaline phosphatase in, 150-3, 157, 340
    aminotransferases in, 150-3, 157, 339
    extrahepatic, causes of, 151
    intrahepatic, causes of, 151
    liver function tests and, 150-3, 156-61
    the neonate and, 337-40
Cholesterol,
    absorption of, 192, 215-6, *F15.3*
    bile acids and, 192
    dietary, 192, 215
    esterified, 192
    free, 192
    high density lipoprotein, 194
    laboratory analysis of, 204, 207
    low density lipoprotein, 194
    metabolism of, 192, 198-200
    nephrotic syndrome and, 84, *F8.4*
    plasma levels of, clinical significance of,
        increased (hypercholesterolaemia), 208
            primary, 208
            secondary, 208
    thyroid disease and, 239
Cholesterol ester transfer complex, 195-200
Cholic acid, 158
Cholinesterase,
    dibucaine number and, 187
    liver disease and, 187
    organophosphate poisoning and, 187, 350
    suxamethonium sensitivity and, 187
    pseudo-, 187
    variants of, 187, 299
Choriocarcinoma, 287, 321
Chorionic gonadotrophin, human (HCG),
    as a pregnancy test, 321
    as a tumour marker, 287-8, 321
    β-subunit of, 227, 287
    ectopic production of, 288
    germ cell carcinomas and, 288, 321
    increased, causes of, 287-8
    trophoblastic tumours and, 288, 321

Creatine kinase,
    muscular dystrophy and, 185
    myocardial infarction and, 185, 188
    rhabdomyolysis and, 52, *F3.11, 352*
Creatinine,
    clearance, 75
    renal disease and, 75
    paediatric values of, 75, 330
Cretinism, 240
Crigler-Najjar syndrome, 146
Crohn's disease,
    malabsorption and, 220
Cryptorrchidism, 327
CSF (see cerebrospinal fluid)
Cushing's disease, 257
Cushing's syndrome, 257
    diagnosis of, 258
Cutaneous forms of porphyria, 280
Cyanocobalamin, 317
Cyclophosphamide,
    antidiuretic hormone and, 15
Cyclosporine,
    acute renal failure and, 79
Cystathione β-synthase deficiency, 302
Cystic fibrosis, 220, 307-9
    detection of carriers of, 307
    malabsorption and, 219
    molecular testing and, 309
    prenatal diagnosis of, 307
    restriction fragment length polymorphism and,
        309
    sweat electrolytes and, 220
Cystinuria, 219
Cytokines, 175
Cytotoxic drugs,
    antidiuretic hormone and, 15
    liver disease and, 155

Dehydration,
    hypertonic, 14
    hypotonic, 13
    isotonic, 13
    laboratory evaluation of, 14
    sodium and, 13-4, 16-9
Dehydroepiandrosterone sulphate (DHEAS),
    congenital adrenal hyperplasia and, 250
Deoxycholic acid, 158
11-Deoxycorticosterone, 63, *F4.1*
11-Deoxycortisol, 64, *F4.1*
    metyrapone test and, 256
Deoxyhaemoglobin,
    acid-base balance and, 39

Depression,
    cortisol and, 257
Desferrioxamine, 277
Dexamethasone suppression test,
    Cushing's syndrome and, 259-60
    types of, 259-60
        low and high-dose, prolonged, short, 259-60
Diabetes insipidus,
    central (neurogenic), 20
    diagnosis of, 21-2
    hypernatraemia and, 16-7, *T1.5*
    nephrogenic, 21
    polyuria and, 20-2
    urine osmolality and, 21-3, *F1.12, F1.13*
    water deprivation test and, 22
Diabetes mellitus, 126-32
    acidosis and, 128
    anion gap and, 129, 137
    classification of, 127
    coma and, 129-30
    complications of, 129-30
    definition of, 126
    diagnostic tests for, 131-3
    gestational, 127
    glucose tolerance test and, 131
    pregnancy and, 127
    insulin-dependent,
        diagnostic features of, 127
    hyperlipidaemia and, 130
    hyperosmolar coma and, 130
    ketosis and, 129, 137
    lactic acid and, 130
    liver function in, 128
    non-insulin-dependent, 127
        evaluation of, 131-3
    osmotic diuresis and, 128
    phosphate and, 128
    potassium and, 31, 128
    renal function in, 130
    sodium and, 129
Diabetic ketoacidosis,
    anion gap and, 52, 137
Diabetic nephropathy, 76, 132
    proteinuria and, 132
Diarrhoea,
    chloride, congenital, 43, 218, 333
    magnesium and, 109
    malabsorption syndromes and, 219-20
    metabolic acidosis and, 32, 42, 219
    metabolic alkalosis and, 43, 219
    osmotic, 218
    potassium and, 32, 219
    secretory, 218

Gastric acid, 212-3, *T15.1*
    bicarbonate formation in, 212
    secretion of, control of, 212
Gastric inhibitory polypeptide, 217
Gastrin, plasma,
    big, 217
    little, 217
    stimulation of gastric secretion and, 212, 217
    Zollinger-Ellison syndrome and, 217, 222
Gastrinomas, 217, 222
G-cells, 217, 222
Gastrointestinal tract,
    enzymes of, 213-4
    hormones of, 213, 217, 222-3
Gaucher's disease, 181, 307
Genotyping, apolipoprotein E, 205
Gentamicin, 348
    magnesium and, 110
    pharmacokinetic parameters of, 348
    potassium and, 33
Gestational diabetes, 127
GGT or γGT (see γ-glutamyltransferase)
Gigantism, pituitary, 230
Gilbert's disease,
    liver function tests and, 146, 338
Globulins,
    acute phase reaction and, 174
    α_1-antitrypsin, 159, 163, 166, 174, 340
    α_1-fetoprotein, 159, 290, 325
    α-lipoprotein, 163, 206, 210
    C-reactive protein, 174
    caeruloplasmin, 159, 163, 167
    complement, 163, 174
    cortisol-binding globulin, 247
    acute infections and changes in, 173
    chronic infections and changes in, 168, 170
    cirrhosis and, 160
    fibrinogen, 163, 174-5
    α_1-globulins, 163
    α_2-globulins, 163
    β-globulins, 163
    γ-globulins, 163
    autoantibodies and, 168, 170
    immunoglobulins and, 167-8
    increased,
        polyclonal, causes of, 170-1
        monoclonal, causes of, 171
    haptoglobin, 163, 174
    β-lipoprotein, 163, 206, 210
    α_2-macroglobulin, 163, 174-5
    paraproteins and, 170-2
    myeloproliferative disorders and, 168, *T12.2*
    nephrotic syndrome and, 169, *T12.3,* 171, *T12.4*

Globulins (contd),
    rheumatoid arthritis and, 171, 175
    sex-hormone binding globulin, 269
    transferrin, 163, 174, 271-3, 275
    thyroxine-binding globulin, 234, 236
Glomerular filtration rate,
    age and, 330
    plasma creatinine and, 75, 330
Glomerular proteinuria, 83
Glomerulonephritis, 76, 79
Glucagon, 125, 217, 223
    effect of, on blood glucose concentrations, 125
    ketosis and, 125, 136-7, *F10.7*
Glucagonoma, 223
Glucocorticoids, 64, 126, 247, 257
    effect of, on blood glucose concentrations, 126
    exogenous, Cushings syndrome and, 257
    thyroxine binding globulin and, 242
Gluconeogenesis, 122
    ethanol inhibition of, 138, 352
    enzymes of, 123
    fasting and, 122
    inborn errors of, 305
Glucose,
    adrenaline and, 126, 295
    blood, hormones regulating, 125-6, *F10.1*
    blood, decreased, (see also hypoglycaemia),
        laboratory evaluation of, 135-6, *F10.6*
    blood, increased, (see also hyperglycaemia),
        laboratory evaluation of, 129-32
    C-peptide and, 125
    CSF, 175
    glucagon and, 125
    glucocorticoids and, 125
    growth hormone and, 126
    insulin and, 125
    intolerance, types of, 127
    metabolism of, 122
    osmolality and, 1, 2
    plasma, fasting, 126, 131
    plasma, random, 126, 131
    renal handling of, 73, 81
    renal threshold of, 73
    tolerance tests and, 131
    urine, 73, 80, 128, 293, 323
Glucose-galactose absorption, 214
Glucose load, response to,
    in acromegaly, 231
Glucose-6-phosphate dehydrogenase deficiency, 116
Glucose tolerance test,
    intravenous, 131
    oral, 131
        interpretation of results, 131

Indomethacin,
 aldosterone and, 70
 antidiuretic hormone and, 15
 cholestasis and, 155
 potassium and, 29
Infarction, myocardial,
 myoglobin and, 185
 aminotransferases and, 188
 creatine kinase, CK-MB isoenzyme and, 188
 lactate dehydrogenase and, 188
 suspected, enzyme tests in, 188
 sequential increases of enzymes after, 189, *F13.6*
Infectious mononucleosis, 150, 160
Infertility, 269, 327
 female, causes of, 269, 327
 male, causes of, 269, 328
 laboratory investigation of, 328, *F26.3, F26.4*
Infiltrations, lung,
 acidosis and, 46
Inflammation, acute, 173
 acute phase reactants and, 174
 serum protein electrophoresis and, 174
Inherited metabolic diseases, (see also names of
 specific disorders), *Chapter 24,* 297-310
 autosomal, 297
 classification of, 298
 sex-linked, 298
Inhibin, 262
Insecticide poisoning, 187, 349-50
Insulin,
 antibodies to, 127
 counterregulatory hormones of, 125
 C-peptide and, 133, 136
 magnesium and, 110
 measurement of, clinical applications of, 134-6
 potassium and, 25
 prolonged oral glucose tolerance test and, 136
 receptors of, antibodies to, 135
Insulin-induced hypoglycaemia test, 232, 255
 growth hormone response to, 232, 255
 cortisol response to, 232, 255-6
Insulin-dependent diabetes mellitus (see diabetes
 mellitus), 127
Insulin-like growth factors, 135, 228
Insulin resistance, 127
Insulinoma, 134, 335
Intercritical gout, 119
Intermediate density lipoproteins, 192
 defective clearance of, 210
Intermittent porphyria, acute, 279-80
Interstitial fluid, 3
 volume, 3
 volume changes, 11

Interstitial lung fibrosis, 56
 alveolar-arterial oxygen gradient and, 56
 diffusion and, 56
Intestinal malabsorption, 219
 causes of, 219, *T15.3*
 diagnosis of, 220-2
Intracellular fluid, 3
 sodium in, 7
 volume, 3
 volume changes, 6-7
Intrahepatic cholestasis, 152-3
Intrauterine growth retardation,
 biochemical monitoring of, 323
Intrinsic factor,
 lack of, 215, *T15.2,* 219
 Schilling test and, 221
 vitamin B_{12} and, 215-6, 219
Inulin clearance, 75
Iodine, 233
 deficiency of, goitre and, 240
 recyling of, 233
 thyroid hormone synthesis and, 233-4, *F17.1,* 242
 uptake of, 233
Iron, *Chapter 20,* 271-7
 absorption, 271
 binding capacity of, serum total, 273
 deficiency of, 274
 metabolism of, 271
 overload, 276
 storage forms of, 272
 transport in plasma of, 272
Iron-deficiency anaemia, 274
 serum ferritin and, 275
 serum protein changes in, 275
 serum transferrin and, 275
 transferrin saturation and, 275
Iron-binding capacity, total, 273
Iron overload (see also haemochromatosis), 276
Isoenzymes,
 acid phosphatase, 181
 alkaline phosphatase, 179
 amylase, 181
 creatine kinase, 184
 lactate dehydrogenase, 186
Isosthenuria, 77

Jaffé reaction, 75
 interferences by ketones and cyclosporine, 75
Jaundice, 147
 cholestatic, 151
 classification of, 148
 investigation of, 147-8, 151

Index of Tables in Text

Index of Figures in Text

393

394

395